Textbook of Clinical Management of Club Drugs and Novel Psychoactive Substances

Textbook of Clinical Management of Club Drugs and Novel Psychoactive Substances

NEPTUNE Clinical Guidance

Dima Abdulrahim
Programme Manager and Principal Researcher for the NEPTUNE Project, Central and North West London NHS Foundation Trust

Owen Bowden-Jones
Consultant Addiction Psychiatrist, Central and North West London NHS Foundation Trust

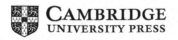

CAMBRIDGE
UNIVERSITY PRESS

CAMBRIDGE
UNIVERSITY PRESS

University Printing House, Cambridge CB2 8BS, United Kingdom

One Liberty Plaza, 20th Floor, New York, NY 10006, USA

477 Williamstown Road, Port Melbourne, VIC 3207, Australia

314–321, 3rd Floor, Plot 3, Splendor Forum, Jasola District Centre,
New Delhi – 110025, India

103 Penang Road, #05–06/07, Visioncrest Commercial, Singapore 238467

Cambridge University Press is part of the University of Cambridge.

It furthers the University's mission by disseminating knowledge in the pursuit of
education, learning, and research at the highest international levels of excellence.

www.cambridge.org
Information on this title: www.cambridge.org/9781009182133
DOI: 10.1017/9781009182126

First published 2022

A catalogue record for this publication is available from the British Library.

ISBN 978-1-009-18213-3 Paperback

Contents

Acknowledgements

The authors would like to express their gratitude to the EU Action Against Drugs and Organised Crime (EU-ACT) (a project funded by the European Union and implemented by FIIAPP International and Ibero-American Foundation for Administration and Public Policy) for an unrestricted quality improvement grant used to produce this publication.

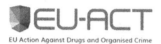

EU Action Against Drugs and Organised Crime

The authors would like to thank the Health Foundation for supporting the development of the NEPTUNE work through unrestricted educational grants.

The authors would also like to thank the multi-disciplinary groups of experts and experts by experience for their invaluable support in the development of work. The authors would like to extend particular thanks to Paul Dargan, David Wood, Jonathan Dewhurst, Sarah Finley, Fabrizio Schifano, Christopher Whitely, and Luke Mitcheson.

An Introduction to Club Drugs and Novel Psychoactive Substances

1.1 Introduction and Background

This document provides a new edition and an update to the 2015 NEPTUNE guidance on the clinical management of harms resulting from acute intoxication and from the harmful and dependent use of 'club drugs' and 'novel psychoactive substances' (NPS).

The guidance is evidence-based and is a response to the gap in knowledge and experience in the management of these drugs. There is evidence that clinicians often feel poorly equipped to assess and manage the harms of NPS and report that more education on emerging drugs and misuse patterns is needed.[1] It has also been noted that continued education on NPS is fundamental for the provision of improved harm reduction services, which can enhance overall care for NPS service users.[2]

Patterns of drug use continue to be dynamic. At the time of publication of this second edition, the quantity and range of drugs available to people is wider than ever. Recreational users typically use a wide repertoire of substances:

- 'Traditional' drugs continue to be the most used (depending on country, but e.g. cannabis, cocaine, amphetamines).
- Novel psychoactive substances (NPS) are used along with these traditional drugs, but have not replaced them.
- Increase of non-medical use of prescription drugs.

This document focuses on the health-related harms of club drugs and NPS and their clinical management.

The use of substances referred to as 'club drugs' has been well established for many decades. It includes illicit substances, e.g. cocaine and amphetamine, as well as NPS.

The use of NPS is a relatively more recent global phenomenon, with 120 countries and territories from all regions of the world having reported one or more NPS to the United Nations Office on Drugs and Crime (UNODC) Early Warning Advisory on New Psychoactive Substances.[3]

Novel psychoactive substances have been found in most of Europe and North America, as well as Oceania, Asia and South America, and in a number of African countries. To some extent, however, NPS are primarily a North American and European phenomenon. Although NPS affects all regions of the world, there are diverse regional patterns, in terms of both the type and number of NPS reported by individual countries. The NPS situation also differs by country from one year to the next.[4]

1.2 NEPTUNE Aims and Guidance Development

1.2.1 Objectives of NEPTUNE

This document is the 2022 update of the 2015 guidance on the harms and management of NPS and club drugs, developed by NEPTUNE (Novel Psychoactive Treatment UK Network). This edition has been funded and supported by *EU-Action Against Drugs and Organised Crime* (EU-Act).[5]

The aim of the guidance is to improve confidence, competence, and skills of clinicians in the detection, assessment, and management of the harms associated with the use of NPS.

Specific areas addressed include:

- **Detection/identification**. Recognising the significant psychological, physical, and social risks which can be associated with club drugs and NPS, and equipping professionals to be able to recognise problematic use, associated harms, and dependence.
- **Assessment**. Assessment of the problems related to the use of club drugs and NPS, including the assessment of both direct and indirect harms.
- **Management**. Clinical management of acute and chronic harms related to the use of club drugs and NPS – based on the best available evidence.

- **Harmr eduction**. Interventions aimed at preventing morbidity and mortality among individuals presenting to clinical settings, including measures to reduce the harms of club drugs and NPS for individuals and communities and to help patients achieve and sustain recovery and well-being.

This document provides guidance, not guidelines. The implementation of NEPTUNE at national levels must take place within the principles of national and international guidelines, national and local protocols, as well as the international standards and broad principles for the treatment of substance misuse disorders.[6,7]

The implementation of NEPTUNE learning into clinical practice must adapt the learning to take into account factors specific to the region, country or sector where they are implemented. This includes the needs, priorities, legislation, policies, systems of healthcare delivery and resources of the various countries. Adaptation should be carried out without undermining the validity of the evidence-based training. Local and national protocols, including prescribing protocols, should be used.

For up-to-date information, it is also recommended that clinicians contact the Poisons Centres in their region, where available. These are specialised units that advise on, and assist with, the prevention, diagnosis, and management of poisoning. Their structure and function varies around the world; however, at a minimum, a poisons centre is an information service. Some centres may also include a toxicology laboratory and/or a clinical treatment unit.[8]

1.2.2 Why Produce Guidance on Club Drugs and Novel Psychoactive Substances?

The underlying principles of good clinical practice in relation to the users of club drugs and NPS are the same as for harmful and dependent drug misuse in general.

Clinicians' existing experience of the treatment of other commonly used drugs (such as heroin, alcohol or cannabis for example) is very relevant to the treatment of club drugs and NPS.

However, good assessment and management of the harms of club drugs and NPS must also consider the particular challenges posed by novel drugs and address them directly. These include challenges posed by:

- New drugs (rapidly changing profile and ever-increasing numbers of substances, with poorly understood harms);
- New populations in treatment (including new patterns of drug use and contexts of harm);
- New harms (some club drugs are associated with harms not previously linked to illicit drug use, e.g. ketamine-related ulcerative cystitis);
- New manifestation of drug-related harms which are familiar to clinicians (e.g. dependence and withdrawal associated with gamma-hydroxybutyrate (GHB).

NEPTUNE therefore aims to improve clinicians' knowledge of the specific issues relating to NPS and to support evidence-based practice at local levels. It also aims to help improve clinicians' confidence in working with patients who use NPS, by providing the following:

- 'Technical' knowledge (what the drugs are and how they work);
- 'Cultural' knowledge (who is using them, and how);
- 'Clinical' knowledge (how to clinically manage both acute and chronic presentations).

1.3 Target Audience for the Guidance

1.3.1 Primary Audience

This guidance is aimed primarily at a clinical audience and most specifically clinicians who manage physical and mental health problems associated with harmful or/and dependent drug use and ensuing acute or chronic problems.

These will include clinicians working in specialist drug treatment and recovery services, as well as in emergency departments. The document is also relevant to professionals working with populations at risk of drug-related harms and associated poorer treatment outcomes, such as mental health services, prison health services, primary care, sexual health services, HIV treatment, hepatology and others.

1.3.2 Other Audiences

Although not directly aimed at them, this document is also a resource for funders/commissioners and policy-makers in developing local, national or regional services. It also provides patients and carers with information on what interventions should be available.

1.4 The Process of Developing the Guidance

1.4.1 Method for the Literature Review

This document is based on a comprehensive review of the English language literature on the harms and the clinical management of a range of club drugs and NPS, using systematic methods. A multi-disciplinary group of people were involved in developing the NEPTUNE framework and the guidance document was independently peer reviewed.

The first edition of this guidance was published in March 2015.This edition also includes a review of the research literature published until 2021.

For the review of the evidence, studies were identified using electronic searches of *Medline, Medline Plus*, the *Cochrane Library, CINAHL, Current Content, Embase, PUBMED, PsychINFO, Google Scholar* and the *Science Citation Index*. In addition, bibliographies of articles were screened for additional relevant studies.

The outputs of searches were considered against sets of inclusion and exclusion criteria. The citations produced by these searches were then screened via their abstract. Those considered relevant were identified and subjected to critical assessment.

The critical assessment of the evidence was based on the framework developed by the British Association for Psychopharmacology for the development of guidelines for the management of substance misuse.[9] This classifies the strength of evidence as follows:

- Strong research evidence (e.g. Cochrane reviews, meta-analyses, high-quality randomised controlled trials);
- Research evidence (e.g. controlled studies or semi-experimental studies);
- Emerging research evidence (e.g. descriptive or comparative studies, correlation studies, evaluations or surveys and non-analytic studies, e.g. case reports, case series);
- Expert panel evidence/consensus;
- Expert by experience evidence (service users/patients);
- Lack of evidence (no evidence, for or against);
- Conflicting evidence.

The 2021 update of the 2015 NEPTUNE guidance document continues to suggest that the evidence base on NPS remains relatively small, albeit expanding.[10]

In particular, studies on the toxicity and management of the harms of NPS and risks associated with long-term use and dependence liability are few, partly because most NPS have limited or no medical use, and partly because some of these substances have only recently emerged.

Overall, a review of the evidence shows that there continues to be limited robust evidence, in particular from meta-analyses or high-quality randomised controlled trials, and even controlled and semi-experimental studies are few. The bulk of the research available provides what is referred to as emerging research evidence, as it is based principally on non-experimental descriptive studies, consisting mainly of case reports and series and a small number of prospective observational studies, retrospective cohort studies and analysis of patient records.

This document therefore does not give definitive answers on the clinical management of NPS, but broad guidance based on the current best available evidence.

1.4.2 Substances and Drug Groups Covered by This Guidance

1.4.2.1 Classifying Novel Psychoactive Substances

Just over psychoactive drugs (NPS) have been reported for the first time in the last decade or so. Because of the very large number of NPS that have been detected and those that will emerge in the future, it is not possible to cover them all in any detail within the confines of this work. Nor is it realistic for clinicians to remember information on all NPS.

In order to deal with these large numbers of NPS and to future-proof this guidance, a two-pronged approach has been adopted.

Categorising Groups of Novel Psychoactive Substances

In order to understand the harms of NPS and how to manage them, it is useful to be able to classify them into different categories. Classification of NPS could be achieved using a variety of approaches, including chemical structure or pharmacological effect.

However, a useful method of categorising NPS is according to their primary psychoactive, physical and psychiatric effects and to use categories that clinicians working with the effects of substance misuse are already familiar with (see Figure 1.1).

3

Primarily STIMULANT Cathinones piperazines Phenethylamines (including amphetamines, methamphetamine, mephedrone, MDMA, 2C series, D series, benzodifurans, PMMA, PMA)	**Primarily DEPRESSANTS** GHB/GBL Ketamine Methoxetamine Nitrous oxide
Primarily HALLUCINOGENS (Agonists at 5H2A receptor) Tryptamines DMT, psilocybin, AMT LSD phenethylamines NBOMe, 2CB *Salvia divinorum* Amanita mushrooms	**SYNTHETIC CANNABONOID RECEPTOR AGONISTS** CB1 and CB2 receptor agonists including JWH and CP (classical, non-classical and hybrid)

Figure 1.1 Categorising substances by their primary psychoactive effects

A drug's primary effects will provide a conceptual framework for NPS, which will help clinicians navigate the hundreds of new substances detected in recent years, while allowing them to draw on their existing experience of substance misuse.

This classifies NPS and club drugs into the following groups:

- Primarily stimulants
- Primarily depressants
- Primarily hallucinogens
- Synthetic Cannabinoid Receptor Agonists (SCRAs) are put in a category of their own and are classified as a fourth separate category, as they do not fit easily into the other groups. This is because they are such a chemically and pharmacologically diverse group that their specific harms and clinical management also varies widely.

Although these classifications provide a useful framework for this guidance, it is important to note that they are not rigid categories. In reality, many drugs have a combination of effects, often dose-related, e.g. a primarily depressant drug can have stimulant effects at low doses. In addition, people will sometimes use NPS as part of a wider repertoire of illegal drugs and alcohol. The co-ingestion of more than one drug is common.

Most NPS are designed to provide legal alternatives to controlled substances, and have harms similar to those associated with the controlled drugs they have been manufactured to mimic.

The proximal mechanisms of most of these effects (as far as they are known) are shown in Table 1.1.

1.4.2.2 Focus on Particular Substances

The second prong of our approach is to focus in more detail on some commonly used NPS drugs (as well as their derivatives and related compounds) and those that potentially cause most harm.

Where a particular NPS is not discussed in this document, clinicians can refer to the broad groups to which it belongs and can extrapolate information on the management of its acute and chronic harms, while taking into account potential differences in potency, toxicity, half-life and length of effect.

1.5 Background: What Are Club Drugs and Novel Psychoactive Substances?

1.5.1 What Is a Club Drug?

'Club drugs' is a short-hand term used for convenience to refer to a group of psychoactive substances typically used in dance venues, house parties, music festivals and sometimes in a sexual context. The term therefore describes a diverse group of substances with different actions.

Table 1.1 Proximal mechanisms of drug effects

Drug	Primary (proximal) target	Brain effect
Alcohol	Agonist at GABA and antagonist at glutamate receptors	Increases GABA; blocks NMDA glutamate receptors
Benzodiazepines	Agonists at benzodiazepine site on GABA-A receptor	Increase GABA
GHB	GHB and GABA-B receptor agonist	Mimics GABA; inhibits dopamine release
Ketamine	NMDA glutamate receptor antagonist	Blocks glutamate
Khat (natural cathinone)	Releases ephedrine, a dopamine releaser	Mild increase in noradrenaline and dopamine
Mephedrone (synthetic cathinone)	Releases dopamine and blocks reuptake	
Natural cannabis	Cannabis CB1 receptor agonist	Stimulates endo-cannabinoid signalling, leading to a change in cortical and memory function
Cocaine	Blocks dopamine reuptake site	Greatly increases dopamine
Amphetamines (dexamphetamine and methyl)	Release dopamine and block reuptake	Greatly increase dopamine and noradrenaline
MDMA	Blocks serotonin and dopamine reuptake	Increases serotonin and dopamine functioning
Hallucinogens	Agonists at serotonin 5-HT2A receptors	Change across-cortex signalling
Opioids	Agonists at endorphin receptors	Produce euphoria, reduce pain

Agonist = drug that activates or stimulates a receptor; Antagonist = drug that blocks a receptor.

1.5.2 What Is a Novel Psychoactive Substance?

The term 'novel psychoactive substance' (NPS) has been used to describe a diverse group of substances that rapidly emerged from the early to mid-2000s.[11]

The UNODC defines NPS as 'substances of abuse, either in a pure form or a preparation, that are not controlled by the 1961 Single Convention on Narcotic Drugs or the 1971 Convention on Psychotropic Substances, but which may pose a public health threat'.

Most NPS are thought to be manufactured to mimic the effects of controlled drugs. NPS were developed initially as 'legal' replacements to established controlled drugs such as cannabis, heroin, cocaine and MDMA. They are sold openly, in some countries at least, as well as on the Internet in branded products advertised as 'legal highs' or 'research chemicals' or as 'food supplements', in attempts to make these substances attractive to users.

Many hundreds of NPS have been reported for the first time in the last decade. There is no doubt that the producers of novel NPS and 'legal highs' are well aware of the legal framework surrounding illicit substances and are continuously replacing controlled compounds with an array of compounds, which are modified to avoid legal control. Given the very numerous possibilities for altering the structure of chemicals, the list of substances produced is likely to grow continuously.[12] New substances are produced very quickly to replace those that are placed under legal control by various states.[13]

As the number of NPS grew rapidly, by 2013 the number of NPS already exceeded the number of psychoactive substances controlled at the international level.[14] By December 2021, a total of 1,124 unique new substances have been reported to the UNODC Early Warning Advisory (EWA) on NPS by Governments, laboratories and partner organisations. These can be grouped as follows: stimulants 36%, SCRAs 29%, classic hallucinogens 15%, opioids 9%, dissociatives 3%, sedatives/hypnotics 3% and not yet assigned 5%.[15,16]

In Europe, 830 new psychoactive substances were being monitored by the end of 2020 by the European Monitoring Centre for Drugs and Drug Addiction (EMCDDA), 46 of which were detected for the first time in Europe in 2020.[17]

Not all NPS detected continue to be available over time, as some appear for the first time and then disappear from the market. The World Drug Reports suggest that the overall number of NPS present on the market has stabilised at approximately 500 substances per year over the period 2015–2019.

In terms of the use of NPS and despite the continuing increase in the emergence of new NPS, one study suggested that a core group of over 80 NPS have become established as recreational drugs, supplementing traditional drugs that are misused and becoming part of the repertoire of substances available for consumption.[18]

Currently, most NPS are stimulants, followed by synthetic cannabinoid receptor agonists and a smaller number of hallucinogenics and opioids.[19,20] It has been noted that the increase in the number of opioid NPS and benzodiazepine NPS potentially signals that new psychoactive substances are increasingly more targeted at the long-term and more problematic drug users.[21]

Novel psychoactive substances are generally produced in bulk quantities by chemical and pharmaceutical companies often in China or India, or in clandestine laboratories in Europe. They are then shipped to Europe, where they are processed into products, packaged and marketed.[22]

It has been argued that these substances are not 'legal' but are instead 'not prohibited'. Their non-controlled status does not reflect their safety, but rather the lack of regulation over their production, distribution and use.[23,24] Many are untested and have unknown psychological and toxicological effects.[25,26]

Not all NPS are 'novel'. 'New' does not always mean a new invention but could refer to substances that have recently been made available for recreational use, e.g. mephedrone was reportedly first synthesised in 1929, but emerged as a recreational substance of misuse as late as 2007.[27] Other 'new' substances were synthesised and patented in the 1970s or earlier, but recently their chemistry has been modified slightly to produce psychoactive effects similar to those of well-established illicit substances.

1.5.3 Changes in Legal Control of Novel Psychoactive Substances

The legal position of some NPS has changed over time. At the international level, up to March 2019, the Commission on Narcotic Drugs placed 48 NPS under international control. These control measures have to be implemented into the national legal framework of each country.[28]

Other NPS continue to be outside International Drug Control Conventions. However, their legal status differs widely from country to country. To date, approximately 60 countries have implemented legal responses to control NPS by amending existing legislation or through innovative legal instruments.

Some countries have adopted controls on entire substance groups of NPS using a so-called generic approach, or have introduced analogue legislation that invokes the principal of 'chemical similarity' to an already controlled substance to control substances not explicitly mentioned in the legislation.[29]

These controls have limited the open sale of these products. They may also have played a role in reducing the number of NPS detected for the first time. However, challenges remain.

1.5.4 Development and Spread of Large Numbers of Novel Psychoactive Substances

Although the number of NPS has been growing at a very fast pace, it has been noted that this yearly increase appears to be slowing down in recent years. In Europe, it has been reported that the number of new substances identified for the first time each year peaked in 2014–2015, but has since stabilised at levels comparable to 2011–2012.[30]

The causes of this are unclear, however may reflect the results of sustained efforts to control new substances in Europe and legislation in some countries. This may have resulted in reducing the incentive for producers to keep ahead of legal controls and develop new compounds. In addition, control measures and law enforcement operations in China targeting laboratories producing NPS may also have played a role.[31,32]

Nonetheless, and despite reduction in yearly number of NPS detected, challenges continue and new ones emerge. NPS continue to appear at the rate of one per week. There is also no evidence that the overall availability of NPS has reduced and the drugs may still be available more covertly on the illicit market.[33]

Some NPS are also now well-established in the drugs market, most particularly SCRAs and synthetic cathinones.[34] There is also some evidence the tightening of regulation may have sometimes led to the decrease in the number of people using NPS, but users instead switched to other types of drugs.[35]

There are also changes in the type of substances being detected for the first time globally, with new substances increasingly targeted at long-term and more problematic drug users, particularly NPS synthetic opioids and benzodiazepines.[36,37,38,39,40] Problematic NPS use is also increasingly found in some vulnerable groups in Europe, e.g. people who inject drugs and homeless people, and has been associated with increased levels of physical and mental health problems.[41]

1.6 Club Drug and Novel Psychoactive Substance Use

1.6.1 Overall Drug Use

Novel psychoactive substances have not replaced traditional illicit drugs, but exist alongside them.

Data from European countries on NPS are available from half the countries, but are often not comparable. Existing information suggests that use of NPS is overall low in comparison to traditional illicit club drugs. NPS nonetheless are consumed and are more likely to be used by some population sub-groups.

1.6.2 Club Drug Users and Contexts of Use

Different people will use substances for different reasons and each chapter in this text will look at the subjective effects of a substance desired by people who use it.

There is some research that has looked at why people use NPS specifically, which includes the fact that users turn to NPS as a substitute to traditional drugs when these are prohibited or when there is reduced supply or perceived drop in quality.[42]

There is also evidence that the motives for using NPS are curiosity, enhancement of social situations, the enjoyable effects, a desire to 'get high', and a belief that NPS are safer and more convenient.[43,44,45,46]

Novel psychoactive substances were also used because they were seen as facilitating a novel and exciting adventure, as promoting self-exploration and personal growth, functioning as coping agents, enhancing abilities and performance, fostering social bonding and belonging, and acting as a means for recreation and pleasure.[47]

It has been argued that the motives for NPS use may be associated with both the groups of users and the specific types of NPS being consumed. Benshop et al.'s (2020) exploratory and confirmatory factor analysis identified five factors across a number of countries: coping, enhancement, social, conformity and expansion motives. Overall, marginalised users scored higher on coping and conformity motives. Nightlife groups showed higher endorsement of social motive, whereas online community users showed higher scores on expansion motives. Various types of NPS were also associated with different motives. Motives for use of the specific substances are also discussed in the relevant sections throughout this chapter.[48,49,50,51,52,53,54]

Some NPS, e.g. mephedrone, are also used for sexual enhancement, including by gay and bisexual men who use it in the context of 'chemsex'.[55]

1.6.3 Population Groups Most Likely to Use Novel Psychoactive Substances

There is evidence that levels of NPS- and drug use are higher among particular populations. These are the following:

1.6.3.1 Young People

The use of club drugs and NPS occurs in nearly all age groups, but studies have also shown that young people are more likely to use them than older people and that they are mainly used by young males.[56,57,58]

In general, clubbing and club drug use, as part of a socially active lifestyle, has been associated with elevated sexual health risks[59] and a history of promiscuous sexual activity.[60]

1.6.3.2 Poly-drug Use

The users of club drugs and NPS will typically use a wide repertoire of substances. The co-ingestion of more than one substance (simultaneous use), including alcohol, increases the risk of adverse effects,[61] as is discussed in greater detail in later chapters of this text.

In comparison to other drug users, NPS users have higher levels of poly-drug use, and a history of overdose on any drug in the past year.[62]

1.6.3.3 'Clubbers' and People Who Frequent Night-Time Economy Leisure Venues

Studies have consistently shown that drug use is more commonly reported in surveys carried out in nightlife settings (like clubs, bars or music festivals) than among the general population.[63] There is evidence that people who use the night-time economy, and dance clubs or nightclubs in particular, are more likely to use club drugs than the general population.[64,65] Young adults attending nightlife events in pubs and discos are also more prone to poly-substance use, mainly combining NPS with alcohol and cocaine.[66] There is also some evidence that the use of club drugs and NPS is higher among people who attend electronic dance music parties at nightclubs, festivals and 'raves' than those who do not.[67,68,69,70,71,72]

Other targeted surveys have also shown variations by user of different types of venues in the night-time economy, e.g. those attending nightclubs reporting significantly higher levels of drug use than bar/pub attenders.[73]

There is some evidence that increased levels of drug use were associated with a higher frequency of visits to pubs, bars and nightclubs. E.g., in the UK, use of any Class A drug (including MDMA and cocaine) in the last year was around 11 times higher among those who had visited a nightclub at least four times in the past month (22.4%) compared with those who had not visited a nightclub (2.1%).[74]

1.6.3.4 Lesbian, Gay, Bisexual and Transgender Populations (LGBT+)

There is evidence that levels of club drug use among men who have sex with men (MSM) and among lesbian, gay, bisexual and transexual (LGBT) people, are higher than in the general population.[75,76,77,78,79,80,81] Club drugs have been described as a popular aspect of socialisation.[82]

There are concerns over associations between club drug and NPS use and high-risk sexual behaviours among a minority of MSM. This includes concern over 'chemsex', a term used to describe sex between men that occurs under the influence of drugs immediately preceding and/or during the sexual session,[83,84] with methamphetamine, GHB/GBL and mephedrone the drugs most often reported.

A combination of factors, including high-risk sexual practices and injecting drug use, have been described as 'a perfect storm for transmission of both HIV and hepatitis C (HCV), as well as a catalogue of ensuing mental health problems'.[85] Whereas not all individuals involved in 'chemsex' practice engage in high-risk behaviours, 'chemsex' has been associated with risk and adverse effects.[86,87,88,89,90,91,92,93,94,95,96,97,98]

1.6.3.5 Problem Drug Users

As mentioned previously, NPS are increasingly targeted at established long-term drug users, such as people dependent on opioids or benzodiazepines. In addition, in some European countries, stimulant NPS and most particularly synthetic cathinones are one of the main substances injected by problem drug users. This will be discussed in further detail below.

1.6.3.6 Homeless Populations and Prison Inmates

In some countries, synthetic cannabinoid receptor agonists (SCRAs), in particular, have been associated with homeless people and with prison populations. This will be discussed in further detail in the following.

1.6.3.7 'Psychonauts'

'Psychonaut' is a term given to a group of people who have been described as having a relatively good understanding of how NPS work, based on them experimenting with a wide variety of traditional and new substances. Psychonauts will document their experience. NPS are typically consumed in a familiar and relatively controlled environment, with dosages often carefully measured and timed. Their experiences are often made available to other psychonauts through online fora.[99]

Internet sites and moderated discussion fora and blogs are used to share information about newer compounds, feedback on the effects of drugs and harm reduction advice developed through experience.[100] The Internet and sites such as *Drugs Forum*, *Bluelight* and *Erowid*, provide platforms for sharing experience and information.[101] These user sites have also provided researchers with some understanding of these drugs in instances where scientific evidence was not available and it is suggested that they are a good source of information for researchers for the better understanding of NPS.[102]

1.6.4 New Markets and User Communication about Drugs

'Traditional' methods remain the most common ways to acquire drugs (dealers, friends, family), both classic drugs and NPS. However, the Internet now occupies a growing role in the sale of drugs, with significant drug sales on the darknet and the potential to grow.

Novel psychoactive substances can sometimes be bought on the 'clearnet' (a part of the Internet accessible to standard search engines) or from the 'dark web' (a part of the Internet only accessible through specialist anonymising web browsers), with the 'darknet' also selling controlled substances.[103,104,105,106,107] It has been reported that when compared with current estimates of the annual retail value of the overall EU drug market, sales volumes on darknet markets are currently modest, but growing.[108]

For a growing number of people, the Internet is now the first place they look when searching for recreational drugs and their related information, especially when faced with the rapid and baffling proliferation of NPS.[109] A study carried out in the Netherlands has shown that online customers are sometimes willing to pay more for the convenience of purchasing drugs online.[110]

The Internet has also had an impact on drug use patterns and behaviours. A UNODC 2020 publication has reported that more than a quarter of people who started using drugs before they began buying drugs on the darknet, then consumed a wider range of drugs, and approximately 10% reported that that they consumed a different class of drugs.[111]

Especially when not controlled, NPS have been marketed as 'plant food', 'bath salts', 'research chemicals', 'incense' or 'herbal highs' and are typically labelled as 'not for human consumption'.[112,113]

There is also some evidence that NPS, as well as traditional drugs, are sometimes acquired through social media. The most commonly used technology to acquire drugs is that of mobile phones. Phone-based drug delivery services, sometimes known as 'ring and bring drug phone lines' or 'dial-a-drug' are increasingly common. This is true for NPS as well as traditional illicit substances, and the European market for cocaine has been described as undergoing a process of 'Uberisation', where more sellers provide 'fast delivery anywhere at any time'.[114]

1.7 Brief Overview of the Effects and Harms of Club Drugs

1.7.1 How Drugs Work

Most NPS are designed to provide legal alternatives to controlled substances, and have effects similar to those associated with the controlled drugs they have been manufactured to mimic.

As mentioned previously, drugs can be classified in various ways – according to chemical structure, pharmacological activity or psychological effects.[53,54,115,116]

1.7.2 Toxicity and Other Acute Harms

The harms associated with club drugs and NPS can, as with 'traditional' drugs including alcohol, be ranked based on the relative harms.[117]

'Toxicity' generally refers to the extent to which a substance causes functional or systemic damage to a living organism.[118,119]

Our knowledge of the effects and toxicity of many NPS remains limited, as it is often mainly based on user reports and clinical intoxication cases, with very limited pharmacological and toxicological data available.[120]

There is nonetheless enough evidence to show that club drugs and NPS are associated with a range of harms.[121] The growing market for new substances has been linked to an increase in the number of serious adverse events – particularly non-fatal and fatal poisonings.[122,123,124]

There are wide variations in the toxicity of the various club drugs and NPS, including their single-dose lethal toxicity.[125] An index for fatal toxicity has been developed, showing differences between the various NPS and demonstrating that GHB/GBL, AMT, synthetic cannabinoid receptor agonists (SCRAs) and benzofurans had a higher fatal toxicity than other NPS.[126] In recent years, benzodiazepine NPS have also been linked with fatalities, such as the case of etizolam and other 'street' benzodiazepines.[127] Similarly, new opioids including fentanyl NPS have been associated with high levels of acute toxicity.

The harm associated with any drug of potential misuse may include: the physical and mental health harms to the individual user caused by the drug; overdose; the dependence-inducing potential of the drug; and the effects of drug use on families, communities and society.[128] All aspects need to be considered when assessing the impact of a drug.

In addition, individuals vary greatly with respect to metabolism and vulnerability to physical and mental health problems. A number of other factors are also linked to acute toxicity:

- The consumption of more than one substance will increase the chances of acute toxicity, particularly when drugs with similar physiological effects are combined (e.g. sedatives such as GHB and alcohol, or stimulants such as cocaine and amphetamine).
- The risk of overdose is increased by repeated administration of the drug.

- The safety ratio of drugs does not reflect the metabolic or functional tolerance that a user may have developed.
- Non-drug variables can alter toxic reactions significantly (e.g. the psychological effects of the environment, diet, stress, expectation etc.).[58,129]
- The mode of administration, with injecting not only exposing the user to the risk of bacterial infections but also increasing the risk of overdose and dependence.[130]
- Drug purity and adulterants can affect toxicity.

Club drugs and NPS pose a particular challenge to clinicians and constitute a public health challenge for the following reasons:[131]

- these substances are not approved for human consumption;
- they are associated with a number of unknown adverse effects;
- insufficient information is available in peer-reviewed scientific journals on harms;
- they appear in increasingly sophisticated (i.e. non-powder) forms and remain unregulated;
- they are often synthesised in underground laboratories by modifying the molecular structure of controlled drugs, raising concerns over the presence of contaminating agents;
- they are largely available online to everyone, 'just a click away'.

Whereas all users of club drugs face the risk of acute toxicity, the harms caused by club drugs encompass a wide range of different patterns. Club drugs are associated with harmful use, which can be physical harms (e.g. ketamine can lead to ulcerative cystitis) or mental (e.g. psychosis associated with synthetic cannabinoids).

Although still limited, we have an increasing understanding of the harms associated with NPS through animal and human studies.[132]

Recently, information has been provided through the Tox-Portal, an online tool developed in collaboration with The International Association of Forensic Toxicologists (TIAFT) that collects data on toxicology and harm related to the use of NPS at a global level.[133] This has shown the following:

- synthetic cannabinoids, synthetic opioids and synthetic stimulants account for the majority of NPS reported to the UNODC EWA Toxicology Portal.
- Synthetic cannabinoids in particular remain harmful, persistent and prevalent.

- Poly-drug use continues to be a factor and an important consideration in NPS fatalities.
- Benzodiazepine-type NPS feature highly in cases of driving under the influence of drugs.[134]

Some NPS have also been shown to have a liability to produce dependence and some have been associated with a withdrawal syndrome, which can be severe, for example in the case of GHB/GBL.

1.7.3 Particular Challenges of Novel Psychoactive Substances

1.7.3.1 Unpredictability of Novel Psychoactive Substances: Products Which Are Not What They Claim to Be

The non-regulated production techniques involved in manufacturing NPS create large variation in dosage, potency or even the content of an NPS product, making it difficult to predict effects on users. There are, of course, no regulations concerning content, potency, point of sale and purchase age[135], and even branded products that look the same and have similar lists of chemical content, may in fact be very different.

Although unpredictability of the content of a product was also a factor with traditional substances to an extent, it is argued that what is distinctive about NPS is that this is significantly more so than with traditional drugs.[136]

People using NPS often have poor knowledge of what they are consuming. The reasons for this include:

- Research has shown that there is significant variation in the content of 'legal high' products bought over the Internet.[137,138,139,140,141,142]
- NPS preparations and products sold for recreational purposes can include a combination of different NPS and/or traditional drugs. Products can contain a mixture of two or three different active compounds (including controlled compounds).[143] This can increase the risk of adverse effects, as well as potentially altering clinical presentations.

For example, the analysis of samples seen by the Home Office Forensic Early Warning System (FEWS) – 2016/2017 showed that 35% of the samples analysed contained a mixture of two or more substances .[144]

- Branded products of the same name can contain different active compounds, depending on time, place and batch purchased.[145,146,147,148,149,150] One study found that six out of seven products analysed did not contain the advertised active ingredients but, rather, some controlled traditional drugs.[151]
- Research to shed light on the purity and price of 10 NPS in the European Union (France, United Kingdom (UK), the Netherlands, Czech Republic and Poland) investigated the products in each of these countries purchased from different webshops. The study found that a considerable proportion of NPS were mislabelled by the webshops. In most instances, highly similar NPS analogues were sold instead of the specific compounds advertised. However, in some cases, the contents were entirely different to those advertised, the consequences of which could cause serious harm. For instance, α-PVP is a much more potent stimulant than 4-FA and it was present in one sample advertised as 4-FA.[152]
- In some cases, studies have shown that NPS analogues similar to more commonly used substances were sold instead of the specific compounds advertised.[153] Sometimes much stronger substances were used than the one advertised. For example, NPS drugs with hallucinogenic effects such as 25I-NBOMe have been sold as LSD to users who were not aware that they have consumed other substances, with a considerably higher dose than equivalent doses of LSD.[154]
- Similarly, NPS are sometimes substituted in place of traditional drugs or other NPS and consumed by users who are not aware of the substitution. In some cases, much more potent substitutions are made. Later chapters will look for example at substitution of MDMA by PMA/PMMA, LSD by 25I-NBOMe,[155,156,157,158] or fentanyl substituted for, or used to adulterate, heroin.[159,160,161,162,163,164,165] As will be discussed later, this can be associated with severe harm and overdose.

1.7.3.2 New Generations of Substances and Novel Psychoactive Substances Over the Years

The 'market' for club drugs and NPS appears to have gradually become more sophisticated. For example, a Spanish study of 2C-B reported that samples collected appeared to change over time from poorly elaborated forms such as powder, to tablets, which become the most common form.[166]

Importantly, new formulations of various NPS have become available over time. They are often more potent than earlier forms and may be associated with greater harms. For example,

- **Four generations of synthetic cannabinoid receptor agonists ((SCRA).** Newer generations appear to be associated with severe adverse reactions, such as catatonia, serious toxicity and death. (For more information see Chapter 13)
- **New generation synthetic cathinones.** E.g. compounds such as α-PVP and MDPHP (also known as 'monkey dust') are associated with more severe effects than previous cathinones. (For more information see Chapter 11)
- **Hallucinogens.** For example, 25B-NBOMe is a highly potent 2C-B derivative even at microgram-level doses. (For more information see Chapter 14.)

1.7.3.3 Limited Drug Testing

One of the attractions of NPS to people who use them is the limited ability of standard drug tests to identify them. This may lead the user to feel that they can use NPS without risk of detection by occupational services or law enforcement.

This, however, can pose challenges to clinicians. There are currently very limited accurate clinic-based testing devices for most of the NPS, despite continued developments in the area of chemical standards, analytical capability and forensic detection of compounds.

It has been argued that although toxicological screening tests are not routinely used in most hospitals across Europe, they can be helpful, mostly in cases of use of unknown agents and unclear clinical presentations, provided that the results are rapidly available and interpreted correctly.[167]

In addition, not all laboratories have the capacity to detect the more uncommon substances. Reference standards are essential for forensic and toxicological investigations for new psychoactive substances; however, these are not available in many laboratories.[168]

The diagnosis of acute toxicity associated with NPS will in most cases be made by clinical assessment. As rapid urine or serum field tests are not commonly available, analytical assessment should not be considered a component of routine diagnosis of NPS.

Assessment should be based on the recognition of the clinical toxidrome associated with the NPS used and the potentially harmful modes of use, with other causes of presentation excluded.

1.8 Response to Club Drug and Novel Psychoactive Substance Use

1.8.1 Novel Psychoactive Substance and Drug-Related Presentations to Hospital Emergency Departments

Accurate data on emergency hospital admissions resulting from club drug and NPS use in the UK were difficult to obtain for a variety of reasons, not least because ICD-10 codes did not include specific codes for NPS[169,170,171] and because coding is generally based on clinical condition at presentation.[172]

More recently, the new classification of substance use disorders and problems in ICD-11 includes a range of diagnostic categories that cover a broad spectrum of health conditions reflecting different levels and patterns of substance use.[173] ICD-11 also covers some NPS and club drugs, for example synthetic cathinones,[174] SCRAs[175] and MDMA.[176]

It has been suggested that these changes may in part help with some of the coding issues, enabling better understanding of the burden of healthcare utilisation related to the use of a wider range of substances.[177] However, in clinical practice, clinicians may not record drug-related codes, but codes based on clinical presentation. In addition, the rapidly emerging number of NPS means that some may not codeable under existing ICD-10 and even ICD-11 codes.

Data on acute drug-related hospital presentations associated with NPS continue to be limited,[178] but have been improving. Interventions have taken place in Europe for a number of years now, including the European Drug Emergencies Network (Euro-Den), in order to address this current paucity of reliable data.[179]

Euro-Den data from 31 sentinel sites in 21 countries reported that there were 23,947 acute drug toxicity presentations reported by the Euro-DEN Plus centres over the four-year period between January 2014 and December 2017. These represented a median of 0.3% of all emergency presentations to the sentinel hospitals. Amongst those, NPS were seen in 9% of presentations over the four-year period, with significant geographical variation in the involvement of NPS in presentations.[180]

Data on deaths associated with club drugs and NPS also remain limited, and it has been argued that the absence of European forensic toxicology guidelines for drug-related death investigations is a barrier to improving monitoring and practice in this area.[181]

However, there is evidence that NPS, including synthetic opioids, synthetic cannabinoid receptor agonists and synthetic cathinones continue to be associated with acute intoxications and deaths. As with all drug-related deaths, fatalities often involve the use of more than one substance (poly-drug use).[182]

Emergency medicine physicians and other clinicians should seek advice on the diagnosis, treatment and care of patients who may have been poisoned with a club drug or an NPS, including from national or regional poisons information services. Interventions provided must be based on local, national and international protocols and guidelines.

1.8.2 Sexual Health Services

The association between substance misuse, including alcohol use, and high-risk sexual behaviours is well established, although evidence of a causal relationship is limited.

There is also some evidence from some countries that the prevalence of drug use is higher among the patients of sexual health services than the general population and most particularly patients who identify as men who have sex with men (MSM). For example, one study of patients at a London sexual health clinic reported significantly higher rates of past month drug use than in the general adult population in England and Wales. This was particularly so among MSM.[183]

Patients of sexual health services who misuse alcohol and drugs have also been identified as higher-risk groups for poor sexual health outcomes. Substance misuse interventions in these settings have been recommended.[184,185,186,187]

It has therefore been argued that sexual health services may provide opportunistic encounters to identify patterns of recreational drug use, explore motivations for use and implement strategies to reduce harms related to drug use.[188,189,190,191] It has been suggested that patient assessment in sexual health services should include a history of alcohol and recreational drug use.[192] Integrated services have also been suggested.[193]

Table 1.2 The role of particular settings and the aims of interventions provided

	Detection	Assessment	Brief intervention	Complex intervention (acute)	Complex intervention (chronic)
Primary care	✓	✓	✓		
Emergency department	✓	✓	✓	✓	
Sexual health	✓	✓	✓		
Substance misuse treatment	✓	✓	✓	Some	✓

1.8.3 Substance Misuse Treatment Services

International Standards for Treatment of Drug Use Disorders have been developed by the UNODC-WHO, and provide the rules and minimum requirements for clinical practice and the generally accepted principles of patient management in any healthcare system.[194]

A set of best practice principles that should underlay drug dependence treatment has been identified and defined by the United Nations Office for Drugs and Crime (UNODC) and the World Health Organization (WHO), and are listed in Box 1.1.[195]

Box 1.1 Outline of the Key Principles and Standards for the Treatment of Drug Use Disorders

- Principle 1: Availability and accessibility of drug dependence treatment
- Principle 2: Screening, assessment, diagnosis and treatment planning
- Principle 3: Evidence-informed drug dependence treatment
- Principle 4: Drug dependence treatment, human rights, and patient dignity
- Principle 5: Targeting special subgroups and conditions
- Principle 6: Addiction treatment and the criminal justice system
- Principle 7: Community involvement, participation and patient orientation
- Principle 8: Clinical governance of drug dependence treatment services
- Principle 9: Treatment systems: policy development, strategic planning and coordination of services

---

Building on these principles, at a practical level, drug treatment services and systems can consider the following to improve their understanding:

- Amending data recording tools to ensure NPS use and associated adverse health effects are accurately recorded
- Engaging in research to build the evidence base for treatment interventions

1.8.4 Overview of the Interventions for the Screening, Identification and Management of Drug Harms in the Target Settings

The different target organisations (treatment settings) of the NEPTUNE guidance have different roles in the detection, identification and management of chronic harms and/or dependence resulting from the use of club drugs and NPS. This is determined by the competence of clinicians to deliver substance misuse treatment and particular pharmacological, psychosocial and recovery interventions.

Table 1.2 provides a summary of the role of each of the target settings and the aims of the interventions provided in terms of the screening, identification, assessment and management of the harms linked to the use of club drugs. Further information on the level of intervention needed is also presented in Chapter 2.

1.9 Reducing Drug-Related Harms

The reduction of the harms associated with the use of club drugs and NPS are to a very large extent based on the same principles that must be adopted for the reduction of harms associated with traditional drugs.

A number of measures are adopted by users or recommended by professionals, including regulating the quantity of drugs used, spacing out doses within a session of substance use, and not combining multiple stimulants or depressants.[196,197,198,199]

A study has shown that polysubstance-using festival attendees who frequently adopt dosing-related harm reduction strategies frequently experience less drug-related harm. However, whereas many users will adopt harm reduction strategies frequently, others will rarely carry out protective strategies, suggesting that there is still a need to encourage use of these strategies among this population.[200]

References

1. Lank P, Pines E, Mycyk M. Emergency physicians' knowledge of cannabinoid designer drugs. *West J Emerg Med* 2013;**14**:467–470.

2. Ramos C, Guirguis A, Smeeton N, et al. Exploring the baseline knowledge and experience of healthcare professionals in the United Kingdom on novel psychoactive substances. *Brain Sci* 2020;**10**:142. https://doi.org/10.3390/brainsci10030142

3. United Nations Office on Drugs and Crime (UNODC). Early Warning Advisory on New Psychoactive Substances. www.unodc.org/LSS/Page/NPS [last accessed 9 February 2022].

4. United Nations Office on Drugs and Crime (UNODC). Global SMART Update Understanding the Synthetic Drug Market: The NPS Factor. Volume 19, March. Appears to be missing the year

5. The EU Action against Drugs and Organised Crime (EU-ACT) funded by the European Commission and implemented by FIIAPP.

6. World Health Organization (WHO) and United Nations Office on Drugs and Crime (UNODC). International standards for the treatment of drug use disorders: revised edition incorporating results of field-testing. Geneva, 2020. License: CC BY-NC-SA 3.0 IGO.

7. European Monitoring Centre for Drugs and Drug Addiction. Action framework for developing and implementing health and social responses to drug problems. Available from: www.emcdda.europa.eu/printpdf/publications/mini-guides/action-framework-for-developing-and-implementing-health-and-social-responses-to-drug-problems_en

8. The World Health Organization has developed guidance and training materials on poisons centres. For more information see: https://apps.who.int/iris/handle/10665/331635; www.unodc.org/documents/drug-prevention-and-treatment/UNODC-WHO_International_Standards_Treatment_Drug_Use_Disorders_April_2020.pdf. For a directory of poisons centres, see: www.who.int/gho/phe/chemical_safety/poisons_centres/en/.

9. Lingford-Hughes AR, Welch S, Peters L, Nutt DJ; British Association for Psychopharmacology, Expert Reviewers Group. BAP updated guidelines: evidence-based guidelines for the pharmacological management of substance abuse, harmful use, addiction and comorbidity: recommendations from BAP. *J Psychopharmacol* 2012;**26**(7):899–952. https://doi.org/10.1177/0269881112444324

10. See e.g. Santos-Toscano R, Guirguis A, Davidson D. How preclinical studies have influenced novel psychoactive substance legislation in the UK and Europe. *Br J Clin Pharmacol*, Special Issue: New Psychoactive Substances 2020;**86**(3):452–481.

11. Peacock A, Bruno R, Gisev N, et al. New psychoactive substances: challenges for drug surveillance, control, and public health responses. *Lancet* 2019;**394**:1668–1684.

12. United Nations Office on Drugs and Crime (UNODC). The Challenge of New Psychoactive Substances. Global SMART Programme 2013.

13. United Nations Office on Drugs and Crime (UNODC). Global SMART Update Understanding the Synthetic Drug Market: The NPS Factor, Volume 19.

14. United Nations Office on Drugs and Crime (UNODC). World Drug Report 2014.

15. World Drug Report 2021 (United Nations publication, Sales No. E.21.XI.8).

16. United Nations Office on Drugs and Crime (UNODC). Early Warning Advisory on New Psychoactive Substances. www.unodc.org/LSS/Announcement?type=NPS [last accessed 21 February 2022].

17. European Monitoring Centre for Drugs and Drug Addiction (2021), European Drug Report 2021: Trends and Developments, Publications Office of the European Union, Luxembourg

18. Corkery JM, Guirguis A, Papanti DG, Orsolini L, Schifano F. Synthetic cathinones: prevalence and motivations for use. In: Zawilska J (ed.), *Synthetic Cathinones: Current Topics in Neurotoxicity*, volume **12**. Springer, Cham, 2018.

19. World Drug Report 2021 (United Nations publication, Sales No. E.21.XI.8).

20. World Drug Report 2020 (United Nations publication, Sales No. E.20.XI.6).

21. The United Nations Office on Drugs and Crime (UNODC) World Drug Report 2019 (United Nations publication, Sales No. E.19.XI.8). Available at: https://wdr.unodc.org/wdr2019/prelaunch/WDR19_Booklet_1_EXECUTIVE_SUMMARY.pdf [last accessed 15 February 2022].

22. European Monitoring Centre for Drugs and Drug Addiction and Europol. EU Drug Markets Report: In-Depth Analysis, EMCDDA–Europol Joint publications. Publications Office of the European Union, Luxembourg, 2016.

23. Reuter P. Options for Regulating New Psychoactive Drugs: A Review of Recent Experiences. UK Drug Policy Commission (UKDPC), 2011.

24. McNabb CB, Russell BR, Caprioli D, Nutt DJ, Gibbons S, Dalley JW. Single chemical entity legal highs: assessing the risk for long term harm. *Curr Drug Abuse Rev* 2012;**5**(4):304–319.

25. Peters FT, Martinez-Ramirez JA. Analytical toxicology of emerging drugs of abuse. *Ther Drug Monit* 2010;**32**(5):532–539. https://doi.org/10.1097/FTD.0b013e3181f33411

26. Maurer HH. Chemistry, pharmacology, and metabolism of emerging drugs of abuse. *Ther Drug Monit* 2010;**32**(5):544–549. https://doi.org/10.1097/FTD.0b013e3181eea318

27. United Nations Office on Drugs and Crime (UNODC). The Challenge of New Psychoactive Substances. Global SMART Programme 2013.

28. United Nations Office on Drugs and Crime (UNODC). Early Warning Advisory on New Psychoactive Substances. www.unodc.org/LSS/Page/NPS [last accessed 9 February 2022].

29. United Nations Office on Drugs and Crime (UNODC). Early Warning Advisory on New Psychoactive Substances. www.unodc.org/LSS/Page/NPS [last accessed 9 February 2022].

30. European Monitoring Centre for Drugs and Drug Addiction. European Drug Report 2019: Trends and Developments. Publications Office of the European Union, Luxembourg, 2019.

31. European Monitoring Centre for Drugs and Drug Addiction. European Drug Report 2017: Trends and Developments. Publications Office of the European Union, Luxembourg, 2017.

32. European Monitoring Centre for Drugs and Drug Addiction. European Drug Report 2019: Trends and Developments. Publications Office of the European Union, Luxembourg, 2019.

33. Home Office. Review of the Psychoactive Substances Act 2016. Available from: https://assets.publishing.service.gov.uk/government/uploads/system/uploads/attachment_data/file/756896/Review_of_the_Psychoactive_Substances_Act__2016___web_.pdf

34. European Monitoring Centre for Drugs and Drug Addiction. European Drug Report 2017: Trends and Developments. Publications Office of the European Union, Luxembourg, 2017.

35. Tanibuchi Y, Matsumoto T, Shimane T, Funada D. The influence of tightening regulations on patients with new psychoactive substance-related disorders in Japan. *Neuropsychopharmacol Rep* 2018;**38**(4):189–196. https://doi.org/10.1002/npr2.12035

36. The United Nations Office on Drugs and Crime (UNODC). World Drug Report 2019 (United Nations publication, Sales No. E.19.XI.8). Available at: https://wdr.unodc.org/wdr2019/prelaunch/WDR19_Booklet_1_EXECUTIVE_SUMMARY.pdf

37. European Monitoring Centre for Drugs and Drug Addiction. European Drug Report 2019: Trends and Developments. Publications Office of the European Union, Luxembourg, 2019.

38. European Monitoring Centre for Drugs and Drug Addiction. Fentanils and synthetic cannabinoids: driving greater complexity into the drug situation. An update from the EU Early Warning System (June 2018). Publications Office of the European Union, Luxembourg, 2018.

39. www.unodc.org/LSS/announcement/Details/4977098d-62f0-4966-a23e-4eaab99c0dfc [last accessed 9 February 2022].

40. World Drug Report 2019 (United Nations publication, Sales No. E.19.XI.8).

41. European Monitoring Centre for Drugs and Drug Addiction European Drug Report 2021: Trends and Developments, Publications Office of the European Union, Luxembourg. 2021

42. Measham F, Moore K, Newcombe R, & Welch Z. Tweaking, bombing, dabbing and stockpiling: the emergence of mephedrone and the perversity of prohibition. *Drugs and Alcohol Today* 2010;**10**(1):14–21.

43. Corazza O, Simonato P, Corkery J, Trincas G, & Schifano F. 'Legal highs': safe and legal 'heavens'? A study on the diffusion, knowledge and risk awareness of novel psychoactive drugs among students in the UK. *Rivista Di Psichiatria* 2014;**49**(2):89–94. https://doi.org/10.1708/1461.16147

44. Sande M. Characteristics of the use of 3-MMC and other new psychoactive drugs in Slovenia, and the perceived problems experienced by users. *Int J Drug Policy* 2016;**27**:65–73. https://doi.org/10.1016/j.drugpo.2015.03.005

45. Winstock AR, Lawn W, Deluca P, Borschmann R. Methoxetamine: an early report on the motivations for use, effect profile and prevalence of use in a UK clubbing sample. *Drug Alcohol Rev* 2016;**35**(2):212–217. https://doi.org/10.1111/dar.12259

46. Measham F, Moore K, Newcombe R, Welch Z. Tweaking, bombing, dabbing and stockpiling: the emergence of mephedrone and the perversity of prohibition. *Drugs Alcohol Today* 2010;**10**(1):14–21. https://doi.org/10.5042/daat.2010.0123

47. Soussan C, Andersson M, Kjellgren A. The diverse reasons for using novel psychoactive substances: a qualitative study of the users' own perspectives. *Int J Drug Policy* 2018;**52**:71–78.

48. Benschop A, Urbán R, Kapitány-Fövény M, et al. Why do people use new psychoactive substances? Development of a new measurement tool in six European countries. *J Psychopharmacol* 2020;**34**(6):600–611. https://doi.org/10.1177/0269881120904951

49. Corazza O, Simonato P, Corkery J, Trincas G, Schifano F. Legal highs: safe and legal heavens? A study on the diffusion, knowledge and risk awareness of novel psychoactive drugs among students in the UK. *Rivista Di Psichiatria* 2014;**49**(2):89–94. http://dx.doi.org/10.1708/1461.16147

50. Johnson LA, Johnson RL, Portier RB. Current legal highs. *J Emerg Med* 2013;**44**(6):1108–1115. http://dx.doi.org/10.1016/j.jemermed.2012.09.147

51. Measham F, Moore K, Newcombe R, Welch Z. Tweaking, bombing, dabbing and stockpiling: the emergence of mephedrone and the perversity of prohibition. *Drugs Alcohol Today* 2010;**10**(1):14–21. http://dx.doi.org/10.5042/daat.2010.0123

52. Sande M. Characteristics of the use of 3-MMC and other new psychoactive drugs in Slovenia, and the perceived problems experienced by users. *Int J Drug Policy* 2016;**27**:65–73. http://dx.doi.org/10.1016/j.drugpo.2015.03.005

53. Werse B, Morgenstern C. How to handle legal highs? Findings from a German online survey and considerations on drug policy issues. *Drugs Alcohol Today* 2012;**12**(4):222–231. http://dx.doi.org/10.1108/17459261211286636

54. Winstock AR, Lawn W, Deluca P, Borschmann R. Methoxetamine: an early report on the motivations for use, effect profile and prevalence of use in a UK clubbing sample. *Drug Alcohol Rev* 2016;**35**:212–217. https://doi.org/10.1111/dar

55. Maxwella S, Shahmanesh M, Gafos M. Chemsex behaviours among men who have sex with men: a systematic review of the literature. *Int J Drug Policy* 2019;**63**:74–89.

56. Soussan C, Andersson M, Kjellgren A. The diverse reasons for using novel psychoactive substances: a qualitative study of the users' own perspectives. *Int J Drug Policy* 2018;**52**:71–78.

57. Soussan C, Kjellgren A. The users of novel psychoactive substances: online survey about their characteristics, attitudes and motivations. *Int J Drug Policy* 2016;**32**:77–84. http://dx.doi.org/10.1016/j.drugpo.2016.03.007

58. Bonaccorso S, Metastasio A, Ricciardi A, et al. Synthetic cannabinoid use in a case series of patients with psychosis presenting to acute psychiatric settings: clinical presentation and management issues. *Brain Sci* 2018;**8**(7):133. https://doi.org/10.3390/brainsci8070133

59. Mitcheson L, McCambridge J, Byrne A, Hunt N, Winstock A. Sexual health risk among dance drug users: cross-sectional comparisons with nationally representative data. *Int J Drug Policy* 2008;**19**(4):304–310. https://doi.org/10.1016/j.drugpo.2007.02.002

60. Sutherland R, Peacock A, Whittaker E, et al. New psychoactive substance use among regular psychostimulant users in Australia, 2010–2015. *Drug Alcohol Depend* 2016;**161**:110–118.

61. Singh AK. Alcohol interaction with cocaine, methamphetamine, opioids, nicotine, cannabis, and γ-hydroxybutyric acid. *Biomedicines* 2019;**7**:16. https://doi.org/10.3390/biomedicines7010016

62. Sutherland R, Peacock A, Whittaker E, et al. New psychoactive substance use among regular psychostimulant users in Australia, 2010–2015. *Drug Alcohol Depend* 2016;**161**:110–118.

63. European Monitoring Centre for Drugs and Drug Addiction. European Drug Report 2019: Trends and Developments. Publications Office of the European Union, Luxembourg, 2019.

64. Measham F, Moore K. Repertoires of distinction: exploring patterns of weekend poly-drug use within local leisure scenes across the English night-time economy. *Criminal Justice* 2009;**9**(4):437–464.

65. Hoare R, Flatley J. Drug Misuse Declared: Findings from the 2007/2008 British Crime Survey (Home Office Statistical Bulletin 13/10). Home Office, 2008.

66. Vento AE, Martinotti G, Cinosi E, et al. Substance use in the club scene of Rome: a pilot study. *Biomed Res Int* 2014;2014:617546. https://doi.org/10.1155/2014/617546

67. Fernández-Calderóna F, Cleland CM, Palamar JJ. Polysubstance use profiles among electronic dance music party attendees in New York City and their relation to use of new psychoactive substances. *Addict Behav* 2018;**78**:85–93. https://doi.org/10.1016/j.addbeh.2017.11.004

68. Fernández-Calderón F, Lozano OM, Vidal C, et al. Polysubstance use patterns in underground rave attenders: a cluster analysis. *J Drug Educ* 2011;**41**:183–202. http://dx.doi.org/10.2190/DE.41.2.d

69. Palamar JJ, Griffin-Tomas M, Ompad DC. Illicit drug use among rave attendees in a nationally representative sample of US high school seniors. *Drug Alcohol Depend* 2015a;**152**:24–31. http://dx.doi.org/10.1016/j.drugalcdep.2015.05.002

70. Palamar JJ, Acosta P, Ompad DC, Cleland CM. Self-reported ecstasy/MDMA/"Molly" use in a sample of nightclub and dance festival attendees in New York City. *Subst Use Misuse* 2016;**52**(1):82–91. http://dx.doi.org/10.1080/10826084.2016.1219373

71. Palamar JJ, Acosta P, Sherman S, Ompad DC, Cleland CM. Self-reported use of novel psychoactive substances among attendees of electronic dance music venues. *Am J Drug Alcohol Abuse* 2016;**42**:624–632. http://dx.doi.org/10.1080/00952990.2016.1181179

72. Palamar JJ, Barratt MJ, Ferris JA, Winstock AR. Correlates of new psychoactive substance use among a self-selected sample of nightclub attendees in the United States. *Am J Addict* 2016c;**25**:400–407. http://dx.doi.org/10.1111/ajad.12403

73. Measham F, Moore K. Repertoires of distinction: exploring patterns of weekend poly-drug use within local leisure scenes across the English night-time economy. *Criminal Justice* 2009;**9**(4):437–464.

74. Home Office and Office for National Statistics. Drug Misuse: Findings from the 2017/2018 Crime Survey for England and Wales Statistical Bulletin 14/18 July 2018.

75. Schuler MS, Stein BD, Collins RL. Differences in substance use disparities across age groups in a national cross-sectional survey of lesbian, gay, and bisexual adults. *LGBT Health* 2019;**6**(1):68–76.

76. Newcomb ME, Birkett M, Corliss HL, Mustanski B. Sexual orientation, gender, and racial differences in illicit drug use in a sample of US high school students. *Am J Public Health* 2014;**104**:304–310.

77. Corliss HL, Rosario M, Wypij D, et al. Sexual orientation and drug use in a longitudinal cohort study of US adolescents. *Addict Behav* 2010;**35**:517–521.

78. Mereish EH, Goldbach JT, Burgess C, DiBello AM. Sexual orientation, minority stress, social norms, and substance use among racially diverse adolescents. *Drug Alcohol Depend* 2017;**178**:49–56.

79. Seil KS, Desai MM, Smith MV. Sexual orientation, adult connectedness, substance use, and mental health outcomes among adolescents: findings from the 2009 New York City Youth Risk Behavior Survey. *Am J Public Health* 2014;**104**:1950–1956.

80. Goldbach JT, Tanner-Smith EE, Bagwell M, Dunlap S. Minority stress and substance use in sexual minority adolescents: a meta-analysis. *Prev Sci* 2014;**15**:350–363.

81. Marshal MP, Dermody SS, Shultz ML, et al. Mental health and substance use disparities among urban adolescent lesbian and bisexual girls. *J Am Psychiatr Nurses Assoc* 2013;**19**:271–279.

82. Halkitis PN, Palamar JJ. GHB use among gay and bisexual men. *Addict Behav* 2006;**31**(11):2135–2139.

83. Bourne A, Reid D, Hickson F, et al. Illicit drug use in sexual settings ('chemsex') and HIV/STI transmission risk behaviour among gay men in South London: findings from a qualitative study. *Sex Transm Infect* 2015;**91**:564–568.

84. Abdulrahim D, Whiteley C, Moncrieff M, Bowden-Jones O. Club Drug Use among Lesbian, Gay, Bisexual and Trans (LGBT) People. Novel Psychoactive Treatment UK Network (NEPTUNE). London, 2016.

85. Kirby T, Thornber-Dunwell M. High-risk drug practices tighten grip on London gay scene. *Lancet* 2013;**381** (9861):101–102.

86. Ahmed AK, Weatherburn P, Reid D, et al. Social norms related to combining drugs and sex ('chemsex') among gay men in South London. *Int J Drug Policy* 2016;**38**:29–35.

87. Evers YJ, Hoebe CJPA, Dukers-Muijrers NHTM, et al. Sexual, addiction and mental health care needs among men who have sex with men practicing chemsex: a cross-sectional study in the Netherlands. *Prev Med Rep* 2020;**18**:101074.

88. Frankis J, Flowers P, McDaid L, Bourne A. Low levels of chemsex amongst men who have sex with men, but high levels of risk among men who engage in chemsex: analysis of a cross-sectional online survey across four countries. *Sex Health* 2018;**15**(2): 144–150. https://doi.org/10.1071/SH17159

89. Giorgetti R, Tagliabracci A, Schifano F, et al. When 'chems' meet sex: a rising phenomenon called 'chemsex'. *Curr Neuropharmacol* 2017;**15**(5):762–770.

90. Graf N, Dichtl A, Deimel D, Sander D, Stöver H. Chemsex among men who have sex with men in Germany: motives, consequences and the response of the support system. *Sex Health* 2018;15(2):151–156. https://doi.org/10.1071/SH17142

91. Hammoud MA, Bourne A, Maher L, et al. Intensive sex partying with gamma-hydroxybutyrate: factors associated with using gamma-hydroxybutyrate for chemsex among Australian gay and bisexual men – results from the Flux Study. *Sex Health* 2018;15(2):123–134. https://doi.org/10.1071 /SH17146

92. Hegazi A., Lee MJ, Whittaker W, et al. Chemsex and the city: sexualised substance use in gay bisexual and other men who have sex with men attending sexual health clinics. *Int J STD AIDS* 2017;28(4):423.

93. Hibbert MP, Brett CE, Porcellato LA, Hope VD. Psychosocial and sexual characteristics associated with sexualised drug use and chemsex among men who have sex with men (MSM) in the UK. *Sex Transm Infect* (online). Available at: https://sti .bmj.com/content/sextrans/early/2019/04/12/sextrans-2018-0 53933.full.pdf [last accessed 15 February 2022].

94. Hockenhull J, Murphy KG, Paterson S. An observed rise in g-hydroxybutyrate-associated deaths in London: evidence to suggest a possible link with concomitant rise in chemsex. *Forensic Sci Int* 2017;270:93–97.

95. O'Reilly M. Chemsex case study: is it time to recommend routine screening of sexualised drug use in men who have sex with men? *Sex Health* 2018;15(2):167–169. https://doi.org/10 .1071/SH17156

96. Pollard A, Nadarzynski T, Llewellyn C. Syndemics of stigma, minority-stress, maladaptive coping, risk environments and littoral spaces among men who have sex with men using chemsex. *Cult Health Sex* 2018;**20**:411–427.

97. Pufall EL, Kall M, Shahmanesh M, et al. Sexualized drug use ('chemsex') and high-risk sexual behaviours in HIV positive men who have sex with men. *HIV Med* 2018;**19**(4):261–270.

98. Stevens O, Forrest JI. Thinking upstream: the roles of international health and drug policies in public health responses to chemsex. *Sex Health* 2018;**15**(2):108–115. https:// doi.org/10.1071/SH17153

99. Ruane D. Field experiments: psychonauts' efforts to reduce the harm of old and new drugs at music festivals. *Drugs Educ Prevent Policy* 2018;**25**(4):337–344. https://doi.org/10.1080/09 687637.2017.1418836

100. European Monitoring Centre for Drugs and Drug Addiction (EMCDDA). EMCDDA–Europol 2012 Annual Report on the Implementation of Council Decision 2005/387/JHA. Publications Office of the European Union, Luxemburg, 2012.

101. Schifano F, Deluca P, Baldacchino A, et al. Drugs on the web; the Psychonaut 2002 EU project. *Prog Neuropsychopharmacol Biol Psychiatry* 2006;**30**(4):640–646.

102. Schifano F. Analyzing the open/deep web to better understand the new/novel psychoactive substances (NPS) scenarios: suggestions from CASSANDRA and NPS Finder Research Projects. *Brain Sci* 2020;10:146. https://doi.org/10.3390 /brainsci10030146

103. European Monitoring Centre for Drugs and Drug Addiction. European Drug Report 2017: Trends and Developments. Publications Office of the European Union, Luxembourg, 2017.

104. Corazza O, Schifano F, Farre M, et al. Designer drugs on the internet: a phenomenon out-of-control? The emergence of hallucinogenic drug Bromo-Dragonfly. *Curr Clin Pharmacol* 2011;**6**(2):125–129.

105. Corazza O, Schifano F, Simonato P, et al. Phenomenon of new drugs on the internet: the case of ketamine derivative methoxetamine. *Hum Psychopharmacol Clin Exp* 2012;**27** (2):145–149.

106. Corazza O, Valeriani G, Bersani FS, et al. "Spice," "Kryptonite," "Black Mamba": an overview of brand names and marketing strategies of novel psychoactive substances on the web. *J Psychoactive Drugs* 2014;**46**(4):287–294.

107. Orsolini L, Papanti D, Corkery J, Schifano F. An insight into the deep web; why it matters for addiction psychiatry? *Hum Psychopharmacol Clin Exp* 2017;32:e2573. https://doi.org/10 .1002/hup.2573

108. European Monitoring Centre for Drugs and Drug Addiction and Europol. Drugs and the Darknet: Perspectives for Enforcement, Research and Policy. EMCDDA–Europol Joint publications. Publications Office of the European Union, Luxembourg, 2017.

109. Orsolini L, Papanti D, Corkery J, Schifano F. An insight into the deep web; why it matters for addiction psychiatry? *Hum Psychopharmacol Clin Exp* 2017;32:e2573. https://doi.org/10.1002/hup.2573

110. van der Gouwe D, Brunt TM, van Laar M, van der Pol P. Purity, adulteration and price of drugs bought on-line versus off-line in the Netherlands (online). https://doi.org/10.1111/add.13720

111. In Focus: Trafficking over the Darknet – World Drug Report 2020. www.unodc.org/documents/Focus/WDR20_Booklet_4_Darknet_web.pdf [last accessed 9 February 2022].

112. European Monitoring Centre for Drugs and Drug Addiction (EMCDDA). EMCDDA–Europol 2012 Annual Report on the Implementation of Council Decision 2005/387/JHA. Publications Office of the European Union, Luxembourg, 2012.

113. Van Hout MC. Nod and wave: an Internet study of the codeine intoxication phenomenon. *Int J Drug Policy* 2015;26:67–77.

114. European Monitoring Centre for Drugs and Drug Addiction (EMCDDA). Recent Changes in Europe's Cocaine Market. Results from an EMCDDA Trendspotter Study. Publications Office of the European Union, Luxembourg, 2018.

115. Schifano F. Novel psychoactive substances (NPS): clinical and pharmacological issues. *Drugs Alcohol Today* 2015;15(1):21–27.

116. Schifano F, Orsolini L, Duccio Papanti G, Corkery JM. Novel psychoactive substances of interest for psychiatry. *World Psychiatry* 2015;14(1):15–26.

117. van Amsterdam J, Nutt D, Phillips L, van den Brink W. European rating of drug harms. *J Psychopharmacology* 2015;29(6):655–660. https://doi.org/10.1177/0269881115581980

118. Gable RS. Acute toxic effects of club drugs. *J Psychoactive Drugs* 2004;36(3):303–313.

119. Gable RS. Comparison of acute lethal toxicity of commonly abused psychoactive substances. *Addiction* 2004;99(6):686–696.

120. Luethia D, Kolaczynskaa KE, Doccia L, Krähenbühla S, Hoenerb MC, Liechti ME. Pharmacological profile of mephedrone analogs and related new psychoactive substances. *Neuropharmacology* 2018;134(Part A):4–12.

121. Centre for Public Health, Faculty of Health and Applied Social Science, Liverpool John Moore's University, on behalf of the Department of Health and National Treatment Agency for Substance Misuse. A Summary of the Health Harms of Drugs. Department of Health, 2011.

122. Elliott S, Sedefov R, Evans-Brown M. Assessing the toxicological significance of new psychoactive substances in fatalities. *Drug Test Anal* 2018;10:120–126.

123. European Monitoring Centre for Drugs and Drug Addiction. European Drug Report: Trends and Developments. Published 2016. Available at: https://dx.doi.org/10.2810/

124. Evans-Brown M, Sedefov R. New psychoactive substances: driving greater complexity into the drug problem. *Addiction* 2017;112:36.

125. Gable RS. Acute toxic effects of club drugs. *J Psychoactive Drugs* 2004;36(3):303–313.

126. King LA, Corkery JM. An index of fatal toxicity for new psychoactive substances. *J Psychopharmacol* 2018; 32(7):793–801.

127. National Records of Scotland Drug-related Deaths in Scotland in 2019. Published on 15 December 2020.

128. Nutt D, King LA, Saulsbury W, Blakemore C. Development of a rational scale to assess the harm of drugs of potential misuse. *Lancet* 2007;369(9566):1047–1053.

129. Gable RS. Comparison of acute lethal toxicity of commonly abused psychoactive substances. *Addiction* 2004;99(6):686–696.

130. Centre for Public Health, Faculty of Health and Applied Social Science, Liverpool John Moore's University, on behalf of the Department of Health and National Treatment Agency for Substance Misuse. A Summary of the Health Harms of Drugs. Department of Health, 2011.

131. Corazza O, Schifano F, Farre M, et al. Designer drugs on the Internet: a phenomenon out-of-control? The emergence of hallucinogenic drug Bromo-Dragonfly. *Curr Clin Pharmacol* 2011;6(2):125–129.

132. Costa G, De Luca MA, Piras G, Marongiu J, Fattore L, Simola N. Neuronal and peripheral damages induced by synthetic psychoactive substances: an update of recent findings from human and animal studies. *Neural Regen Res* 2020;15(5):802–816. https://doi.org/10.4103/1673-5374.268895

133. United Nations Office on Drugs and Crime (UNODC). Current NPS Threats, Volume I. Published March 2019. Available at: www.unodc.org/pdf/opioids-crisis/Current_NPS_Threats_-_Volume_I.pdf [last accessed 9 February 2022].

134. United Nations Office on Drugs and Crime (UNODC). Current NPS Threats, Volume I. Published March 2019. www.unodc.org/pdf/opioids-crisis/Current_NPS_Threats_-_Volume_I.pdf [last accessed 9 February 2022].

135. Guirguis A, Girotto S, Berti B, Stair JL. Identification of new psychoactive substances (NPS) using handheld Raman Spectroscopy employing both 785 and 1064 nm laser sources. *Forensic Sci Int*, published online 4 February 2017. https://doi.org/10.1016/j.forsciint.2017.01.027

136. Addison M, Stockdale K, McGovern R, et al. Exploring the intersections between novel psychoactive substances (NPS) and other substance use in a police custody suite setting in the north east of England. *Drugs Educ Prevent Policy* 2018;25(4):313–319. https://doi.org/10.1080/09687637.2017.1378620

137. Brandt SD, Sumnall HR, Measham F, Cole J. Analyses of second-generation 'legal highs' in the UK: initial findings. *Drug Test Anal* 2010;2(8):377–382. https://doi.org/10.1002/dta.155

138. Brandt SD, Sumnall HR, Measham F, Cole J. Second generation mephedrone. The confusing case of NRG-1. *BMJ* 2010;341:c3564. https://doi.org/10.1136/bmj.c3564

139. Davies S, Wood DM, Smith G, et al. Purchasing 'legal highs' on the Internet: is there consistency in what you get? *QJM* 2010;**103**(7):489–493. https://doi.org/10.1093/q jmed/hcq056.

140. Ramsey J, Dargan PI, Smyllie M, et al. Buying 'legal' recreational drugs does not mean that you are not breaking the law. *QJM* 2010;**103**(10):777–783. https://doi.org/10.1093/q jmed/hcq132

141. Ayres TC, Bond JW. A chemical analysis examining the pharmacology of novel psychoactive substances freely available over the Internet and their impact on public (ill) health. Legal highs or illegal highs? *BMJ Open* 2012;**2**(4): e000977. https://doi.org/10.1136/bmjopen-2012-000977. 2012

142. Baron M, Elie M, Elie L. An analysis of legal highs: do they contain what it says on the tin? *Drug Test Anal* 2011;**3** (9):576–581. https://doi.org/10.1002/dta.274

143. World Drug Report 2016.

144. Home Office Annual Report on the Home Office Forensic Early Warning System (FEWS) 2016/17. A system to identify New Psychoactive Substances (NPS) in the UK November 2018. Available from: https://assets.publishing.service.gov.uk/govern ment/uploads/system/uploads/attachment_data/file/757040/FE WS_Annual_Report_2016-17_STH.pdf

145. See for example: Baron M, Elie M, Elie L. An analysis of legal highs: do they contain what it says on the tin? *Drug Test Anal* 2011;**3**(9):576–581. https://doi.org/10.1002/dta.274

146. James DA, Potts S, Thomas SHL, et al. Clinical features associated with recreational use of 'Ivory Wave' preparations containing desoxypipradrol. *Clin Toxicol* 2011;**49**:201.

147. Kalasinsky KS, Hugel J, Kish SJ. Use of MDA (the 'love drug') and methamphetamine in Toronto by unsuspecting users of ecstasy (MDMA). *J Forensic Sci* 2004;**49**(5):1106–1112.

148. Parrott AC. Is ecstasy MDMA? A review of the proportion of ecstasy tablets containing MDMA, their dosage levels, and the changing perceptions of purity. *Psychopharmacology* 2004;**173**:234–241.

149. Cole JC, Bailey M, Sumnall HR, Wagstaff GF, King LA. The content of ecstasy tablets: implications for the study of their long-term effects. *Addiction* 2002;**97**:1531–1536.

150. Tanner-Smith EE. Pharmacological content of tablets sold as 'ecstasy': results from an online testing service. *Drug Alcohol Depend* 2006;**83**(3):247–254.

151. Baron M, Elie M, Elie L. An analysis of legal highs: do they contain what it says on the tin? *Drug Test Anal* 2011;**3** (9):576–581. https://doi.org/10.1002/dta.274

152. Brunt TM, Atkinson AM, Nefau T, et al. Online test purchased new psychoactive substances in five different European countries: a snapshot study of chemical composition and price. *Int J Drug Policy* 2017;**44**:105–114. https://doi.org/10.1016/j .drugpo.2017.03.006

153. Brunt TM, Atkinson AM, Nefau T, et al. Online test purchased new psychoactive substances in five different European countries: a snapshot study of chemical composition and price. *Int J Drug Policy* 2017;**44**:105–114.

154. Brunt TM, Atkinson AM, Nefau T, et al. Online test purchased new psychoactive substances in five different European countries: a snapshot study of chemical composition and price. *Int J Drug Policy* 2017;**44**:105–114.

155. Kalasinsky KS, Hugel J, Kish SJ. Use of MDA (the 'love drug') and methamphetamine in Toronto by unsuspecting users of ecstasy (MDMA). *J Forensic Sci* 2004;**49**(5):1106–1112.

156. Parrott AC. Is ecstasy MDMA? A review of the proportion of ecstasy tablets containing MDMA, their dosage levels, and the changing perceptions of purity. *Psychopharmacology* 2004;**173**:234–241.

157. Cole JC, Bailey M, Sumnall HR, Wagstaff GF, King LA. The content of ecstasy tablets: implications for the study of their long-term effects. *Addiction* 2002;**97**:1531–1536.

158. Tanner-Smith EE. Pharmacological content of tablets sold as 'ecstasy': results from an online testing service. *Drug Alcohol Depend* 2006;**83**(3):247–254.

159. Ciccarone D, Ondocsin J, Mars SG. Heroin uncertainties: exploring users' perceptions of fentanyl-adulterated and - substituted 'heroin'. *Int J Drug Policy* 2017;**46**:146–155.

160. Unick GJ, Ciccarone D. US regional and demographic differences in prescription opioid and heroin-related overdose hospitalizations. *Int J Drug Policy* 2017;**46**:112–119. https://doi .org/10.1016/j.drugpo.2017.06.003

161. Tomassoni AJ. Multiple fentanyl overdoses—New Haven, Connecticut, June 23, 2016. *Morb Mort Wkly Rep* 2017;**66**:107–111.

162. Fairbairn N, Coffin PO, Walley AY. Naloxone for heroin, prescription opioid, and illicitly made fentanyl overdoses: challenges and innovations responding to a dynamic epidemic. *Int J Drug Policy* 2017;**46**:172–179. https://doi.org/10.1016/j .drugpo.2017.06.005

163. Krause D, Plörer D, Koller G, et al. High concomitant misuse of fentanyl in subjects on opioid maintenance treatment. *Subst Use Misuse* 2017;**52**(5):639–645.

164. Cicero TJ, Ellis MS, Kasper ZA. Increases in self-reported fentanyl use among a population entering drug treatment: the need for systematic surveillance of illicitly manufactured opioids. *Drug Alcohol Depend* 2017;**177**:101–103. https://doi .org/10.1016/j.drugalcdep.2017.04.004

165. Ciccarone D, Ondocsin J, Mars SG. . Heroin uncertainties: exploring users' perceptions of fentanyl-adulterated and - substituted 'heroin'. *Int J Drug Policy* 2017;**46**:146–155.

166. Caudevilla-Gálligo F, Riba J, Ventura M, et al. 4-bromo-2,5-dimethoxyphenethylamine (2C-B): presence in the recreational drug market in Spain, pattern of use and subjective effects. *J Psychopharmacol* 2012;**26**(7):1026–1035. https://doi.org/10.1177/0269881111431752

167. Liakoni E, Yates C, Dines, AM, et al. Acute recreational drug toxicity. *Medicine* 2018;**97**(5):e9784. https://doi.org/10.1097/ MD.0000000000009784

168. European Monitoring Centre for Drugs and Drug Addiction. European Drug Report 2019: Trends and Developments.

Publications Office of the European Union, Luxembourg, 2019.

169. Wood DM, De La Rue L, Hosin AA, et al. Dargan poor identification of emergency department acute recreational drug toxicity presentations using routine hospital coding systems: the experience in Denmark, Switzerland and the UK. *J Med Toxicol* 2019;**15**:112–120. https://doi.org/10.1007/s131 81-018-0687-z

170. Wood DM, Conran P, Dargan PI. ICD- 10 coding: poor identification of recreational drug presentations to a large emergency department. *Emerg Med* 2011;**28**:387–389.

171. Shah AD, Wood DM, Dargan PI. Survey of ICD-10 coding of hospital admissions in the UK due to recreational drug toxicity. *QJM* 2011;**104**:779–784.

172. Wood DM, De La Rue L, Hosin AA, et al. Darganpoor identification of emergency department acuterecreational drug toxicity presentations using routine hospital coding systems: the experience in Denmark, Switzerland and the UK. *J Med Toxicol* 2019;**15**:112–120. https://doi.org/10.1007/s131 81-018-0687-z

173. Poznyak V, Reed GM, Medina-Mora ME. Aligning the ICD-11 classification of disorders due to substance use with global service needs. *Epidemiol Psychiatr Sci* (online). https://doi.org /10.1017/S2045796017000622

174. International Classification of Diseases for Mortality and Morbidity Statistics, 11th edn., v2019-04 6C47. Disorders due to use of synthetic cathinones. Available at: https://icd .who.int/browse11/l-m/en#/http://id.who.int/icd/entity/1605 818663 [last accessed 15 February 2022].

175. International Classification of Diseases for Mortality and Morbidity Statistics, 11th edn., v2019-04 6C42. Disorders due to use of synthetic cannabinoids. Available at: https://icd .who.int/browse11/l-m/en#/http://id.who.int/icd/entity/8048 33492 [last accessed 15 February 2022].

176. International Classification of Diseases for Mortality and Morbidity Statistics, 11th ed., v2019-04 6C4C. Disorders due to use of MDMA or related drugs, including MDA. Available at: https://icd .who.int/browse11/l-m/en#/http://id.who.int/icd/entity/1218 193465[lastaccessed15February2022].

177. Wood DM, De La Rue L, Hosin AA, et al. Dargan poor identification of emergency department acute recreational drug toxicity presentations using routine hospital coding systems: the experience in Denmark, Switzerland and the UK. *J Med 673 Col:311Toxicol* 2019;**15**:112–120. https://doi.org/10 .1007/s13181-018-0687-z

178. European Monitoring Centre for Drugs and Drug Addiction. European Drug Report 2019: Trends and Developments. Publications Office of the European Union, Luxembourg, 2019.

179. Wood DM, Heyerdahl F, Yates CB, et al. The European Drug Emergencies Network (Euro-DEN). *Clin Toxicol* 2014;**52** (4):239–241. https://doi.org/10.3109/15563650.2014.898771

180. European Monitoring Centre for Drugs and Drug Addiction. Drug-related hospital emergency presentations in Europe: update from the Euro-DEN Plus expert network, technical report. Publications Office of the European Union, Luxembourg, 2020.

181. European Monitoring Centre for Drugs and Drug Addiction. European Drug Report 2019: Trends and Developments. Publications Office of the European Union, Luxembourg, 2019.

182. European Monitoring Centre for Drugs and Drug Addiction. European Drug Report 2019: Trends and Developments. Publications Office of the European Union, Luxembourg, 2019.

183. Hunter LJ, Dargan PI, Benzie A, White JA, Wood DM. Recreational drug use in men who have sex with men (MSM) attending UK sexual health services is significantly higher than in non-MSM. *Postgrad Med J* 2014;**90**(1061):133–138. https:// doi.org/10.1136/postgradmedj-2012-131428

184. Scottish Government. The Sexual Health and Blood Borne Virus Framework 2011–2015.

185. Department of Health. A Framework for Sexual Health Improvement in England. Published 2013.

186. Royal College of Physicians. Alcohol and Sex: A Cocktail for Poor Sexual Health (Report of the Alcohol and Sexual Health Working Party). Published 2011.

187. British HIV Association. Standards of Care for People Living with HIV in 2013. Available at: www.bhiva.org/file/WSheCF ExXGBRK/BHIVAStandardsA4.pdf [last accessed 15 February 2022].

188. Hunter LJ, Dargan PI, Benzie A, White JA, Wood DM. Recreational drug use in men who have sex with men (MSM) attending UK sexual health services is significantly higher than in non-MSM. *Postgrad Med J* 2014;**90**(1061):133–138. https:// doi.org/10.1136/postgradmedj-2012-131428

189. Bowden-Jones O. Joining up sexual health and drug services to better meet client needs. Background paper commissioned by the EMCDDA for Health and social responses to drug problems: a European guide. Available at: www .emcdda.europa.eu/system/files/attachments/6239/European ResponsesGuide2017_BackgroundPaper-Sexual-health-and-drug-use.pdf [last accessed 15 February 2022].

190. National Institute for Health and Care Excellence. Alcohol-Use Disorders: Preventing Harmful Drinking (PH24). Published 2010.

191. British Association of Sexual Health and HIV. Standards for the management of sexually transmitted infections (STIs). Published 2019. Available at: www.bashh.org/about-bashh/pu blications/standards-for-the-management-of-stis/ [last accessed 15 February 2022].

192. British Association of Sexual Health and HIV. Standards for the management of sexually transmitted infections (STIs). Published 2019. Available at: www.bashh.org/about-bashh/pu blications/standards-for-the-management-of-stis/ [last accessed 15 February 2022].

193. Department of Health and Social Care, Public Health England. Integrated Sexual Health Services. A suggested national service specification. Published August 2018. Available at: https://ass ets.publishing.service.gov.uk/government/uploads/system/up loads/attachment_data/file/731140/integrated-sexual-health-services-specification.pdf [last accessed 15 February 2022].

194. World Health Organization. International Standards for the Treatment of Drug Use Disorders. Revised edition incorporating results of field-testing. 31 March 2020. Available from: www.who.int/publications/i/item/inter national-standards-for-the-treatment-of-drug-use-disorders

195. United Nations Office for Drugs and Crime, World Health Organization. Principles of Drug Dependence Treatment. Published March 2008. Available at: www.unodc.org/docu ments/drug-treatment/UNODC-WHO-Principles-of-Drug-Dependence-Treatment-March08.pdf [last accessed 15 February 2022].

196. Panagopoulos I, Ricciardelli LA. Harm reduction and decision making among recreational ecstasy users. *Int J Drug Policy* 2005;**16**:54–64.

197. Fernández-Calderón F, Lozano-Rojas Ó, Rojas-Tejada A, et al. Harm reduction behaviors among young polysubstance users at raves. *Subst Abuse* 2014;**35**:45–50.

198. Greenspan NR, Aguinaldo JP, Husbands W, et al. "It's not rocket science, what I do": self-directed harm reduction strategies among drug using ethno-racially diverse gay and bisexual men. *Int J Drug Policy* 2011;**22**:56–62.

199. Cruz OS. Non problematic illegal drug use: drug use management strategies in a Portuguese sample. *J Drug Issues* 2015;**45**:133–150.

200. Fernández-Calderón F, Díaz-Batanero C, Barratt MJ, Palamar JJ. Harm reduction strategies related to dosing and their relation to harms among festival attendees who use multiple drugs. *Drug Alcohol Rev* 2019;**38**:57–67. https://doi.org/10.1111/dar.12868

Psychosocial Interventions for Club Drugs and Novel Psychoactive Substances

2.1 Introduction

There is a large body of evidence on the effectiveness of psychosocial interventions (PSIs) for the management of substance misuse problems, including national guidelines. It is therefore possible to make specific and robust recommendations.

Effective treatment for all substance misuse problems includes PSIs. These in fact are the primary form of treatment intervention for the misuse of, and dependence on, the majority of substances, as only a small number of substances of misuse have recognised pharmacological interventions, such as opiate substitutes for opiate dependence.[1] Where pharmacological interventions do have a role, for instance in opioid dependence, PSIs are generally associated with enhanced treatment outcomes.[2] PSIs are important in helping people prepare for planned, medically assisted detoxification and are essential following detoxification, to sustain positive changes.

Psychological interventions for substance misuse problems focus on supporting behaviour change to achieve desired outcomes. PSIs may aim to support people to achieve abstinence from use of specific or multiple substances, or a reduction in use to a less harmful level or in a less harmful manner. Psychological interventions are also used to help with co-occurring psychological, social or physical problems, again with the aim of contributing to sustained change in substance misuse.

There is evidence for the effectiveness of PSIs including brief interventions, motivational interviewing, self-help groups, behavioural couples therapy, contingency management, CBT-based relapse prevention, community reinforcement approaches, social behaviour network therapy, family therapy and psychodynamic therapy.[3,4,5,6,7,8,9,10] However, in what Orford terms the 'outcome equivalence paradox', no single approach is regarded as universally superior.[11] See Box 2.1 for the key principles for health and social responses to drug problems in Europe, according to the EMCDDA.

Box 2.1 *European Monitoring Centre for Drugs and Drug Addiction (EMCDDA): Key Principles for Health and Social Responses to Drug Problems*[12]

According to the EMCDDA, the key principles for health and social responses to drug problems in Europe should be the following:

- *Be respectful of human rights, including:*
  - o *The right to the enjoyment of the highest attainable standard of physical and mental health;*
  - o *The right of the drug user to give informed consent to treatment;*
- *Respect ethical principles, including informed consent, confidentiality and equity of access;*
- *Promote service user and peer involvement in service design and delivery;*
- *Take a public health approach;*
- *Be based on an assessment of needs and tailored to the specific requirements of the target population;*
- *Respond to cultural and social characteristics, including gender issues and health inequalities; and*
- *Be properly designed and based on evidence, duly monitored and evaluated.*

2.2 Psychosocial Interventions for Novel Psychoactive Substances

Very limited research has so far been published relating specifically to PSIs for the treatment of NPS. Where this exists, it has been summarised in the relevant chapters in this publication. It is argued that the large number of NPS, their diversity and the speed at which they appear, is challenging both for monitoring and developing effective and timely responses.

Many NPS are stimulant in nature and this chapter therefore draws heavily on research for the treatment of stimulant misuse and also draws on the broader literature on PSIs for health behaviour change in general.[6] Reference is also made to commonly accepted good practice for effective psychological interventions in general.

Patterns of NPS use show a close parallel to recognised patterns of alcohol use. The most common pattern is infrequent, non-dependent use, with lower risk of severity and likelihood of harm. A much smaller proportion of users engage in entrenched dependent use with the potential for more significant associated harm. The chapter therefore also draws on the much more extensive literature on PSIs for alcohol problems.[7]

Recent developments in the NPS market, such as opioid and benzodiazepine NPS and potent synthetic cannabinoid receptor agonists (SCRAs), appear to be targeted primarily at the long-term and more problematic drug users.[13] This means that existing recommendations and guidelines for relevant interventions in these groups of users must be considered.

Specialist treatment for problems caused by new and emerging substances is not well developed in most countries. It has been noted that many of the health and social responses to new substances in Europe and elsewhere are adaptations of programmes for 'established' or 'traditional' drugs. Existing interventions often target particular groups. These vary by country but include: recreational stimulant users, psychonauts, men who have sex with men, people avoiding drug tests, and high-risk drug users. Specific guidance on responding to the use of these substances in prisons and custodial settings is also being developed in some countries.[14]

In developing club drug and NPS-specific interventions, adjustments to existing protocols need to take account of specific drug effects, socio-cultural characteristics of risk groups (e.g. party-goers, men who have sex with men) or particular risk behaviours (e.g. high injecting frequency). Multi-disciplinary responses and collaborations between health providers in different settings (e.g. sexual health clinics, custodial settings and drug treatment centres) are needed to reduce these harms. Cultural competence, or an understanding of how cultural issues influence patterns of drug use and associated harms is needed within services, in order to enhance service engagement and uptake.[14]

As the relationship between trauma and substance use is becoming increasingly established, the need for trauma-informed interventions has been identified to facilitate long-term recovery from both addiction and trauma.[15] The link between the harmful use of NPS and club drugs and trauma has not been investigated.

However, evidence supporting a strong association between exposure to childhood adversity and early life trauma and opioid dependence, polydrug use, poor retention in treatment,[16,17,18,19,20,21,22,23] and drug use and imprisonment, suggests that this must be considered in interventions for club drugs and NPS.[24,25,26]

Suggestions have been made on how trauma-informed interventions should be developed.[27,28,29,30,31,32,33,34]

2.3 Stepped Care

Psychosocial interventions for substance use are commonly provided following a stepped care model (Figure 2.1).[35,36]

Within stepped care models, psychological and social interventions are grouped according to the level of specific psychological and social treatment competences required to deliver them effectively. It is therefore common to refer to 'lower-intensity PSIs' and 'higher-intensity PSIs'.

The main principles of a stepped care approach are as follows:

- The least intrusive intervention needed to achieve a required outcome is delivered first.
- If an intervention does not achieve the desired outcome, service users should be offered the option of being 'stepped up' to a more intensive intervention.
- Where a higher level of intensity of treatment is no longer required, 'stepping down' to a less intensive option should be offered.
- Service users should have access to all levels of treatment within a treatment system.
- Service users should have direct access to the intensity of intervention likely to be required to achieve their desired outcomes, and not unnecessarily proceed through lower levels in a stepwise order.

2.4 Identification of Novel Psychoactive Substance Use and Its Severity

The clinical identification of individuals experiencing NPS harmful use or dependence, particularly those less severely affected, is not always easy when regular use may be linked to lifestyle. Determining the need for specific psychosocial interventions to address behaviour change will also be influenced by a wide range of factors.

Many people make substantial changes to their substance misuse without formal treatment.[11]

Substance use or intoxication is not in itself an indication for treatment. Unlike the several robust screening tools for alcohol use, there are no recognised screening tools specifically developed for NPS use and there is no routine screening for NPS use in general health care settings. However, any contact with a health professional where NPS and club drug use is identified can be an opportunity to offer non-judgmental health advice on safety and, potentially, change.

Self-report, incidental or opportunistic enquiry may reveal NPS use and risk but no evidence of harm or need for a treatment intervention. This provides a potentially useful opportunity to offer information and brief advice or to signpost to sources of further information. Other individuals will provide clearer evidence of at least some degree of problematic use. Many such problematic users will be able to change their risky behaviour without assistance and will not require professional help. Some of these problematic users will however benefit from brief advice and information in addition to the offer of referral to formal treatment services. When information and brief advice is used in this way to help address problem use, it forms part of the stepped care 'treatment' pathway shown in Figure 2.1.

Addressing substance misuse problems emphasises approaches based on strengths and needs, for example a 'recovery capital' model, rather than a deficits-based approach[37]. A recovery capital model looks at the strengths and needs a service user has over a range of domains beyond substance use. More resources across the domains would suggest greater likelihood of positive outcomes, and fewer resources suggest an indication for broader and more intensive interventions. Four types of recovery capital are identified:[38]

- **Human capital** – e.g. skills, employment, mental and physical health;
- **Physical capital** – e.g. tangible resources, housing, money;
- **Cultural capital** – e.g. values, beliefs;
- **Social capital** – e.g. relationships with others.

Those who have more strengths and resources (recovery capital) may be more likely to achieve their desired outcomes with little or no professional input.[39] Indicators for more intensive interventions include: longer problem duration, injecting drug use, substance dependence, unsuccessful independent attempts to change, multiple substance misuse problems, multiple co-occurring problems, fewer individual strengths and less access to resources. An additional consideration is that people may have substantial substance misuse problems but at the present time are only ready or able to access and engage with less intensive interventions (e.g. needle exchange interventions for injecting drug use).

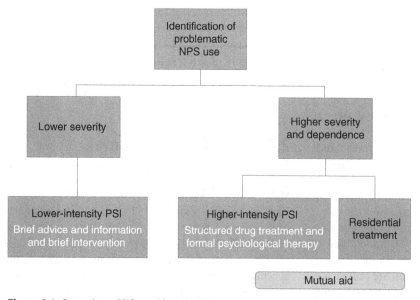

Figure 2.1 *Stepped care PSI for problematic NPS use*

The intensity of the PSI should be more directly related to the severity of the substance misuse problem than to the severity of the health and other consequences of the substance use. For example, someone experiencing an extreme medical consequence of one-off use of a substance may be able to make desired changes without formal treatment.

It seems likely that most NPS use is infrequent, largely remains within the control of the individual and is associated with a low risk of harm.[40] Nonetheless, some NPS are injected and the majority of NPS are associated with reported incidents of serious acute and chronic harms. The repeated use of some NPS can lead to dependence and for some, such as GHB/GBL, acute withdrawal can be a medical emergency.

Box 2.2 lists the recommended pragmatic indicators for a referral to drug treatment services, which will include PSIs.

2.5 Settings for the Delivery of Psychosocial Interventions

The intensity of the psychosocial intervention (PSI) delivered will vary across the settings in which they are offered. Some PSIs require additional or specialist competences to deliver them, whereas mutual aid, for instance, is a peer-led intervention and so is not dependent on particular settings for its delivery (and therefore is not discussed further in this sub-section).

2.5.1 Settings for Lower-Intensity Psychosocial Interventions

In non-drug treatment settings, where NPS use, or problematic use, has been identified during a clinical

---

Box 2.2 *Indicators for a Referral to Drug Treatment Services and Psychosocial Interventions*

- Current injecting of any substance;
- Self-report 2 of inability to make changes to NPS use when attempted;
- Repeated presentation(s) with drug-related harm (psychological, social or physical);
- Self-identification of needing specialist help or request for referral to drug treatment services.

---

interaction with a service user, the offer of brief advice and information may be helpful. Such non-drug treatment settings include primary care, emergency departments, primary and secondary care mental health services, sexual health clinics and HIV services, in addition to other services where people may present with acute problems related to NPS use.

There are a number of non-drug treatment clinical services that work with service user groups with a higher prevalence of NPS use, and these services should consider developing the relevant skills and competences to offer brief interventions (BIs) and referral pathways for additional support if needed. Primary care is the obvious example, but there is evidence that NPS use has a higher prevalence in people attending sexual health services[41] and HIV treatment services.[42] These services (and others with service users with known higher prevalence rates of NPS use) have an appropriate opportunity actively to ask about NPS use as part of their normal clinical assessment process.

Numerous studies report people living with HIV have a higher prevalence of NPS use (as will be discussed later) and there are concerns about the additional health and viral transmission risks NPS use may pose. People living with diagnosed HIV typically have frequent medical review appointments at HIV treatment services. These service contacts provide a valuable opportunity for appropriate questions on NPS use (asked routinely or targeted as appropriate), and the offer of brief advice, information and, if suitable, brief interventions.

Because of high levels of presentations related to substance use, some emergency departments (EDs) may employ staff with skills to provide brief interventions. Similarly, because there are high levels of substance misuse among people accessing mental health services,[43] these services often have staff with additional competences ('dual-diagnosis workers') to provide higher-intensity drug interventions in combination with mental health interventions.

2.5.2 Settings for Higher-Intensity Psychosocial Interventions

Higher-intensity PSIs, structured drug treatment and formal psychological therapy are likely to be delivered in community or residential drug treatment services.

There may be benefits in locating the delivery of higher-intensity PSIs in specific non-drug services where presentation with problematic NPS use is frequent and associated with other health or social problems. This may encourage engagement in drug treatment by minimising any perceived stigma involved in attending drug treatment services. There may also be merit in developing specialist hybrid services for specific populations with co-occurring needs. For example, innovative services where drug treatment and psychological therapy are provided in settings such as sexual health services with a high level of presentation of co-occurring sexual health problems, problematic NPS use and in some cases psychological problems.

These differing levels of intensity of interventions will be reflected in the increasingly specialised competences that the health professionals delivering them will have. All levels of intervention must be delivered within an appropriate governance framework with more intensive PSIs requiring specific supervision.[4]

A stepped care model of interventions for NPS use should be available to service users across a treatment system, with referral pathways between the various services where service users are likely to present. It is recommended that the settings listed in Table 2.1 offer *a minimum* level of PSI. Each intervention is described in greater detail in the following.

All non-drug treatment services should offer referral to drug treatment services, as indicated in Box 2.2.

2.6 Lower-Intensity Psychosocial Interventions

Lower-intensity PSIs can be divided into two main interventions: provision of brief advice and information; and provision of brief interventions. The published evidence that underlies this for drug users mainly relates to the provision of brief interventions. However, recommending the provision of brief advice and information is a considered and pragmatic approach that takes account of wider evidence on brief advice and is based on what is considered a minimum approach to addressing the basic health needs of NPS users attending non-drug treatment services. Brief interventions, derived mainly from the principles of motivational interviewing, have been recommended. They are also opportunistic interventions used in non-drug treatment settings with people who have little or no contact with drug treatment services. Winstock and Mitcheson recommend brief interventions for the majority of NPS users, whose use would

Table 2.1 Minimum recommended levels of psychosocial interventions in health settings dealing with NPS use

Setting	Minimum level of PSI
Primary care/general practice	Availability of brief advice
Emergency department	Availability of brief advice and
Sexual health services	Availability of brief advice and information plus brief intervention
HIV services	Availability of brief advice and information plus brief intervention
Mental health services (including primary and secondary care psychological therapy services)	Availability of brief advice and information plus brief intervention *provide structured*
Drug treatment services	Availability of brief advice and information, brief intervention, structured drug treatment, formal psychological therapy, facilitated access to mutual aid. Access to assessment for residential drug treatment

be in the lower severity range. Provision of brief advice, information and brief interventions is also commonly recommended for risky drinking and alcohol problems.[4,7,44]

Lower-intensity PSIs (brief advice and information, and brief interventions) may be carried out by health professionals outside of the substance misuse treatment field who have identified problematic substance use in the course of a consultation for another problem or after routine or opportunistic screening. Lower-intensity PSIs may take no longer than a few minutes, perhaps forming part of a wider conversation about a health problem. Typically, lower-intensity PSIs for substance use involve:

- Identification of substance use (and any related problems);
- Personalised feedback;
- The offer of information on how changes might be made if the service user decides to take up the advice.

The information may include a short information leaflet or reference to reliable Internet resources. Lower-intensity PSIs can be effective at reducing the risks and harms associated with substance use.[3] The user's desired outcome may be a reduction in drug-related harms rather than drug abstinence. Lower-intensity PSIs are more likely to be effective when users perceive they have a problem (or reason to change) and believe that they can make a change.

All health professionals should already have the competences required to deliver brief advice and information. Clinicians can adopt a key element of motivational interviewing, which has a very strong evidence base for its effectiveness as a substance use intervention, known as the 'elicit, provide, elicit' strategy (see Figure 2.2).[45]

Brief interventions offer structured advice on behaviour change in the context of a warm, reflective, empathic and collaborative approach by the practitioner. While this is likely to require no more than the competences expected of any healthcare professional, a commonly used structure for brief interventions across the substance misuse field is FRAMES (see Box 2.3).[46]

Recommendations from alcohol treatment suggest that simple brief interventions can be enhanced by including goal-setting (e.g. start date and daily or weekly limits of use), written self-help materials for the service user to take away (this may contain more detailed information on consequences of substance use and tips on cutting down) and arrangements for follow-up monitoring.[47]

The World Health Organization has developed a manual on brief interventions in substance misuse for primary care.[48] The manual draws on components of motivational interviewing and the FRAMES model. Although the manual was not developed for, or tested with, NPS specifically, it does cover a range of substances, including amphetamine-type stimulants. The manual provides clear information on how to deliver brief interventions.

Box 2.3 *FRAMES: A Framework for Brief Interventions*

Identification of NPS use (and any related problems) followed by:

- **F** Feedback on personal risk – from screening, medical tests or clinical interviews, give personalised feedback on the person's current and likely substance-related problems
- **R** Responsibility and choice – emphasise the service user's responsibility for and choice in making any changes
- **A** Advice to change – give clear advice to change substance use
- **M** Menu of options – offer a variety of strategies or options
- **E** Empathy – a warm, reflective and understanding style of delivering brief intervention is more effective
- **S** Self-efficacy and optimism – build confidence by affirming what the service user has already done or some aspect of strength

---

An example of a brief intervention based on the FRAMES model is given in Box 2.4.

2.7 Higher-Intensity Psychosocial Interventions

2.7.1 Structured Drug Treatment

Structured drug treatment comprises two or more treatment sessions, each lasting half an hour or longer, applying a single or range of psychosocial

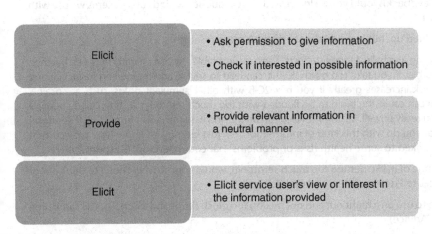

Figure 2.2 *A proposed framework for brief advice and information*

Box 2.4 *Example of a Brief Intervention Based on the FRAMES Model*

HEALTH WORKER (HW): Good news. All of the tests have come back and they are all normal. That means that you are medically fit to be discharged. Before you go, I wonder if you have a few minutes to think about how to avoid something like this from happening again? (**Asking permission**)

SERVICE USER (SU): Yes, okay, if you like.

HW: You mentioned to me earlier you were using 2C-B pretty much every weekend of late? Did I get that right? (**Brief history**)

SU: Yeah, every weekend for a couple of months now, more often than it used to be.

HW: What would a typical weekend be like? (**Open-ended question/brief history**)

SU: Well, no weekend is the same. It depends on who I'm with and where we are going.

HW: Well, maybe you could tell me about this weekend. (**Open-ended question**)

SU: This weekend was a pretty big one: it was my friend's birthday. We were partying then clubbing, then we hooked up with a few other friends and went on to another club.

HW: So you came here to A&E early this morning, Sunday. When did you start?

SU: Early Saturday night, at a friend's place. We had a few drinks then a line or two of cocaine, then just before we all left for the club, we all took 2C-B. I guess before we left I'd had more than usual, but I had decided to wait a couple of hours before taking anything more because I knew it was going to be a long night.

HW: You were thinking ahead, pacing yourself. Good for you. (**Affirmation**)

SU: Then at the club we were having a great time and someone offered me another 2C-B, which hit me quite hard. We were there until about 3am, although things were getting a bit hard to remember by then. I think there were more shots of vodka, but I'm not sure. We left there and went on to another club with these people we met in the first club. They were all really into their 2C-B and had really good quality 2C-B with them. We started taking their 2C-B as we had run out. In the second club things got really messy. I started tripping out. I had never had this with 2C-B before, but I think I had taken too much and that it was much stronger than I was used to. My heart started racing and I was panicking like mad. I went to sit outside with a friend and told him not to let me drink or use any more drugs that night because I had had enough.

HW: So you realized you had taken too much and decided to stop at that point. (**Affirmation**)

SU: I thought things would just settle but they got worse and worse. I'm really confused about what happened next but I remember the ambulance crew arriving and my friends looking really scared.

HW: So, from what you've said, it sounds like your use of 2C-B has been pretty regular over the last few months and may be increasing. This weekend was a big one, as you say. It's likely that you took more and stronger 2C-B than usual and also mixed it with cocaine and alcohol which led to you feeling really ill. It's good someone called an ambulance to get you here. (**Feedback**)Would you be interested to hear about the kinds of problems we see with 2C-B use? (**Asking permission**)

SU: Well, I thought I was pretty clued up, but maybe I should do a bit more research.

HW: 2C-B is a drug causing stimulating and hallucinogenic effects. The dose in a tablet can vary greatly between batches, or even from one tablet to another. If you take too much 2C-B it can lead to severe and frightening hallucinations, confusion and vomiting. This risk increases greatly if you mix 2C-B with other stimulant drugs, such as cocaine, because when combined, they can cause the brain to be flooded with too much serotonin, a stimulating chemical messenger, which can make you really unwell. Mixing with alcohol can also increase the harms from 2C-B. (**Feedback**)
It's of course up to you what you do with this kind of information, I'm just letting you know how your current pattern of 2C-B use might be linked to some health risks or problems that could develop. (**Responsibility**)

SU: I knew a fair bit of that, but some of it, like getting too much serotonin, would concern me. I need to think about how I mix more carefully, because I don't want to end up back here.

HW: Planning what you are going to use on a night out and not mixing too much drugs and alcohol at the same time is a really sensible approach. (**Advice**)

Box 2.4 (cont.)

In terms of being safer, stopping using 2C-B would be the safest option. If that doesn't feel like something you could do just now, not mixing with alcohol or other drugs would make problems like the ones that brought you here less likely. If you do continue use, using less and knowing how much you're using would help. Some people take a very small test dose of 2C-B to judge how strong it is, before deciding how much of the tablet they need for the desired effect without taking too much. It's good that you use with friends and you take care of each other if needed. (**Menu of options**)

SU: I'm not sure stopping taking it is what I want to do right now, but I'd already been a bit concerned about using so often.

HW: You could try having some weekends not using? It sounds like that's something you've managed before. (**Self-efficacy**)

SU: Yes, I've got friends who don't use, but I've not been spending much time with them lately, which isn't what I want.

HW: Is there anything more you'd like me to help with? I have the details of a website that has the information I just spoke about if you'd like it? I'll leave you this card with the details of a local service just in case you want some more expert help. I've heard good things about them.

approaches, commonly including motivational interviewing. Structured drug treatment may range from an extended form of brief intervention, sometimes known as extended brief intervention, to a more ongoing, regular set of treatment sessions. Structured drug treatment of any duration includes the setting and evaluation of specific goal(s) relating to a change in substance use.

Structured drug treatment should follow from a more comprehensive assessment of needs and resources that has led to intervention based on a care plan.[49] More advanced competences, of accreditation standard, in these approaches will be required for effective delivery, along with supervision and an appropriate governance framework. Structured drug treatment may be delivered as individual psychological therapy or as group-based interventions. There is evidence that the outcomes of drug treatment (all drug treatment, not only PSIs) can be enhanced with the use of mapping tools.[50] Mapping tools are not in themselves a psychosocial intervention but an approach that can enhance the effective delivery of treatment. Mapping tools employ a structure known as 'node link mapping' to visually convey key elements for a structured conversation derived from evidence-based PSIs.[51] The most relevant research findings relate to PSIs for various forms of stimulant use. Knapp et al., in a Cochrane review, reported that interventions based on cognitive behavioural therapy and contingency management approaches appear to be effective.[52] Knapp et al. argued that a comprehensive treatment package drawing on these three models may be required for better outcomes,

given the multi-dimensional nature of stimulant dependence. They further argued that for sustained outcomes, treatment needs to support service users to make effective changes to their lives, including abstinence from stimulant use, the ability to work and the ability to maintain successful relationships. A focus on narrow, short-term goals such as reductions in amount or frequency of use is of little benefit in achieving sustained change.[9] The intervention will draw on evidence-based psychosocial approaches and is likely to include motivational interviewing.[8]

As a minimum, structured drug treatment should include: goal setting and planning, feedback and monitoring, and developing social support.[6] The largest amount of reported evidence for structured drug treatment is for cognitive behavioural therapy (CBT), contingency management (CM) and the community reinforcement approach (CRA) as mentioned earlier.[9] Specific competences to deliver such interventions, supervision and an appropriate governance framework are required.

2.7.2 Formal Psychological Treatment

More intensive treatment and formal psychological treatment is likely to be effective for people with higher-severity and dependent use. Formal psychological treatment is particularly relevant where a service user has a co-occurring common mental health problem[3] or other psychological problems. Formal psychological treatment usually consists of a planned, time-limited series of sessions. The intervention will be grounded in a psychological formulation, derived from a process of assessment and evaluated using formal or informal outcome measures. The competences required to deliver this intensity of intervention will be more advanced – of professional registration standard – and a governance and supervision structure will be needed.[53]

Formal psychological treatment may be delivered as individual therapy or as a group-based intervention. It is likely to draw on one or more of the evidence-based psychological therapy models listed below and may be combined with other evidence-based interventions for psychological problems.

The aims of formal psychological treatment are likely to be a combination of changes: to the substance use, to the psychological problems, but also in related domains (e.g. health, social functioning, criminal justice).

There are high levels of co-occurring mental health problems in drug treatment populations[32], and it can be assumed this will be similar for dependent users of NPS.

Some NPS users may have other co-occurring psychological difficulties; for example, there are reports of problematic NPS use associated with psycho-sexual problems.

Treatment services need to be able to screen, assess and provide treatment for these co-occurring difficulties.

Whilst some[3] recommend CBT to treat co-occurring mental health problems, the complexity of the presenting psychological difficulties may limit the impact of these approaches. Other approaches may be required for psycho-sexual problems.

For patients with complex needs, formal psychological treatment may be complemented by a formulation-based approach.[40]

A psychological formulation is a hypothesis about a person's difficulties and integrates a broad range of biopsychosocial causal factors which link theory with practice to guide the intervention. It is individually determined and may draw upon a range of psychological models to achieve an effective treatment plan.

A psychological formulation can integrate both the substance use behaviour and the co-occurring mental distress in a way that seeks to reveal the function of the substance use for the service user. It can also include consideration of other psychological and behavioural factors, such as sexual behaviour.

A formulation-based approach can incorporate personal meaning and be constructed collaboratively with service users and their care teams.

Some key features of a formulation are that it:

- Summarises the service user's core problems;

- Suggests how the service user's difficulties may relate to one another, by drawing on psychological theories and principles;
- Aims to explain, on the basis of psychological theory, the development and maintenance of the service user's difficulties, at this time and in these situations;
- Indicates a plan of intervention which is based in the psychological processes and principles identified;
- Is open to revision and reformulation.

A distinguishing characteristic of psychological formulation is its multiple-model perspective – it integrates theory and evidence from a range of psychological models as well as biological, social/societal and cultural domains.

The incorporation of this multiple-model perspective may have particular value in working with service users from marginalised and stigmatised populations, as it explicitly incorporates culture-specific issues.

For example, a recent report[54] describes the association of NPS use and sexual behaviours, often referred to as 'chemsex'. As detailed in Part III of this publication, contemporary research has highlighted the frequent use of NPS by men who have sex with men (MSM) in the context of sex. A proportion of this behaviour has also been linked to drug-related and sex-related harms. Sex under the influence or intoxication of substances with the potential for associated harm is by no means a new phenomenon, however.

Bourne et al.[55] suggest some NPS offer a specific range of psychological and physical sex-enhancing effects. Where problematic sex and NPS use have over time become powerfully associated for an individual, a combined approach to treatment is likely to be required. By identifying motivations, meanings and values associated with sexualised drug use, individualised for that service user, a psychological formulation can be developed, leading to proposed psychological interventions. A small number of studies in the US have looked at the impact of psychological interventions on condom-less sex among methamphetamine-using MSM. Combined cognitive behavioural and contingency management (CM) interventions have shown a positive impact on changing drug use and sexual behaviours among this population.[55,56]

Working with the same population, however, Rajasingham et al.[57] suggest that CM fails to address service users' mental health needs or to develop post-intervention relapse prevention plans. A review of three randomised controlled trials (RCTs) examining the outcomes of CBT interventions and HIV risk behaviours among substance-misusing MSM found that while CBT did reduce unprotected anal intercourse in this group, it was unclear whether CBT was more effective than less intensive interventions or mere assessment.[58]

It is good practice that higher-intensity PSIs (structured drug treatment and/or formal psychological therapy) are offered to service users where medically assisted detoxification is part of the recommended treatment. Unless detoxification is undertaken as an emergency, higher-intensity PSIs, including motivational interviewing, should be offered before detoxification. Following detoxification, it is essential that higher-intensity PSIs, typically including a relapse prevention model, are offered. Service users completing detoxification may also benefit from formal psychological therapy for any co-occurring psychological problems such as common mental health problems or psycho-sexual problems.

2.8 Residential Psychosocial Treatment

Residential treatment is defined by the controlled environment where treatment takes place. It generally involves one or more evidence-based high-intensity psychological interventions and requires the same level of competence and governance as the higher-intensity PSIs described in Section 2.7. Residential treatment may be preceded by medically assisted detoxification for safe withdrawal from specific substances.

Service users live within the treatment service (or very nearby) for the duration of the treatment. Residential treatment is considered a more intense form of treatment, often requiring several hours per day of treatment engagement over a minimum period of typically 12 weeks. The location of the treatment service is generally a distance away from the service user's usual home. Residential treatment is recognised as an important option; however, there is debate around the precise indications for its use and the evidence base is currently far from clear. Almost without exception, the explicit aim of residential treatment is long-term or lifetime abstinence from all substances. Residential treatment is therefore not appropriate for people who are not prepared for this treatment aim.

Broadly, the indications for residential treatment are:

- Multiple co-existing psychological, physical and/or social problems;
- Poly-drug dependence;
- Optimised community treatment has not been effective;
- The service user has a treatment goal of long-term abstinence.[3]

It is good practice that service users with significant physical, psychological and/or social problems associated with NPS dependence (or use of high severity), who are aiming for long-term abstinence and who have been unable to achieve this in effective community treatment (or who would be highly unlikely to be able to do so), have access to residential treatment, including, where necessary, prior medically assisted detoxification. On successful completion of residential treatment, relapse prevention support should be offered to help service users maintain changes. Service users who leave residential treatment before its completion should be promptly offered support to minimise any return to substance use and the risk of overdose.

2.9 Mutual Aid

There is a long tradition of mutual aid in the substance misuse field. Perhaps the best-known are Alcoholics Anonymous (AA) and Narcotics Anonymous (NA), sometimes known as 12-step groups. More recently, other forms of mutual aid have been developed, including SMART groups where the approach is derived from CBT. There is a strong evidence base for the outcomes from mutual aid (the research has primarily been with 12-step groups).[59]

Mutual aid is not a professionally delivered treatment. There is, though, evidence of the benefit of health professionals proactively supporting service users' engagement with mutual aid, often referred to as facilitating access to mutual aid (FAMA).[3,7,60]

2.10 Models for Specific Psychosocial Approaches

Higher-intensity PSIs for the treatment of substance misuse problems, in the form of structured drug treatment, formal psychological therapy and many of the approaches used in residential treatment, are derived from specific psychological therapy models. The main evidence-based models are described only briefly here, but references are given to sources of more detailed information and to treatment manuals.

2.10.1 Motivational Interviewing

Ambivalence about changing substance use behaviour is common, even for people actively seeking treatment. Motivational interviewing as an approach offers a framework for helping people resolve ambivalence to changes in their substance use. Motivational interviewing and its more manualised variant motivational enhancement therapy (MET) have a robust evidence base across a wide range of substances.[3,4,7] The use of motivational interviewing is likely to be a part of brief interventions and the early part of structured treatment.[61]

2.10.2 Network and Environmental Therapies

Network and environmental therapies are a range of psychological approaches which seek to utilise social contextual reinforcers to promote and sustain change in substance use. This often involves enlisting the support of (non-using) partners, families or peers. Behavioural couples therapy (BCT) has been shown to be effective in the treatment of drug misuse[3,7] including lesbian and gay people.[62] Similarly, studies have shown the positive impact of network and environmental therapies,[3,7] social behaviour network therapy (SBNT), the community reinforcement approach (CRA) and behavioural couples therapy (BCT).[63,64,65]

2.10.3 CBT-Based Relapse Prevention

Relapse prevention (RP) is a commonly used psychological approach in substance misuse treatment[66], and is recommended for the treatment of alcohol problems.[3,7]

It has been argued that CBT focused on drug misuse only is not recommended.[3] RP aims to help people make and sustain changes to substance misuse through the identification of thinking and behavioural patterns that typically precede an individual's substance use. RP is considered particularly relevant in helping people sustain changes to substance misuse once they have achieved them, including following medically assisted detoxification, a phase of treatment often referred to as aftercare. For a description of CBT-based RP models, see Marlatt and Donovan[67] and Mitcheson et al.[12]

Inevitably, innovative developments may take time to be included in high-level meta-analyses. It is worth noting the current attention to what are often referred to as 'third-wave CBT models'. These contemporary developments include mindfulness-based interventions (MBIs), acceptance and commitment therapy (ACT) and dialectical behaviour therapy (DBT). In a systematic review of evidence, Chiesa and Serretti report that MBIs can reduce the use of a range of substances, including stimulant drugs.[68] Zgierska and Marcus[69] note that the combined findings of early studies of MBIs suggest these may be efficacious for substance misuse problems. Of note, Smout et al.[70] conducted a preliminary RCT of ACT for methamphetamine use disorders. While it had no advantage over CBT, Smout et al. described it as a viable intervention for this population. Zgierska and Marcus noted the strength of positive evidence for MBIs with common mental health problems and concluded that they are therefore of value for service users with co-occurring substance misuse and mental health problems.[54]

2.10.4 Contingency Management

Contingency management has a strong evidence base from numerous research trials, carried out primarily in the US, focusing on stimulant use. CM is used to reduce substance use by the provision of tangible (often monetary or material) rewards for the achievement of verifiable behavioural goals, such as negative biological drug screen tests.[13]

2.10.5 Social Re-integration

Psychological interventions must often be accompanied by those that focus on social re-integration. It is well recognised that social exclusion is experienced by many high-risk drug and chronic users, and that interventions addressing these issues, with a focus on the social re-integration of drug users, including improving a person's ability to gain and maintain employment, may be needed. Interventions include vocational training programmes and housing support.[71] It is widely recognised that social support is important in achieving positive outcomes for drug problems.[6]

References

1. Strang J, Chair of the Expert Group. Recovery-Orientated Drug Treatment. An Interim Report. National Treatment Agency for Substance Misuse, 2011.

2. Amato L, Minozzi S, Davoli M, Vecchi S. Psychosocial and pharmacological treatments versus pharmacological treatments for opioid detoxification. *Cochrane Database Syst Rev* 2011;7(9):CD005031. https://doi.org/10.1002/14651858 .CD005031.pub4

3. National Institute for Health and Clinical Excellence. Drug Misuse: Psychosocial Interventions (Clinical Guideline 51). Published 2007.

4. National Institute for Health and Clinical Excellence. Quality Standard for Drug Use Disorders (Quality Standard 23). Published 2012.

5. Department of Health (England) and the Devolved Administrations. Drug Misuse and Dependence: UK Guidelines on Clinical Management. Department of Health, the Scottish Government, the Welsh Assembly Government and Northern Ireland Executive, 2007.

6. National Institute for Health and Clinical Excellence. Behaviour Change: Individual Approaches (PH 49). Published 2014.

7. National Institute for Health and Clinical Excellence. Alcohol Use Disorders: Harmful Drinking and Alcohol Dependence (Clinical Guidance 115: Evidence Update). Published 2013.

8. Smedslund G, Berg RC, Hammerstrøm KT, et al. Motivational interviewing for substance abuse. *Cochrane Database Syst Rev* 2011;11(5):CD008063. https://doi.org/10.1002/14651858 .CD008063.pub2

9. Knapp WP, Soares BG, Farrel M, Lima MS. Psychosocial interventions for cocaine and psychostimulant amphetamines related disorders. *Cochrane Database Syst Rev* 2007;18(3): CD003023.

10. National Treatment Agency for Substance Misuse. The Effectiveness of Psychological Therapies on Drug Misusing Clients. Published 2005.

11. Orford J. Asking the right questions in the right way: the need for a shift in research on psychological treatments for addiction. *Addiction* 2008;103(6):875–885; discussion 886–892. https://doi .org/10.1111/j.1360-0443.2007.02092.x

12. European Monitoring Centre for Drugs and Drug Addiction. Health and Social Responses to Drug Problems: A European Guide. Publications Office of the European Union, Luxembourg, 2017.

13. The United Nations Office on Drugs and Crime (UNODC). World Drug Report 2019 (United Nations publication, Sales No. E.19.XI.8). Available at: https://wdr.unodc.org/wdr2019/p relaunch/WDR19_Booklet_1_EXECUTIVE_SUMMARY.pdf

14. European Monitoring Centre for Drugs and Drug Addiction. Health and Social Responses to Drug Problems: A European Guide. Publications Office of the European Union, Luxembourg, 2017.

15. Tompkins CN, Neale J. Delivering trauma-informed treatment in a women-only residential rehabilitation service: qualitative study. *Drugs Educ Prevent Policy* 2018;25(1):47–55.

16. Carlyle M, Broomby R, Simpson G, et al. A randomised, double-blind study investigating the relationship between early childhood trauma and the rewarding effects of morphine. *Addict Biol* 2021:e13047 (online). https://doi.org/10.1111/adb.13047.

17. Dube SR, Felitti VJ, Dong M, Chapman DP, Giles WH, Anda RF. Childhood abuse, neglect, and household dysfunction and the risk of illicit drug use: the adverse childhood experiences study. *Pediatrics* 2003;111(3):564–572.

18. Kristjansson S, McCutcheon VV, Agrawal A, et al. The variance shared across forms of childhood trauma is strongly associated with liability for psychiatric and substance use disorders. *Brain Behav* 2016;6(2):e00432.

19. Naqavi MR, Mohammadi M, Salari V, Nakhaee N. The relationship between childhood maltreatment and opiate dependency in adolescence and middle age. *Addict Health* 2011;3(3–4):92–98.

20. Taplin C, Saddichha S, Li K, Krausz MR. Family history of alcohol and drug abuse, childhood trauma, and age of first drug injection. *Subst Use Misuse* 2014;49(10):1311–1316.

21. Vogel M, Dursteler-Macfarland KM, Walter M, et al. Prolonged use of benzodiazepines is associated with childhood trauma in opioid-maintained patients. *Drug Alcohol Depend* 2011;119(1–2):93–98.

22. Kumar N, Stowe ZN, Han X, Mancino MJ. Impact of early childhood trauma on retention and phase advancement in an outpatient buprenorphine treatment program. *Am J Addict* 2016;25(7):542–548.

23. Mandavia A, Robinson GG, Bradley B, Ressler KJ, Powers A. Exposure to childhood abuse and later substance use: indirect effects of emotion dysregulation and exposure to trauma. *J Trauma Stress* 2016;29(5):422–429.

24. European Monitoring Centre for Drugs and Drug Addiction. Prison and Drugs in Europe: Current and Future Challenges. Publications Office of the European Union, Luxembourg, 2021.

25. Fuentes CM. Nobody's child: the role of trauma and interpersonal violence in women's pathways to incarceration and resultant service needs. *Med Anthropol Q* 2014;28(1):85–104.

26. Jones MS, Worthen MGF, Sharp SF, McLeod DA. Life as she knows it: the effects of adverse childhood experiences on intimate partner violence among women prisoners. *Child Abuse Negl* 2018;85:68–79.

27. Fallot RD, Harris M. *Trauma-Informed Services: A Self-Assessment and Planning Protocol.* Washington, DC: Community Corrections, 2002.

28. Bateman J, Henderson C, Kezelman C. Trauma-Informed Care and Practice: Towards a Cultural Shift in Policy Reform across Mental Health and Human Services in Australia. Mental Health Coordinating Council, 2013.

29. Brown VB, Harris M, Fallot R. Moving toward trauma-informed practice in addiction treatment: a collaborative model of agency assessment. *J Psychoactive Drugs* 2013;45(5):386–393.

30. Harris M, Fallot R. *Using Trauma Theory to Design Service Systems.* San Francisco: Jossey-Bass, 2001.

31. Harris M. *Trauma Recovery and Empowerment: A Clinician's Guide for Working with Women in Groups*. New York: The Free Press, 1998.

32. Fallot R, Harris M. *Creating Cultures of Trauma-Informed Care (CCTIC): A Self-Assessment and Planning Protocol*. Washington, DC: Community Corrections, 2009.

33. Tompkins CNE, Neale J. Delivering trauma-informed treatment in a women-only residential rehabilitation service: qualitative study. *Drugs Educ Prevent Policy* 2018;25(1):47–55. https://doi.org/10.1080/09687637.2016.1235135

34. Hales TW, Green SA, Bissonette S, et al. Trauma-informed care outcome study. *Res Soc Work Pract* 2019;**29**(5):529–539. https://doi.org/10.1177/1049731518766618

35. Mitcheson L, Maslin J, Meynen T, Morrison T, Hill R, Wanigaratne S. *Applied Cognitive and Behavioural Approaches to the Treatment of Addiction: A Practical Treatment Guide*. Wiley-Blackwell, 2010.

36. Pilling S, Hesketh K, Mitcheson L. Routes to Recovery: Psychosocial Interventions for Drug Misuse. A Framework and Toolkit for Implementing NICE-Recommended Treatment Interventions. National Treatment Agency for Substance Misuse and British Psychological Society, 2010.

37. Marsden J, Eastwood B, Ali R, et al. Development of the Addiction Dimensions for Assessment and Personalised Treatment (ADAPT). *Drug Alcohol Depend* 2014;**139**:121–131. https://doi.org/10.1016/j.drugalcdep.2014.03.018

38. HM Government. The Drug Strategy: 'Reducing Demand, Restricting Supply, Building Recovery: Supporting People to Live a Drug Free Life'. Published 2010.

39. Orford J. *Power, Powerlessness and Addiction*. Cambridge: Cambridge University Press, 2013.

40. Winstock AR, Mitcheson L. New recreational drugs and the primary care approach to patients who use them. *BMJ* 2012;**344**:e288. https://doi.org/10.1136/bmj.e288

41. Hunter LJ, Dargan PI, Benzie A, White JA, Wood DM. Recreational drug use in men who have sex with men (MSM) attending UK sexual health services is significantly higher than in non-MSM. *Postgrad Med J* 2014;**90**(1061):133–138. https://doi.org/10.1136/postgradmedj-2012-131428

42. Colfax G, Guzman R. Club drugs and HIV infection: a review. *Clin Infect Dis* 2006;**42**(10):1463–1469.

43. Weaver T, Madden P, Charles V, et al. Comorbidity of substance misuse and mental illness in community mental health and substance misuse services. *Br J Psychiatry* 2003;**183**:304–313.

44. Heather N, Lavoie D, Morris J. Clarifying Alcohol Brief Interventions: 2013 Update. Alcohol Academy, 2013.

45. Miller WR, Rollnick S. *Motivational Interviewing: Helping People Change* (3rd edition). Guilford, 2013.

46. Miller WR, Sanchez VC. Motivating young adults for treatment and lifestyle change. In: Howard G, ed. *Issues in Alcohol Use and Misuse in Young Adults*. University of Notre Dame Press, 1993.

47. National Treatment Agency for Substance Misuse. Care Planning Practice Guide. Published 2006.

48. Humeniuk RE, Henry-Edwards S, Ali RL, Poznyak V, Monteiro M. *The ASSIST-Linked Brief Intervention for Hazardous and Harmful Substance Use: Manual for Use in Primary Care*. Geneva, World Health Organization, 2010.

49. Independent Expert Working Group. Drug Misuse and Dependence: UK Guidelines on Clinical Management. London: Department of Health, 2017. Available from: https://assets.publishing.service.gov.uk/government/uploads/system/uploads/attachment_data/file/673978/clinical_guidelines_2017.pdf

50. National Treatment Agency for Substance Misuse. The International Treatment Effectiveness Project: Implementing Psychosocial Interventions for Adult Drug Misusers. Published 2007.

51. Day E. *Routes to Recovery via the Community*. Public Health England, 2013.

52. National Institute for Health and Care Excellence. *Drug Misuse in Over 16s: Psychosocial Interventions. NICE Clinical Guideline 51*. London: NICE, 2007.

53. Division of Clinical Psychology, British Psychological Society. Good Practice Guidelines on the Use of Psychological Formulation. Published 2011.

54. Bourne A, Reid D, Hickson F, Torres-Rueda S, Weatherburn P. Illicit drug use in sexual settings ('chemsex') and HIV/STI transmission risk behaviour among gay men in South London: findings from a qualitative study. *Sex Transm Infect* 2015;91(8):564–568.

55. Lee NK, Rawson RA. A systematic review of cognitive and behavioural therapies for methamphetamine dependence. *Drug Alcohol Rev* 2008;27(3):309–317. https://doi.org/10.1080/09595230801919494

56. Reback CJ, Larkins S, Shoptaw S. Changes in the meaning of sexual risk behaviors among gay and bisexual male methamphetamine abusers before and after drug treatment. *AIDS Behav* 2004;8(1):87–9

57. Rajasingham R, Mimiaga MJ, White JM, Pinkston MM, Baden RP, Mitty JA. A systematic review of behavioral and treatment outcome studies among HIV-infected men who have sex with men who abuse crystal methamphetamine. *AIDS Patient Care STDS* 2012;**26**(1):36–52. https://doi.org/10.1089/apc.2011.0153

58. Melendez-Torres GJ, Bonell C. Systematic review of cognitive behavioural interventions for HIV risk reduction in substance-using men who have sex with men. *Int J STD AIDS* 2013;25(9):627–635

59. Weiss RD, Griffin ML, Gallop RJ, et al. The effect of 12-step self-help group attendance and participation on drug use outcomes among cocaine-dependent patients. *Drug Alcohol Depend* 2005;**77**(2):177–184.

60. Public Health England. Facilitating Access to Mutual Aid: Three Essential Stages for Helping Clients Access Appropriate Mutual Aid Support. Published 2013. www.nta.nhs.uk/uploads/mutua laid-fama.pdf

61. Pilling S, Hesketh K, Mitcheson L. Routes to Recovery: Psychosocial Interventions for Drug Misuse. A Framework and Toolkit for Implementing NICE-Recommended Treatment Interventions. National Treatment Agency for Substance Misuse and British Psychological Society, 2010.

62. Fals-Stewart W, O'Farrell TJ, Lam W. Behavioural couples therapy for gay and lesbian couples with alcohol use disorders. *J Subst Abuse Treat* 2009;**37**(4):379–387. https://doi.org/10.1016/j.jsat.2009.05.001

63. Copello A, Orford J, Hodgson R, Tober G. *Social Behaviour Network Therapy for Alcohol Problems*. Routledge, 2009.

64. Miller WR, Meyers RT, Hiller-Strumhofel S. The community reinforcement approach. *Alcohol Research Health* 1999;**23**:116–121.

65. O'Farrell TJ, Fals-Stewart W. *Behavioural Couples Therapy for Alcoholism and Drug Abuse*. Guilford, 2006.

66. National Institute for Clinical Excellence. Drug Misuse – Psychosocial Interventions. Issued: July 2007. NICE Clinical Guideline 51; guidance.nice.org.uk/cg51.

67. Marlatt GA, Donovan DM, eds. *Relapse Prevention: Maintenance Strategies in the Treatment of Addictive Behaviors* (2nd ed.). Guilford Press, 2005.

68. Chiesa A, Serretti A. Are mindfulness-based interventions effective for substance use disorders? A systematic review of the evidence. *Subst Use Misuse* 2014;**49**(5):492–512. https://doi.org/10.3109/10826084.2013.770027

69. Zgierska A, Marcus MT. Mindfulness-based therapies for substance use disorders: part 2. *Subst Abus* 2010;**31**(2):77–78. https://doi.org/10.1080/08897071003641248

70. Smout MF, Longo A, Harrison S, Minniti R, Wickes W, White JM. Psychosocial treatment for methamphetamine use disorders: a preliminary randomized controlled trial of cognitive behavior therapy and acceptance and commitment therapy. *Subst Abus* 2010;**31**(2):98–107. https://doi.org/10.1080/08897071003641578

71. Kletter E. Counseling as an intervention for cocaine-abusing methadone maintenance patients. *J Psychoactive Drugs* 2003;**35**(2):271–277.

Chapter

3

Gamma-Hydroxybutyrate (GHB) and Gamma-Butyrolactone (GBL)

3.1 Introduction

This chapter discusses gamma-hydroxybutyrate (GHB) and its precursor gamma-butyrolactone (GBL). Other precursors of GHB are 1,4-butanediol (1,4-BD) and gamma-valerolactone (GVL).

In some European countries such as the UK, it is GBL rather than GHB that is mainly used for recreational purposes. However, it seems that elsewhere too, GBL appears to be replacing GHB, in part because of its lower cost and the fact that it is easier to obtain.[1] There are also a small number of reports on acute toxicity linked to 1,4-butanediol.[2,3]

3.2 Legal Status

GHB was placed in Schedule IV of the 1971 Convention on Psychotropic Substances of the UN Commission on Narcotic Drugs. It was classified as a controlled substance in the US in 2000 (Schedule I) and in EU nations in 2001 (Schedule III or IV).

GBL and 1,4-butanediol are available for legitimate use in industry, but some countries in Europe (Italy, Latvia and Sweden) now control one or both precursors under drug control or equivalent legislation.

3.3 Quality of the Research Evidence

The international evidence on the management of the acute and chronic harms related to the use of GHB and GBL is emerging. A small number of randomised control trials have been conducted, but the evidence mainly consists of case reports and series together with a small number of prospective observational studies, retrospective cohort studies and analysis of patient records.

Despite these limitations, data/evidence from these sources is relatively consistent.

3.4 Brief Summary of Pharmacology

GHB acts primarily as a CNS depressant, but at low doses can also produce euphoric effects and effects that appear to be like those of stimulants. GHB is both a metabolite and a precursor of the inhibitory neurotransmitter gamma-aminobutyric acid (GABA)[4] and acts as a neuromodulator in the GABA system, acting on both GABA-B and its own so-called GHB receptors. GBL and 1,4-BD are converted into GHB after they are absorbed.[5]

A number of studies have looked at GHB pharmacokinetics in healthy volunteers.[6,7,8,9,10] GHB is absorbed rapidly, is extensively metabolised to carbon dioxide and rapidly eliminated,[11] mainly through the lungs (less than 5% is excreted in the urine as GHB, although this may be greater in overdose). It has a half-life of only 20–30 minutes.[12]

The effects of GHB usually occur 15–20 minutes after ingestion and can last for up to 3–4 hours,[13] with peak effects at 30–60 minutes after ingestion.[12] It is undetectable in urine after approximately 12 hours.[14]

GBL is a precursor of GHB and is non-enzymatically converted in the body into GHB. GBL is absorbed more rapidly than GHB and potentially has a faster onset of action. Its duration of action may also be longer.[14] Some users report that GBL is more potent than GHB.

In contrast, larger doses of GHV may be needed to produce GHB-like effects and therefore GHV toxicity may pose a greater public health concern than GHB.[15]

1,4-BD is another precursor to GHB; it is converted in the liver through a two-step conversion, via hepatic alcohol dehydrogenase to gamma-hydroxybutyraldehyde followed by metabolism into GHB via hepatic acetaldehyde dehydrogenase.[16,17] Animal studies have shown that both ethanol and fomepizole competitively block the metabolism of 1,4-BD to GHB.[18,19]

GHB (and therefore GBL and 1,4-BD) has a steep dose–response curve and narrow therapeutic threshold, whereby even a small increase in dose can cause serious toxic effects, such as impaired consciousness and coma. This steep dose–response relationship differentiates GHB/GBL from other drugs. It can readily cross both the placenta and the blood–brain barrier, leading to profound CNS and respiratory depression.[12,13]

Daily use of GHB/GBL can lead to dependence and the possibility of withdrawal syndrome on cessation of use, which can be severe, with agitation and delirium. Acute GHB/GBL toxicity and acute withdrawal can be life threatening.

Gamma-hydroxyvaleric (GHV) is a 4-methyl-substituted analogue of GHB and a direct GABA receptor agonist. Gamma-valerolactone (GVL) is a precursor of GHV. Larger doses of GHV may be needed to produce GHB-like effects and therefore GHV toxicity may pose a public health concern.[20]

3.5 Clinical and Other Uses

Clinical uses of GHB have included alcohol and opiate detoxification regimens, anti-craving medication after alcohol detoxification,[13] and one study has looked at detoxification from illicit GHB by titration and tapering of pharmaceutical GHB.[21]

GHB is used as an anaesthetic agent in some European countries, although this latter use is now declining. The sodium salt of GHB, sodium oxybate (Xyrem SPC), is approved for the treatment of narcolepsy with problematic catalepsy in specialist sleep centres in the US and Europe. A recent systematic review and meta-analysis of its effectiveness has been conducted.[22]

GHB was sold in US health food stores for weight control and sedation, until over-the-counter sales were banned in 1990 following reports of acute intoxication.[23] It has also been sold for its antidepressant and anxiolytic effects and for its cholesterol-lowering effects. It has also been used in bodybuilding, as it has been thought to release growth hormone; however, its anabolic effects are unproven.[24]

GHB has been implicated as a facilitator in 'date rape' and sexual assaults, but it is not the only substance implicated.[25,26,27] Nonetheless, it has been argued that it is important to consider GHB and its precursors with any cases of sexual assault and non-consensual sex,[28,29,30] and GHB/GBL should be included with any drugs screen that is done in these cases.[31]

There is also some evidence from a study from Hungary that GHB can also be implicated in drug-facilitated acquisitive crimes.[32]

GBL and 1,4-BD are used extensively by the chemical industry as precursors for the synthesis of plastics and industrial solvents. They are found in floor-cleaning products, nail polish (previously nail polish removers) and superglue removers.

3.6 Prevalence and Patterns of Use

At population levels, the use of GHB/GBL is relatively low. However, the health costs of GHB/GBL misuse are relatively high compared with other drugs,[33] because of its intrinsic toxicity, high dependence liability and potentially life-threatening withdrawal syndrome, as discussed in Section 3.12.2.

Although its use is limited in comparison to other drugs used for recreational purposes, the use of GHB and GBL has increased in the last decade in some European Countries, Australia and the US.[34,35,36] Nonetheless, national estimates, where they exist, of the prevalence of GHB in adult and school populations remain low. For example, in their 2017 survey, Norway reported prevalence of GHB use at 0.1% for adults (age 16–64 years).[37]

In Europe in 2017, seizures of GHB or GBL were reported by 14 EU countries as well as Norway and Turkey, with Norway accounting for over a quarter of the total number of seizures. Seizures amounted to almost 127 kilograms and 1,300 litres of the drug. Belgium seized almost half of the total quantity, mainly as GBL.[38]

There is evidence that GHB/GBL users are most likely to be male.[39] The use of GHB appears to be concentrated among some sub-groups, often in specific contexts. In the UK, mainland Europe, the US, Australia and elsewhere, GHB/GBL use is popular among some gay men and other men who have sex with men; it is often one of the drugs used in 'chemsex'.[30,40,41,42,43,44,45,46,47,48] For example, an Australian study reported that 5.4% of gay and bisexual men had used GHB in the past 6 months.[49]

However, although it seems that rates of use among women are much lower than men, and in particular men who have sex with men, there are reports of women using GHB/GBL.[50]

Due to its pro-sexual effects and muscle relaxant properties, GHB/GBL is often used by men who have sex with men in a sexual context.[50] GHB is one of the drugs commonly implicated in 'chemsex' and it has been associated with high-risk sexual behaviours. Drug surveys have also consistently found higher GHB use rates in people socialising on the gay club scene, primarily gay males, but also other LGBT people, as well as by heterosexual people.[50]

GHB/GBL use has been associated with 'clubbing' and visiting the night time economy.[50,51] A number of European surveys conducted in dance music venues and other targeted settings suggest that the lifetime prevalence of use of GHB/GBL ranges from 3% to 19%.[30]

The demographic and socio-economic profile of people who use GHB/GBL shows conflicting results, possibly differing by country. Data from Australia and the UK suggest that GHB/GBL users tend to be well-educated and well-functioning people.[36,52] Conversely, a study in the Netherlands showed that heavy, high-risk GHB consumption is primarily found among what the study describes as 'poorly educated young adolescents in economically less privileged provincial communities'.[53]

3.7 Routes of Ingestion and Frequency of Dosing

The routes of administration of GHB/GBL include:

- Oral use (this route is the most common, when it is typically diluted in a beverage);
- Insufflation (snorting);
- Injection (although this is rare);
- Mucosal (e.g. previously from absorption of nail polish removal pads).

GHB/GBL used for recreational purposes is most usually sold in the form of a liquid formulation, often in bottles or vials. Its taste is described as unpleasant and salty and it is therefore typically diluted in a beverage. It is more rarely used as a powder, usually GHB sodium salt (capsules or loose) or a waxy substance to which water can be added.[30] The 'irritant' nature of GHB/GBL has been described, with a case report of a user syringing the liquid into capsules to make it easier to swallow.[54]

GBL for recreational use is usually bought from street dealers or via the Internet in amounts ranging from 125 ml to 10 litres. Usually, 1 ml of liquid contains 1 g of GHB, although purity and concentration may vary.[30,55,56,57] Miotto et al. suggest that single doses of GHB can range from 0.5 g to 5 g and those who develop tolerance and dependence will use in the range of more than 25 g per day.[50] GBL is far more lipophilic than GHB; hence, typical ingested dosages of GBL are lower than those of GHB.[58,59]

GHB/GBL dose is often measured by users in imprecise 'capfuls', teaspoons, eye droppers or vials. This imprecise dose measurement is one of the main suggested causes of the acute GHB/GBL-related harms, as users risk overdose because of its steep dose–response curve, which is discussed in greater detail in this chapter.

Recreational users will typically use small doses frequently, in the context of binges, or sometimes at night to assist with sleep. Dependent users will ingest GHB/GBL frequently and at regular intervals over prolonged periods. They will generally use multiple daily doses, including at night.[50] The mean frequency of dosing in cases of dependence was reported by McDonough et al. to be every 4.4 hours,[60] although case reports and series show a wide range, from hourly to daily.[51,61,62]

There is evidence that GHB/GBL is often used as part of a wider poly-drug repertoire (see Section 3.10.2). An Internet survey of 189 GHB/GBL users reported that a third had taken GHB/GBL during the last month and that two-thirds reported mixing GHB/GBL with other drugs.[35]

GHB/GBL is reportedly co-ingested with other drugs, including cannabis, ecstasy, stimulants and sildenafil (Viagra).[36,37] Polydrug use increases the risk of acute toxicity, most significantly when another CNS depressant has been consumed.

3.8 Desired and Unwanted Effects of GHB/GBL

GHB/GBL affects people in different ways and a euphoric dose for one person may be a sedative dose for another.[63] GHB/GBL tends to produce euphoric and pleasurable effects[64] without hangover or other subacute adverse effects, which helped popularise it as a 'club drug'.[5] The desired effects of GHB/GBL include euphoria, relaxation, increased sociability and confidence, social and sexual disinhibition, enhanced libido, increased sexual arousal and enhancement of sexual encounters, with effects being dose dependent.[12,30,65,66,67]

The use of GHB/GBL for its stimulant, dissociative and sedating effects has also been reported.[50,68,69] In addition, some individuals use GHB/GBL after using other drugs (generally stimulants), to help 'come down'[36] or to enhance and modify the effects of drugs.[50] GHB/GBL is also used as self-medication for sleep problems and anxiety. There are reports of people using GHB/GBL in the hope that it will improve cognitive ability, reduce the effects of ageing, reduce depression and anxiety, or make them feel more energised.[70]

There are a number of unwanted effects associated with GHB/GBL. GHB/GBL use is often associated with 'blackout' and loss of consciousness. This can be a risk factor for users for becoming involved in unwanted sexual activity or enduring sexual or acquisitive crimes.[71]

Concerns have also been voiced about the potential role of GHB/GBL in reducing safe sex practices because of its links to disinhibition and unconsciousness.[72,73] GHB is associated with high-risk sexual behaviour and thus with an increased risk of sexually transmitted infections. Studies have shown that GHB/GBL use is associated with increased sexual risk, with HIV-positive men more likely to use GHB/GBL and more likely to use it in a sexual context[40,74,75] than those not known to be infected.[76]

A study based on data from 16,065 UK-based respondents to the European MSM Internet Survey (2010), showed that men who have sex with men who reported using methamphetamine and GHB/GBL in the previous year had 1.92- and 2.23-fold higher odds of gonorrhoea, respectively, over the same period after adjusting for age, recruitment website, HIV status, residence and use of other 'chemsex' drugs. Another study showed that multi-partner encounters and condom-unprotected anal intercourse have been associated with GHB use in the previous 6 months.[77]

The role of 'chemsex' in problematic GHB use has been observed with recommendations for the need for public health providers to engage with novel psychoactive substance use and the health and well-being effects of 'chemsex' and the provision of sensitive, culturally competent interventions.[78] It has been suggested that the routine screening for sexualised drug use in men who have sex with men should be implemented so that healthcare professionals can provide better-informed and higher-quality health care to this population.[79] Models for the joining up of sexual health and drug services to better meet client needs have also been proposed.[80]

The effects of the drugs, which include drowsiness, reduced consciousness and coma, make individuals vulnerable to sexual assault, rape and administration of further substances. GHB and related products have been implicated in cases of sexual assault and victims of acquisitive crime.[81]

3.9 Mortality

Acute GHB/GBL toxicity and a severe withdrawal syndrome have been associated with profound CNS and respiratory depression and death.[82,83,84,85,86] Studies have shown that the co-use of alcohol and other drugs, especially CNS depressants, was implicated in many GHB-related deaths.[87,88]

A study of 74 Australian cases in which GHB contributed to death found that typical cases were young males who swallowed GHB and used it with other substances, most commonly at home. Other substances were also found in 92.2% of cases, most commonly psychostimulants (64.1%), hypnosedatives (28.2%) and alcohol (20.3%). Resuscitation was attempted in 20.3% of cases. Acute pneumonia (36.7%) and aspiration of vomitus (30.6%) were common. The study shows that acute drug toxicity was the most common cause of death, but there was a substantial minority due to trauma or suicide.[89]

It has been suggested that the rise in the number of deaths reported in some countries may be associated with increased participation in 'chemsex'.[90] A study of death of LGBT people associated with the use of GHB/GBL based on data from the UK's National Programme on Substance Abuse Deaths database has suggested that typical victims were: male (100%); white (67%); young (mean age 34 years); employed (90%) and with a drug misuse history (81%). Most deaths were accidental (67%) or related to recreational drug use (19%), the remaining were (potential) suicides. GHB/GBL alone was implicated in 10% of fatalities, with others involving the additional use of at least one other substance.[91]

3.10 Acute Harms

3.10.1 Acute GHB/GBL Toxicity

As mentioned above, GHB/GBL affects people in different ways and a euphoric dose for one person could be a sedative dose for another.[58] The adverse effects of GHB/GBL happen at a variety of doses, indicating the variable individual responses to the drug[92] and are also influenced by the dose ingested, individual variation and other substances ingested. Clinical effects are potentiated by ethanol, benzodiazepines, antipsychotics and other CNS depressants, including some co-ingested recreational drugs.[93] In addition to the GHB-related adverse effects, the adulterant compounds may also have serious toxic effects.[30]

There are potential acute harms relating to any use of GHB/GBL. All GHB/GBL users risk acute toxicity and overdose; tolerance is not fully protective of overdose and people dependent on GHB/GBL are also at risk of acute toxicity.[94]

In terms of acute single-dose systemic toxicity, GHB/GBL appears to be a physiologically toxic club drug, with overdoses typically occurring as a consequence of using repeatedly over a short period, or when GHB/GBL is used in combination with other CNS depressants, such as alcohol or benzodiazepines.[13] The hazard profile of GHB has been described as less favourable than that of many other psychoactive substances. One study concluded that GHB is the most physiologically hazardous drug, partly because of the narrow safe dosage range[95] and because its effects vary between individuals and whether other substances have also been used. The imprecise dosing of illicit GHB or GBL can be associated with acute harms and overdose.[85]

The effects of GHB are dose-dependent, as summarised in a recent review (Table 3.2).8

Loss of consciousness and coma associated with GHB/GBL intoxication is common and recurrent coma is a common experience of people who use this drug even recreationally.[101] Unconsciousness or reduced consciousness are the most common symptoms of GHB overdose.[102,103] However, it seems that despite the fact that regular GHB users may experience GHB-induced coma repeatedly, many still consider its use to be safe.[104,105,106,107]

This is sometimes referred to by users as 'blackouts', with one study showing that 14% of participants experienced blackouts 'nearly always' or 'always', and 24% experienced blackouts in at least half of their GHB-using episodes.[108]

Table 3.1 Dose-dependent effects of GHB

Dose	Effects
Below 10 mg/kg	Mild clinical effects: short term anterograde amnesia, hypotonia and euphoria[96]
20–30 mg/kg	Drowsiness, sleep and myoclonus can happen[86,97]
50 mg/kg and over	May cause coma.[98,99,100] May lead to the onset of coma, bradycardia and/or respiratory depression and death[86,88,90]

The usual clinical course after overdose – if other CNS depressants (including alcohol) have not been used – is rapid, spontaneous awakening from drug-induced loss of consciousness or coma and uneventful recovery.[109]

Temporary GHB-induced coma generally lasts between 1 and 4 hours, but could be much briefer. It often reaches the most severe classification on the Glasgow Coma Scale,[110,111,112] but it has been noted that often no side effects are apparent after sudden awakening from this coma. CNS depression usually persists for 1–3 hours, with patients typically, but not always, making a full recovery within 4–8 hours.[82,113,114,115] Thus, patients with acute intoxication typically develop signs of intoxication rapidly but then improve quickly.

Overdoses are common among all users – dependent users as well as inexperienced, intermittent and regular users. Tolerance and dependence do not protect against overdose.[36]

In an Australian study of 76 GHB users, half reported a history of overdose during which they had lost consciousness.[36] In another study, 66% reported some degree of loss of consciousness.[50] Similarly, a study of 505 consecutive GHB cases in emergency departments in Barcelona showed that the motive for seeking medical treatment in all cases was reduced consciousness.[60]

As with alcohol, and unlike with benzodiazepines, there is no antagonist or antidote. Because of GHB's short elimination half-life, people can progress from deep coma to wakefulness over about 30 minutes. A 30-month review of an Australian emergency department reported that if ventilation was not required, the great majority improved rapidly and were discharged straight from the emergency department, without a need for further medical treatment.[116,117] A study of presentation to hospital associated with GHB intoxications, for example, reported sudden recovery in one third of the cases presenting to hospital with impaired consciousness, and the majority of the patients were discharged home directly from the emergency department, despite the characterisation of their intoxication as 'severe' at the time of presentation.[118]

In European cities, accidental GHB/GBL overdoses in night clubs account for a substantial proportion of drug-related emergencies that require ambulance, emergency or hospital services.[30]

A study of GHB/GBL overdose in Norway based on ambulance records suggested that patients were male, in their mid-20s, and found unconscious at the scene. The temporal patterns suggest party use, being most frequent during late-night and weekends.[119] The GHB/GBL victims are younger than opioid overdose victims, and are hospitalised more often.[120]

3.10.1.1 The Features of Acute GHB/GBL Toxicity

Overall, the reported effects of acute GHB/GBL toxicity are summarised as follows (see also Boxes 3.1, 3.2 and 3.3):

- Mild/moderate effects include nausea, hypersalivation, vomiting, diarrhoea, drowsiness, headache, ataxia, dizziness, confusion, amnesia, urinary incontinence, tremor, myoclonus, hypotonia, agitation, euphoria and hypothermia.

- Severe effects include coma, convulsions, bradycardia, ECG abnormalities (e.g. U waves), in rare cases hypertension after intravenous use, Cheyne–Stokes respiration and respiratory depression leading to respiratory arrest. Metabolic acidosis has been reported.

GHB/GBL produces CNS and respiratory depression of relatively short duration. Laboratory investigations may also indicate hypernatraemia, hypokalaemia, hyperglycaemia and metabolic acidosis. High anion gap metabolic acidosis (HAGMA) has been associated with GHB/GBL and 1,4-BD intoxication.[121,122]

Psychotic episodes may occur. It has also been suggested that GHB/GBL intoxication should be

---

Box 3.1 Reported Neurological and Psychiatric Effects

Effects are dose-related. Patients may therefore present with CNS symptoms ranging from sudden drowsiness through to unresponsive coma, depending on dose.[60,82–84,97,98,100,101,123–134]

- Amnesia[135,136]
- Ataxia[61,63,88,98,113,119,120, 137–171]
- Hypotonia[88,108,116,121,172]
- Disorientation[60,98,120,126,151]
- Hyporeflexia[133,142,148,152]
- Dizziness[61,110,119,134,135,136,153]
- Tremor[88,122]
- Confusion[110,120,121,135,136]
- Myoclonus[82,88,89,97,119,132,173,174,175]
- Hallucination[125,126,135,136]
- Somnolence[120,124,132,154]
- Agitation,[63] bizarre behaviour and combativeness, either at presentation or when waking[60,63,86,87,97,98,100,108,110,113,117,118,119,120,122,123,126,127,130,134,135,136,138,140,143,148,150,152,156,157]
- Slurred speech[122,125,126]
- Miosis[60,110]
- Dysarthria[60,119]
- Confusion[110,126,108]
- Mydriasis (wide pupils)[60,110,114,122,127,128,132,134,135]
- Headache[60,127]
- Horizontal and vertical gaze nystagmus[121,122,125,126,127]
- Reduced coordination[122,135]
- Pupils may be sluggish and non-reactive[108,114,136,149]
- Euphoria
- Convulsions (seizures or seizure-like activity) have been reported,[50,88,97,98,100,101,107,110,111,114,116,120,129,131,135,136,139,150,155,156] but most studies have shown them to be uncommon. They may occur secondary to hypoxia or due to other substances used[12]
- Less common neurological effects include bruxism,[140] vertigo,[88] delusion,[152] extrapyramidal side effects,[125] dystonia[125] and athetoid posturing[140]

Box 3.2 Cardiovascular Effects

- Bradycardia[60,88,97,98,107,110,114,118,119,120,122,126,131,134,135,137,138,140,142,144,148,149,150,151,154,156,157]
- Mild bradycardia without haemodynamic compromise is the most common cardiovascular effect and has been noted in recreational drug users[82]
- Chest tightness[60,136]
- Tachycardia and hypertension[60,98,100,114,119,120,121,123,135,148]
- Hypotension[60,88,100,110,116,119,126,131,140,143,144,149,154,176] is rare when GHB/GBL is used on its own; generally, it occurs only when GHB/GBL is co-ingested with other substances [54,68]
- ECG abnormalities occur occasionally[100]

Box 3.3 Central Nervous System and Respiratory Effects

- Dose-related respiratory depression [87,88,97,98,107,110,113,114,117,119,120,123,130,134,135,149]
  Respiratory failure is normally the cause of death from GHB/GBL
- Tachypnoea[100]
- Bradypnea[60,100,101,108,119,126,133,134,140,142,143,146,149]
- Pneumothorax[151]
- Periodic (Cheyne–Stokes) respirations[156,177,178]
- Cyanosis[108,114]
- Pulmonary aspiration[98,108,109,110,112,115,149]
- Pulmonary oedema[119,130,147,179,180]
- Apnoea and respiratory failure[82,84,135]

---

considered a differential diagnosis for patients presenting to an emergency department with acute agitation.[63]

Reported features of GHB/GBL intoxication are listed in Boxes 3.1 and 3.2. It is important to note that other additional symptoms or features may occur due to co-use of alcohol (ethanol) or other drugs.

The CNS symptoms of acute toxicity can vary, depending on ingested dose, from sudden drowsiness to unresponsiveness and profound coma. CNS depression typically persists for 1–3 hours, with patients making a complete recovery typically within 4–8 hours.

Coma accounts for a significant proportion of GHB-/GBL-related presentations to emergency departments, with a reported range of 16–33%.[110] For example, a third of cases in a Swiss study[110] presented to hospital with coma, 28% of cases of a US study[82] and 16% of cases in a study conducted in Spain.[97] In a case series of presentations to a London emergency department, approximately 16% of cases had severe coma at presentation, with a score on the Glasgow Coma Scale (GCS) of 3. In this study, 47% of patients had a GCS

score ≤8, which is the usual cut-off for intubation.[107] A case series of 88 patients presenting to medical services after taking GHB reported a GCS score of 3 and 33% had a score of 4–8.[82]

Acute GHB/GBL toxicity can cause amnesia, which increases the risk of relapse because users do not remember the experience of acute intoxication and overdose.[181] As mentioned above, GHB can cause profound unconsciousness and the steep dose–response curve puts the user at risk of death. The co-ingestion of alcohol is a significant added risk factor, but GHB/GBL intoxication alone can cause death.[5] Other reported effects of GHB/GBL use include one observational case report of acute central serous chorioretinopathy.[182]

Vomiting

Vomiting during acute intoxication is common. The London-based study mentioned above reported that vomiting occurred in 17% of presentations,[107] while Garrison et al. reported vomiting in 22% of presentations.[183] Other studies have reported higher rates including vomiting in 30% of the presentations to a US emergency department study[82] and in more than half of cases of GHB/GBL overdose in an Australian study.[36] Vomiting in individuals with reduced consciousness (especially when the GCS score is less than 8 out of 15) is believed to increase the risk of aspiration due to the lack of protective airway reflexes.[184] Indeed, aspiration in patients intoxicated with GHB/GBL needs to be considered a significant risk, particularly in those with reduced consciousness. Local clinical protocols should include steps to assess and reduce the likelihood of vomiting and subsequent aspiration.

Seizures or seizure-like activity are associated with GHB/GBL consumption and have been widely reported,[50,97,100,107,110,114,129,135,155,185] especially when intoxication is severe. Studies suggest however that seizures are uncommon,[12] although it has been argued that it is difficult to determine the true frequency of 'seizures', as GHB and its analogues have been shown to cause myoclonic jerks, which – in pre-hospital settings in particular – may be misinterpreted as a seizure.[168]

Hypothermia is usually not severe, but can be common. For example, in a series of 88 cases of GHB/GBL overdose, 55% were assessed to have an initial temperature of 36°C or less and 25% an initial temperature of 35°C or less.[82]

Bradycardia is also common. In the same case series of 88 GHB overdose patients, over one-third (36%) developed bradycardia, although only one case was severe enough to require atropine.[82]

3.10.1.2 Acute Withdrawal

People who use at least daily may commonly develop tolerance and dependence. Withdrawal syndrome following abstinence or dose reduction after prolonged use can be severe and must be treated as a medical emergency. For more details on withdrawal see Section 3.12.2.

3.10.2 Poly-drug Use and Drug Interactions

The co-ingestion of alcohol (ethanol) and/or other recreational drugs may contribute to some of the other clinical features seen in patients presenting with GHB/GBL and or GHB/GBL toxicity.[186] A number of authors have suggested that GHB users who co-ingest alcohol are more likely to develop severe complications related to GHB use.

A double-blind, placebo-controlled, cross-over volunteer study that investigated the potential for toxicity associated with GHB alone compared with GHB and alcohol co-ingestion showed that GHB plus ethanol was associated with more adverse effects, in particular hypotension and hypoxia; there were no differences in GHB/GBL concentrations between the groups.[187]

Co-ingestion of GHB/GBL and alcohol has been associated with increased agitation[110] and aggressive behaviour. Patients who used alcohol were also more likely to vomit.[110] There is evidence that when GHB/GBL is taken in combination with other drugs (including alcohol or stimulants), the duration and depth of coma is greater than when it is consumed alone, and recovery times are longer.[60,110,188]

3.10.2.1 GHB and HIV Antiretroviral Therapy (ART)

There is evidence that men who have sex with men who are living with HIV are one of the population groups likely to use GHB/GBL.[189] Many will be receiving antiretroviral therapy (ART).

While clearance of GHB from the systemic circulation occurs rapidly by oxidation to succinic acid,[190,191] animal data suggest that GHB is also a substrate of first-pass metabolism (which may involve the enzymes CYP2D6 and CYP3A4). Therefore, co-administration of GHB with CYP2D6 inhibitors (i.e. cobicistat) or CYP3A4 inhibitors (i.e. ritonavir, cobicistat) may lead to raised systemic exposures of GHB and increased toxicity. It has been recommended that GHB/GBL should be used with caution by people receiving ART with predisposing seizure disorders or with opportunistic infections that may lower seizure threshold (i.e. toxoplasmosis, cryptococcal meningitis), as GHB/GBL may precipitate seizure-like activity.

There is a case study of a patient taking saquinavir/ritonavir and experiencing extreme sedation, myoclonus and bradycardia after taking a small dose of GHB. These severe manifestations of GHB toxicity were thought to be due to CYP isoenzyme inhibition with resultant drug accumulation.[192]

GHB/GBL use may cause severe nausea, vomiting and gastrointestinal tract irritation, and adversely affect absorption of ART.[193] There are also concerns about compliance with HIV medication while intoxicated, especially during prolonged binges, which may complicate ART and affect adherence.[177]

It has also been noted that the co-administration of EVG/COBI (Elvitegravir; Cobicistat) may potentially increase concentration of phencyclidine (PCD) or methamphetamine, cocaine, GABA-mimetics (e.g. lorazepam, midazolam, triazolam, alprazolam and GHB). EVG/COBI via inhibition of P-gp could potentially increase the effects of opiates in the CNS.[194,195]

3.11 Clinical Management of Acute Toxicity

3.11.1 Identification and Assessment

Diagnosis of acute GHB/GBL toxicity should be made on clinical assessment. Urine and serum tests are not routinely available[196] in frontline clinical settings so analytical assessment should not be considered a component of routine diagnosis. It has been suggested that the diagnosis of acute GHB/GBL toxicity be based on the recognition of the clinical toxidrome associated with the overdose of GHB/GBL.[168]

Standard medical assessment is always indicated, so that other causes of the presentation can be excluded.

Problems relating to the identification of GHB/GBL intoxication are linked to the similarities in clinical features to alcohol, opiate and/or benzodiazepine intoxication,[12,197,198] or similarities to other clinical presentations, such as hypoglycaemia. Given the similarity to acute opioid toxicity, it is recommended that where there is clinical uncertainty, it may be worth considering a trial of the opioid antagonist naloxone, although it is not effective in managing acute GHB/GBL intoxication.[199]

Diagnosis is also complicated by frequency of other co-intoxicants[200] and by the diversity of clinical presentation.[63] Some or all of the clinical features of acute GHB/GBL toxicity may be 'masked' by other co-ingested substances (e.g. an individual may present with drowsiness and normal heart rate due to co-ingestion of GHB/GBL and a stimulant such as cocaine or amphetamine).

3.11.2 Clinical Management of Overdose and Acute Toxicity

For up-to-date guidance on the management of GHB/GBL acute toxicity, it is recommended that information be sought from national or regional poisons information services.

Clinicians should also consult their local or national guidelines and protocols.

There is consistency in the evidence reviewed that the treatment of GHB/GBL acute toxicity should consist of symptom-directed supportive care with an emphasis on respiratory support.[201] Wood et al. suggest that the duration of reduced consciousness (particularly non-responsive coma) is generally short-lived, with the majority of patients recovering fully within 2–3 hours of the onset of coma.[168]

The protection of airways and proper airway management is recommended because vomiting is common.[98,117,151,162,202]

It has been argued that routine intubation of patients with acute GHB/GBL toxicity is not recommended unless patients exhibit vomiting, seizures or other clinical indications for intubation.[168] Clinical consensus suggests that there does not appear to be a need to intubate purely on the basis of GCS score, as in other medical presentations and trauma. On the other hand, others have recommended that if the patients are unconscious then intubation should be considered for the first few hours of recovery.[203]

Reports in the literature indicate that intubation is needed in 3–13% of cases.[82,97,100,110,204] One study found a greater requirement for mechanical ventilation for patients who had ingested GHB/GBL with other drugs or alcohol, as the duration and depth of coma were greater than when GHB/GBL was taken alone.[60]

In addition, is it recommended that in cases of GHB overdose, clinicians should monitor vital signs and cardiac rhythm and check the capillary blood sugar. A 12-lead ECG should be performed in all patients who require assessment and it is recommended that 12-lead ECGs are repeated, especially in symptomatic patients or in those who have co-ingested other sustained release preparations. Clinicians should also check cardiac rhythm, QRS duration and QT interval. It is also recommended that clinicians check U&Es and creatinine, blood glucose and CK in all patients who require assessment. It is also recommended that clinicians consider arterial blood gas analysis in patients who have a reduced level of consciousness (e.g. GCS less than 8; AVPU scale P or U) or have reduced oxygen saturation on pulse oximetry.[205]

Symptom-directed supportive care might include the management of seizures, bradycardia, hypotension, hypertension, metabolic acidosis, hyperthermia, rhabdomyolysis, agitation and delirium.[206] Cardiovascular symptoms resulting from overdosing with GHB don't normally require invasive therapy.[207]

It has been recommended that all patients who require assessment should be observed for at least 4 hours after exposure. Asymptomatic patients can then be considered for discharge with advice to return if symptoms develop.[208]

Expert consensus has highlighted the need to fully investigate unconscious patients, particularly when the diagnosis is unclear. CT scanning may be indicted, particularly when convulsions occur, although there is no robust evidence on the routine use of CT scanning specifically for GHB/GBL overdoses.

Some patients may have a fluctuating course on recovery, where they have periods of agitation alongside periods of drowsiness or coma. These patients can sometimes be difficult to manage, since they require appropriate sedation for their periods of agitation, which may worsen the degree of sedation when it occurs. Should this occur, there may be a need for appropriate respiratory support until the patient has fully recovered. Dependent users may begin to go into withdrawal on recovery from the overdose – see Section 3.12.2.

Gastric decontamination (e.g. activated charcoal) is not recommended, as its effects are uncertain. There are no antidotes for GHB/GBL poisoning.[12]

A study has suggested that treatment with inhibitors of monocarboxylate transporter 1 (MCT1) (a transporter that mediates many of the processes involved in the absorption, distribution, including brain uptake and elimination of GHB/GBL), has been shown to prevent GHB-induced respiratory depression by increasing the renal clearance of GHB. Overall, this study indicates that inhibition of MCT1 is an effective treatment of GHB/GBL overdose.[209]

Outside clinical settings, in night clubs for example, harm reduction information should stress the need to put people in the recovery position and call for an ambulance. GHB/GBL users should similarly be told to put people with signs of acute intoxication in the recovery position (see also Section 3.15).

3.11.3 Treatment Outcome

Patients with GHB/GBL acute toxicity will typically develop symptoms quickly, but will generally also improve rapidly. Even in more severe cases, patients will usually make a full recovery, provided they are hospitalised and receive appropriate supportive care.[12,210]

Studies have shown that patients will regain a GCS score of 15 in a short time after presentation (a median of 76 minutes in one study), albeit this is longer for those with severely reduced consciousness, typically resulting from poly-substance use.[60,100] They also show a rapid rate of discharge from hospital,[60,100] although people presenting to hospital with a low GCS may have a longer recovery period.[107]

A retrospective study of patients presenting to a large London inner-city emergency department with acute poisoning with self-reported GHB/GBL toxicity reported on the disposition of patients with acute GHB/GBL intoxication. The majority (92.2%) were discharged directly or self-discharged from the department or required only a short period of observation in the emergency department observation ward. Fewer than 1 in 10 (7.8%) required admission to hospital. Among those, the majority were admitted to critical care facilities, usually because of significant neurological or respiratory compromise and the need for airway protection and intubation. The study also looked at length of stay and reported an overall median stay of 2.8 hours: discharged or self-discharged directly from the emergency department 2.4 hours (range 1.7–3); admitted to the emergency department observation ward 5.6 hours (range 3.6–8.6); admitted to general medical ward 15.6 hours; admitted to a critical care facility 18.7 hours (range 10.1–39.2).[107]

As amnesia is a direct effect of GHB/GBL, patients may recover with no recall of GHB/GBL intoxication or overdose.[50] In a study of 42 users, 13% had amnesia during GHB use and 45% after GBL use.[50] It has been noted that because they do not remember their experience of overdose, people may put themselves at risk of overdosing in another GHB use episode or may delay treatment.[165]

3.11.4 Acute Withdrawal Following Detoxification

In GBL-/GHB-dependent people, rapid improvement from acute toxicity may be followed by deterioration as withdrawal symptoms develop (for details on withdrawal see Section 3.12.2). Withdrawal symptoms may manifest quickly, or up to 24–48 hours later, and the potential for delayed onset of withdrawal symptoms in those with GHB/GBL dependence must be considered in the management of acute toxicity.[211] A vital part of discharge instructions from hospital to GHB-/GBL-dependent patients, their friends and carers after recovery from overdose, is to inform them about the potential for withdrawal symptoms to occur after discharge.[196]

In the majority of published cases of GHB/GBL withdrawal, detoxification was unplanned and started after the patient presented in crisis, usually to an emergency department.[55] Acute withdrawal is potentially life threatening and it is recommended that cases are considered a medical emergency. It is also recommended that all dependent users of GHB/GBL are advised not to stop use abruptly or to attempt self-detoxification. Medical assistance should always be sought.

3.12 Harms Associated with Chronic Use

3.12.1 Dependence

The regular, prolonged use of GHB/GBL and its analogues can lead to physiological dependence.[12] Its typical features include difficulty controlling the amount used, neglect of other activities and withdrawal symptoms, which in the case of GHB/GBL can be severe.

Part of the dependence syndrome is tolerance, in which larger doses are needed over time to produce the same psychoactive effects. Long-term users therefore typically use higher doses than naïve users.[30] Users have reported taking larger doses in order to achieve previous effects or use just 'to normalise' themselves rather than to experience acute intoxication.[56] Cross-tolerance between GHB/GBL and alcohol may exist.

At a social level, dependence has been described by patients to be the opposite to why they chose to use GHB/GBL in the first place: rather than enhancing sociability, GHB/GBL dependence leads to introversion, lack of motivation and failing to maintain contact with family and non-using friends; other concerns included absenteeism and loss of employment.[47]

3.12.2 The GHB/GBL Withdrawal Syndrome

The potential of GHB/GBL to produce dependence is well recognised. Dependent users will consume GHB/GBL at regular intervals during the day and at night, sometimes as often as every 1–3 hours,[13] in order to avoid withdrawal.

Abrupt decrease or discontinuation of heavy GHB use may result in a severe and life-threatening withdrawal syndrome, characterised by autonomic instability, delirium and aggression.[212]

GHB/GBL withdrawal can appear clinically similar to withdrawal from opioids, benzodiazepines and alcohol,[12] and problems relating to the identification of GHB/GBL intoxication and withdrawal are linked to the similarities in clinical features.[182] Symptoms are often more prolonged than in alcohol withdrawal (up to 2 weeks, occasionally longer) and are typically more resistant to treatment with benzodiazepines.

GHB/GBL withdrawal can also have similarities to clinical presentations such as hypoglycaemia or sympathomimetic toxicity, typically associated with stimulant use.

3.12.2.1 Predictors of Withdrawal

Dependent users will develop withdrawal symptoms on reduction or cessation of use, which can be severe and life threatening.[55,213,214,215] GHB/GBL withdrawal symptoms occur on a spectrum that varies in clinical severity.

Withdrawal symptoms have typically been observed after prolonged use of high doses of GHB but can be seen after as little as 2–3 months of use,[55] or even a shorter time after high-frequency use.

There is increasing evidence that daily use of GHB/GBL is a predictor of withdrawal.[55] People who consume GHB doses at short intervals (e.g. every 2–3 hours) appear to have the highest risk of severe withdrawal symptoms when stopping GHB use. It is suggested that GHB users who consume the drug at regular intervals during the day and night (every 1–3 hours) appear to be particularly at risk to develop dependence.[216] Less-frequent users may experience mild withdrawal symptoms upon cessation.[217]

In their review, McDonough et al. report a minimum daily dose associated with withdrawal is approximately 18 g for GHB and 10 g for GBL,[55] but it is possible that it occurs at lower daily doses.

3.12.2.2 Onset and Duration of Withdrawal Syndrome

One distinctive feature of GHB/GBL dependence is the quick onset of withdrawal symptoms. These can occur 30 minutes after the last dose, but more typically after a few hours. GHB/GBL withdrawal symptoms have been reported to last from 48 hours to 21 days,[12,55] with one review reporting a mean of 9 days.[55] Longer term withdrawal symptoms tend to include psychiatric symptoms such as delirium, psychosis or depression.[218,219,220]

Wood et al. report that in their clinical experience, 50% of those who present to hospital with acute GHB/

GBL withdrawal will require barbiturates and admission to intensive care, as they typically present with delirium.[221]

3.12.2.3 Individual Variations and Unpredictability of the Withdrawal Syndrome

Although there are similarities between cases of GHB/GBL withdrawal reported in the literature, there are also wide variations in both the withdrawal symptoms and the clinical responses between patients.[222] Withdrawal symptoms can be self-limiting in some patients, but others can present with more severe withdrawal that can progress rapidly and require acute medical intervention.

3.12.2.4 GHB/GBL Withdrawal Symptoms

The symptoms of GHB/GBL withdrawal seem to vary between people, and may depend on the amount and duration of use of GHB. Withdrawal symptoms typically start a few hours after the last GHB ingestion.[223]

Withdrawal symptoms reported in the literature are summarised in Box 3.4.

It is not possible to determine accurately how common these symptoms are. A review of 36 emergency department presentations reported that the early symptoms of withdrawal were tremor (67%), hallucinations (63%), tachycardia (63%), insomnia (58%), seizures (7%) and rhabdomyolysis (7%).[200]

McDonough et al. in their review reported that an eight-hourly dosing was the minimum frequency associated with withdrawal delirium.[55] There are indications that heavy, frequent users are most likely to progress to severe delirium. It has been proposed that withdrawal in cases of co-dependence on GHB/GBL and another CNS depressant (opiates or other sedatives) or CNS stimulant are likely to be more severe, but such cases have not been widely described in the literature.[55] Seizures associated with GHB/GBL withdrawal appear to be less common than with alcohol and are reported in fewer than 10% of cases.

The early symptoms of GHB/GBL withdrawal typically include insomnia, tremor, confusion, nausea and vomiting. Over the next 12–48 hours, tachycardia, hypertension, agitation, seizures and/or myoclonic jerks and hallucinations may develop.

Box 3.4 GHB Withdrawal Symptoms

Commonly Reported Symptoms

- Hallucinations – visual and auditory[13,23,57,198,200,224,225,226,227,228,229,230,231,232,233,234,235,236,237,238]
- Anxiety[23,37,50,56,57,90,198,208,209,215,239,240,241]
- Tremors[37,52,56,57,90,182,207–210,213,215,216,218–223]
- Paranoia[13,23,56,57,198,212–215,218,221]
- Tachycardia[23,50,57,198,200,207–210,212,215–218,222,223]
- Insomnia[23,37,52,57,90,207,208,210,212,215,217,221]
- Hypertension[57,198,207,208,217,218,223]
- Disorientation[23,198,200,208,209,212,215,217,221]
- Sweating[52,56,57,198,207,208,210,213–216,218,222]
- Confusion[23,198,182,208,212,215,219]
- Agitation[50,198,182,200,212,214,216,217,219,242]
- Aggression/combativeness[56,198,209,211,218]

Other Reported Symptoms

- Depression[52,57,215]
- Tachypnoea[213]
- Miosis[212]
- Nausea and vomiting[198,222]
- Nystagmus[23,216,221,223]
- Diarrhoea[198,224]
- Cardiac palpitations[51,219,223]

- Abdominal pain (less common)[223]
- Dyspnoea[219]
- Myoclonic jerks[168]

Severe Withdrawal

- Delirium[37,50,57,182,200,207,216,217,219]
- Seizures[56,182,198,200,212] – may become life-threatening
- Psychosis[109,210,212,215,218,219,220]
- Withdrawal mimicking schizophrenia[243]
- Rhabdomyolysis[200,208,220]

Medical complications reported during withdrawal include sepsis, myoglobinuria, Wernicke's encephalopathy without alcohol dependence, catatonic stupor and mutism have also been reported[244]

Life-threatening complications include seizures, bradycardia, cardiac arrest and renal failure[245,246]

It has been suggested that although GHB/GBL withdrawal syndrome does not always follow a predictable pattern, it can be broadly divided into three phases[247]:

- The first stage, which typically lasts 1–3 hours, is characterised by severe craving, profuse sweating – mostly of the palms and feet, tachycardia, irritability, anxiety and nausea.
- The second stage, lasting for up to 3 days, is characterised by psychiatric symptoms such as confusion, delirium, and visual, auditory and tactile hallucinations. The physical symptoms include autonomic dysregulation (e.g. raised blood pressure) and motor symptoms, which can include muscle spasms, convulsions, choreatic movements of extremities and restlessness of the tongue.[248,249,250]
- The last phase can last for days to months. It is characterised by dysphoria, anxiety, lethargy and apathy, lack of concentration, sleep problems and loss of libido. Over the longer term, symptoms of withdrawal may include persisting depression, apathetic state and cognitive problems including memory problems.[251,252,253]

3.13 Harms from Chronic Use

GBL has been described as a mild skin irritant and a strong mucous membrane irritant. It can penetrate the epidermis and cause rashes and eczema.[5]

Little is known about the long-term harms of GHB/GBL that are secondary to acute harms or dependence. It is recommended that more research be carried out on the long-term effects of GHB/GBL,

including psychiatric (and cognitive), physical and teratogenicity-related harms. This includes the recommendation by Miotto et al. to study the possibility of persistent problems with memory acquisition as a result of GHB/GBL use.[254]

Among men who have sex with men in particular, GHB/GBL is often used in a sexual context and in a context of potential high-risk sexual behaviour. Studies have shown that GHB/GBL use is associated with increased sexual risk and potential transmission of HIV, as well as other sexually transmitted and blood-borne infections[255,256,257]

3.13.1 Clinical Management of Dependence

3.13.1.1 Identification and Assessment of GHB/GBL Dependence and Withdrawal

Signs suggesting GHB/GBL dependence include:

- Multiple daily dosing;
- Waking at night to dose;
- Using other drugs to prevent withdrawal symptoms overnight;
- Withdrawal symptoms on days when not using or after periods of reduction or cessation;
- Not able to go a day without use.

There are no validated GHB/GBL withdrawal scales. In the absence of a specific scale, it may be reasonable to use alcohol or benzodiazepine withdrawal scales. However, in cases of emergency acute withdrawal, many would recommend focusing treatment on the basis of symptomatic control, since non-GHB-specific scales do not always pick up the degree of neuro-psychiatric symptoms, which could lead to inappropriate clinical management and subsequent escalation of withdrawal symptoms including delirium.

In specialist drug treatment clinical practice, the Clinical Institute Withdrawal Assessment of Alcohol Scale (CIWA-Ar) has been used,[258] as well as the Alcohol Withdrawal Scale (AWS). Other scales used include the Subjective Withdrawal Scale, where staff record standard observations, such as heart rate and blood pressure.[259]

There are no validated tools for the identification of or screening for harmful GHB/GBL use in non-drug specific settings. Winstock and Mitcheson have provided helpful guidance for addressing substance misuse issues in general practice.[260]

3.13.1.2 Psychosocial and Pharmacological Support

Chapter 2 discusses in general terms the psychosocial interventions for the use of club drugs. These are applicable to the management of the chronic harms of GHB use, as well as aftercare and support, and so are not discussed further here. The pharmacological interventions are discussed below. GHB treatment should be based on a bio-psycho-social model as discussed below.

3.13.2 Clinical Management of Withdrawal

GHB detoxification can be challenging for frontline clinicians because of the rapid onset and potentially life-threatening symptoms that can occur during withdrawal. It has been argued that the focus of the treatment should be to prevent complications such as delirium, psychosis, extreme anxiety and hypertension.[261]

The research evidence on the management of GHB/GBL withdrawal is still emerging and it is therefore not possible to draw robust recommendations.

It is, though, consistently suggested that symptomatic treatment is indicated for GHB/GBL withdrawal syndrome. The review of the evidence shows that benzodiazepines are most typically used for this purpose.[23,198,208,212,213,217,222,224] There is one case report, which shows the challenges associated with detoxification during pregnancy.[262]

There are no consistently recommended benzodiazepine titration regimens in the literature, with studies recommending a wide range of intervals of dosing and of benzodiazepine doses. In the UK, Toxbase of

the National Poisons Information Service suggests in excess of 100 mg in divided doses of 10–20 mg at 2–4 hourly intervals[263] in severe cases or when treatment is delayed. Some studies have suggested that for the treatment of severe withdrawal, high dosages of up to 300 mg diazepam or 130–200 mg lorazepam may be necessary.[264,265,266,267,268,269]

Combined evidence suggests that benzodiazepines are the first line of treatment, but adjuncts may be helpful to control symptoms,[208] especially where there is benzodiazepine-resistance or poor response.

Baclofen and barbiturates have been described as second-line adjuncts.[55,57,86,198,168,200] The use of a combination of diazepam and baclofen has been used successfully in clinical practice, as part of medically assisted detoxification[37,270] and to prevent relapse.[271]

One study has suggested 10 mg of baclofen three times a day as an adjunct to benzodiazepine prescribing, with the addition of a two-day preload of baclofen 10 mg three times a day in elective detoxifications.[272]

The use of Baclofen on its own has also been suggested,[273,274] as baclofen might be an adequate substitute for GHB due to its high-affinity for the GABA-B receptor. Baclofen's GABA-B agonism is similar to GHB,[14,15] but with a longer half-life (T = 2–6 h).[275]

Detoxification by titration and tapering (DeTiTap) with pharmaceutical GHB in an open-label consecutive case series of 23 GHB-dependent patients was shown to be feasible, effective and safe. However, the high relapse rates warrant further investigation.[276,277]

There is limited evidence that patients receiving baclofen after detoxification showed reduced relapse rates compared with patients receiving treatment as usual.[278,279,280] However, one study has suggested that baclofen 45–60 mg/day for 3 months might be effective in preventing relapse and increasing treatment adherence in patients with GHB use disorder.[281] The use of baclofen up to 60 mg daily in patients with GHB use disorder appears safe, when prescribed according to the protocol. Mild tiredness, sleepiness and depressed feelings were reported in the baclofen group as the most relevant side effects. Future studies with longer follow-up and a randomised double-blind design should be conducted to confirm these findings before recommendations for clinical practice can be made.[282,283]

There is some evidence that patients receiving baclofen after detoxification showed reduced relapse rates compared with patients receiving treatment as usual. Studies have shown the potential effectiveness of baclofen in preventing relapse in patients with GHB dependence after detoxification. However, more research is needed.

Baclofen may play a role in relapse prevention, as shown in a case series of GHB-dependent patients. However, controlled studies on the effectiveness of baclofen to prevent relapse in GHB-dependent patients are still limited.[284]

A wide range of medications have been used and described as potentially helpful in GHB/GBL withdrawal management. However, supporting evidence for any of these medications is mainly based on a small number of case reports and case series. The decision on which additional agent to use depends on the clinical presentation. Antipsychotics should be used with caution due to the risk of neuroleptic malignant syndrome and the lowering of the seizure threshold. Medications reported by the literature and which have

been used to manage acute withdrawal are listed in Box 3.5.

It is worth noting that some individuals self-medicate with baclofen, ethanol or benzodiazepines to prevent GHB/GBL withdrawal. There is some evidence from Internet fora that baclofen is consumed without medical supervision by GHB/GBL users to treat GHB withdrawal.[289] Clinicians must be aware of the risks of patients taking baclofen in addition to GHB/GBL, as the combination can lead to respiratory distress and coma.[290] Self-detoxification from GHB/GBL can be dangerous and should be avoided, as withdrawal symptoms can be severe and potentially life threatening. GHB/GBL users who wish to stop should be encouraged to seek medical assistance. If they want to reduce GHB/GBL use on their own, they should do so in very small increments and with the support of health professionals. Consumption diaries are suggested as a useful tool to assist in gradual withdrawal.

Box 3.5 Medications Used to Manage Acute GHB/GBL Withdrawal

Benzodiazepines are safe and effective in managing most cases

Diazepam[198,196,224,285]

Baclofen[37,182,215]

Barbiturates[57,90,216,218,220]

Barbiturates can be used in benzodiazepine refractory cases[55]

Carbamazepine[215]

Gabapentin[215]

Chloral hydrate[210,215]

Clonidine[51,215]

Paroxetine[51]

Beta blockers[51,286]

Bromocriptine[200]

Trazadone[57,209,215]

Propofol[64,119,220]

Antipsychotics[23,198,209,210,212,214,218,219,220,221,225]

- Antipsychotics, including haloperidol, should be administered with caution.[210,216,219,287] Typical antipsychotics should be avoided due to the risk of developing NMS type syndromes.[215]
- It is suggested that intramuscular typical antipsychotics in GHB withdrawal should be used with caution.[220] Antipsychotics are not indicated unless delirium is present.[226]

Also reported:

Lorazepam and/or droperiol for the management of agitation.[63]

Olanzapine 160 and Pentobarbital have been reported in an inpatient setting.[57]

Propranolol[51] and pharmaceutical GHB.[51]

Some argue that a serious withdrawal syndrome can be prevented by titration tapering with pharmaceutical GHB. This alternative to benzodiazepines was shown to be effective and safe, especially in patients who have developed resistance to benzodiazepines.[288]

Attempts at self-detoxification from GHB/GBL can be ineffective. In one study of 56 GHB/GBL users recruited via the Internet, respondents had unsuccessfully attempted to cease using GHB/GBL on average 4.07 times. Only 30% had been previously treated for GHB/GBL misuse by health services.[65]

3.13.3 Medically Assisted Elective or Planned Withdrawal and Detoxification

It has been argued that it is best if medically assisted GHB/GBL detoxification is carried out on an elective basis,[37] planned in advance so that withdrawal symptoms can be identified and treated early. Most patients presenting to emergency services symptomatically following enforced abstinence have presented with more severe symptoms and increased risk of delirium.[57] An elective approach to detoxification also enables planning of post-withdrawal support and recovery.

There is limited evidence on the provision of elective medically assisted withdrawal of GHB/GBL, as most case reports and series are concerned with unplanned withdrawal in acute medical settings.[37,291,292,293,294,295] However, where elective withdrawal has taken place, the management of withdrawal in most cases is by titration with high doses of benzodiazepines and successive tapering off.[296]

For planned detoxification and based on existing evidence, Kamal et al. (2017)[297] suggested an algorithm for the treatment of GHB withdrawal, using benzodiazepines as follows:[298,299]

- For patients using less than 30–32 g of GHB in 24 hours, daily doses of diazepam up to 20–60 mg could be administered.[300]
- When 30–32 g or more of GHB is used in 24 hours, daily doses of diazepam from 80 to 150 mg daily may be needed.[301]
- Stabilisation for 2–3 days followed by tapering diazepam by 5–10 mg per day over 7–21 days has been suggested.[302,303]
- The presence of symptoms of delirium might require higher dosages of diazepam, and it has been suggested that benzodiazepine resistance may require administration of oral long-acting phenobarbital after 24 hours.[304,305]

There is no consensus on what the best clinical setting for elective detoxification from GHB/GBL should be. Intensive care, hospital inpatient basis or in outpatient specialist drug treatment centres have all been suggested.

Some have recommended that GHB/GBL withdrawal symptoms in the context of a planned, medically assisted detoxification should be monitored in an intensive care unit (ICU) along with continuous monitoring of vital parameters because of the severity of associated symptoms.[12,306,307] Others have described successful outpatient detoxification.[37] There have been some attempts to identify the parameters and to develop algorithms for the management of GHB/GBL detoxification in specialist drug treatment or acute centres on an inpatient or outpatient basis,[55] as well as to define the medication and monitoring required.[37,55]

An algorithm was developed based on a study of the bio-psychosocial state of 20 vignette patients, whereby addiction physicians and psychiatrists established the criteria and conditions recommended for the indication of an outpatient GHB detoxification. Criteria for identification of the setting included intensity of addiction in terms of daily dose and frequency of dosing as well as the complexity of any comorbid psychiatric disorders. The importance of a stable support system for the person undergoing detoxification was emphasised.[308]

Rosenberg et al. suggest that all cases of GHB withdrawal delirium be considered medical emergencies and be managed in critical care settings, rather than psychiatric settings. The involvement of both disciplines, however, may be required.[220]

3.13.4 Treatment Outcome: Aftercare and Supporting Recovery

Epidemiological data from the Netherlands show that GHB patients stay longer in inpatient care and show high relapse rates (60% within 3 months after detoxification) compared with other substance-dependent patients.[309] There is some evidence that heavier GHB/GBL use predicted poor treatment retention.[310]

A Dutch study compared patients with GHB dependence with those dependent on other drugs and behavioural addictions. It found that of all patients in addiction care, GHB-dependent patients showed the highest treatment intensity, as indicated by high admission rates, long admissions and high number of treatment contacts. In addition, GHB-dependent patients had the highest risk of re-enrolment into a new treatment episode in addiction care. In addition, duration of admission was higher in GHB-dependent patients as compared with other patients, as well as high re-enrolment rates.[311]

A number of studies have examined the high relapse rates following GHB/GBL detoxification and found that anxiety, cognitive problems, unsupportive living environments and lack of daily activities are often mentioned as reasons for rapid relapse.[312,313,314] It has been argued that the lack of evidence-based relapse prevention strategies specifically for GHB/GBL may be contributing to the high relapse rate following detoxification. There is little evidence available to support GHB/GBL users who do not identify abstinence as their goal but instead request support with stabilisation. This is an area which requires further research.[315]

3.14 Public Health and Safety

GHB/GBL use can have a negative impact on public health and safety. Studies have shown that it is associated with increased sexual risk and potential transmission of HIV, as well as other sexually transmitted infections and blood-borne infections.[233,234,235] The links between GHB/GBL use and increased aggression (especially in combination with alcohol) should also be kept in mind, as should the possibility that GHB/GBL is used in drug-facilitated sexual assaults.

GHB/GBL has been commonly associated with drug-facilitated sexual assaults.[316,317,318,319,320] This is due to their properties of causing retrograde amnesia, sedation, ease to dissolve in drinks, rapid onset of action and rapid elimination from the body.

GHB/GBL is associated with the abrupt onset of sleep, which can have dangerous consequences if driving or operating heavy machinery.[13] However, the lack of hangover or sub-acute effects may encourage some to drive under the influence. One study also reported arrests for driving under the influence of GHB/GBL.[321]

3.15 Harm Reduction

3.15.1 Supporting Patients Undergoing Outpatient Medically Assisted GHB/GBL Withdrawal

Patients undergoing outpatient medically assisted GHB/GBL withdrawal should be provided with a proforma letter describing their detoxification and medication regimen, to be presented to the emergency department in case of severe withdrawal.

References

1. Busardò FP, Gottardi M, Tini A, et al. Replacing GHB with GBL in recreational settings: a new trend in chemsex. *Curr Drug Metab* 2018;**19**(13):1080–1085. https://doi.org/10.2174/1389200219666180925090834

2. See for example Castro AL, Dias AS, Melo P, Tarelho S, Franco JM, Teixeira HM. Quantification of GHB and GHB-GLUC in an 1,4-butanediol intoxication: a case report. *Forensic Sci Int* 2019;**297**:378–382. https://doi.org/10.1016/j.forsciint.2019.01.035

3. Stefani M, Roberts DM. 1,4-Butanediol overdose mimicking toxic alcohol exposure. *Clin Toxicol* 2020;**58**(3):204–207. https://doi.org/10.1080/15563650.2019.1617419

4. Office for National Statistics. Deaths Related to Drug Poisoning in England and Wales, 2013 (Statistical Bulletin). Home Office, September 2014.

5. Advisory Council on the Misuse of Drugs (ACMD). GBL and 1,4-BD: Assessment of Risk to the Individual and Communities in the UK. Published 2008.

6. Palatini P, Tedeschi L, Frison G, Padrini R, Zordan R, Orlando R, et al. Dose-dependent absorption and elimination of gamma-hydroxybutyric acid in healthy volunteers. *Eur J Clin Pharmacol* 1993;**45**:353–356.

7. Borgen LA, Okerholm R, Morrison D, Lai A. The influence of gender and food on the pharmacokinetics of sodium oxybate oral solution in healthy subjects. *J Clin Pharmacol* 2003;**43**:59–65.

8. Brenneisen R, Elsohly MA, Murphy TP, Passarelli J, Russmann S, Salamone SJ, et al. Pharmacokinetics and excretion of gamma-hydroxybutyrate (GHB) in healthy subjects. *J Anal Toxicol* 2004;**28**:625–630.

9. Helrich M, Mcaslan TC, Skolnik S, Bessman SP. Correlation of blood levels of 4-hydroxybutyrate with state of consciousness. *Anesthesiology* 1964;**25**:771–775.

10. Abanades S, Farre M, Segura M, Pichini S, Barral D, Pacifici R, et al. Gamma-hydroxybutyrate (GHB) in humans: pharmacodynamics and pharmacokinetics. *Ann NY Acad Sci* 2006;**1074**:559–576.

11. Brailsford AD, Cowan DA, Kicman AT. Pharmacokinetic properties of g-hydroxybutyrate (GHB) in whole blood, serum, and urine. *J Anal Toxicol* 2012;**36**(2):88–95. https://doi.org/10.1093/jat/bkr023

12. Schep LJ, Knudsen K, Slaughter RJ, Vale JA, Mégarbane B. The clinical toxicology of γ-hydroxybutyrate, γ-butyrolactone and 1,4-butanediol. *Clin Toxicol* 2012;**50**(6):458–470. https://doi.org/10.3109/15563650.2012.702218

13. González A, Nutt D. Gamma hydroxy butyrate abuse and dependency. *J Psychopharmacol* 200;519(2):195–204.

14. European Monitoring Centre for Drugs and Drug Addiction (EMCDDA). Report on the Risk Assessment of GHB in the Framework of the Joint Action on New Synthetic Drugs. Published 2002.

15. Carter LP, Chen W, Wu H, et al. Comparison of the behavioral effects of gamma-hydroxybutyric acid (GHB) and its 4-methyl-substituted analog, gamma-hydroxyvaleric acid (GHV). *Drug Alcohol Depend* 2005;**78**(1):91–99.

16. Bessman SP, Fishbein WN. Gamma-hydroxybutyrate, a normal brain metabolite. *Nature* 1963;**200**:1207–1208.

17. Poldrugo F, Snead OC. 1,4-butanediol and ethanol compete for degradation in rat brain and liver in vitro. *Alcohol* 1986;**3**(6):367–370.

18. Poldrugo F, Snead OC. 1,4-butanediol, gamma-hydroxybutyric acid and ethanol: relationships and interactions. *Neuropharmacology* 1984;**23**(1):109–113.

19. Quang LS, Desai MC, Shannon MW, Woolf AD, Maher TJ. 4-methylpyrazole decreases 1,4-butanediol toxicity by blocking its in vivo biotransformation to gamma-hydroxybutyric acid. *Ann NY Acad Sci* 2004;**1025**:528–537.

20. Carter LP, Chen W, Wu H, et al. Comparison of the behavioral effects of gamma-hydroxybutyric acid (GHB) and its 4-methyl-substituted analog, gamma-hydroxyvaleric acid (GHV). *Drug Alcohol Depend* 2005;**78**(1):91–99.

21. Dijkstra BAG, Kamal R, van Noorden MS, de Haan H, Loonen AJM, De Jong CAJ. Detoxification with titration and tapering in gamma-hydroxybutyrate (GHB) dependent patients: The Dutch GHB monitor project. *Drug Alcohol Depend* (online) 2017:170164–170173. https://doi.org/10.1016/j.drugalcdep.2016.11.014

22. Xu X-M, Wei Y-D, Liu Y, Li Z-X. Gamma-hydroxybutyrate (GHB) for narcolepsy in adults: an updated systematic review and meta-analysis. *Sleep Med* 2019;**64**: 62–70. https://doi.org/10.1016/j.sleep.2019.06.017

23. Craig K, Gomez HF, McManus JL, Bania TC. Severe gamma-hydroxybutyrate withdrawal: a case report and literature review. *J Emerg Med* 2000;**18**:65–70.

24. Nicholson KL, Balster RL. GHB: a new and novel drug of abuse. *Drug Alcohol Depend* 2001;**63**:1–22.

25. Grela A, Gautam L, Cole MD. A multifactorial critical appraisal of substances found in drug-facilitated sexual assault cases. *Forensic Sci Int* 2018;**292**:50–60. https://doi.org/10.1016/j.forsciint.2018.08.034

26. See www.medicinescomplete.com/mc/bnf/current/PHP2146-sodium-oxybate.htm; www.medicines.org.uk/emc/medicine/17364/SPC/Xyrem+500+mg+ml+oral+solution; www.xyrem.com/images/Xyrem_Med_Guide.pdf; as well as the manufacturer's website.

27. Bertol E, Di Milia MG, Fioravanti A, et al. Proactive drugs in DFSA cases: toxicological findings in an eight-years study. *Forensic Sci Int* 2018;**291**:207–215.

28. Busardò FP, Varì MR, Di Trana A, Malaca S, Carlier J, Di Luca NM. Drug-facilitated sexual assaults (DFSA): a serious underestimated issue. *Eur Rev Med Pharmacol Sci* 2019;**23**:10577–10587.

29. Pettigrew M. Somnophilia and sexual abuse through the administration of GHB and GBL. *J Forensic Sci* 2019;**64**(1):302–303. https://doi.org/10.1111/1556-4029.13812

30. Paul A, Mahesan A. Date rape drugs in Las Vegas: detection after the fact. *Obstet Gynecol* 2019;**133**:98S. https://doi.org/10.1097/01.AOG.0000558790.02961.d9

31. Varela M, Nogue S, Oro M. Gamma hydroxybutyrate use for sexual assault. *Miro Emerg Med J* 2004;**21**:255–256. https://doi.org/10.1136/emj.2002.002402

32. Kapitány-Fövény M, Zacher G, Posta J, Demetrovics Z. GHB-involved crimes among intoxicated patients. *Forensic Sci Int* 2017;**275**:23–29. https://doi.org/10.1016/j.forsciint.2017.02.028

33. European Monitoring Centre for Drugs and Drug Addiction (EMCDDA). GHB and Its Precursor GBL: An Emerging Trend Case Study (Thematic Paper). Published 2008. Available at: www.emcdda.europa.eu/system/files/publications/505/TP_GHB_and_GBL_107300.pdf [last accessed 19 February 2022].

34. van Noorden MS, Mol T, Wisselink J, Kuipers W, Dijkstra BAG. Treatment consumption and treatment re-enrollment in GHB-dependent patients in the Netherlands. *Drug Alcohol Depend* 2017;**176**:96–101.

35. Kamal RM, van Noorden MS, Wannet W, Beurmanjer H, Dijkstra BA, Schellekens A. Pharmacological treatment in γ-hydroxybutyrate (GHB) and γ-butyrolactone (GBL) dependence: detoxification and relapse prevention. *CNS Drugs* 2017;**31**(1):51–64.

36. Heliodore C, Malissin I, Megarbane B, Gourlain H, Labat L. Gamma-hydroxybutyrate (GHB) and gamma-butyrolactone (GBL) poisonings admitted to the ICU: features and usefulness of plasma GHB concentration measurement. *Clin Toxicol* 2019;**57**(6);472. Httos://doi.org/10.1080/15563650.2019.1598646

37. European Monitoring Centre for Drugs and Drug Addiction. European Drug Report 2019: Trends and Developments. Publications Office of the European Union, Luxembourg, 2019.

38. European Monitoring Centre for Drugs and Drug Addiction. European Drug Report 2019: Trends and Developments. Publications Office of the European Union, Luxembourg, 2019.

39. Miró Ò, Galicia M, Dargan P, et al. Intoxication by gamma hydroxybutyrate and related analogues: clinical characteristics and comparison between pure intoxication and that combined with other substances of abuse. *Toxicol Lett* 2017;**277**:84–91. https://doi.org/10.1016/j.toxlet.2017.05.030

40. Sumnall H, Woolfalla K, Edward S, Cole J, Beynon C. Use, function, and subjective experiences of gammahydroxybutyrate (GHB). *Drug Alcohol Depend* 2008;**92**(1–3):286–290.

41. Degenhardt L, Darke S, Dillon P. GHB use among Australians: characteristics, use patterns and associated harm. *Drug Alcohol Depend* 2002;**67**(1):89–94.

42. Guasp A. Gay and Bisexual Men's Health Survey. Stonewall 2012.

43. Wood DM, Measham F, Dargan PI. 'Our favourite drug': prevalence of use and preference for mephedrone in the London night-time economy 1 year after control. *J Substance Use* 2012;**17**(2):91–97. https://doi.org/10.3109/14659891 .2012.661025

44. Measham F, Wood DM, Dargan PI, Moore KA. The rise of legal highs: prevalence and patterns in the use of illegal drugs and first- and second-generation 'legal highs' in south London gay dance clubs. *J Substance Use* 2011;**16**(40):263–272.

45. Halkitis PN, Palamar JJ. GHB use among gay and bisexual men. *Addict Behav* 2006;**31**:2135–2139.

46. Giorgetti R, Tagliabracci A, Schifano F, Zaami S, Marinelli E, Busardò FP. When 'chems' meet sex: a rising phenomenon called 'chemsex'. *Curr Neuropharmacol* 2017;**15**(5): 762–770.

47. Hibbert MP, Brett CE, Porcellato LA, Hope VD. Psychosocial and sexual characteristics associated with sexualised drug use and chemsex among men who have sex with men (MSM) in the UK. *Sex Transm Infect* 2019;**95**(5):1368–4973.

48. Trombley TA, Capstick RA, Lindsle CW. DARK classics in chemical neuroscience: gamma-hydroxybutyrate (GHB). *ACS Chem Neurosci* 2019 (online). https://doi.org/10.1021/acsche mneuro.9b00336

49. Hammoud MA, Bourne A, Maher L, et al. Intensive sex partying with gamma-hydroxybutyrate: factors associated with using gamma-hydroxybutyrate for chemsex among Australian gay and bisexual men – results from the Flux Study. *Sex Health* 2018;**15**(2):123–134. https:// doi.org/10.1071/SH17146

50. Joyce N, MacNeela P, Sarma K, Ryall G, Keenan E. The experience and meaning of problematic 'G' (GHB/GBL) use in an Irish context: an interpretative phenomenological analysis. *Int J Ment Health Addict* 2018;**16**:1033–1054. https://doi.org/ 10.1007/s11469-017-9851-y

51. Giorgetti R, Tagliabracci A, Schifano F, Zaami S, Marinelli E, Busardò FP. When chems meet sex: a rising phenomenon called ChemSex. *Curr Neuropharmacol* 2017;**15**(5):762–770.

52. Bell J, Collins R. Gamma-butyrolactone (GBL) dependence and withdrawal. *Addiction* 2011;**106**(2):442–447. https://doi .org/10.1111/j.1360-0443.2010.03145.x

53. Grund J-P, de Bruin D, Van Gallen S. Going knock: recurrent comatose GHB intoxication in the Netherlands. *Int J Drug Policy* 2018;**58**:137–148.

54. Evans R, Sayal K. Gammabutyrolactone: withdrawal syndrome resembling delirium tremens. *J Substance Use* 2012;**17** (4):384–387.

55. Miotto K, Darakjian J, Basch J, Murray S, Zogg J, Rawson R. Gamma-hydroxybutyric acid: patterns of use, effects and withdrawal. *Am J Addict* 2001;**10**(3):232–241.

56. de Jong CA, Kamal R, Dijkstra BA, de Haan HA. Gamma-hydroxybutyrate detoxification by titration and tapering. *Eur Addict Res* 2012;**18**(1):40–45. https://doi.org/10.1159 /000333022

57. Herold AH, Sneed KB. Treatment of a young adult taking gamma-butyrolactone (GBL) in a primary care clinic. *J Am Board Fam Pract* 2002;**15**(2):161–163.

58. Drug Enforcement Agency.

59. Couper FJ, Marinetti LJ. Gamma-hydroxybutyrate (GHB) – effects on human performance and behavior. *Forensic Sci Rev* 2002;**14**(1):101–121.

60. McDonough M, Kennedy N, Glasper A, Bearn J. Clinical features and management of gamma- hydroxybutyrate (GHB) withdrawal: a review. *Drug Alcohol Depend* 2004; **75**:3–9.

61. Chew G, Fernando A. Epileptic seizure in GHB withdrawal. *Australas Psychiatry* 2004;**12**:410–411.

62. Sivilotti MLA, Burns MJ, Aaron CK, Greenberg MJ. Pentobarbital for severe gamma-butyrolactone withdrawal. *Ann Emerg Med* 2001;**38**:660–665.

63. Kam P, Yoong F. Gamma-hydroxybutyric acid: an emerging recreational drug. *Anaesthesia* 1998;**53**:1195–1198.

64. Abanades S, Farré M, Barral D, Torrens M, Closas N, Langohr K, et al. Relative abuse liability of [gamma]-hydroxybutyric acid, flunitrazepam, and ethanol in club drug users. *J Clin Psychopharmacol* 2007;**27** (6):625–638.

65. Galicia M, Nogue S, Miro O. Liquid ecstasy intoxication: clinical features of 505 consecutive emergency department patients. *Emerg Med J* 2011;**28**(6):462–466. https://doi.org/10 .1136/emj.2008.068403

66. Luby S, Jones J, Zalewski A. GHB use in South Carolina. *Am J Public Health* 1992;**82**(1):128.

67. Henderson DL, Ginsberg JP. Withdrawal, recovery, and long-term sequelae of gamma- butyrolactone dependence: a case report. *Am J Addict* 2008;**17**(5):456–457. https://doi.org /10.1080/10550490802266193

68. Zvosec DL, Smith SW. Agitation is common in gamma-hydroxybutyrate toxicity. *Am J Emerg Med* 2005;**23** (3):316–320.

69. Oliveto A, Gentry WB, Pruzinsky R, et al. Behavioral effects of gamma-hydroxybutyrate in humans. *Behav Pharmacol* 2010;**21**(4):332–342. https://doi.org/10.1097/ FBP.0b013e32833b3397

70. Stein LA, Lebeau R, Clair M, et al. A web-based study of gamma hydroxybutyrate (GHB): patterns, experiences, and functions of use. *Am J Addict* 2011;**20**(1):30–39. https://doi.org /10.1111/j.1521-0391.2010.00099.x

71. Kapitány-Fövény M, Mervó B, Corazza O, et al. Enhancing sexual desire and experience: an investigation of the sexual correlates of gamma-hydroxybutyrate (GHB). *Hum Psychopharmacol Clin Exp* 2015;**30**:276–284. https://doi.org/1 0.1002/hup.2491

72. Bourne A, Reid D, Hickson F, Torres-Rueda S, Weatherburn P. Illicit drug use in sexual settings ('chemsex') and HIV/STI transmission risk behaviour among gay men in South London: findings from a qualitative study. *Sex Transm Infect* (online). https://doi.org/10.1136/sextrans-2015-052052

73. Daskalopoulou M, Rodger A, Thornton A, et al. Sexual behaviour, recreational drug use and hepatitis C

co-infection in HIV-diagnosed men who have sex with men in the United Kingdom: results from the ASTRA study. *J Int AIDS Soc* 2014b;**17**(4 Suppl. 3). https://doi.org /10.7448/IAS.17.4.19630

74. Colfax GN, Mansergh G, Guzman R, et al. Drug use and sexual risk behaviour among gay and bisexual men who attend circuit parties: a venue-based comparison. *J Acquir Immune Defic Syndr* 2001;**28**(4):373–379.

75. Mattison AM, Ross MW, Wolfson T, Franklin D, San Diego HIV Neurobehavioral Research Center Group. Circuit party attendance, club drug use and unsafe sex in gay men. *J Subst Abuse* 2001;**13**(1–2):119–126.

76. Keogh P, Reid D, Bourne A, et al. Wasted Opportunities: Problematic Alcohol and Drug Use Among Gay Men and Bisexual Men. Sigma Research, 2009. Available at: http://sig maresearch.org.uk/files/report2009c.pdf [last accessed 19 February 2022].

77. Hammoud MA, Bourne A, Maher L, et al. Intensive sex partying with gamma-hydroxybutyrate: factors associated with using gamma-hydroxybutyrate for chemsex among Australian gay and bisexual men – results from the Flux Study. *Sex Health* 2018;**15**(2):123–134. https:// doi.org/10.1071/ SH17146

78. Bourne A, Ong J, Pakianathan M. Sharing solutions for a reasoned and evidence-based response: chemsex/party and play among gay and bisexual men. *Sex Health* 2018;**15**:99–101. https://doi.org/10.1071/SH18023

79. O'Reilly M. Chemsex case study: is it time to recommend routine screening of sexualised drug use in men who have sex with men? *Sex Health* 2018;**15**(2):167–169. https://doi.org/10 .1071/SH17156

80. Bourne A, Reid D, Hickson F, Torres-Rueda S, Weatherburn P. Illicit drug use in sexual settings ('chemsex') and HIV/STI transmission risk behaviour among gay men in South London: findings from a qualitative study. *Sex Transm Infect* 2015;**91**(8):564–568.

81. Advisory Council on the Misuse of Drugs: An assessment of the harms of gamma-hydroxybutyric acid (GHB), gamma-butyrolactone (GBL), and closely related compounds. Published 2020.

82. Schep LJ, Knudsen K, Slaughter RJ, Vale JA, Mégarbane B. The clinical toxicology of γ-hydroxybutyrate, γ-butyrolactone and 1,4-butanediol. *Clin Toxicol* 2012;**50**(6):458–470. https:// doi .org/10.3109/15563650.2012.702218

83. Caldicott DG, Chow FY, Burns BJ, Felgate PD, Byard RW. Fatalities associated with the use of gamma-hydroxybutyrate and its analogues in Australasia. *Med J Aust* 2004;**181**:310–313.

84. Couper FJ, Thatcher JE, Logan BK. Suspected GHB overdoses in the emergency department. *J Anal Toxicol* 2004;**28**:481–484.

85. Corkery JM, Loi B, Claridge H, et al. Gamma hydroxybutyrate (GHB), gamma butyrolactone (GBL) and 1,4 butanediol (1,4-BD; BDO): a literature review with a focus on UK fatalities related to non-medical use. *Neurosci Biobehav Rev* 2015 (online). http://dx.doi.org/10.1016/j.neubiorev.2015.03.012

86. Küting T, Krämer M, Bicker W, Madea B, Hess C. Case report: another death associated to γ-hydroxybutyric acid intoxication. *Forensic Sci Int* 2019;**299**:34–40.

87. Corkery JM, Loi B, Claridge H, et al. Gamma hydroxybutyrate (GHB), gamma butyrolactone (GBL) and 1,4 butanediol (1,4-BD; BDO): a literature review with a focus on UK fatalities related to non-medical use. *Neurosci Biobehav Rev* (online) 2015. https://doi.org/10.1016/j .neubiorev.2015.03.012

88. National Programme on Substance Abuse Deaths (NPSAD). Drug-Related Deaths Reported by Coroners in England, Wales, Northern Ireland, Guernsey, Jersey and the Isle of Man; Police Forces in Scotland; and the Northern Ireland Statistics and Research Agency Annual Report 2013 on Deaths Between January–December 2012.

89. Darke S, Peacock A, Duflou J, Farrell M, Lappin J. Characteristics and circumstances of death related to gamma hydroxybutyrate (GHB). *Clin Toxicol* 2020 (online). https:// doi.org/ 10.1080/15563650.2020.1726378

90. Hockenhulla J, Murphy KG, Paterson S. An observed rise in g-hydroxybutyrate-associated deaths in London: evidence to suggest a possible link with concomitant rise in chemsex. *Forensic Sci Int* 2017;**270**:93–97.

91. Corkery JM, Loi B, Claridge H, Goodair C, Schifano F. Deaths in the lesbian, gay, bisexual and transgender United Kingdom communities associated with GHB and precursors. *Curr Drug Metab* 2017 (online). https://doi.org/10.2174 /1389200218666171108163817

92. Chin RL, Sporer KA, Cullison B, Dyer JE, Wu TD. Clinical course of gamma-hydroxybutyrate overdose. *Ann Emerg Med* 1998;**31**(6):716–722.

93. Miróa O, Galiciaa M, Darganb P, et al. Euro-DEN Research Group: Intoxication by gamma hydroxybutyrate and related analogues: clinical characteristics and comparison between pure intoxication and that combined with other substances of abuse. *Toxicol Lett* 2017;**277**(5):84–91. https://doi.org/10.1016 /j.toxlet.2017.05.030

94. Morse BL, Chadha GS, Felmlee MA, Follman KE, Morris ME. Effect of chronic γ-hydroxybutyrate (GHB) administration on GHB toxicokinetics and GHB-induced respiratory depression. *Am J Drug Alcohol Abuse* 2017;**43**(6):686–693. https://doi.org/10.1080/00952990 .2017.1339055

95. Gable RS. Acute toxic effects of club drugs. *J Psychoactive Drugs* 2004;**36**(3):303–313.

96. Snead OC, Gibson KM. Gamma-hydroxybutyric acid. *N Engl J Med* 2005;**352**(26):2721–2732.

97. Li J, Stokes SA, Woeckener A. A tale of novel intoxication: a review of the effects of gamma-hydroxybutyric acid with recommendations for management. *Ann Emerg Med* 1998;**31**:729–736.

98. Centers for Disease Control (CDC). Multistate outbreak of poisonings associated with illicit use of gamma hydroxy butyrate. *Morb Mortal Wkly Rep* 1990;**39**:861–863.

99. Vickers MD. Gamma-hydroxybutyric acid. *Int Anesthesiol Clin* 1969;7:75–89.

100. Galloway GP, Frederick SL, Staggers FE, et al. Gamma-hydroxybutyrate: an emerging drug of abuse that causes physical dependence. *Addiction* 1997;**92**:89–96.

101. Grund JP, de Bruin D, van Gaalen S. Going knock: recurrent comatose GHB intoxication in the Netherlands. *Int J Drug Policy* 2018;**58**:137–148. https://doi.org/10.1016/j.drugpo.2018.06.010

102. Madah-Amiri D, Myrmel L, Battebø G. Intoxication with GHB/GBL: characteristics and trends from ambulance-attended overdoses. *Scand J Trauma Resusc Emerg Med* 2017;**25**:98. https://doi.org/10.1186/s13049-017-0441-6

103. Schep LJ, Knudsen K, Slaughter RJ, Vale JA, Mégarbane B. The clinical toxicology of gamma-hydroxybutyrate, gamma-butyrolactone and 1,4-butanediol. *Clin Toxicol (Phila)* 2012;**50**:458–470.

104. Korf DJ, Nabben T, Benschop A, Ribbink K, Van Amsterdam JGC. Risk factors of γ-hydroxybutyrate overdosing. *Eur Addict Res* 2014;**20**:66–74.

105. Liechti ME, Kunz I, Greminger P, Speich R, Kupferschmidt H. Clinical features of gamma-hydroxybutyrate and gamma-butyrolactone toxicity and concomitant drug and alcohol use. *Drug Alcohol Depend* 2006;**81**:323–326.

106. Miró Ò, Galicia M, Dargan P, et al. Intoxication by gamma hydroxybutyrate and related analogues: clinical characteristics and comparison between pure intoxication and that combined with other substances of abuse. *Toxicol Lett* 2017;**277**:84–91.

107. Van Amsterdam JGC, Brunt TM, McMaster MTB, Niesink RJM. Possible long-term effects of γ-hydroxybutyric acid (GHB) due to neurotoxicity and overdose. *Neurosci Biobehav Rev* 2012;**36**:1217–1227.

108. Kapitány-Fövény M, Mervó B, Corazza O, et al. Enhancing sexual desire and experience: an investigation of the sexual correlates of gamma-hydroxybutyrate (GHB) use. *Hum Psychopharmacol Clin Exp* 2015;**30**:276–284. https://doi.org/10.1002/hup.2491

109. Lopez Nunez OF, Rymer JA, Tamama K, Case of sudden acute coma followed by spontaneous recovery. *J Appl Lab Med* 2018;**3**(3):507–510. https://doi.org/10.1373/jalm.2017.025718

110. Korf DJ, Nabben T, Benschop A, Ribbink K, Van Amsterdam JGC. Risk factors of γ-hydroxybutyrate overdosing. *Eur Addict Res* 2014;**20**:66–74.

111. Liechti ME, Kunz I, Greminger P, Speich R, Kupferschmidt H. Clinical features of gamma-hydroxybutyrate and gamma-butyrolactone toxicity and concomitant drug and alcohol use. *Drug Alcohol Depend* 2006;**81**:323–326.

112. Miró Ò, Galicia M, Dargan P, et al. Intoxication by gamma-hydroxybutyrate and related analogues: clinical characteristics and comparison between pure intoxication and that combined with other substances of abuse. *Toxicol Lett* 2017;**277**:84–91.

113. Miró O, Nogué S, Espinosa G, To-Figueras J, Sánchez M. Trends in illicit drug emergencies: the emerging role of gamma-hydroxybutyrate. *J Toxicol Clin Toxicol* 2002;**40**(2):129–135.

114. Louagie HK, Verstraete AG, DeSoete CJ, Baetens DG, Calle PA. A sudden awakening from a near coma after combined intake of gamma-hydroxybutyric acid (GHB) and ethanol. *J Toxicol Clin Toxicol* 1997;**35**:591–594.

115. Ingels M, Rangan C, Bellezzo J, Clark RF. Coma and respiratory depression following the ingestion of GHB and its precursors: three cases. *J Emerg Med* 2000;**9**(1):47–50.

116. Munir VL, Hutton JE, Harney JP, Buykx P, Weiland TJ, Dent AW. Gamma-hydroxybutyrate: a 30-month emergency department review. *Emerg Med Australas* 2008;**20**(6):521–530. https://doi.org/10.1111/j.1742-6723.2008.01140.x

117. Van Sassenbroeck DK, De Neve N, De Paepe P, Belpaire FM, Verstraete AG, Calle PA, et al. Abrupt awakening phenomenon associated with gamma-hydroxybutyrate use: a case series. *Clin Toxicol* 2007;**45**:533–538.

118. Liakoni E, Walther F, Nickel CH, Liechti ME. Presentations to an urban emergency department in Switzerland due to acute γ-hydroxybutyrate toxicity. *Scand J Trauma Resusc Emerg Med* 2016;**24**:107. https://doi.org/10.1186/s13049-016-0299-z

119. Madah-Amiri D, Myrmel L, Battebø G. Intoxication with GHB/GBL: characteristics and trends from ambulance-attended overdoses. *Scand J Trauma Resusc Emerg Med* 2017;**25**:98. https://doi.org/10.1186/s13049-017-0441-6

120. Madah-Amiri D, Clausen T, Myrmel L, Battebø G, Lobmaier P. Circumstances surrounding non-fatal opioid overdoses attended by ambulance services. *Drug Alcohol Rev* 2017;**36**:288–294.

121. Carlier L, Van Belleghem V, Croes K, Hooft F. Gamma-hydroxybutyrate (GHB), an unusual cause of high anion gap metabolic acidosis. *Can J Emerg Med* 2018;**20**(S2):S2–S5.

122. Stefani M, Roberts DM. 1,4-Butanediol overdose mimicking toxic alcohol exposure. *Clin Toxicol* 2020;**58**(3):204–207. https://doi.org/10.1080/15563650.2019.1617419

123. Wood DM, Warren-Gash C, Ashraf T, et al. Medical and legal confusion surrounding gamma-hydroxybutyrate (GHB) and its precursors gamma-butyrolactone (GBL) and 1,4-butanediol (1,4BD). *QJM* 2008;**101**:23–29.

124. Rambourg-Schepens MO, Buffet M, Durak C, Mathieu-Nolf M. Gamma-butyrolactone poisoning and its similarities to gamma-hydroxybutyric acid: two case reports. *Vet Hum Toxicol* 1997;**39**(4):234–235.

125. Knudsen K, Greter J, Verdicchio M. High mortality rates among GHB abusers in Western Sweden. *Clin Toxicol* 2008;**46**:187–192.

126. Liechti ME, Kunz I, Greminger P, Speich R, Kupferschmidt H. Clinical features of gamma-hydroxy-butyrate and gamma-butyrolactone toxicity and concomitant drug and alcohol use. *Drug Alcohol Depend* 2006;**81**:323–326.

127. Dietze PM, Cvetkovski S, Barratt MJ, Clemens S. Patterns and incidence of gamma-hydroxybutyrate (GHB)-related

ambulance attendances in Melbourne, Victoria. *Med J Aust* 2008;**188**:709–711.

128. Theron L, Jansen K, Skinner A. New Zealand's first fatality linked to use of 1,4-butanediol (1,4-B, Fantasy): no evidence of coingestion or comorbidity. *N Z Med J* 2003;**116**:U650.

129. Couper FJ, Thatcher JE, Logan BK. Suspected GHB overdoses in the emergency department. *J Anal Toxicol* 2004;**28**:481–484.

130. Roberts DM, Smith MW, Gopalakrishnan M, Whittaker G, Day RO. Extreme gamma-butyrolactone overdose with severe metabolic acidosis requiring hemodialysis. *Ann Emerg Med* 2011;**58**:83–85.

131. Anderson IB, Kim SY, Dyer JE, et al. Trends in gamma-hydroxybutyrate (GHB) and related drug intoxication: 1999 to 2003. *Ann Emerg Med* 2006;**47**:177–183.

132. Ryan JM, Stell I. Gamma hydroxybutyrate: a coma inducing recreational drug. *J Accid Emerg Med* 1997;**14**:259–291.

133. Centers for Disease Control and Prevention (CDC). Gamma hydroxy butyrate use – New York and Texas, 1995–1996. *Morb Mortal Wkly Rep* 1997;**46**:281–283.

134. Schneidereit T, Burkhart K, Donovan JW. Butanediol toxicity delayed by preingestion of ethanol. *Int J Med Toxicol* 2000;**3**:1.

135. Zvosec DL, Smith SW, McCutcheon JR, Spillane J, Hall BJ, Peacock EA. Adverse events, including death, associated with the use of 1,4-butanediol. *N Engl J Med* 2001;**344**:87–94.

136. Centers for Disease Control and Prevention (CDC). Adverse events associated with ingestion of gamma-butyrolactone – Minnesota, New Mexico, and Texas, 1998–1999. *Morb Mortal Wkly Rep* 1999;**48**:137–140.

137. Stephens BG, Baselt RC. Driving under the influence of GHB? *J Anal Toxicol* 1994;**18**:357–358.

138. Al-Samarraie MS, Karinen R, Morland J, Opdal MS. Blood GHB concentrations and results of medical examinations in 25 car drivers in Norway. *Eur J Clin Pharmacol* 2010;**66**:987–998.

139. Ross TM. Gamma hydroxybutyrate overdose: two cases illustrate the unique aspects of this dangerous recreational drug. *J Emerg Nurs* 1995;**21**:374–376.

140. Ortmann LA, Jaeger MW, James LP, Schexnayder SM. Coma in a 20-month-old child from an ingestion of a toy containing 1,4-butanediol, a precursor of gamma-hydroxybutyrate. *Pediatr Emerg Care* 2009;**25**:758–760.

141. Price PA, Schachter M, Smith S, Baxter RC, Parkes JD. Gamma-hydroxybutyrate in narcolepsy. *Ann Neurol* 1981;**9**:198.

142. Couper FJ, Logan BK. Determination of gamma-hydroxybutyrate (GHB) in biological specimens by gas chromatography–mass spectrometry. *J Anal Toxicol* 2000;**24**:1–7.

143. Eckstein M, Henderson SO, DelaCruz P, Newton E. Gamma hydroxybutyrate (GHB): report of a mass intoxication and review of the literature. *Prehosp Emerg Care* 1999;**3**:357–361.

144. Bosman IJ, Lusthof KJ. Forensic cases involving the use of GHB in the Netherlands. *Forensic Sci Int* 2003;**133**:17–21.

145. Mégarbane B, Fompeydie D, Garnier R, Baud FJ. Treatment of a 4-butanediol poisoning with fomepizole. *J Toxicol Clin Toxicol* 2002;**40**:77–80.

146. Piastra M, Tempera A, Caresta E, et al. Lung injury from 'liquid ecstasy': a role for coagulation activation? *Pediatr Emerg Care* 2006;**22**:358–360.

147. Gunja N, Doyle E, Carpenter K, et al. Gamma-hydroxybutyrate poisoning from toy beads. *Med J Aust* 2008;**188**:54–55.

148. Hefele B, Naumann N, Trollmann R, Dittrich K, Rascher W. Fast-in, fast-out. *Lancet* 2009;**373**:1398.

149. Ragg M. Gamma hydroxy butyrate overdose. *Emerg Med* 1997;**9**:29–31.

150. Williams H, Taylor R, Roberts M. Gamma-hydroxybutyrate (GHB): a new drug of misuse. *Ir Med J* 1998;**91**:56–57.

151. Dyer JE. Gamma-hydroxybutyrate: a health-food product producing coma and seizure-like activity. *Am J Emerg Med* 1991;**9**:321–324.

152. Chin MY, Kreutzer RA, Dyer JE. Acute poisoning from gamma-hydroxybutyrate in California. *West J Med* 1992;**156**:380–384.

153. Viswanathan S, Chen C, Kolecki P. Revivarant (gamma-butyrolactone) poisoning. *Am J Emerg Med* 2000;**18**:358–359.

154. Osterhoudt KC, Henretig FM. Comatose teenagers at a party: what a tangled 'Web' we weave. *Pediatr Case Rev* 2003;**3**:171–173.

155. Shannon M, Quang LS. Gamma-hydroxybutyrate, gamma-butyrolactone, and 1,4-butanediol: a case report and review of the literature. *Pediatr Emerg Care* 2000;**16**:435–440.

156. Caldicott DG, Kuhn M. Gamma-hydroxybutyrate overdose and physostigmine: teaching new tricks to an old drug? *Ann Emerg Med* 2001;**37**:99–102.

157. Runnacles JL, Stroobant J. Gamma-hydroxybutyrate poisoning: poisoning from toy beads. *BMJ* 2008;**336**:110.

158. Yates SW, Viera AJ. Physostigmine in the treatment of gamma-hydroxybutyric acid overdose. *Mayo Clin Proc* 2000;**75**:401–402.

159. Libetta C. Gamma hydroxybutyrate poisoning. *J Accid Emerg Med* 1997;**14**:411.

160. Savage T, Khan A, Loftus BG. Acetone-free nail polish remover pads: toxicity in a 9-month-old. *Arch Dis Child* 2007;**92**:371.

161. Robert R, Eugène M, Frat JP, Rouffineau J. Diagnosis of unsuspected gamma hydroxy-butyrate poisoning by proton NMR. *J Toxicol Clin Toxicol* 2001;**39**:653–654.

162. Winickoff JP, Houck CS, Rothman EL, Bauchner H. Verve and jolt: deadly new Internet drugs. *Pediatrics* 2000;**106**:829–831.

163. Lenz D, Rothschild MA, Kroner L. Intoxications due to ingestion of gamma-butyrolactone: organ distribution of gamma-hydroxybutyric acid and gamma-butyrolactone. *Ther Drug Monit* 2008;**30**:755–761.

164. Lora-Tamayo C, Tena T, Rodriguez A, Sancho JR, Molina E. Intoxication due to 1,4-butanediol. *Forensic Sci Int* 2003;**133**:256–259.

165. Higgins TFJ, Borron SW. Coma and respiratory arrest after exposure to butyrolactone. *J Emerg Med* 1996;**14**:435–457.

166. Yambo CM, McFee RB, Caraccio TR, McGuigan M. The inkjet cleaner 'Hurricane' – another GHB recipe. *Vet Hum Toxicol* 2004;**46**:329–330.

167. Suner S, Szlatenyi CS, Wang RY. Pediatric gamma hydroxybutyrate intoxication. *Acad Emerg Med* 1997;**4**:1041–1045.

168. Krul J, Girbes AR. Gamma-hydroxybutyrate: experience of 9 years of gamma-hydroxybutyrate (GHB)-related incidents during rave parties in the Netherlands. *Clin Toxicol* 2011;**49**:311–315.

169. Elliott S. Nonfatal instances of intoxication with gamma-hydroxybutyrate in the United Kingdom. *Ther Drug Monit* 2004;**26**:432–440.

170. Tancredi DN, Shannon MW. Case records of the Massachusetts General Hospital. Weekly clinico-pathological exercises. Case 30-2003. A 21-year-old man with sudden alteration of mental status. *N Engl J Med* 2003;**349**:1267–1275.

171. Cisek J. Seizure associated with butanediol ingestion. *Int J Med Toxicol* 2001;**4**:12.

172. Harraway T, Stephenson L. Gamma hydroxybutyrate intoxication: the Gold Coast experience. *Emerg Med* 1999;**11**:45–48.

173. Hardy CJ, Slifman NR, Klontz KC, Dyer JE, Coody GL, Love LA. Adverse events reported with the use of gamma butyrolactone products marketed as dietary supplements. *Clin Toxicol* 1999;**37**:649–650.

174. Mahon KD, Tomaszewski CA, Tayal VS. Emergency department presentation of serum confirmed GHB ingestions. *Acad Emerg Med* 1999;**6**:395–396.

175. Vickers MD. Gamma hydroxybutyric acid. *Proc R Soc Med* 1968;**61**:821–824.

176. Geldenhuys FG, Sonnendecker EW, De Kirk MC. Experience with sodium-gamma-4-hydroxybutyric acid (gamma-OH) in obstetrics. *J Obstet Gynaecol Br Commonw* 1968;**75**(4):405–413.

177. Tunstall ME. Gamma-OH in anesthesia for caesarean section. *Proc R Soc Med* 1968;**61**:827–830.

178. Laborit H. Soduim 4-hydroxybutyrate. *Int J Neuropharmacol* 1964;**3**:433–445.

179. Piastra M, Barbaro R, Chiaretti A, Tempera A, Pulitanò S, Polidori G. Pulmonary oedema caused by 'liquid ecstasy' ingestion. *Arch Dis Child* 2002;**86**:302–303.

180. Jones C. Suspicious death related to gamma-hydroxybutyrate (GHB) toxicity. *J Clin Forensic Med* 2001;**8**:74–76.

181. Doyon S. The many faces of ecstasy. *Curr Opin Pediatr* 2001;**13**(6):170–176.

182. Bamonte G, de Hoog J, Van Den Biesen PR. A case of central serous chorioretinopathy occurring after γ-hydroxybutyric acid (liquid ecstasy) ingestion. *Retin Cases Brief Rep* 2013;**7**(4):313–314. https://doi.org/10.1097/ICB.0b013e31828ef073

183. Garrison G, Mueller P. Clinical features and outcomes after unintentional gamma hydroxybutyrate (GHB) overdose. *J Toxicol Clin Toxicol* 1998;**35**:503–504.

184. Wood DM, Brailsford AD, Dargan PI. Acute toxicity and withdrawal syndromes related to gamma-hydroxybutyrate (GHB) and its analogues gamma-butyrolactone (GBL) and 1,4-butanediol (1,4-BD). *Drug Test Anal* 2011;**3**(7–8):417–425. https://doi.org/10.1002/dta.292

185. Entholzner E, Mielke L, Pichlmeier R, Weber F, Schneck H. EEG changes during sedation with gamma-hydroxybutyric acid. *Anaesthesist* 1995;**44**:345–350.

186. Okun MS, Boothby LA, Bartfield RB, Doering PL. GHB: an important pharmacological and clinical update. *J Pharm Pharm Sci* 2001;**4**(2):167–175.

187. Thai D, Dyer JE, Benowitz NL, Haller CA. Gamma-hydroxybutyrate and ethanol effects and interactions in humans. *J Clin Psychopharmacol* 2006;**26**(5):524–529.

188. Department of Health. A Summary of the Health Harms of Drugs. Published August 2011.

189. Hammoud MA, Bourne A, Maher L, et al. Intensive sex partying with gamma-hydroxybutyrate: factors associated with using gamma-hydroxybutyrate for chemsex among Australian gay and bisexual men – results from the Flux Study. *Sex Health* 2018;**15**(2):123–134. https://doi.org/10.1071/SH17146

190. Lettieri J, Fung HL. Absorption and first-pass metabolism of 14C-gamma-hydroxybutyric acid. *Res Commun Chem Pathol Pharmacol* 1976;**13**:425–437.

191. Harrington RD, Woodward JA, Hooton TM, Horn JR. Life-threatening interactions between HIV-1 protease inhibitors and the illicit drugs MDMA and gamma-hydroxybutyrate. *Arch Intern Med* 1999;**159**(18):2221–2224.

192. Harrington RD, Woodward JA, Hooton TM, Horn JR. Life-threatening interactions between HIV-1 protease inhibitors and the illicit drugs MDMA and gamma-hydroxybutyrate. *Arch Intern Med* 1999;**159**(18):2221–2224.

193. Romanelli F, Smith KM, Pomeroy C. Use of club drugs by HIV-seropositive and HIV-seronegative gay and bisexual men. *Top HIV Med* 2003;**11**(1):25–32.

194. Staltari O, Leporini C, Caroleo B, et al. Drug-drug interactions: antiretroviral drugs and recreational drugs. *Recent Pat CNS Drug Discov* 2014;**9**:153–163.

195. Psichogiou M, Poulakou G, Basoulis D, Paraskevis D, Markogiannakis A, Daikos GL. Recent advances in antiretroviral agents: potent integrase inhibitors. *Curr Pharmaceut Des* 2017;**23**:1–16.

196. Drogies T, Willenberg A, Ramshorn-Zimmer A, et al. Detection of gamma hydroxybutyrate in emergency

department: nice to have or a valuable diagnostic tool? *Hum Exp Toxicol* 2015;**35**(7):1–8.

197. Busardò FP, Jones AW. GHB pharmacology and toxicology: acute intoxication, concentrations in blood and urine in forensic cases and treatment of the withdrawal syndrome. *Curr Neuropharmacol* 2015;**13**(1):47–70.

198. LeTourneau JL, Hagg DS, Smith SM. Baclofen and gamma-hydroxybutyrate withdrawal. *Neurocrit Care* 2008;**8**(3):430–433. https://doi.org/10.1007/s12028-008-9062-2

199. LeTourneau JL, Hagg DS, Smith SM. Baclofen and gamma-hydroxybutyrate withdrawal. *Neurocrit Care* 2008;**8**(3):430–433.

200. Mason PE, Kerns WP. Gamma hydroxybutyric acid (GHB) intoxication. *Acad Emerg Med* 2002;**9**(7):730–739.

201. Busardò FP, Jones AW. GHB pharmacology and toxicology: acute intoxication, concentrations in blood and urine in forensic cases and treatment of the withdrawal syndrome. *Curr Neuropharmacol* 2015;**13**(1):47–70.

202. Thomas G, Bonner S, Gascoigne A. Coma induced by abuse of gamma-hydroxybutyrate (GHB or liquid ecstasy): a case report. *BMJ* 1997;**314**:35–36.

203. Busardò FP, Jones AW. GHB pharmacology and toxicology: acute intoxication, concentrations in blood and urine in forensic cases and treatment of the withdrawal syndrome. *Curr Neuropharmacol* 2015;**13**(1)47–70.

204. Liechti ME, Kupferschmidt H. Gamma-hydroxybutyrate (GHB) and gamma-butyrolactone (GBL): analysis of overdose cases reported to the Swiss Toxicological Information Centre. *Swiss Med Wkly* 2004;**134**:534–537.

205. TOXBASE www.toxbase.org [accessed 3 February 2020].

206. TOXBASE www.toxbase.org [accessed 3 February 2020].

207. Busardò FP, Jones AW. GHB pharmacology and toxicology: acute intoxication, concentrations in blood and urine in forensic cases and treatment of the withdrawal syndrome. *Curr Neuropharmacol* 2015;**13**(1):47–70.

208. TOXBASE www.toxbase.org [accessed 3 February 2020].

209. Follman KE, Morris M. Treatment of gamma-hydroxybutyric acid and gamma-butyrolactone overdose with two potent monocarboxylate transporter 1 inhibitors, AZD3965 and AR-C155858. *J Pharmacol Exp Ther* 2019;**370**(1):84–91. https://doi.org/10.1124/jpet.119.256503

210. Lopez Nunez OF, Rymer JA, Tamama K. Case of sudden acute coma followed by spontaneous recovery. *J Appl Lab Med* 2018;**3**(3):507–510.

211. Reeves J, Duda R. GHB/GBL intoxication and withdrawal: a review and case presentation. *Addict Disord Treatment* 2003;**2**:25–28.

212. van Noordena MS, Mol T, Wisselink J, Kuijpers W, Boukje AG. Dijkstra Treatment consumption and treatment re-enrollment in GHB-dependent patients in the Netherlands. *Drug Alcohol Depend* 2017;**176**:96–101.

213. Dyer JE, Roth B, Hyma BA. Gamma-hydroxybutyrate withdrawal syndrome. *Ann Emerg Med* 2001;**37**:147–153.

214. Galloway GP, Frederick SL, Staggers F. Physical dependence on sodium oxybate. *Lancet* 1994;**343**:57.

215. Wojtowicz JM, Yarema MC, Wax PM. Withdrawal from gamma-hydroxybutyrate, 1,4-butanediol and gamma-butyrolactone: a case report and systematic review. *CJEM* 2008;**10**(1):69–74.

216. Kamal RM, van Noorden MS, Wannet W, Beurmanjer H, Dijkstra BAG, Schellekens A. Pharmacological treatment in c-hydroxybutyrate (GHB) and c-butyrolactone (GBL) dependence: detoxification and relapse prevention. *CNS Drugs* 2017;**31**:51–64. https://doi.org/10.1007/s40263-016-0402-z

217. Kamal RM, van Noorden MS, Wannet W, Beurmanjer H, Dijkstra BAG, Schellekens A. Pharmacological treatment in c-hydroxybutyrate (GHB) and c-butyrolactone (GBL) dependence: detoxification and relapse prevention. *CNS Drugs* 2017;**31**:51–64. https://doi.org/10.1007/s40263-016-0402-z

218. Wojtowicz J. Withdrawal from gamma-hydroxybutyrate,1,4-butanediol and gamma-butyrolactone: a case report and systematic review. *CJEM* 2008;**10**(1):69–74.

219. Mahr G, Bishop CL, Orringer DJ. Prolonged withdrawal from extreme gamma-hydroxybutyrate (GHB) abuse. *Psychosomatics* 2001;**42**(5):439–440.

220. Kamal RM, van Noorden MS, Wannet W, et al. Pharmacological treatment in c-hydroxybutyrate (GHB) and c-butyrolactone (GBL) dependence: detoxification and relapse prevention. *CNS Drugs* 2017;**31**:51–64. https://doi.org/10.1007/s40263-016-0402-z

221. Wood DM, Dargan PI. Development of a protocol for the management of acute gamma-hydroxy- butyrate (GHB) and gamma-butyrolactone (GBL) withdrawal. *Clin Toxicol* 2010;**48**:306.

222. Glasper A, McDonough M, Bearn J. Within-patient variability in clinical presentation of gamma- hydroxybutyrate withdrawal: a case report. *Eur Addict Res* 2005;**11**(3):152–154.

223. Kamal RM, van Noorden MS, Wannet W, Beurmanjer H, Dijkstra BAG, Schellekens A. Pharmacological treatment in c-hydroxybutyrate (GHB) and c-butyrolactone (GBL) dependence: detoxification and relapse prevention. *CNS Drugs* 2017;**31**:51–64. https://doi.org/10.1007/s40263-016-0402-z

224. Snead OC. Gamma-hydroxybutyrate. *Life Sci* 1977;**20**:1935–1944.

225. van Noorden MS, van Dongen L, Zitman FG, Vergouwen T. Gamma-hydroxybutyrate withdrawal syndrome: dangerous but not well-known. *Gen Hosp Psychiatry* 2009;**31**:394–396.

226. Miglani JS, Kim KY, Chahil R. Gamma-hydroxy butyrate withdrawal delirium: a case report. *Gen Hosp Psychiatry* 2000;**22**:213–215.

227. Hutto B, Fairchild A, Bright R. Gamma-hydroxybutyrate withdrawal and chloral hydrate. *Am J Psychiatry* 2000;**157**:1706.

228. Hernandez M, McDaniel CH, Costanza CD, Hernandez OJ. GHB-induced delirium: a case report and review of the

literature of gamma hydroxybutyric acid. *Am J Drug Alcohol Abuse* 1998;**24**:179–183.

229. Catalano MC, Glass JM, Catalano G, Burrows S, Lynn W, Weitzner BS. Gamma butyrolactone (GBL) withdrawal syndromes. *Psychosomatics* 2001;**42**:83–88.

230. Bowles TM, Sommi RW, Amiri M. Successful management of prolonged gamma-hydroxybutyrate and alcohol withdrawal. *Pharmacotherapy* 2001;**21**:254–257.

231. Mahr G, Bishop CL, Orringer DJ. Prolonged withdrawal from extreme gamma-hydroxybutyrate (GHB) abuse. *Psychosomatics* 2001;**42**:439–440.

232. McDaniel CH, Miotto KA. Gamma hydroxybutyrate (GHB) and gamma butyrolactone (GBL) withdrawal: five case studies. *J Psychoactive Drugs* 2001;**33**:143–149.

233. Schneir AB, Ly HT, Clark RF. A case of withdrawal from the GHB precursors gamma-butyrolactone and 1,4-butanediol. *J Emerg Med* 2001;**21**:31–33.

234. Perez E, Chu J, Bania T. Seven days of gamma-hydroxybutyrate (GHB) use produces severe withdrawal. *Ann Emerg Med* 2006;**48**:219–220.

235. Zepf FD, Holtmann M, Duketis E, et al. A 16-year-old boy with severe gamma-butyrolactone (GBL) withdrawal delirium. *Pharmacopsychiatry* 2009;**42**:202–203.

236. Bennett WRM, Wilson LG, Roy-Byrne PP. Gamma-hydroxybutyric acid (GHB) withdrawal: a case report. *J Psychoactive Drugs* 2007;**39**:293–296.

237. Rosenberg MH, Deerfield LJ, Baruch EM. Two cases of severe gamma-hydroxybutyrate withdrawal delirium on a psychiatric unit: recommendations for management. *Am J Drug Alcohol Abuse* 2003;**29**:487–496.

238. Friedman J, Westlake R, Furman M. 'Grievous bodily harm': gamma hydroxybutyrate abuse leading to a Wernicke–Korsakoff syndrome. *Neurology* 1996;**46**:469–471.

239. Addolorato G, Caputo F, Capristo E, Bernardi IM, Stefanini GF, Gasbarrini G. A case of gamma-hydroxybutyric acid withdrawal syndrome during alcohol addiction treatment: utility of diazepam administration. *Clin Neuropharmacol* 1999;**22**:60–62.

240. Mycyk MB, Wilemon C, Aks SE. Two cases of withdrawal from 1,4-butanediol use. *Ann Emerg Med* 2001;**38**:345–346.

241. Price G. In-patient detoxification after GHB dependence. *Br J Psychiatry* 2000;**177**:181.

242. Mullins ME, Fitzmaurice SC. Lack of efficacy of benzodiazepines in treating gamma-hydroxybutyrate withdrawal. *J Emerg Med* 2001;**20**:418–420.

243. Constantinides P, Vincent P. Chronic gamma-hydroxybutyric acid use followed by gamma-hydroxybutyric acid withdrawal mimic schizophrenia: a case report. *Cases J* 2009;**2**:7520. https://doi.org/10.4076/1757-1626-2-7520

244. Claussen M, Hassanpour K, Jenewein J, Boettger S. Catatonic stupor secondary to gamma-hydroxy-butyric acid

245. Chien J, Ostermann G, Turkel SB. Sodium oxybate-induced psychosis and suicide attempt in an 18-year-old girl. *J Child Adolesc Psychopharmacol* 2013;**23**(4):300–301.

246. Kamal RM, Dijkstra BAG, de Weert-van Oene GH, van Duren JAM, De Jong CAJ. Psychiatric comorbidity, psychological distress and quality of life in gamma-hydroxybutyrate (GHB) dependent patients. *J Addict Dis* 2016 (online). https://doi.org/10.1080/10550887.2016.1214000

247. Kamal RM, van Noorden MS, Wannet W, Beurmanjer H, Dijkstra BAG, Schellekens A. Pharmacological treatment in c-hydroxybutyrate (GHB) and c-butyrolactone (GBL) dependence: detoxification and relapse prevention. *CNS Drugs* 2017;**31**:51–64. https://doi.org/10.1007/s40263-016-0402-z

248. Kamal RM, van Noorden MS, Wannet W, Beurmanjer H, Dijkstra BAG, Schellekens A. Pharmacological treatment in c-hydroxybutyrate (GHB) and c-butyrolactone (GBL) dependence: detoxification and relapse prevention. *CNS Drugs* 2017;**31**:51–64. https://doi.org/10.1007/s40263-016-0402-z

249. Constantinides P, Vincent P. Chronic gamma-hydroxybutyric -acid use followed by gamma-hydroxybutyric-acid withdrawal mimic schizophrenia: a case report. *Cases J* 2009;**2**:7520.

250. Kuiper MA, Peikert N, Boerma EC. Gamma-hydroxybutyrate withdrawal syndrome: a case report. *Cases J* 2009;**2**:6530. https://doi.org/10.1186/1757-1626-2-6530

251. Snead O, Gibson KM. g-hydroxybutyric acid. *N Engl J Med* 2005;**352**(26):2721–2732.

252. Freese TE, Miotto K, Reback CJ. The effects and consequences of selected club drugs. *J Subst Abuse Treat* 2002;**23**(2):151–156.

253. Domınguez I, Bruguera P, Balcells-Olivero´ M, Batalla A. Depression following c-hydroxybutyrate withdrawal: a case report. *J Clin Psychopharmacol* 2015;**35**(5):618–619.

254. Miotto K, Darakjian J, Basch J, Murray S, Zogg J, Rawson R. Gamma-hydroxybutyric acid: patterns of use, effects and withdrawal. *Am J Addict* 2001;**10**(3):232–241.

255. Heiligenberg M, Wermeling PR, van Rooijen MS, et al. Recreational drug use during sex and sexually transmitted infections among clients of a city sexually transmitted infections clinic in Amsterdam, the Netherlands. *Sex Transm Dis* 2012;**39**(7):518–527. https://doi.org/10.1097/OLQ.0b013e3182515601

256. Carey JW, Mejia R, Bingham T, et al. Drug use, high-risk sex behaviors, and increased risk for recent HIV infection among men who have sex with men in Chicago and Los Angeles. *AIDS Behav* 2009;**13**(6):1084–1096. https://doi.org/10.1007/s10461-008-9403-3

257. Grov C, Parsons JT, Bimbi DS, Sex and Love v3.0 Research Team. In the shadows of a prevention campaign: sexual risk behavior in the absence of crystal methamphetamine. *AIDS Educ Prev* 2008;**20**(1):42–55. https://doi.org/10.1521/aeap.2008.20.1.42

258. Liao P-C, Chang H-M, Chen Y-L. Clinical management of gamma-hydroxybutyrate (GHB) withdrawal delirium with

CIWA-Ar protocol. *J Formos Med Assoc* 2018;117(12):1124–1127.

259. Handelsman L, Cochrane KJ, Aronson MJ, Ness R, Rubinstein KJ, Kanof PD. Two new rating scales for opiate withdrawal. *Am J Drug Alcohol Abuse* 1987;**13**:293–308.

260. Winstock AR, Mitcheson L. New recreational drugs and the primary care approach to patients who use them. *Br Med J* 2012;**344**:e288. https://doi.org/10.1136/bmj.e288

261. Kamal RM, van Noorden MS, Wannet W, Beurmanjer H, Dijkstra BAG, Schellekens A. Pharmacological treatment in c-hydroxybutyrate (GHB) and c-butyrolactone (GBL) dependence: detoxification and relapse prevention. *CNS Drugs* 2017;**31**:51–64. https://doi.org/10.1007/s40263-016-0402-z

262. van Mechelen JC, Dijkstra BAG, Vergouwen ACM. Severe illicit gamma-hydroxybutyric acid withdrawal in a pregnant woman: what to do? *BMJ Case Rep* 2019;**12**:e230997. https://doi.org/10.1136/bcr-2019-230997

263. www.toxbase.org/poisons-index-a-z/g-products/ghb-and-analogues/ [last accessed 23 February 2022].

264. Craig K, Gomez HF, McManus JL, Bania T. Sever gamma-hydroxybutyrate witdrawal: a case report and literature review. *J Emerg Med* 2000;**18**(1):65–70.

265. McDonough M, Kennedy N, Glasper A, Bearn J. Clinical features and management of gamma-hydroxybutyrate (GHB) withdrawal: a review. *Drug Alcohol Depend* 2004;**75**(1):3–9.

266. McDaniel C, Miotto KA. Gamma hydroxybutyrate (GHB) and gamma butyrolactone (GBL) withdrawal: five case studies. *J Psychoactive Drugs* 2001;**33**:143–149.

267. de Jong C, Kamal R, Dijkstra BA, de Haan HA. Gamma-hydroxybutyrate detoxification by titration and tapering. *Eur Addict Res* 2012;**18**(1):40–45.

268. Chin R. A case of severe withdrawal from gamma-hydroxybutyrate. *Ann Emerg Med* 2001;**37**(5):551–552.

269. van Mechelen JC, Dijkstra BAG, Vergouwen ACM. Severe illicit gamma-hydroxybutyric acid withdrawal in a pregnant woman: what to do? *BMJ Case Rep* 2019;12:e230997. https://doi.org/10.1136/bcr-2019-230997

270. Floyd CN, Wood DM, Darganm PI. Baclofen in gamma-hydroxybutyrate withdrawal: patterns of use and online availability. *Eur J Clin Pharmacol* 2018;**74**:349–356. https://doi.org/10.1007/s00228-017-2387-z

271. Beurmanjer H, Kamal RM, de Jong CAJ, Dijkstra BAG, Schellekens AFA. Baclofen to prevent relapse in gamma-hydroxybutyrate (GHB)-dependent patients: a multicentre, open-label, non-randomized, controlled trial. *CNS Drugs* 2018;**32**:437–442. https://doi.org/10.1007/s40263-018-0516-6

272. Lingford-Hughes A, Patel Y, Bowden-Jones O, et al. Improving GHB withdrawal with baclofen: study protocol for a feasibility study for a randomised controlled trial. *Trials* 2016;**17**:472. https://doi.org/10.1186/s13063-016-1593-9

273. Beurmanjer H, Kamal RM, de Jong CAJ, Dijkstra BAG, Schellekens AFA. Baclofen to prevent relapse in gamma-hydroxybutyrate (GHB)-dependent patients: a multicentre, open-label, non-randomized, controlled trial. *CNS Drugs* 2018;**32**:437–442. https://doi.org/10.1007/s40263-018-0516-6

274. Habibian S, Ahamad K, McLean M, Socias M. Successful management of gamma-hydroxybutyrate (GHB) withdrawal using baclofen as a standalone therapy: a case report. *J Addiction Med* 2019;**13**(5):415–417. https://doi.org/10.1097/ADM.0000000000000514

275. Beurmanjer H, Kamal RM, de Jong CAJ, Dijkstra BAG, Schellekens AFA. Baclofen to prevent relapse in gamma-hydroxybutyrate (GHB)-dependent patients: a multicentre, open-label, non-randomized, controlled trial. *CNS Drugs* 2018;**32**:437–442. https://doi.org/10.1007/s40263-018-0516-6

276. Dijkstra BAG, Kamal R, van Noorden MS, de Haan H, Loonen AJM, De Jong CAJ. Detoxification with titration and tapering in gamma-hydroxybutyrate (GHB) dependent patients: the Dutch GHB monitor project. *Drug Alcohol Depend* 2017;170164–170173. https://doi.org/10.1016/j.drugalcdep.2016.11.014

277. Kamal RM, van Noorden MS, Wannet W, et al. Pharmacological treatment in c-hydroxybutyrate (GHB) and c-butyrolactone (GBL) dependence: detoxification and relapse prevention. *CNS Drugs* 2017;**31**:51–64. https://doi.org/10.1007/s40263-016-0402-z

278. Beurmanjer H, Kamal RM, de Jong CAJ, Dijkstra BAG, Schellekens AFA. Baclofen to prevent relapse in gamma-hydroxybutyrate (GHB)-dependent patients: a multicentre, open-label, non-randomized, controlled trial. *CNS Drugs* 2018;**32**:437–442. https://doi.org/10.1007/s40263-018-0516-6

279. Lingford-Hughes A, Patel Y, Bowden-Jones O, et al. Improving GHB withdrawal with baclofen: study protocol for a feasibility study for a randomised controlled trial. *Trials* 2016;**17**:472. https://doi.org/10.1186/s13063-016-1593-9

280. Beurmanjer H, Kamal RM, de Jong CAJ, Dijkstra BAG, Schellekens AFA. Baclofen to prevent relapse in gamma-hydroxybutyrate (GHB)-dependent patients: a multicentre, open-label, non-randomized, controlled trial. *CNS Drugs* 2018;**32**:437–442. https://doi.org/10.1007/s40263-018-0516-6

281. Beurmanjer H, Kamal RM, de Jong CAJ, Dijkstra BAG, Schellekens AFA. Baclofen to prevent relapse in gamma-hydroxybutyrate (GHB)-dependent patients: a multicentre, open-label, non-randomized, controlled trial. *CNS Drugs* 2018;**32**:437–442. https://doi.org/10.1007/s40263-018-0516-6

282. Beurmanjer H, Kamal RM, de Jong CAJ, Dijkstra BAG, Schellekens AFA. Baclofen to prevent relapse in gamma-hydroxybutyrate (GHB)-dependent patients: a multicentre, open-label, non-randomized, controlled trial. *CNS Drugs* 2018;**32**:437–442. https://doi.org/10.1007/s40263-018-0516-6

283. Habibian S, Ahamad K, McLean M, Socias M. Successful management of gamma-hydroxybutyrate (GHB) withdrawal

using baclofen as a standalone therapy: a case report. *J Addict Med* 2019;**13**(5):415–417.

284. Beurmanjer H, Kamal RM, de Jong CAJ, Dijkstra BAG, Schellekens AFA. Baclofen to prevent relapse in gamma-hydroxybutyrate (GHB)-dependent patients: a multicentre, open-label, non-randomized, controlled trial. *CNS Drugs* 2018;**32**:437–442. https://doi.org/10.1007/s40263-018-0516-6

285. Addolorato G, Caputo F, Capristo E, et al. Diazepam in the treatment of GHB dependence. *Br J Psychiatry* 2001;**178**:183 (letter).

286. Dyer JE, Andrews KM. Gamma hydroxybutyrate withdrawal. *J Toxicol Clin Toxicol* 1997;**35**:553–554.

287. Eiden C, Capdevielle D, Deddouche C, Boulenger JP, Blayac JP, Peyrière H. Neuroleptic malignant syndrome-like reaction precipitated by antipsychotics in a patient with gamma-butyrolactone withdrawal. *J Addict Med* 2011;**5** (4):302–303. https://doi.org/10.1097/ADM.0b013e3182236730

288. Veerman Selene ATE, Veerman RT. Current developments regarding GHB and GBL incidents, treatment and detection: a qualitative review. *World J Pharm Res* 2019;**8**(7):11–26.

289. Floyd CN, Wood DM, Dargan PI. Baclofen in gamma-hydroxybutyrate withdrawal: patterns of use and online availability. *Eur J Clin Pharmacol* 2018;**74**:349–356. https://doi.org/10.1007/s00228-017-2387-z

290. Kamal RM, Qurishi R, De Jong CA. Baclofen and γ-hydroxybutyrate (GHB), a dangerous combination. *J Addict Med* 2015;**9**(1):75–77. https://doi.org/10.1097/ADM.0000000000000084

291. de Jong C, Kamal R, Dijkstra BA, de Haan HA. Gamma-hydroxybutyrate detoxification by titration and tapering. *Eur Addict Res* 2012;**18**(1):40–45.

292. van Raay MEJ. GHB-onttrekkingsverschijnselen behandeled met diazepam, baclofen en propranolol. *Psyfar* 2012;**2**:22–25.

293. Bell J, Collins R. Gamma-butyrolactone (GBL) dependence and withdrawal. *Addiction* 2011;**106**(2):442–447.

294. de Weert-van Oene GH, Schellekens AF, Dijkstra BA, Kamal R, de Jong CA. Detoxification of patients with GHB dependence. *Tijdschr Psychiatr Dutch* 2013;**55**(11):885–890.

295. Stalcup J, Wylie B, Stalcup SA. Outpatient treatment for GHB dependence. In: T Porrata, ed. *"G'd Up" 24/7: The GHB Addiction Guide*. Sam Clemente, CA: LawTech Publishing, 2007.

296. Kamal RM, van Noorden MS, Wannet W, Beurmanjer H, Dijkstra BA, Schellekens A. Pharmacological treatment in γ-hydroxybutyrate (GHB) and γ-butyrolactone (GBL) dependence: detoxification and relapse prevention. *CNS Drugs* 2017;**31**(1):51–64.

297. Kamal RM, van Noorden MS, Wannet W, Beurmanjer H, Dijkstra BA, Schellekens A. Pharmacological treatment in γ-hydroxybutyrate (GHB) and γ-butyrolactone (GBL) dependence: detoxification and relapse prevention. *CNS Drugs* 2017;**31**(1):51–64.

298. McDonough M, Kennedy N, Glasper A, Bearn J. Clinical features and management of gamma-hydroxybutyrate (GHB) withdrawal: a review. *Drug Alcohol Depend* 2004;**75**(1):3–9.

299. Kamal RM, van Iwaarden S, Dijkstra BA, de Jong CA. Decision rules for GHB (c-hydroxybutyric acid) detoxification: a vignette study. *Drug Alcohol Depend* 2014;**135**:146–151.

300. Kamal R, De Jong CAJ. *Practice-Based Recommendations for the Detoxification of Patients with GHB Abuse Disorders in an Outpatient Setting*. Nijmegen, Nijmegen Institute for Scientist Practitioners in Addiction (NISPA), 2013.

301. McDonough M, Kennedy N, Glasper A, Bearn J. Clinical features and management of gamma-hydroxybutyrate (GHB) withdrawal: a review. *Drug Alcohol Depend* 2004;**75** (1):3–9.

302. McDonough M, Kennedy N, Glasper A, Bearn J. Clinical features and management of gamma-hydroxybutyrate (GHB) withdrawal: a review. *Drug Alcohol Depend* 2004;**75** (1):3–9.

303. Bell J, Collins R. Gamma-butyrolactone (GBL) dependence and withdrawal. *Addiction* 2011;**106**(2):442–447.

304. McDonough M, Kennedy N, Glasper A, Bearn J. Clinical features and management of gamma-hydroxybutyrate (GHB) withdrawal: a review. *Drug Alcohol Depend* 2004;**75** (1):3–9.

305. Ghio L, Cervetti A, Respino M, Belvederi Murri M, Amore M. Management and treatment of gamma butyrolactone withdrawal syndrome: a case report and review. *J Psychiatr Pract* 2014;**20**(4):294–300.

306. Project GHB. 2002.

307. Zepf FD, Holtmann M, Duketis E, et al. Withdrawal syndrome after abuse of GHB (gamma-hydroxybutyrate) and its physiological precursors – its relevance for child and adolescent psychiatrists. *Z Kinder Jugendpsychiatr Psychother* 2009;**37**(5):413–420. https://doi.org/10.1024/1422-4917.37.5.413

308. Kamal RM, Iwaarden S, de Jong CAJ. Decision rules for GHB (gamma-hydroxybutyric acid) detoxification: a vignette study. *Drug Alcohol Depend* 2014;**135**:146–151. https://doi.org/10.1016/j.drugalcdep.2013.12.003

309. Dijkstra B, De Weert-van Oene GH, Verbrugge CAG, De Jong C. End report GHB detoxification with pharmaceutical GHB DeTiTap monitor, in the Netherlands addiction care. Nijmegen, Nijmegen Institute for Scientist-Practitioners in Addiction, 2013.

310. Cappetta M, Murnion BP. In-patient management of gamma-hydroxybutyrate withdrawal. *Australas Psychiatry* 2019;**27**(3):284–287. https://doi.org/10.1177/1039856218822748

311. van Noordena MS, Mol T, Wisselink J, Kuijpers W, Dijkstra BAG. Treatment consumption and treatment re-enrollment in GHB-dependent patients in the Netherlands. *Drug Alcohol Depend* 2017;**176**:96–101.

312. Dijkstra BAG, DeWeert-Van Oene GH, Verbrugge CAG, De Jong CAJ. *GHB-Detoxification Using Pharmaceutical GHB;*

Report from DeTiTap®-Monitoring in Dutch Addiction Care. NISPA, Nijmegen, The Netherlands, 2013.

313. Beurmanjer H, Verbrugge CAG, Schrijen S, Schellekens AFA, De Jong CAJ, Dijkstra BAG. *Treatment of GHB-Dependence after Detoxification; Report NISPA GHB Monitor 2.0.* NISPA, Nijmegen, The Netherlands.

314. Beurmanjer H, Asperslag EM, Verbrugge CAG, et al. *GHB-Dependence: Disease Perceptions and Need for Treatment.* NISPA, Nijmegen, The Netherlands.

315. van Noordena MS, Mol T, Wisselink J, Kuijpers W, Dijkstra BAG. Treatment consumption and treatment re-enrollment in GHB-dependent patients in the Netherlands. *Drug Alcohol Depend* 2017;**176**:96–101.

316. Busardò FP, Varì MR, Di Trana A, Malaca S, Carlier J, Di Luca NM. Drug-facilitated sexual assaults (DFSA): a serious underestimated issue. *Eur Rev Med Pharmacol Sci*2019;**23**:10577–10587.

317. Németh Z, Kun B, Demetrovics Z. The involvement of gamma-hydroxybutyrate in reported sexual assaults: a systematic review. *J Psychopharmacol* 2010;**24**(9):1281–1287.

318. Veerman ATE, Veerman SRT. Current developments regarding GHB and GBL incidents, treatment and detection: a qualitative review. *World J Pharm Res* (online) 2019;**8**(7). www.researchgate.net/profile/Selene-Veerman/publication/333565737

319. Pettigrew M. Somnophilia and sexual abuse through the administration of GHB and GBL. *J Forensic Sci* 2019;**64**(1). https://doi.org/10.1111/1556-4029.13812

320. Bracchi M, Stuart D, Castles R, Khoo S, Back D, Boffito M. Increasing use of 'party drugs' in people living with HIV on antiretrovirals: a concern for patient safety. *Aids* 2015;**29**(13):1585–1592.

321. Jones AW, Holmgren A, Kugelberg FC. Driving under the influence of gamma-hydroxybutyrate (GHB). *Forensic Sci Med Pathol* 2008;**4**(4):205–211. https://doi.org/10.1007/s12024-008-9040-1

Chapter 4

New Benzodiazepine Novel Psychoactive Substances

4.1 Introduction

Benzodiazepine misuse is a worldwide public health concern that is associated with a number of concerning consequences.[1] Whereas in the past, the misuse of benzodiazepines was linked to the diversion of medicinal benzodiazepines, currently synthetic processes for benzodiazepine manufacture are freely available, and many illicitly manufactured benzodiazepines have been reported in recent years.

Over the last decade, a number of new benzodiazepines have been developed and marketed, typically in clandestine laboratories in ways very similar to other novel psychoactive substances (NPS). Like other NPS, these new benzodiazepines can evade drug misuse legislation, at least initially.[2] In Europe today, new benzodiazepines, often sold at a very low price, have appeared on illicit drug markets in some countries and have been associated with harm, including an increased risk of overdose. The use of these NPS by high-risk drug users and other marginalised and vulnerable populations also appears to have increased.[3]

Benzodiazepine NPS are sold in their own right. They are also used to make fake versions of medicinal benzodiazepines, which are also sold on the illicit drug market or Internet. A small number of new benzodiazepines may be sourced from companies in some countries such as India for example, typically as finished medicinal products.[4]

4.2 Street Names

Various names for many drugs exist, depending on location and substance. For example, phenazepan is sometimes known as Bonzai or Bonzai Supersleep.

4.3 Legal Status

There are some differences in the way that different European countries control benzodiazepine NPS. For example, in the UK, benzodiazepines are controlled under the Misuse of Drugs Act by the listing of individual substances – rather than by the use of a generic definition. In contrast, the German generic definition was designed to ensure all established and novel analogues of this drug group were brought within the scope of their Narcotics Act. Their generic definition is based on the use of a series of structural diagrams of 16 different benzodiazepine cores, together with a defined range of modifications, coupled with a limit on the molecular weight of the materials controlled.[5]

Etizolam has been listed as an NPS by the World Health Organization (WHO) since 2015.[6] Etizolam, as well as alprazolam, triazolam and flualprazolam, are in Schedule IV of the 1971 Convention on Psychotropic Substances.

4.4 Quality of Research Evidence

There is a wide body of evidence on the efficacy of medically prescribed benzodiazepines as well as the harms associated with their use.

This chapter focuses on the non-medical use of benzodiazepines, where the evidence is much more limited. In particular, information on the new benzodiazepines, their pharmacology, pharmacokinetics, adverse effects and their management is sparse.

4.5 Brief Summary of Pharmacology

Benzodiazepines in general increase the binding of γ-aminobutyric acid (GABA) primarily at the $GABA_A$-receptor, and to a lesser extent at the $GABA_B$-receptor, which causes a sedative-hypnotic effect. They are prescribed on a short-term basis for their anxiolytic, antiepileptic, muscle relaxant and hypnotic effects. They are also used as premedication for anaesthesia and as adjuncts for withdrawal from alcohol and other substances.

The chemical structure and pharmacokinetics of benzodiazepines vary widely. There are differences in their lipid solubility, and this affects how they are processed in the body, including the duration of their psychoactive effects.[7] Benzodiazepines can be categorised based upon their elimination half-life as:[8,9]

- Short acting, with half-lives of less than 6 hours (e.g. midazolam, triazolam);
- Intermediate acting, 6–24 hours (e.g. temazepam, alprazolam);
- Long acting with half-lives of over 24 hours (e.g. diazepam).

4.6 Novel Psychoactive Substances or Designer Benzodiazepines

In recent years, a number of NPS benzodiazepines, sometimes referred to as 'designer' benzodiazepines, are emerging as recreational drugs.[10] A market for non-controlled benzodiazepine-type substances, used alone or in combination with controlled benzodiazepines, is emerging in some Western countries.[11]

Overall, as with other NPS, there is a range of possible modifications which are applicable to several different benzodiazepine core structures, so there is a potential for the development of families of novel, closely related benzodiazepine NPS. This position is similar to that of the synthetic cannabinoids.[12]

The majority of benzodiazepine-type NPS are not registered as medications and have not undergone clinical trials.[13] Most have been synthesised as potential drug candidates by pharmaceutical companies, but were not subsequently marketed as medication. They have not been approved for medicinal use in any country and are sold on the Internet, generally as 'research chemicals'.

It is also possible to purchase benzodiazepine NPS on the illicit market or online. Benzodiazepines such as etizolam or phenazepam, which are licensed in a small number of countries only, appear to be increasingly used recreationally, particularly in Europe where they have been classed as NPS.[14]

Most benzodiazepine NPS are sourced from China as bulk powders. In Europe, they are processed into tablets and other products and sold as legal replacements for commonly prescribed benzodiazepine medicines, such as alprazolam and diazepam. They are also used to make fake versions of these medicines, which are then sold on the illicit drug market.

According to the 2019 European Drug Report, over the last few years there has been an increase in the number, type and availability of the new benzodiazepine class, which are not controlled under international drug control laws. By June 2019, the EMCDDA was monitoring 28 new (NPS) benzodiazepines – 23 of which were first detected in Europe in the last 5 years (European Drug Report 2019). As with opioid NPS discussed in Chapter 5, the appearance and increase in the number of benzodiazepine NPS has been seen as potentially signalling that new psychoactive substances are increasingly more targeted at long-term and more problematic drug users.[15]

The first illicit benzodiazepines identified in Europe to the EMCDDA were phenazepam (fenazepam), nimetazepam and etizolam.[16] Today, the most common are phenazepam, etizolam, diclazepam, flubromazolam and pyrazolam.[17] The most seized new benzodiazepines reported in the EU, Norway and Turkey, are etizolam, clonazolam/clonitrazolam, norfludiazepam, diclazepam and phenazepam.[18] At the time of writing, these and a large number of other benzodiazepine NPS have been detected, with more likely to emerge in the future.[19,20,21,22]

Like pharmaceutical benzodiazepines, they have different core structures which are structurally related to different benzodiazepines. Many benzodiazepine NPS are particularly potent, even at a small dose. For example, flualprazolam is structurally related to alprazolam (Xanax), but more potent. Norfludiazepam is structurally related to diazepam and 4-chlorodiazepam and can be used in the synthesis of midazolam. Fluclotizolam is structurally related to brotizolam and etizolam, and claims have been made that it has an approximately three-fold higher potency and a shorter half-life compared to etizolam.[23]

There are also differences between the various benzodiazepine NPS in their half-life and duration of effects. For example, flubromazepam has a half-life of 106 hours, longer than other benzodiazepines in therapeutic use such as diazepam (20–100 hours) and other NPS-benzodiazepines such as phenazepam (60 hours).[24] Some consumers have suggested that flubromazepam has a greater 'euphoric' effect and has resulted in prolonged fatigue over days.[24]

4.7 Modes of Use

NPS benzodiazepines are sold as tablets, capsules, blotters in various doses (similar to LSD) and as pure powders[25] and pellets.[26] They have also been reported as liquid.[27]

The forms in which benzodiazepine NPS are sold, together with the high potency of some products, can make it difficult for users to measure doses accurately. Tablets can vary greatly in the content of active ingredient, leading to the risk of unintended overdose (see Section 4.11 for details).

4.8 Prevalence and Patterns of Use

In Europe, the 2019 European Drug Report suggested that there seemed to be an increase of reports to the EU Early Warning System for benzodiazepine NPS. Similarly, although police seizures of NPS are typically dominated by synthetic cannabinoids and cathinones, the quantity of benzodiazepines seized in Europe appears to have increased.[28]

The World Drug Report 2018 reported that the non-medical use of the common sedative/hypnotic benzodiazepines and similar substances was one of the main drug use problems in some 60 countries.[29] The 2019 report stated that in 2017, 40 Member States ranked the non-medical use of sedatives and tranquillisers among the three most commonly used substances in their countries, while the non-medical use of benzodiazepines was ranked number one within the broader category of sedatives and tranquillisers.[30]

It has also been noted that recent signs suggest that use of these substances might be growing among young people, and this is an area requiring further investigation, policy consideration and prevention efforts.[31]

Overall, there is significant emerging evidence indicating that the misuse of benzodiazepines is associated with a range of poor outcomes, including increased risk of mortality, HIV/HCV high-risk behaviours, poor self-reported quality of life, criminality, and continued substance use during treatment.[32]

In the UK, population level data from the Office of National Statistics for the year ending in March 2020 reported that 0.5% of the adult population (16–59 years) have used 'tranquillisers' in the past year. Within the 16-to-25-year age group, this rises to 0.8% (tranquillisers can either be classified as Class B (such as barbiturates) or Class C (such as benzodiazepines).[33]

4.9 Desired Effects

There are many reasons why people chose to misuse benzodiazepine, including NPS benzodiazepines. Reports from users on Internet forums suggest that the effects of benzodiazepine NPS resemble those of prescription benzodiazepines.[34]

The effects of benzodiazepines are alcohol-like and they can be used instead of alcohol; more commonly they are used with alcohol to potentiate its effects.[35]

A number of EU countries have expressed concern regarding the availability on the Internet of extremely cheap, often counterfeit, illicit benzodiazepines, leading to the increased use of these drugs by vulnerable teenagers, often in combination with alcohol.[36]

A number of other factors have been identified. For example, a study of 333 posts on discussion groups and forums has shown that people misused NPS benzodiazepine for the following reasons: anxiolysis, tapering benzodiazepines/ management of benzodiazepine withdrawal, sedation/sleep aid, management of stimulant withdrawal, euphoria, ability to function during use and muscle relaxation. Other minor reasons for use reported included use to combat alcohol withdrawal, opioid withdrawal, calm a 'trip', increased sociability, unavailability of preferred benzodiazepine supply, low cost, combat vasoconstriction, chronic pain and solubility.[37]

Benzodiazepines are often used in the context of polydrug use. They are used with other sedatives to potentiate their effects, or to reduce the 'come down' after stimulant use. They are also sometimes used by injection to produce heroin-like effects, and benzodiazepines such as alprazolam ('Xanax') are sometimes found mixed into heroin as 'extenders'.[38] Benzodiazepines have limited potential as euphoriants when administered alone, but euphoric effects appear to be enhanced when taken in combination with opioids.[39]

In comparison to the general population, there is evidence to suggest that the misuse of benzodiazepines is more common among people with psychiatric or physical comorbidity and people with substance misuse disorder. People from low socio-economic backgrounds are also more likely to misuse benzodiazepines as well as young people in general.

In the US for example, research has shown that young people and young adults under 25 years of age are one of the population groups most likely to misuse tranquillisers/sedatives[40] In Europe, the increasing use and availability of sedative drugs amongst young people has been identified as an area of particular concern, requiring further investigation, policy consideration and prevention efforts.

There is some evidence to suggest that rates of non-medical use of benzodiazepines appears to be relatively high among people who use the night time economy and 'clubbers' in particular, in comparison to the general population. A study found that the use of benzodiazepines is prevalent in the club scene and the authors have argued that benzodiazepine dependence appears to be more prevalent in this sample than in other populations described in the literature.[41]

Among young people, factors associated with elevated levels of use are similar to those associated with illicit drugs, including clubbing and high frequency of using the night-time economy. Some studies have also shown that gay clubbers and other young men who have sex with men who attend nightlife venues misuse tranquillisers regularly.[42] Young polydrug users also misuse benzodiazepine and this sometimes occurs in the context of 'coming down' from club drugs and countering the effects of stimulants used.[43,44]

The misuse of benzodiazepines is also common among opiate users, including among people in opioid-substitution treatment (OST) programmes. It is also a strong predictor of a more severe polysubstance use problem, including more harmful patterns of use of benzodiazepines.[45] Benzodiazepines are commonly implicated in opioid-related mortality. Overdoses associated with the ingestion of benzodiazepines are more likely to occur with concomitant use of opioids.[46]

There is a strong association between benzodiazepine use and suicidal ideation in opioid use disorders.[47,48]

Benzodiazepine misuse among opiate substitute treatment (OST) clients presents a serious public health risk as these individuals are at increased risk of overdose[49] and multiple drug overdoses.[50,51]

Amongst this group, benzodiazepine use is also associated with a number of other adverse outcomes,[52] which include:

- People who are prescribed opioids and benzodiazepines were found to take higher opioid doses and for longer periods;[53]
- Reduced likelihood of opioid abstinence;[54]
- Reduced retention in treatment and early withdrawal from treatment;[55,56]
- Increased use of other psychoactive drugs and greater levels of anxiety and depression;[57]
- Increased injecting-related risks;[58]
- Participation in criminal activities.[58]

4.10 Benzodiazepine Acute Harms

The potential harms associated with pharmaceutical benzodiazepines are well known. Guidance and protocols are available on the management of overdose, as well as the management of the adverse effects of long-term and frequent use, including dependence and withdrawal.[59,60,61,62,63,64]

The effects of benzodiazepines are dose-dependent and include drowsiness, lethargy, fatigue, excessive sedation, stupor and 'hangover effects'. Benzodiazepines have effects on memory, concentration and attention, which put people at risk of accidents. The use of benzodiazepines is also linked to nystagmus, hypotonia and ataxia. It can be associated with decreased libido and erectile dysfunction.

Symptoms of benzodiazepine toxicity may range from mild drowsiness to a coma-like state, which is more likely to occur in cases of polydrug use. Similarly, hypotension, bradycardia and respiratory depression may occur occasionally, but tend to be more severe if benzodiazepines are taken with other CNS depressants, including alcohol.

Studies show a dose–response relationship between benzodiazepines and all-cause mortality.[65] Life-threatening respiratory depression can occur with large oral ingestions with or without co-ingestants.[66] However, the co-ingestion of alcohol and other central nervous system depressants potentiates the effects of benzodiazepines and can increase toxicity[67,68] and the likelihood of adverse effects, including the potential of respiratory depression and airway compromise. Severe effects in overdose also include rhabdomyolysis and hypothermia.

4.11 Risks of Untested Benzodiazepine Novel Psychoactive Substances and Counterfeit Medications

The evidence of adverse effects of benzodiazepine NPS is limited, and little is known about their effects. However, it can be assumed that they will be broadly similar to those of currently available pharmaceutical benzodiazepines and will require similar clinical management.

Nonetheless, the limited evidence on benzodiazepine NPS also suggests that clinicians may need to consider issues particular to NPS. In fact, it has been argued that given the limited information on their pharmacology, toxicity, variations in dosage, onset of effects, combination of substances, potency and general patient or individual variability, the concomitant use of these substances with other drugs in particular entails several and unpredictable risks.[69] The fact that some of them are extremely powerful, including at lower dosages, must be considered.

In general, the reported adverse effects of benzodiazepine NPS are typical for a sedative-hypnotic toxidrome, but have also included atypical symptoms in some cases, such as agitation, hyperthermia and tachycardia.[70] A review of the adverse effects of designer benzodiazepines reported fatigue, impairment of thinking, confusion, dizziness, drowsiness, lethargy, amnesia, blurred vision, slurred speech, palpitations and muscle weakness, as well as auditory and visual hallucinations, delirium, seizures, deep sleep and coma at high doses.[71]

Some benzodiazepine NPS have either a higher potency and/or longer duration of action than traditional benzodiazepines, which in turn may lead to increased sedation and/or amnesia.

Some of these benzodiazepine NPS are highly potent, with the potential of producing harm at low dose. For example, etizolam is six to ten times more potent than diazepam. Similarly, due to their high potency, compounds like clonazolam or flubromazolam can cause strong sedation and amnesia at oral doses as low as 0.5 mg.[72] There is emerging evidence of severe intoxication following the use of flubromazolam, resulting in prolonged, severe symptoms including prolonged bradycardia,[73] hypotension, rhabdomyolysis and coma.[73]

It has also been shown that the slow elimination of some benzodiazepine NPS, such as flunitrazolam, causes their accumulation in lipid-based tissues, which can lead to a delayed overdose in case of repeated consumption.[74]

Benzodiazepine NPS can pose a risk of severe life-threatening intoxication,[75,76,77,78,79,80] not only because of the risks of the benzodiazepine itself but because other factors can also increase the risk. As mentioned earlier, dosing for example, poses a risk to people who use benzodiazepine NPS, as it is difficult for users to accurately measure doses, particularly when consumed as a powder.

Tablets can also vary greatly in the content of active ingredients, leading to the risk of unintended overdose. There is also unpredictability in what a product manufactured in a clandestine laboratory contains. As people are buying benzodiazepines from the illicit 'street' market or the Internet, they face the risk of using unknown substances and doses. In the UK, it has been reported that laboratory analyses of police seizures suggests that branded benzodiazepines such as 'Valium' and 'Xanax' often contain other benzodiazepines instead of, or as well as, the product they are claimed to be. For example, out of the 712 samples submitted to WEDINOS[81] in 2020/2021 with purchase intent stated as diazepam, 22 other substances, either in isolation or combination, were identified. Of the 320 samples submitted as alprazolam, 16 other substances, either in isolation or combination, were identified; 58% of samples submitted as alprazolam were found to contain other substances. The most common substitute was flualprazolam.

The dose of benzodiazepine in the product can also be variable and unpredictable. For example, 'Xanax' (alprazolam) sold in the UK is mainly counterfeit[82] and analysis reveals that the majority of pills contain alprazolam, but concentration varies widely, with some which are much stronger than the dose indicates on the tablet or packaging.[85]

Cases of hospital presentations and overdose related to the use of benzodiazepine NPS have been reported. They include presentations involving toxicity from diclazepam[83] and the STRIDA project has also reported on hospital presentations involving etizolam, metizolam, estazolam, pyrazolam, flubromazepam, nifoxipam, diclazepam, meclonazepam, bromazepam, flubromazolam, deschloroetizolam, clonazolam, 3-hydroxyphenazepam, ketazolam and phenazepam. Most cases reported by the study (89%) also involved other drugs.

CNS depression was the most prominent clinical sign, a minority of patients were observed in the intensive care unit, and they responded positively to flumazenil treatment.[84]

There is evidence from some countries that deaths where a benzodiazepine was implicated have increased over the past decade, consistent with an increased role of illicitly manufactured benzodiazepines. In Scotland for example, 'street' or unlicensed benzodiazepines were involved in 85% of the 792 deaths in 2018 where a benzodiazepine was implicated, while medicinal 'prescribed' benzodiazepines were reported in only 30%.[85]

4.12 High-Risk Sexual Behaviours

There is a link between the use of sedatives and hypnotics (including benzodiazepines) and high-risk sexual behaviours. A study of non-medical prescription drug use in five European countries mentioned earlier also reported that sexual health risk factors were associated with an increased likelihood of past-year non-medical prescription drug use.[86]

US studies also suggest that polysubstance use, particularly when it involves prescription drug use, may be associated with high-risk sexual behaviours in young people. This was found among young people within a study, for example, reporting significant relationships between prescription drug misuse and sexual risk behaviours among adolescents and young adults (ages 14–20), with each class of drug (i.e. sedatives, stimulants, opioids/pain relievers) being positively associated with sexual risk behaviours.[87]

Other research showed that students with lifetime prescription medication misuse were more likely to report past-3-month sexual risk behaviours.[90,88] Similarly, in a study among US college students, prescription medication misusers were significantly more likely than others to report having multiple sexual partners, unprotected sex, sex after 'having too much to drink' and sex after using drugs.[91]

Clayton et al.'s [89] data from cross-sectional surveys conducted among nationally representative samples of students also showed that non-medical use of prescription drugs is associated with sexual behaviours that put high school students at risk for sexually transmitted infections.[92]

Non-medical use of prescription drugs (NMUPD) was associated with having sexual intercourse, being currently sexually active having ≥4 lifetime sexual partners, drinking alcohol or using drugs before last sexual intercourse and not using a condom at last sexual intercourse. The authors also reported that as the frequency of NMUPD increased, the association between NMUPD and each of the sexual risk behaviours increased in strength, suggesting a dose–response relationship.[92]

4.13 Aggressive Behaviours

Benzodiazepines in general can cause aggressive behavioural reactions. There is evidence that alprazolam is of particular concern, especially when used with alcohol.[90,91] It is possible that this also applies to benzodiazepine NPS which are structurally related to alprazolam, including flualprazolam, flunitrazolam and clobromazolam.[92]

As well as being self-administered, benzodiazepines have potential for use in drug-facilitated crimes, particularly as some are known to cause amnesia.[93]

4.14 Management of Acute Toxicity

4.14.1 Testing

Whereas rapid bedside testing may not be available to detect benzodiazepine NPS, it is possible to detect these newer benzodiazepines with traditional forensic toxicology laboratory tools and it is important to include these benzodiazepines in the confirmation tests.[94]

Treatment for acute benzodiazepine toxicity must be based on local and national protocols and clinical guidance. Management is mainly supportive care and may include endotracheal intubation to provide definitive airway management.

Flumazenil treatment can be used for the management of benzodiazepine intoxication primarily to reverse the sedative effect of benzodiazepines and prevent respiratory depression. However, there are potential adverse effects associated with its use.[95] There are reports of the effectiveness of flumazenil for NPS benzodiazepines.[96]

4.15 Chronic Harms

Regular and long-term benzodiazepine use has been linked to impaired cognitive functioning[97,98] and an increased risk of accidental falls.[99,100]

People who use benzodiazepines regularly are at risk of developing dependence, including withdrawal symptoms and tolerance. Symptom rebound (i.e. recurrence of the original disorder, most commonly a sleep disorder) after discontinuation has been described.[101,102,103,104,105,106,107,108] It has been suggested that dependence develops in approximately half of patients who use benzodiazepines for longer than 1 month.[109]

4.16 Dependence and Withdrawal

People who become dependent on benzodiazepines and stop using the drug abruptly may experience withdrawal symptoms, which can begin as early as a few hours after the drug was last taken. It has been suggested that dependence develops in approximately half of patients who use benzodiazepines for longer than 1 month.[109] Symptoms of withdrawal after long-term benzodiazepine use usually develop faster with shorter acting agents than with longer-acting agents.[110]

Benzodiazepine withdrawal symptoms include:

- Increased anxiety
- Nervousness

- Sleep disorders
- Inner restlessness
- Depressive symptoms
- Irritability
- Psychosis-like conditions, delirium
- Depersonalisation and derealisation
- Confusion
- Trembling
- Sweating
- Nausea and vomiting
- Motor agitation
- Dyspnea
- Increased heart rate
- Elevated blood pressure
- Headaches
- Muscle tension
- Increased risk of seizures
- Impairment of voluntary movements
- Cognitive impairments
- Impairment of memory
- Pronounced perceptual impairments
- Hyperacusis
- Photophobia
- Hypersomnia
- Dysesthesia, kinaesthetic disorders, muscle twitching and fasciculation[110]

Seizures are associated with benzodiazepine, especially if it is discontinued abruptly. It can be assumed that this is also true for benzodiazepine NPS. Severe withdrawal symptoms include paranoid thoughts, hallucinations, depersonalisation and withdrawal delirium.[110] People dependent on benzodiazepines should not attempt to stop taking them on their own and instead seek medical support. Withdrawal symptoms from these drugs can be severe and can be potentially life-threatening.

The chronic use of benzodiazepine NPS may also lead to the development of tolerance and dependence.[111] Withdrawal symptoms, such as anxiety, panic attacks, restlessness, insomnia, seizures and life-threatening convulsions, may follow the abrupt cessation of chronic benzodiazepine NPS use.[112,113]

4.17 Mental Health Co-morbidity

Bipolar disorder patients with regular use of benzodiazepines show higher levels of treatment resistance to mood stabilisers.[114] They are also at greater risk of both manic and depressive relapses that is independent of the effects of comorbid anxiety and insomnia.[115]

There is also evidence that benzodiazepines have direct depressive effects,[116,117] which may be particularly harmful to individuals with bipolar disorder.

There is an association between benzodiazepine use and dependence and suicide ideation.[118] Benzodiazepine intoxication, high-dose prescription of benzodiazepines and a diagnosis of depression are also considered significant risk factors in reported and completed suicides.[119]

4.18 Treatment of Dependence/Withdrawal

For treatment of benzodiazepine dependence and for benzodiazepine detoxification, clinicians must fellow local protocols and national guidelines and reduction regimens.

Specific information on the management of dependence and detoxification associated with benzodiazepine NPS and clandestinely manufactured benzodiazepines is not available, although it is likely to be broadly similar to that of pharmaceutical benzodiazepines.

Some recommend to first convert sedative-hypnotics into an appropriate dose of diazepam or similar benzodiazepines. This is particularly indicated if the patient is dependent on short-acting, potent benzodiazepines or on preparations that do not easily allow for small reductions in dose.[120]

Clinicians should follow national recommendations on reduction regimens, but keep in mind that an optimal speed or duration of dose reduction is not known.[121] It has been recommended that the medical management of benzodiazepine NPS withdrawal should be individually tailored to the patient. It usually involves prescribing a longer-acting benzodiazepine, prescribing on a slow dose taper, maintaining the dose if symptoms become uncomfortable or increasing the dose if symptoms become intolerable. Additional prescribing for symptomatic relief may be needed.[122] For people with long-term benzodiazepine dependence, the period needed for complete withdrawal may vary from several months to a year or more.[123]

No medication is approved for the treatment of benzodiazepine-use disorders and dependence and there is a paucity of evidence for effective interventions to support withdrawal. A recent review failed to identify evidence of sufficient quality to support any pharmacological interventions.[124]

It is argued that concomitant psychopharmacotherapy for benzodiazepine withdrawal should be symptom-oriented and pragmatic. Reduction regimens using benzodiazepines have been described, and a small number of reports have recommended alternative non-benzodiazepine anxiolytic agents, such as pregabalin, gabapentin, beta-blockers and non-benzodiazepine hypnotic agents.[125] More research is needed.

Short-term symptomatic treatment may include antidepressant agents for depression and sleep problems, as well as mood stabilisers.

A Cochrane review stated that it is currently not possible to draw firm conclusions regarding pharmacological interventions to facilitate benzodiazepine discontinuation in chronic benzodiazepine users. This is because of the low or very low quality of the evidence for the reported outcomes, and the small number of trials identified with a limited number of participants for each comparison.[126]

Anticonvulsants have some efficacy in benzodiazepine withdrawal if the patient is not dependent on other drugs. Carbamazepine has a modest benefit[127] and pregabalin can be effective.[128] Antidepressants and beta-blockers have no proven benefit. Flumazenil has been used as a low-dose intravenous or subcutaneous infusion over four days to help patients rapidly withdraw from benzodiazepines to a lower dose or to abstinence without significant withdrawal symptoms. There are some data showing effectiveness, albeit in small groups of patients.[129] Although relatively uncommon, seizures can occur with low-dose flumazenil infusion and so should only be considered in a specialised unit.[130]

No medication is approved for the treatment of benzodiazepine-use disorders. Psychosocial interventions may be more promising.[131] A meta-analysis of treatment for benzodiazepine discontinuation found that gradual dose reduction combined with psychological treatment was superior to gradual dose reduction alone.[132]

It has been shown that minimal, brief interventions in primary care (provision of simple advice and informational leaflets) can in some cases facilitate an initial reduction in benzodiazepine use.[133,134] Psychotherapeutic interventions for long-term benzodiazepine use have three goals: facilitate the withdrawal itself, facilitate further abstinence and treat the underlying disorder.[135] Cognitive behavioural therapy can play a role in treating benzodiazepine dependence.[136]

References

1. Votaw VR, Geyer R, Rieselbach MM, McHugh RK. The epidemiology of benzodiazepine misuse: a systematic review. *Drug Alcohol Depend* 2019;**200**:95–114. https://doi.org/10.1016/j.drugalcdep.2019.02.033

2. European Monitoring Centre for Drugs and Drug Addiction (EMCDDA). The misuse of benzodiazepines among high-risk opioid users in Europe. Perspectives on Drugs (PODs). EMCDDA, Lisbon, 2018. Available at: www.emcdda.europa.eu/system/files/publications/2733/Misuse%20of%20benzos_POD2015.pdf

3. European Monitoring Centre for Drugs and Drug Addiction and Europol. EU Drug Markets Report 2019. Publications Office of the European Union, Luxembourg, 2019.

4. European Monitoring Centre for Drugs and Drug Addiction and Europol. EU Drug Markets Report 2019. Publications Office of the European Union, Luxembourg, 2019.

5. Advisory Council on the Misuse of Drugs. Novel Benzodiazepines. A Review of the Evidence of Use and Harms of Novel Benzodiazepines. Published April 2020.

6. Busardò FP, Trana A, Montanari E, Mauloni S, Tagliabracci A, Giorgetti R. Is etizolam a safe medication? Effects on psychomotor performance at therapeutic dosages of a newly abused psychoactive substance. *Forensic Sci Int* 2019;**301**:137–141.

7. European Monitoring Centre for Drugs and Drug Addiction (EMCDDA). The misuse of benzodiazepines among high-risk opioid users in Europe. Perspectives on Drugs (PODs). EMCDDA, Lisbon, 2018. Available at: www.emcdda.europa.eu/system/files/publications/2733/Misuse%20of%20benzos_POD2015.pdf

8. Jann M, Kennedy WK, Lopez G. Benzodiazepines: a major component in unintentional prescription drug overdoses with opioid analgesics. *J Pharm Prac* 2014;**27**(1):5–16.

9. Advisory Council on the Misuse of Drugs. Novel Benzodiazepines. A Review of the Evidence of Use and Harms of Novel Benzodiazepines. Published April 2020.

10. Zawilska JB, Wojcieszak J. An expanding world of new psychoactive substances: designer benzodiazepines. *Neuro Toxicology* 2019;**73**:8–16.

11. United Nations Office on Drugs and Crime (UNODC). World Drug Report 2018. Executive Summary Conclusions and Policy Implications. Available at: www.unodc.org/wdr2018/prelaunch/WDR18_Booklet_1_EXSUM.pdf [last accessed 24 February 2022].

12. Advisory Council on the Misuse of Drugs (ACMD). Advice on U-47,700, etizolam and other designer benzodiazepines. Home Office, London, 2016.

13. Zawilska JB, Wojcieszak J. An expanding world of new psychoactive substances: designer benzodiazepines. *NeuroToxicology* 2019;**73**:8–16.

14. European Monitoring Centre for Drugs and Drug Addiction. Fentanils and synthetic cannabinoids: driving greater complexity into the drug situation. An update from the EU Early Warning System (June 2018). Publications Office of the European Union, Luxembourg, 2018.

15. European Monitoring Centre for Drugs and Drug Addiction. European Drug Report 2019: Trends and Developments. Publications Office of the European Union, Luxembourg, 2019.

16. Manchester KR, Lomas EC, Waters L, Dempsey FC, Maskell PD. The emergence of new psychoactive substance (NPS) benzodiazepines: a review. *Drug Test Anal* 2017;**10**(1):37–53.

17. Zawilska JB, Wojcieszak J. An expanding world of new psychoactive substances: designer benzodiazepines. *NeuroToxicology* 2019;**73**:8–16.

18. European Monitoring Centre for Drugs and Drug Addiction and Europol. EU Drug Markets Report 2019. Publications Office of the European Union, Luxembourg, 2019.

19. Manchester KR, Lomas EC, Waters L, Dempsey FC, Maskell PD. The emergence of new psychoactive substance (NPS) benzodiazepines: a review. *Drug Test Anal* 2017;**10**(1):37–53. https://doi.org/10.1002/dta.2211

20. Ameline A, Richeval C, Gaulier J-M, Raul J-S, Kintz P. Detection of the designer benzodiazepine flunitrazolam in urine and preliminary data on its metabolism. *Drug Test Anal* 2019;**11**(2):223–229.

21. Mortelé O, Vervliet P, Gys C, et al. *In vitro* Phase I and Phase II metabolism of the new designer benzodiazepine cloniprazepam using liquid chromatography coupled to quadrupole time-of-flight mass spectrometry. *J Pharm Biomed Anal* 2018;**153**:158–167. https://doi.org/10.1016/j.jpba.2018.02.032

22. Pettersson Bergstrand M, Richter LHJ, Maurer HH, Wagmann L, Meyer MR. *In vitro* glucuronidation of designer benzodiazepines by human UDP-glucuronyltransferases. *Drug Test Anal* 2019;**11**:45–50.

23. Orsolini L, Corkery JM, Chiappini S, et al. 'New/Designer Benzodiazepines': an analysis of the literature and psychonauts' trip reports. *Curr Neuropharmacol* 2020 (online). https://doi.org/10.2174/1570159x18666200110121333

24. Abouchedid R, Gilks T, Dargan PI, Archer JRH, Wood DM. Assessment of the availability, cost, and motivations for use over time of the new psychoactive substances – benzodiazepines diclazepam, flubromazepam, and pyrazolam – in the UK. *J Med Toxicol* 2018;**14**:134–143. https://doi.org/10.1007/s13181-018-0659-3

25. Advisory Council on the Misuse of Drugs (ACMD). Designer Benzodiazepines. A Review of the Evidence of Use and Harms 2016.

26. Abouchedid R, Gilks T, Dargan PI, Archer JRH, Wood DM. Assessment of the availability, cost, and motivations for use over time of the new psychoactive substances – benzodiazepines diclazepam, flubromazepam, and pyrazolam – in the UK. *J Med Toxicol* 2018;**14**:134–143. https://doi.org/10.1007/s13181-018-0659-3

27. Murphy L, Melamed J, Gerona R, Hendrickson RG. Clonazolam: a novel liquid benzodiazepine. *Toxicol Commun* 2019;**3**(1):75–78. https://doi.org/10.1080/24734306.2019.1661568

28. European Monitoring Centre for Drugs and Drug Addiction. European Drug Report 2019: Trends and Developments. Publications Office of the European Union, Luxembourg, 2019.

29. United Nations Office on Drugs and Crime (UNODC). World Drug Report 2018. Executive Summary Conclusions and Policy Implications. Available at: www.unodc.org/wdr2018/prelaunch/WDR18_Booklet_1_EXSUM.pdf [last accessed 24 February 2022].

30. World Drug Report 2019 (United Nations publication, Sales No. E.19.XI.8).

31. United Nations Office on Drugs and Crime (UNODC). World Drug Report 2018. Executive Summary Conclusions and Policy Implications. Available at: www.unodc.org/wdr2018/prelaunch/WDR18_Booklet_1_EXSUM.pdf [last accessed 24 February 2022].

32. Votaw VR, Geyer R, Rieselbach MM, McHugh RK. The epidemiology of benzodiazepine misuse: a systematic review. *Drug Alcohol Depend* 2019;**200**:95–114.

33. Office of National Statistics. Drug misuse in England and Wales: year ending March 2020. An overview of the extent and trends of illicit drug use for the year ending March 2020. Data are from the Crime Survey for England and Wales.

34. El Balkhi S, Monchaud C, Herault F, Geniaux H, Saint-Marcoux F. Designer benzodiazepines' pharmacological effects and potencies: how to find the information. *J Psychopharmacol* 2020;**1**:2. https://doi.org/10.1177/0269881119901096

35. Advisory Council on the Misuse of Drugs. Advice on U-47,700, etizolam and other designer benzodiazepines. London, Home Office, 2016.

36. European Monitoring Centre for Drugs and Drug Addiction and Europol. EU Drug Markets Report 2019. Publications Office of the European Union, Luxembourg, 2019.

37. Abouchedid R, Gilks T, Dargan PI, Archer JRH, Wood DM. Assessment of the availability, cost, and motivations for use over time of the new psychoactive substances – benzodiazepines diclazepam, flubromazepam, and pyrazolam – in the UK. *J Med Toxicol* 2018;**14**:134–143. https://doi.org/10.1007/s13181-018-0659-3

38. Advisory Council on the Misuse of Drugs. Novel Benzodiazepines. A Review of the Evidence of Use and Harms of Novel Benzodiazepines. April 2020

39. Luethi D, Liechti ME. Designer drugs: mechanism of action and adverse effects. *Arch Toxicol* (online). https://doi.org/10.1007/s00204-020-02693-7

40. Schepis TS, Teter CJ, Simoni-Wastila L, McCabe S. Esteban prescription tranquilizer/sedative misuse prevalence and correlates across age cohorts in the US. *Addict Behav* 2018;**87**:24–32.

41. Kurtz SP, Surratt HL, Levi-Minzi MA, Mooss A. Benzodiazepine dependence among multidrug users in the club scene. *Drug Alcohol Depend* 2011;**119**(1–2):99–105.

42. Kecojevic A, Corliss HL, Lankenau SE. Motivations for prescription drug misuse among young men who have sex with men (YMSM) in Philadelphia. *Int J Drug Policy* 2015;**26** (8):764–771. https://doi.org/10.1016/j.drugpo.2015.03.010

43. Kurtz SP, Surratt HL, Levi-Minzi MA, Mooss A. Benzodiazepine dependence among multidrug users in the club scene. *Drug Alcohol Depend* 2011;**119**(1–2):99–105.

44. Inciardi JA, Surratt HL, Kurtz SP, Cicero TJ. Mechanisms of prescription drug diversion among drug-involved club- and street-based populations. *Pain Med* 2007; **8**(2):171–183.

45. Vogel M, Knopfli B, Schmid O, et al.Treatment or 'high': benzodiazepine use in patients on injectable heroin or oral opioids. *Addict Behav* 2013;**38**:2477–2484.

46. Advisory Council on the Misuse of Drugs. Novel Benzodiazepines. A Review of the Evidence of Use and Harms of Novel Benzodiazepines. April 2020.

47. Wines JD, Saitz R, Horton NJ, Lloyd-Travaglini C, Samet JH. Suicidal behaviour, drug use and depressive symptoms after detoxification: a 2-year prospective study. *Drug Alcohol Depend* 2004;**76**:S21–29.

48. Backmund M, Meyer K, Schütz C, Reimer J. Factors associated with suicide attempts among injection drug users. *Subst Use Misuse* 2011;**46**:1553–1559.

49. Sun E, Dixit A, Humphreys K, Darnall B, Baker L, Mackey S. Association between concurrent use of prescription opioids and benzodiazepines and overdose: retrospective analysis. *Br Med J* 2017;**356**:j760.

50. Chen K, Berger C, Forde D, D'Adamo C, Weintraub E, Gandhi D. Benzodiazepine use and misuse among patients in a methadone program. *BMC Psychiatry* 2011;**11**(1):90.

51. Sun E, Dixit A, Humphreys K, Darnall B, Baker L, Mackey S. Association between concurrent use of prescription opioids and benzodiazepines and overdose: retrospective analysis. *Br Med J* 2017;**356**:j760.

52. Deacon RM, Nielsen S, Leung S, et al. Alprazolam use and related harm among opioid substitution treatment clients – 12 months follow up after regulatory rescheduling. *Int J Drug Policy* 2016;**36**:104–111.

53. Kay C, Fergestrom N, Spanbauer C, Jackson J. Opioid dose and benzodiazepine use among commercially insured individuals on chronic opioid therapy. *Pain Med* 2019;**21**(6):1–7.

54. Kamal F, Flavin S, Campbell F, et al. Factors affecting the outcome of methadone maintenance treatment in opiate dependence. *Irish Med J.* 2007;**100**(3):393–397.

55. Meiler A, Mino A, Chatton A, Broers B. Benzodiazepine use in a methadone maintenance programme: patient characteristics and the physician's dilemma. *Schweiz Arch Neurol Psychiatr* 2005;**156**:310–317.

56. Peles E, Schreiber S, Adelsona M. 15-Year survival and retention of patients in a general hospital-affiliated methadone maintenance treatment (MMT) center in Israel. *Drug Alcohol Depend* 2010; **107**:141–148.

57. Lavie E, Fatséas M, Denis C, Auriacombe M. Benzodiazepine use among opiate-dependent subjects in buprenorphine maintenance treatment: correlates of use, abuse and dependence. *Drug Alcohol Depend* 2009; **99**:338–344.

58. Darke S, Hall W, Ross M, Wodak A. Benzodiazepine use and HIV risk-taking behaviour among injecting drug users. *Drug Alcohol Depend* 1992;**31**(1):31–36.

59. NICE hypnotics and anxiolytics. Available at: https://bnf .nice.org.uk/treatment-summary/hypnotics-and-anxiolytics.html [last accessed 24 February 2022].

60. NICE hypnotics. Available at: www.nice.org.uk/advice/KTT6/chapter/Evidence-context [last accessed 24 February 2022].

61. NICE benzodiazepine and z-drug withdrawal. Available at: https://cks.nice.org.uk/topics/benzodiazepine-z-drug-withdrawal/management/benzodiazepine-z-drug-withdrawal/ [last accessed 24 February 2022].

62. Baandrup L, EbdrupBH, Rasmussen JO, Lindschou J, Gluud C, Glenthøj BY. Pharmacological interventions for benzodiazepine discontinuation in chronic benzodiazepine users. Cochrane Systematic Review – Intervention Version published 15 March 2018. https://doi.org/10.1002/14651858 .CD011481.pub2. Available at: www.cochranelibrary.com/cds r/doi/10.1002/14651858.CD011481.pub2/full [last accessed 24 February 2022].

63. Darker CD, Sweeney BP, Barry JM, Farrell MF, Donnelly-Swift E. Psychosocial interventions for benzodiazepine harmful use, abuse or dependence. Cochrane Systematic Review – Intervention Version published 11 May 2015. https:// doi.org/10.1002/14651858.CD009652.pub2

64. Denis C, Fatséas M, Lavie E, Auriacombe M. Pharmacological interventions for benzodiazepine mono-dependence management in outpatient settings. *Cochrane Database Syst Rev* 2006;(**3**):CD005194.

65. Tiihonen J, Mittendorfer-Rutz E, Torniainen M, Alexanderson K, Tanskanen A. Mortality and cumulative exposure to antipsychotics, antidepressants, and benzodiazepines in patients with schizophrenia: an observational follow-up study. *Am J Psychiatry* 2016;**173**:600–606.

66. Kang M, Ghassemzadeh S. Benzodiazepine toxicity. [Updated 8 March 2019.] In *Treasure Island*. StatPearls Publishing, Florida, 2019.

67. TOXBASE www.toxbase.org [last accessed 27 February 2019].

68. TOXBASE www.toxbase.org [last accessed 27 February 2019].

69. Orsolini L, Corkery JM, Chiappini S, et al. 'New/Designer Benzodiazepines': an analysis of the literature and psychonauts' trip reports. *Curr Neuropharmacol* 2020 (online). https://doi.org/10.2174/1570159x18666200110121333

70. Luethi D, Liechti ME. Designer drugs: mechanism of action and adverse effects. *Arch Toxicol* 20200;**94**(4):1085–1133.

71. Zawilska JB, Wojcieszak J. An expanding world of new psychoactive substances: designer benzodiazepines.

NeuroToxicology 2019;**73**:8–16. https://doi.org/10.1016/j
.neuro.2019.02.015

72. Moosmann B, King LA, Auwarter V. Designer
benzodiazepines: a new challenge. *Psychiatry* 2015;**14**:2.

73. Bohnenberger K, Liu MT. Flubromazolam overdose: a review
of a new designer benzodiazepine and the role of flumazenil.
Mental Health Clinician 2019;**9**(3):133–137. https://doi.org/10
.9740/mhc.2019.05.133

74. Ameline A, Richeval C, Gaulier J-M, Raul J-S, Kintz P.
Characterization of flunitrazolam, a new designer
benzodiazepine, in oral fluid after a controlled single
administration. *J Anal Toxicol* 2018;**42**:e58–e60. https://doi
.org/10.1093/jat/bky012

75. O'Brien CP. Benzodiazepine use, abuse, and dependence.
J Clin Psychiatry 2005;**66**:28–33.

76. Moosmann B, Huppertz LM, Hutter M, et al. Detection and
identification of the designer benzodiazepine flubromazepam
and preliminary data on its metabolism and pharmacokinetics.
J Mass Spectrom 2013;**48**:1150–1159.

77. Moodmann B, King AL, Auwa¨rter V. Designer
benzodiazepines: a new challenge. *World Psychiatry*
2015;**14**:2.

78. Moosmann B, Bisel P, Auwa¨rter V. Characterization of the
designer benzodiazepine diclazepam and preliminary data on
its metabolism and pharmacokinetics. *Drug Test Anal*
2014;**6**:757–763.

79. Schifano F, Orsolini L, Papanti GD, et al. Novel psychoactive
substances of interest for psychiatry. *World Psychiatry*
2015;**14**:15–26.

80. Nakamae T, Shinozuka T, Sasaki C, et al. Case report: etizolam
and its major metabolites in two unnatural death cases.
Forensic Sci Int 2008;**20**:182.

81. WEDINOS. PHILTRE Annual Report 2020-2021. Available at:
www.wedinos.org/resources/downloads/Annual-Report-20-2
1-English.pdf [last accessed 23 April 2022].

82. Public Health England. RIDR SUMMARY – MAY 2019. Report
unexpected or severe adverse reactions to illicit drugs. Available
at: www.gov.uk/government/publications/drug-health-harms-
national-intelligence/national-intelligence-network-on-drug-
health-harms-briefing-april-2019?msclkid=216cf526c26
d11ec94c0857fb53f773f [last accessed 23 April 2022].

83. Runnstrom MC, Kalra SS, Lascano J, Patel DC. Designer Drug
Diclazepam: A Journey from Death to Life. C42. Critical Care
Case Reports: Toxicology and Poisonings.

84. Bäckberg M, Pettersson Bergstrand M, Beck O, Helander A.
Occurrence and time course of NPS benzodiazepines in
Sweden – results from intoxication cases in the STRIDA
project. *Clin Toxicol* 2019;**57**(3):203–212. https://doi.org/10
.1080/15563650.2018.1506130

85. National Records of Scotland (NRS). Drug-related deaths in
Scotland in 2018. Edinburgh, National Records of Scotland,
2019.

86. Novak SP, Håkansson A, Martinez-Raga J, Reimer J, Krotki K,
Varughese S. Nonmedical use of prescription drugs in the

European Union. *BMC Psychiatry* 2016;**16**:274. https://doi.org
/10.1186/s12888-016-0909-3

87. Bonar EE, Cunningham RM, Chermack ST, et al.
Prescription drug misuse and sexual risk behaviors among
adolescents and emerging adults. *J Stud Alcohol Drugs*
2014;**75**(2):259–268.

88. Benotsch EG, Koester S, Luckman D, Martin AM, Cejka A.
Non-medical use of prescription drugs and sexual risk
behavior in young adults. *Addict Behav* 2011;**36**:152–155.

89. Clayton HB, Lowry R, August E, Everett Jones S. Nonmedical
use of prescription drugs and sexual risk behaviors. *Pediatrics*
2016;**137**(1).

90. Jones KA, Nielsen S, Bruno R, Frei M, Lubman DI.
Benzodiazepines: their role in aggression and why GPs should
prescribe with caution. *Aust Fam Physician* 2011;40(11):862–
865.

91. Albrecht B, Staiger P, Hall K, Miller P, Best D, Lubman D.
Benzodiazepine use and aggressive behaviour: a systematic
review. *Aust N Z J Psychiatry* 2014;**48**(12):1096–1114.

92. Advisory Council on the Misuse of Drugs. Novel
Benzodiazepines. A Review of the Evidence of Use and Harms
of Novel Benzodiazepines. April 2020.

93. Advisory Council on the Misuse of Drugs. NPS Committee
Meeting Paper: Benzodiazepines. Published 2015.

94. O'Connor LC, Torrance HJ, McKeown DA. ELISA detection
of phenazepam, etizolam, pyrazolam, flubromazepam,
diclazepam and delorazepam in blood using Immunalysis®
benzodiazepine kit. *J Anal Toxicol* 2016;**40**:159–161. https://
doi.org/10.1093/jat/bkv122

95. Penninga EI, Graudal N, Ladekarl MB, Jurgens G. Adverse
events associated with flumazenil treatment for the
management of suspected benzodiazepine intoxication –
a systematic review with meta-analyses of randomised trials.
Basic Clin Pharmacol Toxicol 2016;**118**:37–44. https://doi.org/
10.1111/bcpt.12434

96. Bäckberg M, Pettersson Bergstrand M, Beck O, Helander A.
Occurrence and time course of NPS benzodiazepines in
Sweden – results from intoxication cases in the STRIDA
project, *Clin Toxicol* 2019;**57**(3):203–212. https://doi.org/10
.1080/15563650.2018.1506130

97. Barker MJ, Greenwood KM, Jackson M, Crowe SF. Cognitive
effects of long-term benzodiazepine use: a meta-analysis. *CNS
Drugs* 2004;**18**:37–48.

98. McAndrews PM, Weiss RT, Sandor P, Taylor A, Carlen PL,
Shapiro CM. Cognitive effects of long-term benzodiazepine
use in older adults. *Hum Psychopharmacol* 2003;**18**:51–57.

99. French DD, Chirikos TN, Spehar A, Campbell R, Means H,
Bulat T. Effect of concomitant use of benzodiazepines and
other drugs on the risk of injury in a veteran population. *Drug
Saf* 2005;**28**:1141–1150.

100. Airagnes G, Pelissolo A, Lavallee M, Flament M, Limosin F.
Benzodiazepine misuse in the elderly: risk factors,
consequences, and management. *Curr Psychiatry Rep*
2016;**18**:89.

101. Lader MH. Limitations on the use of benzodiazepines in anxiety and insomnia: are they justified? *Eur Neuropsychopharmacol* 1999;**9**(Suppl. 6):S399–S405.

102. Pariente A, de Gage SB, Moore N, Bégaud B. The benzodiazepine-dementia disorders link: current state of knowledge. *CNS Drugs* 2016;**30**:1–7.

103. Buffett-Jerrott SE, Stewart SH. Cognitive and sedative effects of benzodiazepine use. *Curr Pharm Des* 2002;**8**:45–58.

104. Lader M, Tylee A, Donoghue J. Withdrawing benzodiazepines in primary care. *CNS Drugs* 2009;**23**:19–34.

105. Mura T, Proust-Lima C, Akbaraly T, et al. Chronic use of benzodiazepines and latent cognitive decline in the elderly: results from the Three-City Study. *Eur Neuropsychopharmacol* 2013;**23**:212–223.

106. Lader M, Tylee A, Donoghue J. Withdrawing benzodiazepines in primary care. *CNS Drugs* 2009;**23**:19–34.

107. Koyama A, Steinman M, Ensrud K, Hillier TA, Yaffe K. Ten-year trajectory of potentially inappropriate medications in very old women: importance of cognitive status. *J Am Geriatr Soc* 2013;**61**:258–263.

108. Pisani MA, Murphy TE, Araujo KL, Slattum P, Van Ness PH, Inouye SK. Benzodiazepine and opioid use and the duration of intensive care unit delirium in an older population. *Crit Care Med* 2009;**37**:177–183.

109. de las Cuevas C, Sanz E, de la Fuente J. Benzodiazepines: more 'behavioural' addiction than dependence. *Psychopharmacology (Berl)* 2003;**167**:297–303.

110. Soyka M. Treatment of benzodiazepine dependence. *N Engl J Med* 2017;**376**:1147–1157. https://doi.org/ 10.1056/ NEJMra1611832

111. Zawilska JB, Wojcieszak J. An expanding world of new psychoactive substances: designer benzodiazepines. *Neurotoxicology* 2019;**73**:8–16. https://doi.org/10.1016/j .neuro.2019.02.015

112. Andersson M, Kjellgren A. The slippery slope of flubromazolam: experiences of a novel psychoactive benzodiazepine as discussed on a Swedish online forum. *Nord Stud Alcohol Drugs* 2017;**34**(3):217–229. https://doi.org/10 .1177/1455072517706304

113. Zawilska JB, Wojcieszak J. An expanding world of new psychoactive substances: designer benzodiazepines. *Neurotoxicology* 2019;**73**:8–16. https://doi.org/10.1016/j .neuro.2019.02.015

114. Parker GB, Graham RK. Clinical characteristics associated with treatment-resistant bipolar disorder. *J Nerv Ment Dis* 2017;**205**:188–191.

115. Bjorklund L, Horsdal HT, Mors O, Ostergaard SD, Gasse C. Trends in the psychopharmacological treatment of bipolar disorder: a nationwide register-based study. *Acta Neuropsychiatr* 2016;**28**:75–84.

116. Hall RC, Joffe JR. Aberrant response to diazepam: a new syndrome. *Am J Psychiatry* 1972;**129**:738–742.

117. Michelini S, Cassano GB, Frare F, Perugi G. Long-term use of benzodiazepines: tolerance, dependence and clinical problems in anxiety and mood disorders. *Pharmacopsychiatry* 1996;**29**:127–134.

118. Schepis TS, Teter CJ, Simoni-Wastila L, McCabe SE. Prescription tranquilizer/sedative misuse prevalence and correlates across age cohorts in the US. *Addict Behav* 2018;**87**:24–33.

119. Advisory Council on the Misuse of Drugs. Novel Benzodiazepines. A Review of the Evidence of Use and Harms of Novel Benzodiazepines. April 2020.

120. Clinical Guidelines on Drug Misuse and Dependence. Update 2017, Independent Expert Working Group. Drug Misuse and Dependence: UK Guidelines on Clinical Management. London, Department of Health, 2017.

121. Clinical Guidelines on Drug Misuse and Dependence. Update 2017, Independent Expert Working Group. Drug Misuse and Dependence: UK Guidelines on Clinical Management. London, Department of Health, 2017.

122. Taylor S, Annand F, Burkinshaw P, et al. Dependence and Withdrawal Associated with Some Prescribed Medicines: An Evidence Review. London, Public Health England, 2019.

123. Fluyau D, Revadigar N, Manobianco BE. Challenges of the pharmacological management of benzodiazepine withdrawal, dependence, and discontinuation. *Ther Adv Psychopharmacol* 2018;8(5):147–168.

124. Baandrup L, Ebdrup BH, Rasmussen JØ, Lindschou J, Gluud C, Glenthøj BY. Pharmacological interventions for benzodiazepine discontinuation in chronic benzodiazepine users. *Cochrane Database Syst Rev* 2018;**3**:CD011481.

125. Soyka M. Treatment of benzodiazepine dependence. *N Engl J Med* 2017;**376**:1147–1157. https://doi.org/ 10.1056/ NEJMra1611832

126. Baandrup L, Ebdrup BH, Rasmussen JØ, Lindschou J, Gluud C, Glenthøj BY. Pharmacological interventions for benzodiazepine discontinuation in chronic benzodiazepine users. *Cochrane Database Syst Rev* 2018;**3**:CD011481. https:// doi.org/10.1002/14651858.CD011481.pub2

127. Denis C, Fatséas M, Lavie E, Auriacombe M. Pharmacological interventions for benzodiazepine mono-dependence management in outpatient settings. *Cochrane Database Syst Rev* 2006;**3**:CD005194.

128. Oulis P, Konstantakopoulos G. Efficacy and safety of pregabalin in the treatment of alcohol and benzodiazepine dependence. *Expert Opin Investig Drugs* 2012;**21**:1019–1029.

129. Hood SD, Norman A, Hince DA, Melichar JK, Hulse GK. Benzodiazepine dependence and its treatment with low dose flumazenil. *Br J Clin Pharmacol* 2014;**77**:285–294.

130. Lugoboni F, Faccini M, Quaglio G, Albiero A, Casari R, Pajusco B. Intravenous flumazenil infusion to treat benzodiazepine dependence should be performed in the inpatient clinical setting for high risk of seizure. *J Psychopharmacol* 2011;**25**:848–849.

131. Hayhoe B, Lee-Davey J. Tackling benzodiazepine misuse. *Br Med J* 2018;**362**:k3208. https://doi.org/10.1136/bmj.k3208

132. Parr JM, Kavanagh DJ, Cahill L, Mitchell G, Young RMcD. Effectiveness of current treatment approaches for benzodiazepine discontinuation: a meta-analysis. *Addiction* 2009;**104**:13–24.

133. Ten Wolde GB, Dijkstra A, van Empelen P, van den Hout W, Neven AK, Zitman F. Long-term effectiveness of computer-generated tailored patient education on benzodiazepines: a randomized controlled trial. *Addiction* 2008;**103**:662–670.

134. Mugunthan K, McGuire T, Glasziou P. Minimal interventions to decrease long-term use of benzodiazepines in primary care: a systematic review and meta-analysis. *Br J Gen Pract* 2011;**61**(590): e573–e578.

135. Soyka M. Treatment of benzodiazepine dependence. *N Engl J Med* 2017;**376**:1147–1157. https://doi.org/ 10.1056/ NEJMra1611832

136. Lader M, Tylee A, Donoghue J. Withdrawing benzodiazepines in primary care. *CNS Drugs* 2009;**23**:19–34.

Chapter 5

Synthetic Opioid Novel Psychoactive Substances (Fentanyl and Non-fentanyl)

5.1 Introduction

New synthetic opioids are an increasing risk for public health across the world. These drugs can be divided into two categories, pharmaceutical and non-pharmaceutical fentanyls, as well as non-fentanyl opioid novel psychoactive substances (NPS). These NPS are easily available on the Internet and are characterised by low price, purity, legality and lack of detection in laboratory tests. However, most have not been approved or are not recommended for human use.[1]

In North America in particular, a crisis linked to the misuse of opioids has been observed for a number of years and has been associated with very high levels of mortality. The origins of the crisis are to some extent associated over-prescription, and unauthorised distribution or the diversion of opioid medications.[2]

Only a relatively limited number of people have required specialised drug treatment for addiction to opioid pain medication in Europe, in contrast to other countries, such as the US for example. However, under-reporting cannot be dismissed and it is possible that the real level of dependence on opioid medication is under-estimated.

There is evidence of some misuse of opioid medication. For example, in a survey of young people in European schools, 4% of students aged 15–16 years reported lifetime use of painkillers to get high.[3] Data from the European Early Warning System has also been reporting a rise in the number of deaths related to synthetic opioids and an increasing number of new synthetic opioids are being reported, including new fentanyls.[4]

In recent years, opioids with structures distinct from those used therapeutically have been emerging, in particular fentanyl derivatives and other substances that are linked with significant risk of acute toxicity and overdose. Although the number of novel synthetic opioid analogues detected is small in comparison with other types of NPS, such as stimulants, the largest percentage increase in recent years has been observed in opioid

NPS. The appearance and increase in the number of these opioid NPS has been seen as potentially signalling that new psychoactive substances are increasingly more targeted at the long-term and more problematic drug users.[5]

These substances have also been described as a global public health threat,[6] with implications for clinical practice.[7] The World Drug Report suggests that this increase in the number of opioid NPS, as well as the increase of benzodiazepine NPS for example, potentially signals that new psychoactive substances are increasingly more targeted at the long-term and more problematic drug users.[8]

In Europe, a large-scale recent study showed that non-medical prescription high-potency opioid use is a public health concern in Europe.[9]

The 2019 European Drugs Report showed that since 2009, 49 opioid NPS have been detected on Europe's drug market – including 11 reported for the first time in 2018. Of the 49 opioid NPS, 34 were fentanyl derivatives (six of which were reported for the first time in 2018), but a small number of other types of opioids (such as U-47,700 and U-51,754) were also reported.[10]

At a global level, the number of new psychoactive substances reported that are opioids have been rising at an unprecedented rate and consists mainly of fentanyl analogues. Numbers rose from just one substance in 2009, to 15 in 2015 and 46 in 2017. Although, the number of opioid NPS is still small, they now form a greater proportion of NPS in general. Opioid NPS accounted for just 2% of the number of NPS identified in 2014, but by 2018 that figure had risen to 9%.[11]

This chapter focuses on the misuse of fentanyl, fentanyl analogues and other non-fentanyl opioid NPS and does not address issues pertaining to their use in legitimate therapeutic and clinical contexts.

5.2 Legal Status

Fentanyl and its pharmaceutical analogues are Schedule I substances according to the United Nations Single

Convention on Narcotic Drugs 1961, amended in 1972 (substances that are highly addictive and liable to abuse). Some non-pharmaceutical analogues are Schedule I–IV substances, while new compounds are being progressively incorporated into the lists.

5.3 Quality of the Research Evidence

Although there is a large body of evidence relating to pharmaceutical opioids including fentanyl and its analogues, the evidence on the novel fentanyls and other opioid NPS, their harms and clinical management, is currently limited and cannot be considered as robust. Nonetheless, the research findings are broadly consistent and this document provides clinically relevant information based on the best evidence currently available. In addition, it is expected that the harms associated with opioid NPS and their management are broadly the same as other opioids.

The harms of new fentanyls and other opioid NPS will be discussed in greater detail in this chapter. New fentanyls in particular are associated with severe adverse effects resulting from their strong potency in comparison to morphine and the length of the effects of some. They are often used in combination with other drugs which can result in toxicity, including respiratory depression. They are also associated with dependence and a withdrawal syndrome.

5.4 New Fentanyl Analogues

5.4.1 Brief Summary of Pharmacology

Fentanyl (N-[1-(2-phenylethyl)-4-piperidinyl]-N-phenylpropanamide) is a potent opioid used in human and veterinary medicine. It has analgesic and sedative effects and is widely used in the management of severe pain and in anaesthesia.[12] Fentanyl is a full agonist at the μ-opioid receptor. It is at least 80 times more potent than morphine[13,14] and when misused is associated with a risk of acute toxicity.

Licensed fentanyl and fentanyl analogues are used in human medicine for pain relief and used regularly in hospitals, especially in intensive care units and operating theatres, for anaesthesia and post-operative pain control. They are also used to provide sedation and pain relief for medical procedures such as fracture manipulation. Some are also used by pre-hospital teams, emergency departments and in primary care, for example, by patients receiving palliative care at home. Some fentanyls are not licensed for human use but may be used in

veterinary practice, for example carfentanil for large animals. However, these drugs also have euphoric effects and most have the potential for misuse.[15]

In recent years, a number of opioid NPS have been reported to the EU Early Warning System on new psychoactive substances and adverse effects associated with their use have been reported. They include carfentanyl, which is intended only for veterinary use on large animals, is not approved for medical use in humans and is estimated to be about 10,000 times more potent than morphine.[13,16,17]

Other new fentanyl derivatives sold on the illicit market include analogues that have been rediscovered by the manufacturers from studies described in the scientific literature but never developed into pharmaceutical products. New fentanyls also include newly designed fentanyl analogues made by new modifications of the fentanyl chemical structure, to avoid legal control, as with other NPS (see Box 5.1). They are produced in clandestine laboratories and are sometimes referred to as non-pharmaceutical fentanyls (NPF) or even 'research chemicals'. It has been argued that as a result of the low cost of clandestine laboratory production and enormous profit potential, opioid NPS and fentanyls in particular are establishing a strong position on the illegal drug market as stand-alone products, adulterants in heroin, or constituents of counterfeit prescription medications.[18]

Box 5.1 Examples of Non-pharmaceutical Fentanyl Analogues

Alpha-methyl-fentanyl, 3-methylfentanyl, acetylfentanyl, butyrylfentanyl, betahydroxy-thio-fentanyl, 4-fluorobuyrylfentanyl, furanylfentanyl, ocfentanil, acrylyolfentanyl, 4-methoxibutyrylfentanyl, tetrahydr ofuranfentanyl, beta-hydroxytihiofentanyl, para-fluoro-isobutyryl fentanyl, cyclopentyfentanyl, 4-fluoroisobutyrylfentanyl, and 4-chloroisobutyrylfentanyl, 3-fluorofentanyl, 4-fluorobutyrfentanyl, 4-methoxybutyrfentanyl, acetylfentanyl, acrylfentanyl, beta-hydroxy-thiofentanyl, butyrfentanyl, despropionylfentanyl, despropionyl-2-fluorofentanyl, furanylfentanyl, isobutyrfentanyl, (iso)butyr-F-fentanyl N-benzyl analog, methoxyacetylfentanyl, ocfentanil, parafluoroisobutyrfentanyl, tetrahydrofuranylfentanyl, and valerylfentanyl.

Published data on the pharmacology of most fentanyl NPS are limited mainly to in vitro and in vivo animal studies. These data suggest that they are selective and potent μ-opioid receptor agonists with a pharmacology that is broadly comparable to fentanyl (e.g. furanylfentanyl) and include:

- Furanylfentanyl, or N-phenyl-N-[1-(2-phenylethyl)piperidin-4-yl]furan-2-carboxamide;
- Acryloylfentanyl, or N-(1phenethylpiperidin-4-yl)-N-phenylacrylamide;
- Acrylofentanyl, or N-(1-phenethylpiperidin-4-yl)-N-phenylacrylamide;
- Para-fluoroisobutyrfentanyl;
- 4-fluorobutyrfentanyl;
- Methoxyacetylfentanyl2-methoxy-N-phenyl-N-[1-(2-phenylethyl)piperidin-4-yl]acetamide (methoxyacetylfentanyl)
- (cyclopropylfentanyl);
- 4-fluoroisobutrylfentanyl, tetrahydrofuranylfentanyl and carfentanil.

Fentanyl has a rapid onset of action, almost immediate, following intravenous administration, but its maximal analgesic and respiratory depressant effect may not be noted for several minutes. Following intramuscular administration, the onset of action is from 7 to 8 minutes and the duration of action is 1–2 hours. The duration of action of fentanyl, when administered intravenously, is 30–60 minutes,[19,20] much shorter than with heroin (4–5 hours). This may lead to frequent redosing.[21]

Overall, reasons for the potency of fentanyl include its high lipophilicity (which allows it easily to cross the blood–brain barrier) and high receptor affinity, with high selectivity and specificity for the μ-opioid receptor over other opioid receptor subtypes.[22] In terms of toxicity, as potent agonists of the μ-opioid receptor, fentanyls are associated with a number of acute physiological effects, including respiratory depression.

Fentanyl analogues developed by pharmaceutical companies, but not sold, have properties similar to fentanyl. Non-pharmaceutical analogues have higher potencies than morphine, for example butyryl-fentanyl (1.5–7), acetylfentanyl and 4-fluorobutyrfentanyl (15.7), alpha-metylfentanyl (56.9), octafentanil (90), 3-methylfentanyl (48.5–569) and beta-hydroxy-3-methylfentanyl (6,300).[23]

Our knowledge of novel non-pharmaceutical analogues is limited, and these drugs may differ in their potency, efficacy and duration of action.[24,25]

There are differences between the various fentanyls. Butyrylfentanyl, for example, is a potent, short-acting synthetic opioid analgesic, around one-quarter of the potency of fentanyl. On the other hand, some fentanyl analogues are more potent than fentanyl and some fentanyl analogues have a longer duration of action.[26]

These new fentanyls have been associated with significant morbidity and mortality, including from illicitly manufactured fentanyls and fentanyl analogues.[27,28]

5.5 Mode and Patterns of Use of Fentanyl Novel Psychoactive Substances

Clandestinely manufactured fentanyl and/or its analogues are sold in solid or liquid forms,[13] including powders, pills, capsules, patches, lozenges and liquid, and on blotting paper. Although less common, furanylfentanyl has also been seized in Europe as a green 'herbal' material, as well as being sold as e-liquids for vaping in electronic cigarettes.[29,30,31]

Fentanyl and its analogues may be consumed by several routes, including injecting (intravenous or intramuscular), orally, trans-dermally, by smoking,[32] intra-nasally or sublingually through a spray or vaporisation.[31] Also worth noting are new forms of pharmaceutical fentanyl, for example oromucosal administration as 'lollipops'. One concern noted in the EMCDDA European Drug Report 2017 was the appearance on the market of nasal sprays containing non-pharmaceutical fentanyls, such as acryloylfentanyl and furanylfentanyl.[33]

The prevalence of use of fentanyl and NPS fentanyl varies significantly between European countries. In Estonia, for example, the majority of treatment entrants reporting an opioid as their primary drug were using fentanyl[34] and an endemic problem with fentanyl has existed since the early 2000s, with high rates of overdose in comparison with other EU countries. Fentanyl and 3-methylfentanyl have also been marketed in 2010–2012 as replacements for heroin in EU countries affected by heroin shortages (e.g. Bulgaria, Slovakia). Fentanyl and its analogues have also been reported in other European countries, for example in Germany, Finland and the UK, where fentanyl-related deaths have been mentioned,[35] as well as in Sweden, Hungary, Belgium, Switzerland and Poland.[36,37] In Estonia, the majority of treatment entrants reporting an opioid as their primary drug were using fentanyl.[38]

Fentanyl, fentanyl analogues and other new synthetic opioids are often also sold on the illicit market as heroin (or mixed with heroin) to people who believe they are receiving heroin. There are in addition reports from elsewhere in the world that they are also sold as, or mixed with, other illicit drugs and counterfeit medicines.[34] International evidence suggests that fentanyl products have also been found in products sold as cocaine or crack cocaine, 'black tar' heroin and MDMA.[13,39] Furthermore, there are reports of individuals purchasing prescription medication, such as oxycodone[40] and alprazolam,[41,42] on the Internet only to be sold counterfeit products that contain new fentanyls.[43,44]

5.6 Desired Effects of Fentanyls

All the fentanyl class drugs are associated with a feeling of warmth and euphoria. These effects can be more intense, but last a shorter time that those of morphine and diamorphine.[45] The effects of fentanyls that are desired by those who use them outside medical supervision are similar to those of other opioids and include analgesia, anxiolysis, euphoria, drowsiness and feelings of relaxation, with some suggestion that the latter are less pronounced than with heroin and morphine.[46,47]

There are reports of heroin users being suspicious that they had unknowingly consumed a new synthetic opioid or fentanyl, as their experience of the drug effect was different from normal.[48] Some research suggests that users who were initially unaware that they had used a fentanyl (initially believing that they were administering heroin) described the effects of fentanyls as stronger and qualitatively different from those of heroin,[49] or describe the experience as like taking heroin but more intense.[50,51,52]

5.7 Acute Harms of Fentanyls

The reported acute harms associated with the use of fentanyls are summarised in Table 5.1.

Intoxication associated with opioid NPS is characterised by a reduced level of consciousness, which can range from drowsiness to stupor, and resembles that produced by more classic opioid agents.[53]

The adverse effects of fentanyls are dose-dependent and are similar to those of other opioids. They include pruritus (itchy skin), constipation and delirium.[54] Adverse effects of fentanyl also include constipation, nausea, vomiting, itching, cough suppression, nasal burn or nasal drip after insufflation, a bitter taste after oral ingestion, anxiety, agitation, sweating, disorientation, orthostatic (or postural) hypotension and urinary urgency or retention, bradycardia and hypothermia. Other adverse effects linked to the use of fentanyls include dysphoria, depression, paranoia and hallucinations.[48,55,56]

The health risks associated with the use of fentanyl and its analogues are linked to the very high potency of the substances, leading to a high risk of overdose and respiratory depression.[57,58,59]

The misuse of fentanyls is associated with a high risk of acute toxicity, or ability to cause harm through a single or short-term exposure to the drug. For fentanyl, the estimated lethal dose in humans could be as low as 2 mg by intravenous injection. The features of opioid overdose include reduced level of consciousness, miosis and respiratory depression associated

Table 5.1 Fentanyl toxicity

Fentanyl toxicity	Fentanyl severe toxicity	Differences between heroin and fentanyl overdoses

• Miosis (pinpoint pupils)
 • Nausea, vomiting
 • Anxiety, agitation
 • Euphoria, dysphoria
 • Depression
 • Paranoia
 • Hallucinations
	• Respiratory and central nervous system depression
	 • Decreased consciousness
	 • Apnoea
	 • Can lead to deep coma, convulsions and respiratory arrest.
	 • Sudden-onset chest wall rigidity may be associated with increased risk of mortality
		• In comparison with heroin, intoxication with fentanyl and analogues presents with:
		    · Increased risk of overdose
		    · More rapid onset of overdose
		    · More rapid progression of signs and symptoms

with loss of respiratory reflexes and risk of aspiration. These may rapidly lead to respiratory arrest and death in the absence of appropriate medical treatment.[60]

Respiratory depression is associated with increasing doses and may occur with fentanyl more quickly after overdose than with heroin, reducing the window of opportunity for effective treatment with naloxone.[61]

Fentanyl causes dose-dependent respiratory depression, which has been reported by one study to be maximal 25 minutes after a single intravenous dose and to last as long as 2–3 hours.[56] Fentanyls can also be linked to apnoea, severe bradycardia, asystole, convulsions, respiratory arrest, deep coma and death.[62]

Fentanyl toxicity has been associated with chest wall rigidity, particularly when injected.[47,48,56,57,63–66] Fentanyl-induced respiratory muscle rigidity (FIRMR), can cause increased stiffness of the chest wall (also known as 'wooden chest') and laryngospasm (vocal cord closure), further restricting breathing. This effect of fentanyls is distinct from the respiratory depression caused by opioids and can occur rapidly after intravenous fentanyl use and occasionally after modest doses.[67,68,69] There are suggestions that sudden-onset chest wall rigidity is a significant factor in deaths from intravenous fentanyl use.[70]

Atypical characteristics in overdoses with fentanyl and analogues have been described to include:

- Immediate blue discolouration of the lips, gurgling sounds with breathing, foaming at the mouth, confusion, stiffening of the body or seizure-like activity, and confusion or strange affect before unresponsiveness;[71,72,73,74,75]
- Lung damage (including alveolar haemorrhage, haemoptysis and acute lung injury, with the NPS butyrfentanyl);[76]
- Toxic leukoencephalopathy characterised by cerebellar white matter;[77]
- Syncope and chest pain mimicking acute coronary syndrome;[78]
- Unusual amnestic syndrome associated with combined fentanyl and cocaine use that included acute, complete and bilateral hippocampal lesions on magnetic resonance imaging.[79]

One of the risks of overdose is directly related to the fact that a substantial number of people who had used fentanyl or its analogue NPS did not know that they had done so when they consumed the drug, but thought they were using heroin or another substance.[54] This can result in a user inadvertently consuming a significantly more potent and more unpredictable substance than intended.[13,44]

In addition to the risks associated with the potency of fentanyl and its analogues, fentanyl products sold online and on the black market pose a threat to public health, because of variable components and erratic adulteration[13,22] or because the potency of the substance is unpredictable.[56]

The risk of overdose is increased by unsafe methods of preparation and administration (especially intravenous injection), imprecise measuring by users, drug potency and users mostly being unaware of what they are consuming.[13] The EMCCDA has reported concerns over the apparent popularity of selling ready-to-use or using home-made nasal sprays containing solutions for the administration of fentanyls, including cyclopropylfentanyl. These typically contain milligram amounts of dissolved substance, but the dosage is imprecise and may lead to solutions with higher (or lower) concentrations.[80]

We do not know much about the adverse effects of the various fentanyl NPS; information, especially in humans, is currently very limited, however it is expected that they are similar to the harms of fentanyl.

There are differences between the various fentanyl NPS, as well as differences between the latter and fentanyl. As shown in Box 5.2, some NPS are less potent than fentanyl while others appear to be more potent.

In addition, it has been argued that the prolongation of effects (for some opioid NPS), and their frequent use in combination with other drugs increases the risk of serious drug interactions which can result in toxicity (e.g. respiratory depression) and opioid withdrawal symptoms (in the case of previously developed opioid tolerance).[81]

There is evidence from Europe that fentanyl NPS have been associated with overdose and deaths. For example, cases of acute intoxication suspected to be due to furanylfentanyl reported in Europe showed clinical features generally consistent with opioid-like toxicity and included life-threatening effects and death.[40,41] There are similar reports regarding acute toxicity and deaths linked to acryloylfentanyl and methoxyacetylfentanyl, including considerable risk of acute toxicity through respiratory depression.[42,82]

Box 5.2 Example of Fentanyl Novel Psychoactive Substances

Acetylfentanyl

Acetylfentanyl is a common novel opioid, with reported deaths from drug toxicity in several European countries and across much of the US. Acetylfentanyl is 5–15 times more potent than heroin, 16 times more potent than morphine, but its potency is one third that of fentanyl.[96] It has been reported that the range between the therapeutic dose as a medication dose and the lethal dose of acetylfentanyl when it is misused is narrower than that of morphine and fentanyl, which increases the risk of a fatal overdose.[97] Acetylfentanyl has been associated with deaths that have occurred when used by insufflation as well as intravenously and orally. Almost all cases are fatalities from poly-drug use or use of multiple drugs.[98]

Furanylfentanyl

Furanylfentanyl is more potent than morphine but approximately five times less potent than fentanyl. Deaths associated with it have been reported in Canada, Sweden and the US.[98]

Acrylfentanyl also known as acryloylfentanyl is slightly more potent than fentanyl in displacing labelled naloxone from the mu-opioid receptor. Deaths have been reported and have included evidence of nasal insufflation of both sprays and crushed tablets.[98]

Butyrylfentanyl: Also Known as Butyrfentanyl

Butyrylfentanyl is a potent short-acting synthetic opioid analgesic, around one-quarter of the potency of fentanyl, but approximately seven times more potent than morphine

Butyrylfentanyl has no current legitimate clinical use. It appears to be in the form of powder, tablets, capsules, blotters, liquids or in injectable formulas. It could be administered orally, nasally (using sprays), by snorting, smoking or by intravenous injection. Butyrylfentanyl has been associated with deaths in Europe and the US.[99,100]

4-Fluorobutyrylfentanyl

It is usually in the form of powder or a nasal spray, liquids, tablets or capsules. It is used orally, nasally (with sprays), by snorting, smoking, by intravenous injection rectally or by heating the drug and inhaling the vapour. It is available on the Internet added to heroin, often without the user's knowledge. Fatalities have been reported.[101]

Ocfentanil

This opioid is about twice as potent as fentanyl, with reported cases of associated deaths when no other drugs were apparently involved.[101]

Methylfentanyls

3-Methylfentanyl is approximately 7,000 times more potent than morphine and has been associated with morbidity and mortality for many years, but first reported in the US in the 1980s. More recently, deaths have been reported in Finland[102] and later in an epidemic in Estonia.[103,104,105]

Carfentanyl

Carfentanyl is an analogue of fentanyl, and is one of the most potent opioids known and used commercially. Carfentanyl has been approved for use in veterinary medicine as a general anaesthetic agent or as a tranquillising agent for large-animal use only.

Carfentanyl is 10,000 times more potent than morphine and 100 times more potent than fentanyl,[106] with activity in humans starting at about 1 microgram. There have been cases of carfentanyl laced with or disguised as heroin, leading to a number of deaths.[107]

The non-medical use of fentanyl has been implicated in a significant and increasing number of deaths in several countries, including some European countries, Australia and Japan.[47,83,84,85,86] In Canada and the US, the problem of opioid-related overdose death has been particularly severe for a number of years.[87,88,89,90,91] In the US, it has been suggested that the increases in the numbers of deaths involving opioid NPS are being driven by increases in the numbers of deaths involving fentanyl, which are likely due to illicitly manufactured fentanyl.[92]

Deaths related to opioid NPS, including fentanyls, have been reported in Europe, albeit at a significantly lower rate. Nonetheless deaths were reported where fentanyl NPS were implicated including acryloylfentanyl, furanylfentanyl methoxyacetylfentanyl and cyclopropylfentanyl.[93,94]

It has been reported by the EMCDDA that highly potent opioid NPS, and the fentanyl derivatives in particular, appear to be playing an increasing role in drug overdose in Europe.[95] Deaths related to a number of fentanyls and analogues have been reported in Sweden and other Nordic countries as well as a small number in the US.[96] Deaths where other fentanyl NPS were implicated include acetyl-fentanyl, acrylfentanyl, butr(yl)fentanyl, carfentanil, 2- and 4-fluorofentanyls, 4-fluorobutyrfentanyl, 4-fluoroisobutyrfentanyl, furanylfentanyl, a- and 3-methylfentanyls, 4-methoxyfentanyl, ocfentanil[96] and 4-methoxybutyrfentanyl.[96]

5.8 Differences between Heroin and Fentanyl Acute Toxicity

The high potency of fentanyls, as well as their rapid onset of action, contributes to making them particularly dangerous in comparison with heroin when used in a non-medical setting.[15,108,109] A report from a drug consumption room in Australia found that, under medical surveillance, the risk of overdose when injecting fentanyl was two times higher than when injecting heroin, and eight times higher than when injecting other prescription opioids.[110]

Fentanyl overdose can begin suddenly, rapidly progress to death and manifest atypical physical symptoms. In comparison with heroin overdose, where death typically does not occur until at least 20–30 minutes after use,[111] fentanyl can be associated with potentially lethal respiratory depression within 2 minutes.[22,43,112]

Fatalities associated with fentanyl often also involve the concurrent use of other substances, such as cocaine and heroin.[113,107,110] The use of fentanyl (and analogues) at the same time as other CNS depressants (e.g. alcohol, benzodiazepine, pregabalin, gabapentin) can have serious adverse effects; poly-drug use has been reported to be common among fentanyl-related fatalities in Europe[31] and elsewhere.[114]

Injecting is the most commonly reported route of administration of fentanyl in fatal overdoses, but deaths linked with other modes of use of fentanyl have also been reported. For example, a study looking at fentanyl-related deaths in the US from July to December 2016 reported that one in five deaths involving fentanyl or fentanyl analogues had evidence of insufflation, smoking or ingestion and no evidence of injecting.[115] This is an important distinction from heroin, whereby deaths are most likely to be associated with intravenous injecting.

5.9 Poly-drug Use

As with other opioids, the combined use of fentanyl with other CNS and respiratory depressants, such as alcohol or benzodiazepines, is linked to increased toxicity. Studies have recommended the ongoing need for targeted messages on risks of synthetic opioids alone, as well as their use in combination with alcohol and other CNS depressants.[116]

In general, the use of opioids with other CNS depressants, such as alcohol or benzodiazepines, increases CNS depression which can lead to respiratory distress, coma and death.

A new trend which has also been reported is fentanyl that is added to cocaine for the purpose of 'speedballing', to combine the rush of the stimulant (cocaine) with a drug that depresses the CNS (fentanyl), thus helping to ease the after effects. People who use drugs may also be inadvertently exposed to fentanyl or other opioid NPS when they are unknowingly taking cocaine or other drugs that are laced with them. In this case, a drug interaction can also occur and the user can have unexpected adverse effects.[117]

Like other opioids, opioid NPS including fentanyls will interact with other illicit substances, as well as medication.[118] Amphetamines in combination with opiates enhance the sense of euphoria.[119] Dexamphetamine and methylphenidate increase the analgesic effects of morphine and other opioids and reduce their sedative and respiratory depressant effects.[120,121] Combinations involving amphetamine-like substances with certain opioids may increase the risk of serotonin syndrome through effects on the serotonin transporter or serotonin receptors (tramadol and fentanyl most frequently implicated).[122]

The use of fentanyl in combination with inhibitors of the isoenzymes CYP450 3A4 and CYP450 3A5 may result in increased plasma concentration of fentanyl (and probably new analogues), thus increasing the risk of poisoning, including potentially fatal respiratory depression. Inhibitors include ritonavir, clarithromycin, erythromycin, fluconazole, indinavir, itraconazole, ketoconazole, nefazodone, saquinavir, verapamil and grapefruit juice.[31]

There is limited evidence that use of fentanyl with serotoninergic agents (prescribed medication including SSRIs, SNRIs or MAOIs, or illicit substances, such as MDMA) may be associated with serotonin syndrome.[123] It is not known if this association is also seen with fentanyl derivatives.[31]

Buprenorphine is predicted to increase the risk of precipitated opioid withdrawal when given with fentanyl.[124]

5.10 Lack of Testing

Analytical methods for detecting fentanyl and other opioid NPS use are very limited at present and it is unlikely that onsite testing is currently available in hospital laboratories.

Standard immunoassay screening tests in the clinical setting do not detect synthetic opioids. More complex methods are required, such as gas chromatography mass spectrometry or liquid chromatography mass spectrometry. Testing is complicated by the fact that tests for fentanyl may not detect all analogues.

5.11 Management of Acute Toxicity

The evidence on the management of acute adverse effects associated specifically with the misuse of fentanyl and its analogue NPS and overdose is limited, but emerging.[22] However, they are broadly similar to other fentanyls and opioids, with effects potentially reversed by naloxone.[125]

There are several documents and guidance issues by international organisations aimed at addressing the prevention of drug-related deaths[126] and the principles they suggest should inform clinical practice. The World Health Organization (WHO) published guidelines for the community management of opioid overdose in 2014.[127] As shown in Table 5.2 below, the use of naloxone for opioid overdose is recommended. This is also recommended by the EMCDDA.[128,129]

Naloxone plays an important role in preventing deaths associated with opioids, including fentanyl. Naloxone reverses the features of opioid toxicity, improving the level of consciousness and respiratory rate. Naloxone is very effective provided it can be administered in adequate doses before irreversible effects occur, such as brain damage resulting from lack of oxygen delivery.[130]

There are clear distinctions between the responses to opioid overdose carried out in community settings and responses in hospital or other acute medical settings. At a global level, access to naloxone is generally limited to health professionals and it is a prescription medicine in almost all countries, although there has been an increase in recent years of 'take home' naloxone schemes.

5.12 Clinical Settings

Clinicians should refer to their national and local protocols and guidelines on naloxone regimens and administration.

WHO guidelines[131] make recommendations on the use of naloxone for the management of opioid overdose. They recommend using a dose of 0.4 mg naloxone and repeating the dose if necessary, and suggest monitoring the person for 4 hours after resuscitation. These guidelines also state that long-acting-opioid overdose may need to be managed in hospital, with assisted ventilation and/or naloxone infusion.

Table 5.2 World Health Organization recommendations

Recommendation	Strength of recommendation	Quality of evidence
People likely to witness an opioid overdose should have access to naloxone and be instructed in its administration to enable them to use it for emergency management of suspected opioid overdose	Strong	Very low
Naloxone is effective when delivered by intravenous, intramuscular, subcutaneous and intranasal routes of administration. Persons using naloxone should select a route of administration based on the formulation available, their skills in administration, the setting and local context	Conditional	Very low
In suspected opioid overdose, first responders should focus on airway management, assisting ventilation and administering naloxone	Strong	Very low
After successful resuscitation following the administration of naloxone, the level of consciousness and breathing of the affected person should be closely monitored until full recovery has been achieved	Strong	Very low

Source: WHO, 2014

It has been suggested that naloxone regimens developed for the reversal of heroin overdose are likely to be effective for the majority of cases of fentanyl toxicity, however, the total dose may be too low, and the rate of administration too slow for the most severe cases.[132] The dose of naloxone required in an emergency is dependent upon many factors. Some patients with fentanyl overdose have required relatively high doses of naloxone, with up to 2.4 mg being reported.[133]

There are a number of naloxone regimens. In the UK for example, current recommended naloxone dosing in the UK for acute treatment of adults with heroin overdose by healthcare professionals is an initial injection of 0.4 mg. If this is ineffective, a further injection should be administered after 1 minute; this can be repeated after another minute if needed (total dose 2.0 mg). If that is ineffective, a further dose of 2.0 mg is advised.[134] This regimen allows the administration of up to 4 mg naloxone within 3 minutes for those patients who need a high dose.[135] A rapid dose titration is also appropriate for those exposed to highly potent analogues such as carfentanil.[136]

Naloxone, however, is not effective for treating fentanyl-induced respiratory muscle rigidity (FIRMR) or laryngospasm triggered by fentanyls, where the use of a muscle relaxant, endotracheal intubation and mechanical ventilation are required.[137] Other potential challenges include the fact that some fentanyl analogues have a prolonged duration of effect, whereas naloxone has a relatively short half-life. Initially effective treatment may be followed by a relapse of the symptoms of opioid overdose, especially if a longer-acting fentanyl has been used. This necessitates longer medical observation.[137]

There are reports of multiple doses of naloxone sometimes being required.[71] Because the length of time is shorter between substance use and potentially life-threatening respiratory depression with fentanyl than with heroin, the reversal of the fentanyl overdose may be less likely than with heroin, as the naloxone can be administered late. There have been reports of unsuccessful attempts to revive with naloxone despite administration of multiple or escalating doses. Despite the standard resuscitation procedures indicating the potential need to administer repeat doses of naloxone, the clinical outcome of fentanyl poisoning may vary from case to case.[138]

There are other challenges. The prompt administration of naloxone in an emergency situation can reverse respiratory depression and can be lifesaving, but giving too much can lead to an acute withdrawal syndrome. It has been noted that the naloxone administration regimen must be based on an appropriate and flexible strategy which balances the risk of delayed reversal of respiratory depression with that of causing acute withdrawal from excessive naloxone use.[139]

However, some people argue for the use of high doses of naloxone, despite the risk of acute withdrawal.[140] For example, Moss et al. (2019) have argued that the benefit of adequately reversing opioid toxicity outweighs the risk of opioid withdrawal syndrome.[140]

It has been argued opioid NPS, including fentanyls, do not require hospital clinical staff to change their approach to the management of acute opioid toxicity and overdose.[141] It has been suggested that initial care of the opioid-intoxicated patient should focus on protecting the airway and maintaining breathing and circulation, as in any emergency. External stimulation should be attempted in all patients, and an external ventilatory support mask device should be provided for those with profound hypoventilation.[148]

- Anticipatory titration of naloxone with the goal of restoring ventilatory drive remains the mainstay for patients who do not respond in a sustained fashion to the above.[148] Overdoses can be reversed through the use of naloxone as in the case of other opioids, together with appropriate supportive care.[142]

- It has been proposed that clinical suspicion may be sufficient to carry out empirical treatment with naloxone, considering that there are no significant side-effects to its use in such circumstances.[149]

- Potent, faster-acting synthetic opioids, such as fentanyls, make it more difficult to balance the need for an effective opioid antidote with the risks of precipitated withdrawal.[143]

5.12.1 Administering Naloxone in Community Settings

It is acknowledged that overdoses are often witnessed by a family member, friend or peer and that increased access to naloxone for people likely to witness an overdose could significantly reduce the high numbers of opioid overdose deaths.[144] There is evidence on the effectiveness of training family members or peers in how to administer the drug.[145]

'Take-home' naloxone (THN) programmes are now increasingly available in Europe. They aim to make naloxone more readily available in places where overdoses might occur and to expand the availability of naloxone to opioid-using peers, family members and other trained laypeople. THN programmes can also target other potential first responders to an overdose, such as healthcare providers, staff in homeless shelters and police and prison officers. As part of these programmes, trainees learn how to correctly recognise and respond to an overdose, including administration of naloxone, before the arrival of emergency medical help.[146]

It has been argued that the same principles of response with THN initiatives apply to the prevention of deaths from fentanyl overdose as with other opioids, although early administration of naloxone is likely crucial.[147]

A number of naloxone products for THN are dispensed in different European countries, including injectable formulation (including ampoules and pre-filled syringes) and nasal sprays. In the case of suspected fentanyl overdose, it is suggested that training for THN should emphasise:

- The importance of calling ambulance or emergency services promptly and transfer to hospital, especially in cases where naloxone is not available in the community, or if there is need for prolonged naloxone administration, which may be the case for fentanyl overdose.
- It has also been suggested that more advanced resuscitation skills (such as chest compressions and automatic defibrillators) may need to be more widely incorporated into community emergency response training to tackle fentanyl overdose, and is vital if responsiveness to naloxone administration is inadequate or delayed.[33]

However, there is growing evidence that higher doses or multiple administrations of naloxone are required to fully reverse the toxicity of illicitly manufactured fentanyl analogues. Recently, the US Food and Drug Administration approved THN kits with a concentrated naloxone dose that produce high bioavailability. However, their accessibility to the general public is limited.[148] There are also some reports that small-scale interventions targeted at fentanyl have been developed based on the assumption that take-home naloxone kits provided to users of opioid NPS may require higher doses of naloxone than those provided to heroin users.[149] There are reports of some naloxone programmes providing more than the standard two doses of naloxone, and others have begun utilising higher-dose devices.[22] More research is needed to assess whether the approach will prove to be effective.

Other interventions to prevent fentanyl-related harm include the use of fentanyl test strips as an opioid overdose prevention strategy by allowing users to test if fentanyl analogues are mixed with heroin and often sold to unwitting consumers.[150,151] A study has demonstrated that devices for fentanyl drug checking are valid.[152]

5.13 Chronic Harms and Dependence

Despite limited evidence, it is assumed that fentanyls, including the novel analogues, have a high potential

---

Box 5.3 Overdose Management: Fentanyl in Comparison with Heroin Overdose

The broad principles of management apply to all opioids, with the following to be taken into account where fentanyl is suspected:

- Where the use of fentanyls is suspected, there is a need to call emergency services and transfer to hospital, especially in cases where naloxone is not available in the community, or if there is need for prolonged naloxone administration.
- A more rapid escalation of additional doses of naloxone may be needed in comparison with heroin or other opioids.
- Overall, higher doses of naloxone may be needed for fentanyl patients than for heroin patients.
- A longer period of clinical observation is advised for fentanyl patients than for heroin patients.
- In cases of heroin overdose, some have suggested that patients with heroin-induced respiratory depression can be safely discharged from hospital after a one-hour observation period.[153] Armenian et al. argued that this is not recommended for opioid NPS, including fentanyls, which may require larger and repeated doses of naloxone and require a longer period of observation because symptoms may recur when the naloxone wears off.[23]
- They also recommend that due to the extremely high potency and lack of human pharmacokinetic and clinical overdose knowledge of carfentanyl, that all carfentanyl cases be monitored for 24 hours in the hospital setting.[23]

for harmful use and a high dependence liability that is similar to, or greater than morphine.

Increasing numbers of people are entering drug treatment for fentanyl-related harmful or dependent use. In the US, where there is currently a significantly higher level of fentanyl use than in the UK, a study of people entering drug treatment reported that fentanyl misuse increased modestly from 2012 to 2016. However, it also showed that whereas the misuse of branded fentanyl products remained stable, the misuse of 'unknown' fentanyls, presumed to be non-pharmaceutical fentanyl, increased significantly.[154] In Estonia, data from specialised drug treatment centres indicate that opioid NPS (mainly non-pharmaceutical fentanyl or 3 methylfentanyl) were the most commonly reported primary substances for first-time clients entering treatment in 2015. In more recent years, fentanyl has become the main injected opioid substance in that country.[155]

Fentanyls are associated with tolerance and withdrawal symptoms. Reports from users suggest the development of tolerance, withdrawal-like symptoms and physiological dependence similar to those with other opioids.[156,157] Characteristic withdrawal symptoms include sweating, anxiety, diarrhoea, bone pain, abdominal cramps and shivers or 'goose flesh'.[47,48]

5.14 Other Long-term Effects

There is some limited evidence that the long-term use of fentanyl has also been associated with: hyperalgesia (opioid-induced abnormal pain sensitivity, also called paradoxical hyperalgesia);[158] gastrointestinal disturbance;[159] immunological dysfunction;[166] hormonal disruption;[166] muscle rigidity and myoclonus.[166] Among older people in particular, long-term use of fentanyl is linked to raised risk of fracture and acute myocardial infarction[160] and generally increased mortality.[161]

5.15 Public Health Risks: Injecting and Other High-Risk Drug-Using Behaviours

It has been argued that fentanyl and its analogues pose distinct risks for the transmission of blood-borne viruses such as hepatitis C and HIV.[162] There is also some evidence that use is associated with high-risk behaviours. Users of illicit fentanyl in Toronto, for example, reported engaging in practices that exposed them to blood-borne viruses.[169] It has also been associated with

bacterial infections and vein damage, with one study showing how fentanyl injecting-related harms are exacerbated by the use of lemon juice or vinegar, which can cause vein damage when injected.[163]

There have been suggestions that fentanyl-specific harm-reduction information be developed. It has been suggested that 'an increase in fentanyl-related overdoses and deaths suggests that information about how to reduce harms associated with injecting fentanyl is lacking'. In their study of the non-medical use of fentanyl patches, users reported lack of knowledge of the drug they were using, including exactly what it was, how to extract it and how to measure the dose. Peer networks were identified as the key source of information in drug-using practices, but information shared was poor, even dangerous.[163]

5.16 Management of Fentanyl and Other Opioid Novel Psychoactive Substances Dependence

There is little published information on the management of dependence and withdrawal specifically for fentanyl misuse or its analogues. Methadone and buprenorphine are listed by the World Health Organization (WHO) as essential medicines for the pharmacological treatment for opioid use disorders to reduce cravings and withdrawal symptoms. Methadone has been used in cases of fentanyl dependence. In Estonia, where the most commonly reported primary substances for first-time clients entering treatment in 2015 were fentanyls, most clients received opioid substitution therapy (OST) and methadone in particular. As with any effective treatment of dependence, pharmacology should be complemented by psycho-social interventions.

The management of dependence associated with fentanyl and analogues is similar to that of other opioids and requires a bio-psycho-social response. It is sometimes appropriate to stabilise opioid-dependent patients on to a prescribed opioid in the context of care-planned treatment and support. While the evidence base is limited for fentanyl and analogue NPS, buprenorphine or methadone are often used and there is a good body of evidence to support pharmacological interventions for relapse prevention or craving management for opiates, although evidence on NPS opioids is limited.

Pharmacological interventions and substitute prescribing must involve a psycho-social component to help support an individual's recovery. As with all drug treatment, a psycho-social response is also required as part of the treatment plan, including assessment of co-occurring physical, mental and social morbidity.

5.17 Other Novel Synthetic Opioids (Non-fentanyl)

In addition to fentanyl and its analogues, in the past years more than a dozen additional opioid NPS have entered the illicit opioid market. These were all first synthesised in the 1970s[163] by pharmaceutical companies, but never progressed to clinical trials or were never used in pharmaceutical or medicinal products. Some have been redis-covered by traffickers from research published between the 1960s and 1990s, when they were described in the scientific literature but never developed into pharmaceutical products.

Newly marketed opioid NPS have appeared with structures distinct from those used in medical practice. Examples include, but are not limited to, AH-7921 (a benzamide), U-47700 (a compound closely related to AH-7921) and MT-45 (a pipera-zine), U448800, U-77891, U-50488, U-51754, and O-desmethyltramadol.[164] See Box 5.4.

5.18 Pharmacology

Opioid NPS have lower potencies than fentanyl, but are more potent than morphine.[166]

Most opioid NPS have mechanisms of action and effects similar to established opioids, with their main effects mediated through activation of μ-opioid receptors (for example, U-47700 is a potent μ-

---

Box 5.4 Chemical Structures of Opioid Novel Psychoactive Substances

Opioid NPS have different chemical structures. For example:

- AH-7921 is 3,4-dichloro-N-(1-(dimethylamino) cyclohexylmethyl)benzamide;
- U-47700 is trans-3,4-dichloro-N-(2-(dimethylamino)cyclohexyl)-N-methylbenzamide;
- MT-45 is 1-cyclohexyl-4-(1,2-diphenylethyl) piperazine;
- U-448800, and U77891 are benzamides;
- U-50488 and U-51754 are acetamides.[165]

---

opioid receptor agonist; AH-7921 is an agonist of μ and κ receptors; and MT-45 is an agonist of μ-, κ- and δ-opioid receptors.). However, some opioid NPS have different mechanisms of action. U-50488 is mainly a κ-opioid receptor agonist that has been studied in animal models as an analgesic, antitussive, diuretic, and anticonvulsant. Its side effects include dysphoria and hallucinations, and it has been reported to present μ-opioid receptor antagonist effects. U-51754 is not as selective for k-opioid receptor.[167]

The pharmacology, availability and modes of use of these three substances are outlined in Table 5.3.

5.19 Availability and Mode of Use

Opioid NPS are generally found on websites selling so-called 'research chemicals'. They are usually con-sumed orally, but can also be used by inhalation/vaporising, nasal insufflation, sub-lingually, intraven-ous injection or rectal administration and are sold as a powder, tablets and capsules.[176,177,178] See Box 5.4. Opioid NPS are marketed as stand-alone products but are also found as adulterants in heroin and in coun-terfeit opioid medications.[179]

5.20 Desired Effects

Based on user reports, the effects of opioid NPS appear to resemble those of classical opioids including mild euphoria and relaxation.[184,185] Some users report self-medicating to relieve pain, others to alleviate withdrawal symptoms due to cessation of other opioids. It has also been noted that the effects are not only the general and expected opioid effects, but some opioid NPS also show other unanticipated effects including increased energy, reduced inhibition and a facilitation of social situations.[186] In one study, people who used opioid NPS reported 'pleasure and enjoyment', 'coping with life challenges' and addictive character of these substances.[187]

The effects desired by users are listed in Table 5.5.

5.21 Unwanted and Adverse Effects of Intoxication

AH-7921, U-47700 and MT-45 have broadly similar profiles of unwanted and adverse effects, as shown in Table 5.6. Signs of intoxication include[196]:

Table 5.3 Non-fentanyl opioid novel psychoactive substances: brief pharmacology

Pharmacology		
AH-7921	**U-47700**	**MT-45**
AH-7921 is an opioid analgesic patented by Allen and Hanburys Ltd in 1976 but has never been used in a pharmaceutical or medicinal product. Thought to be a morphine-like analgesic acting mainly as a μ-opioid receptor agonist. Human data are mostly not available, but animal studies have shown that AH-7921 is approximately as potent as morphine with regard to respiratory depression, antinociception, sedation and miosis (decrease in pupil diameter), decrease in body temperature and inhibition of gut propulsion[168,169,170]	U-47700 is an opioid analgesic and is structurally related to AH-7921. Although U-47700 exhibits some k-opioid receptor agonism, it has far more activity at the μ-opioid receptors.[49] It is a selective μ-opioid receptor agonist, and in animal models has been demonstrated to have ~7.5 times the potency of morphine.[171,172,173] According to user reports, U-47700 acts longer than AH-7921[26]	MT-45, also known as IC-6, was developed in the 1970s as an alternative to morphine for analgesia. It is an N,N-di-substituted 4-(1,2-diphenylethyl) piperazine chemically unrelated to other opioid agonists. The pharmacology of MT-45 is complex and involves opioid and non-opioid receptors that have not been fully characterised; however, it has been demonstrated in animal studies to have approximately the same potency as morphine.[174] It appears that MT-45 has a slow onset of action, greater than 1–2 hours when taken orally, which may increase the risk of toxic overdose from redosing before peak effect is reached[175]

Table 5.4 Availability and Mode of Use

AH-7921	**U-47700**	**MT-45**
AH-7921 has been available in Europe since mid-2012 via websites selling 'research chemicals'. AH-7921 is sold as a free base and as a hydrochloride salt in a white/off-white powder form,[180] but has also been detected in Japan as a co-ingredient in synthetic cannabinoid and cathinones.[181] AH-7921 is usually consumed orally but can also be used by inhalation/vaporising, nasal insufflation, sub-lingually, intravenous injection or rectal administration and is sold as a powder, tablet or capsule	In the recreational drug market, U-47700 is sometimes referred to as 'pink', because it can be slightly pink in colour. The drug is also known as 'U4'.[182] It is taken orally, nasally, rectally, by smoking, intravenous injection or by combinations of these routes[26]	MT-45 is typically sold on the Internet or illicit market as a dihydrochloride salt. Typical routes of administration include oral, insufflation, intravenous and intramuscular. Rectal use has also been reported.[57] It has been found mixed with other drugs, including synthetic cannabinoids and synthetic cathinones[183]

- Miosis (pinpoint pupils), with the exception of MT-45, which has only a small miotic effect
- Nausea, vomiting
- Anxiety, agitation
- Euphoria, dysphoria
- Depression
- Paranoia
- Hallucinations

These opioid NPS have a broadly similar, or higher potential to morphine in inducing analgesia; acute harms include respiratory depression, hypothermia and dependence liability.[194,195,196,197,198]

Severe opioid toxicity produces depression of the respiratory and central nervous systems. If untreated, the depression of the level of consciousness can lead to deep coma, convulsions and respiratory arrest.

5.22 Management of Acute Intoxication and Overdose

Opioid NPS are currently not tested as a routine part of most forensic drug screening. However, it has been argued that the clinical approach in managing opioid toxicity and overdose should not change and should include the management of airways and the administration of naloxone to reverse the overdose.[209]

AH-7921, U-47700 and MT-45 require similar management of acute intoxication and overdose to

Table 5.5 Desired effects of three novel synthetic opioids

AH-7921	U-47700	MT-45
Much of what we know about its effects comes from reports of people who have used it. Based on this, the effects of AH-7921 appear to resemble those of classic opioids Experience with AH-7921 was described as predictable and repetitive. Effects reported by users include nausea and vertigo, 'opiate glow', alertness, occasional itching, nausea and tremors[188] AH-7921 produces relaxation, euphoria, a physical anaesthetic effect, mental relaxation and pleasant mood lift.[189] An interesting finding reported by one study was that the users of AH-7921 (as well as of MT-45) report experiences of increased energy[190] There are reports of its use as self-medication to relieve pain or to alleviate withdrawal symptoms due to cessation of the use of other opioids[197] The dissociative effects of AH-7921 were also reported[191]	Based on animal models, it is expected that U-47700 produces effects similar to those of other potent opioid agonists, including analgesia, sedation, euphoria.[192] It has been suggested that U-47700 induces significant euphoria, which is short-lived and causes an urge to keep 'redosing'[193]	Effects similar to other opioids[57]

Table 5.6 Unwanted and adverse effects of intoxication of three novel synthetic opioids
All opioid NPS are associated with respiratory depression. Other adverse effects and acute harms include the following:

AH-7921	U-47700	MT45
A study found that morphine has a twofold greater safety margin than AH-7921, which suggests readier appearance of toxic effects after AH-7921 use[199,200] The side-effects range from milder symptoms (e.g. stomach upsets, light headache) to more severe conditions (e.g. anxiety and panic)[197] Other reported adverse effects include abdominal pain, constipation, reduced mobility, light-headedness, headache, urinary retention, visual impairment, pain in the mouth Unwanted adverse effects also include vertigo induced by movement.[196] Users also reported itching as one of the side-effects of AH-7921 use, as well as other forms of skin irritation. There are also reports of numbing of different parts of the body[197] Temperature change, tremors, numbness, blister, seizures, hypertension and tachycardia and respiratory depression have also been reported[201]	Based on animal models, it is expected that U-47700 produces effects similar to those of other potent opioid agonists including constipation, itching and respiratory depression[41,199]	MT-45 has only a small miotic effect (restriction of pupils or pinned pupils),[202] in contrast to other commonly used opioid drugs Although MT-45 is structurally unrelated to morphine, it has analgesic and CNS depressant properties similar to those of morphine, including respiratory depression.[203] Some animal studies suggest a higher toxicity than morphine[210] Drug users also report some dissociative-like symptoms.[181] Other reported unwanted effects include nausea, itching, bilateral hearing loss and possible withdrawal symptoms A unique feature of MT-45 toxicity is its association with ototoxicity – that is, it is linked with hearing loss, with a reported case of bilateral hearing loss lasting for 2 weeks[57,182] MT-45 has been associated with bilateral hearing loss, hair depigmentation and loss, folliculitis, dermatitis, dry eyes, liver enzyme alteration and leukonychia striata on the nails. Cataracts have also been observed[204,205,206,207] Other symptoms including dry and scaly skin, angular cheilitis, cracks on the fingers and under the feet, redness and moist

Table 5.6 (cont.)

AH-7921	U-47700	MT45
		maceration of the groin and armpits, and total alopecia, as well as loss of taste, smell and chills almost constantly, elevated levels of the enzymes aspartate transaminase (AST) and alanine transaminase (ALT), sudden hearing loss and deafness, irritated and dry eyes, culminating in loss of vision and almost blindness, imposing the need for cataract surgery performed on both eyes[208]
Deaths		
Overall, it seems that lethal doses for opioid NPS are often variable and deaths associated with these compounds seem to occur at both low and high concentrations, probably due to different levels of tolerance and individual differences. In most cases, opioid NPS associated with death also involves other drugs as well[209]		
AH-7921 has been associated with fatal overdoses, including a small number of deaths in the UK[187,210,211,212,213,214] Deaths associated with AH-7921 seem to occur both at low and high concentrations, possibly a result of different levels of tolerance to the drug[215] As with other overdose deaths, poly-drug use has been involved in many AH-7921 deaths,[175,196] but AH-7921 use alone has also been reported[222]	Deaths reported[199,200,216,217]	Deaths reported in Europe and elsewhere[57,199,218,219,220,221,222,223,224,225]

those required for other opioids (see Section 5.11). It has been suggested that emergency responders may have difficulty in identifying MT-45 overdose because the drug produces a small miotic effect (restriction of pupils) and this is important for clinical staff to be aware of.[209]

As opioid NPS have various potencies, receptor affinities and street concentrations, it has been argued that it is possible only to speculate about the doses of naloxone required for reversal and this should be determined on a case-by-case and drug-by-drug basis.[148]

5.23 Chronic Effects and Dependence

Despite limited evidence, it is assumed that AH-7921 and U-47700 have a high addictive potential similar to or greater than that of morphine.[57,226] Reports from users suggest the development of tolerance and of withdrawal-like symptoms with MT-45, AH-7921 and U-47700 is similar to that with other opioids. Withdrawal symptoms have been described as feelings of depression and mild insomnia and have been classified to be worse than those for morphine.[227]

5.24 Managing Dependence

The management of dependence will be the same as for other opioids and opioid NPS, including fentanyl. See Section 5.16.

References

1. Karila L, Marillier M, Chaumette B, Billieux J, Franchitto N, Benyamina A. New synthetic opioids: part of a new addiction landscape. *Neurosci Biobehav Rev* 2019;**106**:133–140.

2. Stoicea N, Costa A, Periel L, Uribe A, Weaver T, Bergese SD. Current perspectives on the opioid crisis in the US healthcare system: a comprehensive literature review. *Medicine* 2019;**98** (20):e15425. https://doi.org/10.1097/MD.0000000000015425

3. European School Survey Project on Alcohol and Other Drugs. Published 2015. Available at: www.espad.org/sites/espad.org/files/ESPAD_report_2015.pdf [last accessed 28 February 2022].

4. European Monitoring Centre for Drugs and Drug Addiction. European Drug Report 2019: Trends and Developments. Publications Office of the European Union, Luxembourg, 2019.

5. European Monitoring Centre for Drugs and Drug Addiction. European Drug Report 2019: Trends and Developments. Publications Office of the European Union, Luxembourg, 2019.

6. Pichini S, Solimini R, Berretta P, Pacifici R, Busardò FP. Acute intoxications and fatalities from illicit fentanyl and analogues: an update. *Ther Drug Monit* 2018;**40**:38–51. https://doi.org/10.1097/FTD.0000000000 000465

7. Schifano F, Chiappini S, Corkery JM, Guirguis A. Assessing the 2004–2018 fentanyl misusing issues reported to an international range of adverse reporting systems. *Front Pharmacol* 2019;**10**:46.

8. The United Nations Office on Drugs and Crime (UNODC). World Drug Report 2019 (United Nations publication, Sales No. E.19.XI.8). Available at: https://wdr.unodc.org/wdr2019/prelaunch/WDR19_Booklet_1_EXECUTIVE_SUMMARY.pdf; www.unodc.org/wdr2018/prelaunch/WDR18_Booklet_1_EXSUM.pdf [last accessed 28 February 2022].

9. Schifano F, Chiappini S, Corkery JM, Guirguis A. Assessing the 2004–2018 fentanyl misusing issues reported to an international range of adverse reporting systems. *Front Pharmacol* 2019;**10**:46.

10. European Monitoring Centre for Drugs and Drug Addiction. European Drug Report 2019: Trends and Developments. Publications Office of the European Union, Luxembourg, 2019.

11. The United Nations Office on Drugs and Crime (UNODC). World Drug Report 2020 (United Nations publication, Sales No. E.20.XI.6).

12. United Nations Office on Drugs and Crime (UNODC). Fentanyl and its analogues – 50 years on. Global SMART Update, 2017.

13. Ayres WA, Starsiak MJ, Sokolay P. The bogus drug: three methyl and alpha methyl fentanyl sold as 'China White'. *J Psychoactive Drugs* 1981;**13**(1):91–93.

14. Higashikawa Y, Suzuki S. Studies on 1-(2-phenethyl)-4-(N-propionylanilino) piperidine (fentanyl) and its related compounds. VI. Structure–analgesic activity relationship for fentanyl, methyl-substituted fentanyls and other analogues. *Forensic Toxicol* 2008;**26**(1):1–5. https://doi.org/10.1007/s11419-007-0039-1

15. Advisory Council on the Misuse of Drugs (ACMD). Misuse of Fentanyl and Fentanyl Analogues. January 2020.0

16. Lemmens H. Pharmacokinetic-pharmacodynamic relationships for opioids in balanced anaesthesia. *Clin Pharmacokinet* 1995;**29**:231–242.

17. Janssen PA. Potent, new analgesics, tailormade for different purposes. *Acta Anaesthesiol Scand* 1982;**26**(3):262–268.

18. Pichini S, Zaami S, Pacifici R, Tagliabracci A, Busardò FP. The challenge posed by new synthetic opioids: pharmacology and toxicology. *Front Pharmacol* 2019;**10**:563.

19. Pearson J, Poklis J, Poklis A, et al. Post-mortem toxicology findings of acetyl fentanyl, fentanyl, and morphine in heroin fatalities in Tampa, Florida. *Acad Forensic Pathol* 2015;**5**(4):676–689.

20. Pompei P, Micioni Di Bonaventura MV, Cifani C. The 'legal highs' of novel drugs of abuse. *J Drug Abuse* 2016;**2**:2.

21. Fairbairn N, Coffin PO, Walley AY. Naloxone for heroin, prescription opioid, and illicitly made fentanyl overdoses: challenges and innovations responding to a dynamic epidemic. *Int J Drug Policy* 2017;**46**:172–179. https://doi.org/10.1016/j.drugpo.2017.06.005

22. Armenian P, Vo KT, Barr-Walker J, Lynch KL. Fentanyl, fentanyl analogs and novel synthetic opioids: a comprehensive review. *Neuropharmacology* 2017;pii:S0028–3908(17)30484-7. https://doi.org/10.1016/j. neuropharm.2017.10.016

23. Pérez-Mañá C, Papaseit E, Fonseca F, Farré A, Torrens M, Farré M. Drug interactions with new synthetic opioids *Front Pharmacol* 2018 (online). https://doi.org/10.3389/fphar.2018.01145.

24. Labutin AV, Temerdashev AZ, Dukova OA, et al. Identification of furanoylfentanil and its metabolites in human urine. *J Environ Anal Toxicol* 2017;**7**:3. https://doi.org/10.4172/2161-0525.1000456

25. Zawilska JB. An expanding world of novel psychoactive substances: opioids. *Front Psychiatry* 2017;**8**:110. https://doi.org/10.3389/fpsyt.2017.00110

26. Pérez-Mañá C, Papaseit E, Fonseca F, Farré A, Torrens M, Farré M. Drug interactions with new synthetic opioids *Front Pharmacol* 2018 (online). https://doi.org/10.3389/fphar.2018.01145.

27. Pérez-Mañá C, Papaseit E, Fonseca F, Farré A, Torrens M, Farré M. Drug interactions with new synthetic opioids *Front Pharmacol* 2018 (online). https://doi.org/10.3389/fphar.2018.01145.

28. Daniulaityte R, Juhascik MP, Strayer KE, et al. Overdose deaths related to fentanyl and its analogs – Ohio, January–February 2017. *Morb Mortal Wkly Rep* 2017;**66**:904–908. https://doi.org/10.15585/mmwr.mm6634a3

29. Rogers JS, Rehrer SJ, Hoot NR. Acetylfentanyl: an emerging drug of abuse. *J Emerg Med* 2016;**50**(3):433–436. https://doi.org/10.1016/j.jemermed.2015.10.014

30. European Monitoring Centre for Drugs and Drug Addiction (EMCDDA). Report on the Risk Assessment of Nphenyl-N-[1-(2-phenylethyl)piperidin-4-yl]furan-2-carboxamide (Furanylfentanyl) in the Framework of the Council Decision on New Psychoactive Substances. Lisbon, EMCDDA, 2017.

31. Rojkiewicz M, Majchrzak M, Celinski R, Kus P, Sajewicz M. Identification and physicochemical characterization of 4-fluorobutyrfentanyl (1-((4-fluorophenyl)(1- phenethylpiperidin-4-yl)amino)butan-1-one, 4-FBF) in seized materials and postmortem biological samples. *Drug Test Anal* 2017;**9**:405–414.

32. European Monitoring Centre for Drugs and Drug Addiction (EMCDDA). Fentanyl drug profile. Available at: www.emcdda.europa.eu/publications/drug-profiles/fentanyl_en [last accessed 23 April 2022].

33. European Monitoring Centre for Drugs and Drug Addiction (EMCDDA). European Drug Report 2017: Trends and Developments. Luxembourg: Publications Office of the European Union, 2017.

34. European Monitoring Centre for Drugs and Drug Addiction. European Drug Report 2019: Trends and Developments. Publications Office of the European Union, Luxembourg, 2019.

35. Mounteney J, Giraudon I, Denissov G, Griffiths P. Fentanyls: are we missing the signs? Highly potent and on the rise in Europe. *Int J Drug Pol* 2015;**26**:626–631. https://doi.org/10.1016/j.drugpo.2015.04.003

36. Pichini S, Pacifici R, Marinelli E, Busardò FP. European drug users at risk from illicit fentanyls mix. *Front Pharmacol* 2017;31:785. https://doi.org/10.3389/fphar.2017.00785

37. Pichini S, Solimini R, Berretta P, Pacifici R, Busardò FP. Acute intoxications and fatalities from illicit fentanyl and analogues: an update. *Ther Drug Monit* 2018;**40**:38–51. https://10.1097/FTD.0000000000000465

38. European Monitoring Centre for Drugs and Drug Addiction. European Drug Report 2019: Trends and Developments. Publications Office of the European Union, Luxembourg, 2019.

39. Klar SA, Brodkin E, Gibson E, et al. Notes from the field: furanyl-fentanyl overdose events caused by smoking contaminated crack cocaine – British Columbia, Canada, 15–18 July 2016. *Morb Mortal Weekly Rep* 2016;**65**(37):1015–1016. https://doi.org/10.15585/mmwr.mm6537a6

40. Frank RG, Pollack HA. Addressing the fentanyl threat to public health. *N Engl J Med* 2017;**376**(7):605–607. https://doi.org/10.1056/NEJMp1615145

41. Arens AM, van Wijk XMR, Vo KT, et al. Adverse effects from counterfeit alprazolam tablets. *JAMA Intern Med* 2016;**176**(10):1554–1555. https://doi.org/doi:10.1001/jamainternmed.2016.4306

42. Green TC, Gilbert M. Counterfeit medications and fentanyl. *JAMA Inter Med* 2016;176(**10**):1555–1557. https://doi.org/10.1001/jamai-nternmed.2016.4310

43. Stogner JM. The potential threat of acetyl fentanyl: legal issues, contaminated heroin, and acetyl fentanyl 'disguised' as other opioids. *Ann Emerg Med* 2014;**64**(6):637–639. https://doi.org/10.1016/j.annemergmed.2014.07.017

44. Lozier MJ, Boyd M, Stanley C, et al. Acetyl fentanyl, a novel fentanyl analog, causes overdose deaths in Rhode Island, March–May 2013. *J Med Toxicol* 2015;**11**:208–217. https://doi.org/10.1007/s13181-015-0477-9

45. Advisory Council on the Misuse of Drugs (ACMD). Misuse of Fentanyl and Fentanyl Analogues. January 2020.

46. Suzuki J, El-Haddad S. A review: fentanyl and non-pharmaceutical fentanyls. *Drug Alcohol Depend* 2016;171:107–116. https://doi.org/10.1016/j.drugalcdep.2016.11.033

47. Stanley TH. The fentanyl story. *J Pain* 2014;**15**:1215–1226. https://doi.org/10.1016/j.jpain.2014.08.010 10

48. Armenian P, Olson A, Anaya A, et al. Fentanyl and a novel synthetic opioid U-47700 masquerading as street 'Norco' in Central California: a case report. *Ann Emerg Med* 2017;**69**:87–90.

49. Miller JM, Stogner JM, Miller BL, Blough S. Exploring synthetic heroin: accounts of acetyl fentanyl use from a sample of dually diagnosed drug offenders. *Drug Alcohol Rev* 2017;**37**(1):121–127. https://doi.org/10.1111/dar.12502

50. Amlani A, McKee G, Khamis N, et al. Why the FUSS (Fentanyl Urine Screen Study)? A cross-sectional survey to characterize an emerging threat to people who use drugs in British Columbia, Canada. *Harm Reduction J* 2015;**12**:54. https://doi.org/10.1186/s12954-015-0088-4

51. Ciccarone D, Ondocsin J, Mars S. Heroin uncertainties: exploring users' perceptions of fentanyl-adulterated and -substituted heroin. *Int J Drug Policy* 2017;**46**:146–155.

52. Macmadu A, Carroll JJ, Hadland SE, et al. Prevalence and correlates of fentanyl-contaminated heroin exposure among young adults who use prescription opioids non-medically. *Addict Behav* 2017;**68**:35–38. https://doi.org/10.1016/j.addbeh.2017.01.014

53. Prekupec MP, Mansky PA, Baumann MH. Misuse of novel synthetic opioids: a deadly new trend. *J Addict Med* 2017;**11**:256–265.

54. Gill H, Kelly E, Henderson H. How the complex pharmacology of the fentanyls contributes to their lethality. *Addiction* 2019 (online). https://doi.org/10.1111/add.14614

55. McClain DA, Hug CC Jr. Intravenous fentanyl kinetics. *Clin Pharmacol Ther* 1980;**28**(1):106–114.

56. Siddiqi S, Verney C, Dargan P, et al. Understanding the availability, prevalence of use, desired effects, acute toxicity and dependence potential of the novel opioid MT-45. *Clin Toxicol* 2015;**53**(1):54–59.

57. Gladden RM, Martinez P, Seth P. Fentanyl law enforcement submissions and increases in synthetic opioid-involved overdose deaths – 27 states, 2013–2014. *Morb Mortal Wkly Rep* 2016;**65**:837–843.

58. Peterson AB, Gladden RM, Delcher C, et al. Increases in fentanyl-related overdose deaths – Florida and Ohio, 2013–2015. *Morb Mortal Wkly Rep* 2016;**65**:844–849.

59. United Nations Office on Drugs and Crime Early Warning Advisory. Deaths associated with use of emerging synthetic opioids (News announcement). November 2016.

60. Advisory Council on the Misuse of Drugs (ACMD). Misuse of Fentanyl and Fentanyl Analogues. January 2020.

61. Gill H, Kelly E, Henderson H. How the complex pharmacology of the fentanyls contributes to their lethality. *Addiction* 2019 (online). https://doi.org/10.1111/add.14614

62. Bowdle TA. Adverse effects of opioid agonists and agonist-antagonists in anaesthesia. *Drug Saf* 1998;**19**:173–189.

63. Armenian P, Vo KT, Barr-Walker J, Lynch KL. Fentanyl, fentanyl analogs and novel synthetic opioids: a comprehensive review. *Neuropharmacology* 2017;**134**:121–132. https://doi.org/10.1016/j.neuropharm.2017.10.016

64. Prekupec MP, Mansky PA, Baumann MH. Misuse of novel synthetic opioids: a deadly new trend. *J Addict Med*

2017;**11**:256–265. https://doi.org/10.1097/
ADM.0000000000000324

65. Ventura L, Carvalho F, Dinis-Oliveira RJ. Opioids in the frame
of new psychoactive substances network: a complex
pharmacological and toxicological issue. *Curr Mol Pharmacol*
2018;**11**:97–108. https://doi.org/10.2174/
1874467210666170704110146

66. Solimini R, Pichini S, Pacifici R, Busardò FP, Giorgetti R.
Pharmatoxicology of non-fentanyl derived new synthetic
opioids. *Front Pharmacol* 2018;**9**:654. https://doi.org/10.3389
/fphar.2018.00654

67. Kinshella MW, Gauthier T, Lysyshyn M. Rigidity, dyskinesia
and other atypical overdose presentations observed at
a supervised injection site, Vancouver, Canada. *Harm Reduct J*
2018;**15**:64. https://doi.org/10.1186/s12954-018-0271-5

68. Mayer S, Boyd J, Collins A, Kennedy MC, Fairbairn N,
McNeil R. Characterizing fentanyl-related overdoses and
implications for overdose response: findings from a 64 rapid
ethnographic study in Vancouver, Canada. *Drug Alcohol
Depend* 2018;**193**:69–74. https://doi.org/10.1016/j
.drugalcdep.2018.09.006.

69. Torralva PR, Janowsky A. Noradrenergic mechanisms in
fentanyl-mediated rapid death explain failure of naloxone in
the opioid crisis. *J Pharmacol Exp Ther* 2019;**371** (2):453–475.
https://doi.org/10.1124/jpet.119.258566

70. Burns G, DeRienz RT, Baker DD, et al. Could chest wall
rigidity be a factor in rapid death from illicit fentanyl abuse?
Clin Toxicol 2016;**54**(5):420–423.

71. Armenian P, Vo KT, Barr-Walker J, Lynch KL. Fentanyl,
fentanyl analogs and novel synthetic opioids: a comprehensive
review. *Neuropharmacology* 2017;**134**:121–132. https://doi.org
/10.1016/j.neuropharm.2017.10.016

72. Somerville NJ, O'Donnell J, Gladden RM, et al. Characteristics
of fentanyl overdose – Massachusetts, 2014–2016. *Morb
Mortal Wkly Rep* 2017;**66**(14):382–386.

73. Prekupec MP, Mansky PA, Baumann MH. Misuse of novel
synthetic opioids: a deadly new trend. *J Addict Med*
2017;**11**:256–265. https://doi.org/10.1097/
ADM.0000000000000324

74. Ventura L, Carvalho F, Dinis-Oliveira RJ. Opioids in the frame
of new psychoactive substances network: a complex
pharmacological and toxicological issue. *Curr Mol Pharmacol*
2018;**11**:97–108. https://doi.org/10.2174/
1874467210666170704110146

75. Solimini R, Pichini S, Pacifici R, Busardò FP, Giorgetti R.
Pharmatoxicology of non-fentanyl derived new synthetic
opioids. *Front Pharmacol* 2018;**9**:654. https://doi.org/10.3389
/fphar.2018.00654

76. Cole JB, Dunbar JF, McIntire SA, et al. Butyrfentanyl overdose
resulting in diffuse alveolar hemorrhage. *Pediatrics* 2015;**235**
(3). https://doi.org/10.1542/peds.2014-2878

77. Ruzycki S, Yarema M, Dunham M, et al. Intranasal fentanyl
intoxication leading to diffuse alveolar hemorrhage. *J Med
Toxicol* 2016;**12**(1):185–188.

78. Kucuk HO, Kucuk U, Kolcu Z, et al. Misuse of fentanyl
transdermal patch mixed with acute coronary syndrome. *Hum
Exp Toxicol* 2016;**35**(1):51–52.

79. Duru UB, Pawar G, Barash JA, et al. An unusual amnestic
syndrome associated with combined fentanyl and cocaine use.
Ann Intern Med 2018 (online). https://doi.org/10.7326/L17-
0575

80. European Monitoring Centre for Drugs and Drug Addiction
(EMCDDA). Cyclopropylfentanyl. EMCDDA–Europol Joint
Report on a new psychoactive substance: N-phenyl-
N-[1-(2-phenylethyl)piperidin-4-yl]
cyclopropanecarboxamide (cyclopropylfentanyl). Available at:
www.emcdda.europa.eu/system/files/publications/7926/2018
1014_TDAS18001ENN_PDF.pdf [last accessed 23 April 2022].

81. Pérez-Mañá C, Papaseit E, Fonseca F, Farré A, Torrens M,
Farré M. Drug interactions with new synthetic opioids. *Front
Pharmacol* 2018 (online). https://doi.org/10.3389/fphar
.2018.01145

82. Helander A, Bäckberg M, Signell P, Beck O. Intoxications
involving acrylfentanyl and other novel designer fentanyls –
results from the Swedish STRIDA project. *Clin Toxicol* 2017;**55**
(6):589–599.

83. Pichini S, Solimini R, Berretta P, et al. Acute intoxications and
fatalities from illicit fentanyl and analogues: an update. *Ther
Drug Monit* 2018;**40**(1):38–51. https://doi.org/10.1097/FTD
.0000000000000465

84. Roxburgh A, Burns L, Drummer OH, et al. Trends in fentanyl
prescriptions and fentanyl-related mortality in Australia. *Drug
Alcohol Rev* 2013;**32**(3):269–275.

85. Rodda LN, Pilgrim JL, Di Rago, M, et al. A cluster of
fentanyl-laced heroin deaths in 2015 in Melbourne, Australia.
Anal Toxicol 2017;**41**(4):318–324. https://doi.org/10.1093/jat/
bkx013

86. Guerrieri D, Roman M, Thelander G, Kronstrand R.
Acrylfentanyl: another new psychoactive drug with fatal
consequences. *Forensic Sci Int* 2017;**277**:e21–e29. https://doi
.org/10.1016/j.forsciint.2017.05.010

87. Rudd RA, Seth P, David F, et al. Increases in drug and opioid-
involved overdose deaths: United States, 2010–2015. *Morb
Mortal Wkly Rep* 2016;**65**:1445–1452.

88. Warner M, Chen LH, Makuc DM, et al. Drug Poisoning
Deaths in the United States, 1980–2008 (NCHS Data Brief,
No. 81). Hyattsville, MD, National Center for Health Statistics,
2011. Available at www.cdc.gov/nchs/products/databriefs/d
b81.htm [last accessed 28 February 2022].

89. Chen LH, Hedegaard H, Warner M. Drug-poisoning Deaths
Involving Opioid Analgesics: United States, 1999–2011
(NCHS Data Brief, No. 166). Hyattsville, MD, National
Center for Health Statistics, 2014. Available at: www.cdc.gov
/nchs/products/databriefs/db166.htm [last accessed
28 February 2022].

90. Hedegaard H, Chen LH, Warner M. Drug-poisoning Deaths
Involving Heroin: United States, 2000–2013 (NCHS Data
Brief, No. 190). Hyattsville, MD: National Center for Health

Statistics, 2015. Available at: www.cdc.gov/nchs/products/dat abriefs/db190.htm [last accessed 28 February 2022].

91. National Center for Health Statistics. Public-use Data Files: Mortality Multiple Cause Files, 2015.

92. Centre for Disease Control and Prevention. Synthetic Opioid Data Excluding Methadone but Including Drugs Like Tramadol and Fentanyl.

93. European Monitoring Centre for Drugs and Drug Addiction (EMCDDA), Europol. Joint Report on a New Psychoactive Substance: 2-methoxy-N-phenyl-N-[1-(2-phenylethyl) piperidin-4-yl]acetamide (methoxyacetylfentanyl). Available at: www.emcdda.europa.eu/system/files/publications/7925/20 181015_TDAS18002ENN_PDF.pdf [last accessed 28 February 2022].

94. European Monitoring Centre for Drugs and Drug Addiction (EMCDDA), Europol. Joint Report on a New Psychoactive Substance: N-phenyl-N-[1-(2-phenylethyl)piperidin-4-yl] cyclopropanecarboxamide (cyclopropylfentanyl). Available at: www.emcdda.europa.eu/system/files/publications/7926/2018 1014_TDAS18001ENN_PDF.pdf [last accessed 28 February 2022].

95. European Monitoring Centre for Drugs and Drug Addiction (EMCDDA). Prevention of Drug-related Deaths. Available at: www.emcdda.europa.eu/publications/topic-overviews/pr evention-drug-related-deaths [last accessed 28 February 2022].

96. Drummer OH. Fatalities caused by novel opioids: a review. *Forensic Sci Res* 2019;4(2):95–110. https://doi.org/10.1080/20 961790.2018.1460063

97. Lovrecic B, Lovrecic M, Gabrovec B, et al. Non-medical use of novel synthetic opioids: a new challenge to public health. *Int. J. Environ. Res. Public Health* 2019;16:177. https://doi.org/10 .3390/ijerph16020177

98. Drummer OH. Fatalities caused by novel opioids: a review. *Forensic Sci Res* 2019;4(2):95–110. https://doi.org/10.1080/20 961790.2018.1460063

99. Lovrecic B, Lovrecic M, Gabrovec B, et al. Non-medical use of novel synthetic opioids: a new challenge to public health. *Int J Environ Res Public Health* 2019;16:177. https://doi.org/10 .3390/ijerph16020177

100. Drummer OH. Fatalities caused by novel opioids: a review. *Forensic Sci Res* 2019;4(2):95–110. https://doi.org/10.1080/20 961790.2018.1460063

101. Lovrecic B, Lovrecic M, Gabrovec B, et al. Non-medical use of novel synthetic opioids: a new challenge to public health. *Int J Environ Res Public Health* 2019;16:177. https://doi.org/10 .3390/ijerph16020177

102. Hull MJ, Juhascik M, Mazur F, et al. Fatalities associated with fentanyl and co-administered cocaine or opiates. *J Forensic Sci* 2007;52:1383–1388.

103. Drummer OH. Fatalities caused by novel opioids: a review. *Forensic Sci Res* 2019;4(2):95–110. https://doi.org/10.1080/20 961790.2018.1460063

104. Ojanpera I, Gergov M, Liiv M, et al. An epidemic of fatal 3-methylfentanyl poisoning in Estonia. *Int J Legal Med* 2008;122:395–400.

105. Marinetti LJ, Ehlers BJ. A series of forensic toxicology and drug seizure cases involving illicit fentanyl alone and in combination with heroin, cocaine or heroin and cocaine. *J Anal Toxicol* 2014;38:592–598.

106. National Center for Biotechnology Information. PubChem Compound Summary for CID 62156, Carfentanil. Available at: https://pubchem.ncbi.nlm.nih.gov/compound/Carfentanil [last accessed 1 March 2022].

107. Lovrecic B, Lovrecic M, Gabrovec B, et al. Non-medical use of novel synthetic opioids: a new challenge to public health. *Int J Environ Res Public Health* 2019;16:177. https://doi.org/10 .3390/ijerph16020177

108. Bäckberg M, Beck O, Jönsson K-H, Helander A. Opioid intoxications involving butyrfentanyl, 4-fluorobutyrfentanyl, and fentanyl from the Swedish STRIDA project. *Clin Toxicol* 2015;53(7):609–617. https://doi.org/10.3109/15563650 .2015.1054505

109. McIntyre IM, Anderson DT. Post-mortem fentanyl concentrations: a review. *J Forensic Res* 2012;3:157.

110. Latimer J, Ling S, Flaherty I, et al. Risk of fentanyl overdose among clients of the Sydney Medically Supervised Injecting Centre. *Int J Drug Policy* 2016;37:111–114.

111. Darke S, Duflou J. The toxicology of heroin-related death: estimating survival times. *Addiction* 2016;111(9):1607–1613. https://doi.org/10.1111/ add.13429

112. Kim HK, Connors NJ, Mazer-Amirshahi ME. The role of take-home naloxone in the epidemic of opioid overdose involving illicitly manufactured fentanyl and its analogs. *Expert Opin Drug Saf* 2019(online). https://doi.org/ 10.1080/14740338.2019.1613372

113. Henderson GL. Fentanyl-related deaths: demographics, circumstances, and toxicology of 112 cases. *J Forensic Sci* 1991;36(2):422–433.

114. Woodall KL, Martin TL, McLellan BA. Oral abuse of fentanyl patches (Duragesic®): seven case reports. *J Forensic Sci* 2008;53 (1):222–225. https://doi.org/10.1111/j.1556-4029.2007.00597.x

115. O'Donnell JK, Halpin J, Mattson CL, et al. Deaths involving fentanyl, fentanyl analogs, and u-47700 – 10 states, July–December 2016. *Morb Mortal Wkly Rep* 2017;66(43):1197–1202. https://doi.org/10.15585/mmwr .mm6643e1

116. Gomes T, Juurlink DN, Mamdani MM, et al. Prevalence and characteristics of opioid-related deaths involving alcohol in Ontario, Canada. *Drug Alcohol Depend* 2017;179:416–423.

117. Pérez-Mañá C, Papaseit E, Fonseca F, Farré A, Torrens M, Farré M. Drug interactions with new synthetic opioids. *Front Pharmacol* 2018 (online). | https://doi.org/10.3389/fphar .2018.01145

118. Pérez-Mañá C, Papaseit E, Fonseca F, Farré A, Torrens M, Farré M. Drug interactions with new synthetic opioids. *Front Pharmacol* 2018 (online). https://doi.org/10.3389/fphar .2018.01145

119. Atkinson TJ, Fudin J. Interactions between pain medications and illicit street drugs. *Pract Pain Manag* 2014;7:1–4.

120. Mozayani A, Raymon LP. *Handbook of Drug Interactions.* New Jersey, NJ, Humana Press Inc., 2004. https://doi.org/10.1007/ 978-1-59259-654-6

121. Pérez-Mañá C, Papaseit E, Fonseca F, Farré A, Torrens M, Farré M. Drug interactions with new synthetic opioids. *Front Pharmacol* 2018 (online). https://doi.org/10.3389/fphar .2018.01145

122. Rickli A, Liakoni E, Hoener MC, Liechti ME. Opioid-induced inhibition of the human 5-HT and noradrenaline transporters in vitro: link to clinical reports of serotonin syndrome. *Br J Pharmacol* 2018;175:532–543. https://doi.org/10.1111 /bph.14105

123. Greenier E, Lukyanova V, Reede L. Serotonin syndrome: fentanyl and selective serotonin reuptake inhibitor interactions. *AANA J* 2014;82(5):340–345.

124. National Institute for Health and Care Excellence. Fentanyl interactions. Available at: https://bnf.nice.org.uk/interaction/ fentanyl-2.html?msclkid=fc39a64bc2f311ecb6896 b20054e84be [last accessed 23 April 2022].

125. World Health Organization Expert Committee on Drug Dependence, thirty-ninth report. Geneva, WHO, 2018 (WHO Technical Report Series, No. 1009). License: CC BY-NC-SA 3.0 IGO.

126. Available at: www.unodc.org/documents/commissions/CND/ Drug_Resolutions/2010-2019/2012/CND_Res-55-7.pdf; www .unodc.org/docs/treatment/overdose.pdf; https://sustainable development.un.org/sdg3; www.unodc.org/documents/brus sels/News/2017.11_GERRA_S-O-S_initiative_Brochure_13 .pdf [last accessed 1 March 2022].

127. World Health Organization. Community Management of Opioid Overdose, 2014. Available at: https://apps.who.int/iris/ bitstream/handle/10665/137462/9789241548816_eng.pdf;jses sionid=F58F5BF19670B076BDF8B483B062C22F?sequence=1 [last accessed 1 March 2022].

128. Strang J, McDonald R. *Preventing Opioid Overdose Deaths with Take-Home Naloxone.* Publications Office of the European Union, Luxembourg. 2016. Available at: www.emcdda.europa.eu/system/files/publications/2089/T DXD15020ENN.pdf [last accessed 1 March 2022].

129. European Monitoring Centre for Drugs and Drug Addiction. Take-Home Naloxone. Available at: www.emcdda.europa.eu/ publications/topic-overviews/take-home-naloxone_en [last a ccessed 1 March 2022].

130. Advisory Council on the Misuse of Drugs. Misuse of Fentanyl and Fentanyl Analogues 2020. Available at: https://assets .publishing.service.gov.uk/government/uploads/system/uploa ds/attachment_data/file/855893/ACMD_Report_-_Misuse_ of_fentanyl_and_fentanyl_analogues.pdf [last accessed 1 March 2022].

131. World Health Organization. Community Management of Opioid Overdose Guideline, 2014. Available at: www.who.int/p ublications/i/item/9789241548816 [last accessed 23 April 2022].

132. Advisory Council on the Misuse of Drugs. Misuse of Fentanyl and Fentanyl Analogues. January 2020.

133. Mayer S, Boyd J, Collins A, Kennedy MC, Fairbairn N, McNeil R. Characterizing fentanyl-related overdoses and implications for overdose response: findings from a 64 rapid ethnographic study in Vancouver, Canada. *Drug Alcohol Depend* 2018;193:69–74. https://doi.org/10.1016/j .drugalcdep.2018.09.006.

134. NPIS, TOXBASE. www.toxbase.org

135. Advisory Council on the Misuse of Drugs. Misuse of Fentanyl and Fentanyl Analogues. January 2020.

136. Lynn RR, Galinkin JL. Naloxone dosage for opioid reversal: current evidence and clinical implications. *Ther Adv Drug Saf* 2018;9(1):63–88. https://doi.org/10.1177 /2042098617744161

137. Advisory Council on the Misuse of Drugs. Misuse of Fentanyl and Fentanyl Analogues. January 2020.

138. Strang J, McDonald R (eds). *Preventing Opioid Overdose Deaths with Take-Home Naloxone.* Luxembourg, EMCDDA, 2016. Available at: www.emcdda.europa.eu/system/files/publi cations/2089/TDXD15020ENN.pdf [last accessed 23 April 2022].

139. Advisory Council on the Misuse of Drugs. Misuse of Fentanyl and Fentanyl Analogues. January 2020.

140. Moss RB, Carlo DJ. Higher doses of naloxone are needed in the synthetic opioid era. *Subst Abuse Treat Prev Policy* 2019;14:6. https://doi.org/10.1186/s13011-019-0195-4

141. Lucyk SN, Nelson LS. Novel synthetic opioids: an opioid epidemic within an opioid epidemic. *Ann Emerg Med* 2017;69 (1):91–93. https://doi.org/10.1016/j. annemergmed.2016.08.445

142. Ramos-Matos C, López-Ojeda W. China White: clinical insights of an evolving designer underground drug. *Universal J Clin Med* 2015;3(1):6–9. https://doi.org/10.13189/ujcm .2015.030102

143. Neale J, Strang J. Naloxone – does over-antagonism matter? Evidence of iatrogenic harm after emergency treatment of heroin/opioid overdose. *Addiction* 2015;110(10):1644–1652. https://doi.org/10.1111/add.13027

144. Guidelines for the Psychosocially Assisted Pharmacological Treatment of Opioid Dependence (2009). Available at: www .who.int/publications/i/item/9789241547543?msclkid=6d2b2 cadc2f511ec84abaff20e8ad971; WHO: Community management of opioid overdose 2014. Available at: https://ap ps.who.int/iris/bitstream/handle/10665/137462/97892415488 16_eng.pdf [last accessed 23 April 2022].

145. Strang J, McDonald R (eds). Preventing Opioid Overdose Deaths with Take-Home Naloxone. EMCDDA, 2016. Available at: www.emcdda.europa.eu/system/files/publica tions/2089/TDXD15020ENN.pdf [last accessed 23 April 2022].

146. European Monitoring Centre for Drugs and Drug Addiction (EMCDDA). Take-Home Naloxone. Available at: www .emcdda.europa.eu/publications/topic-overviews/take-home-naloxone_en [last accessed 1 March 2022].

147. Strang J, McDonald R, Campbell G, et al. Take-home naloxone for the emergency interim management of opioid overdose: the public health application of an emergency medicine. *Drugs* 2019;**79**:1395–1418. https://doi.org/10.1007/s40265-019-0115 4-5

148. Kim HK, Connors NJ, Mazer-Amirshahi ME. The role of take-home naloxone in the epidemic of opioid overdose involving illicitly manufactured fentanyl and its analogs. *Expert Opin Drug Saf* 2019 (online). https://doi.org/10.1080/14740338 .2019.1613372

149. Schumann H, Erickson T, Thompson TM, et al. Fentanyl epidemic in Chicago, Illinois and surrounding Cook County. *Clin Toxicol (Phila)* 2008;**46**:501–506.

150. Peipera NC, Duhart Clarke S, Vincent LB, Ciccarone D, Krala AH, Zibbella JE. Fentanyl test strips as an opioid overdose prevention strategy: findings from a syringe services program in the Southeastern United States. *Int J Drug Policy* 2019;**63**:122–128.

151. Goldman JE, Waye KM, Periera KA, et al. Perspectives on rapid fentanyl test strips as a harm reduction practice among young adults who use drugs: a qualitative study. *Harm Reduct J* 2019;**16**:3. https://doi.org/10.1186/s12954-0 18-0276-0

152. Green TC, Nyeong J, Park MI, et al. An assessment of the limits of detection, sensitivity and specificity of three devices for public health-based drug checking of fentanyl in street-acquired samples. *Int J Drug Policy* 2020;**77**:102661.

153. Willman MW, Liss DB, Schwarz ES, et al. Do heroin overdose patients require observation after receiving naloxone? *Clin Toxicol* 2017;**55**(2):81–87.

154. Cicero TJ, Ellis MS, Kasper ZA. Increases in self-reported fentanyl use among a population entering drug treatment: the need for systematic surveillance of illicitly manufactured opioids. *Drug Alcohol Depend* 2017;**177**:101–103. https://doi .org/10.1016/j.drugalcdep.2017.04.004

155. European Monitoring Centre for Drugs and Drug Addiction. Estonia, Country Drug Report 2017. Luxembourg, Publications Office of the European Union, 2017.

156. Allan J, Herridge N, Griffiths P, et al. Illicit fentanyl use in rural Australia – an exploratory study. *J Alcohol Drug Depend* 2015;**3**:196. https://doi.org/10.4172/23296488 .1000196

157. Gecici O, Gokmen Z, Nebioglu M. Fentanyl dependence caused by the non-medical use: a case report. *Klinik Psikofarmakoloji Bülteni-Bull Clin Psychopharmacol* 2010;**20**(3):255–257. https://doi.org/10.1080/10177833 .2010.11790668

158. Ossipov MH, Lai J, King T, et al. Underlying mechanisms of pronociceptive consequences of prolonged morphine exposure. *Biopolymers* 2005;**80**(2–3):319–324.

159. Benyamin R, Trescot AM, Datta S, et al. Opioid complications and side effects. *Pain Physician* 2008;**11**(2 Suppl.):S105–S120.

160. Ballantyne JC. 'Safe and effective when used as directed': the case of chronic use of opioid analgesics. *J Med Toxicol* 2012;**8** (4):417–423.

161. Solomon DH, Rassen JA, Glynn RJ, et al. The comparative safety of opioids for nonmalignant pain in older adults. *Arch Intern Med* 2010;**170**(22):1979–1986.

162. Firestone M, Goldman B, Fischer B. Fentanyl use among street drug users in Toronto, Canada: behavioural dynamics and public health implications. *Int J Drug Policy* 2009;**20**(1):90–92. https://doi.org/10.1016/j.drugpo.2008.02.016

163. United Nations Office on Drugs and Crime (UNODC). World Drug Report 2017. Vienna, UNODC, 2017.

164. Advisory Council on the Misuse of Drugs (ACMD). Misuse of Fentanyl and Fentanyl Analogues. January 2020.

165. Solimini R, Pichini S, Pacifici R, Busardò FP, Giorgetti R. Pharmatoxicology of non-fentanyl derived new synthetic opioids. *Front Pharmacol* 2018;**9**:654. https://doi.org/10.3389 /fphar.2018.00654

166. Pérez-Mañá C, Papaseit E, Fonseca F, Farré, Torrens M, Farré M. Drug interactions with new synthetic opioids. *Front Pharmacol* 2018 (online). https://doi.org/10.3389/fphar .2018.01145

167. Pérez-Mañá C, Papaseit E, Fonseca F, Farré, Torrens M, Farré M. Drug interactions with new synthetic opioids. *Front Pharmacol* 2018 (online). https://doi.org/10.3389/fphar .2018.01145

168. Karinen R, Tuv SS, Rogde S, et al. Lethal poisonings with AH-7921 in combination with other substances. *Forensic Sci Int* 2014;**244**:e21–e24.

169. Hayers AG, Tyers MB. Determination of receptors that mediate opiate side effects in the mouse. *Br J Pharmacol* 1983;**79**:731–736. https://doi.org/10.1111/ j.1476-5381.1983 .tb10011.x

170. Ciccarone D. Fentanyl in the US heroin supply: a rapidly changing risk environment. *Int J Drug Policy* 2017;**46**:107–111. https://doi.org/10.1016/j.drugpo.2017.06.010

171. Lovrecic B, Lovrecic M, Gabrovec B, et al. Non-medical use of novel synthetic opioids: a new challenge to public health. *Int J Environ Res Public Health* 2019;**16**:177. https://doi.org/10 .3390/ijerph16020177

172. Cheney BV, Szmuszkovicz J, Lahti RA, Zichi DA. Factors affecting binding of trans-N-[2-(methylamino) cyclohexyl] benzamides at the primary morphine receptor. *J Med Chem* 1985;**28**:1853–1864.

173. Harper NJ, Veitch GB, Wibberley DG. 1-(3,4-dichlorobenzamidomethyl)cyclohexyldimethylamine and related compounds as potential analgesics. *J Med Chem* 1974;**17**:1188–1193.

174. Papsun D, Krywanczyk A, Vose JC, et al. Analysis of MT-45, a novel synthetic opioid, in human whole blood by LC–MS–MS

and its identification in a drug-related death. *J Anal Toxicol* 2016;**40**(4):313–317. https://doi.org/10.1093/jat/bkw012

175. Helander A, Bäckberg M, Beck O. MT-45, a new psychoactive substance associated with hearing loss and unconsciousness. *Clin Toxicol* 2014;**52**(8):901–904.

176. Katselou M, Papoutsis I, Nikolaou P, Spiliopoulou C, Athanaselis S. AH-7921: the list of new psychoactive opioids is expanded. *Forensic Toxicol* 2015;**33**(2):195–201.

177. Coppola M, Mondola R. AH-7921: from potential analgesic medicine to recreational drug. *Int J High Risk Behav Addict* 2017;**6**(2):e22593. https://doi.org/10.5812/ijhrba.22593

178. European Monitoring Centre for Drugs and Drug Addiction (EMCDDA). Technical report on 3,4-dichloro-N-{[1-(dimethylamino)cyclohexyl]methyl}benzamide (AH-7921). Lisbon, EMCDDA, April 2014.

179. Tabarra I, Soares S, Rosado T, et al. Novel synthetic opioids – toxicological aspects and analysis. *Forensic Sci Res* 2019;**4** (2):111–140. https://doi.org/10.1080/20961790 .2019.1588933

180. European Monitoring Centre for Drugs and Drug Addiction. EMCDDA–Europol Joint Report on a New Psychoactive Substance: AH-7921. Luxembourg, Publications Office of the European Union, 2016. Available at: www.emcdda.europa.eu/ publications/joint-report/AH-7921_en [last accessed 23 April 2022].

181. Uchiyama N, Matsuda S, Kawamura M, et al. Two new-type cannabimimetic quinolinyl carboxylates, QUPIC and QUCHIC, two new cannabimimetic carboxamide derivatives, ADB-FUBINACA and ADBICA, and five synthetic cannabinoids detected with a thiophene derivative a-PVT and an opioid receptor agonist AH-7921 identified in illegal products. *Forensic Toxicol* 2013;**31**:223–240.

182. Prekupec MP, Mansky PA, Baumann MH. Misuse of novel synthetic opioids: a deadly new trend. *J Addict Med* 2017;**11** (4):256–265. https://doi.org/10.1097 /ADM.0000000000000324

183. Uchiyama N, Matsuda S, Kawamura M, et al. Identification of two new-type designer drugs, piperazine derivative MT-45 (I-C6) and synthetic peptide noopept (GVS-111), with synthetic cannabinoid A-834735, cathinone derivative 4-methoxy-alpha-PVP, and phenethylamine derivative 4-methylbuphedrine from illegal products. *Forensic Toxicol* 2014;**32**:9–18.

184. Kjellgren A, Jacobsson K, Soussan C. The quest for well-being and pleasure: experiences of the novel synthetic opioids AH-7921 and MT-45, as reported by anonymous users online. *J Addict Res Ther* 2016;**7**(287):2.

185. Elliott S, Brandt S, Smith C. The first reported fatality associated with the synthetic opioid 3,4-dichloro-N-[2-(dimethylamino)cyclohexyl]-Nmethylbenzamide (U-47700) and implications for forensic analysis. *Drug Test Anal* 16-0092–R1. https://doi.org/10.1002/dta .1984

186. Kjellgren A, Jacobsson K, Soussan C. The quest for well-being and pleasure: experiences of the novel synthetic opioids

AH-7921 and MT-45, as reported by anonymous users online. *J Addict Res Ther* 2016;**7**(287):2.

187. Soussan C, Kjellgren A. The users of novel psychoactive substances: online survey about their characteristics, attitudes and motivations. *Int J Drug Policy* 2016;**32**:77–84.

188. Tabarra I, Soares S, Rosado T, et al. Novel synthetic opioids – toxicological aspects and analysis *Forensic Sci Res* 2019;**4** (2):111–140. https://doi.org/10.1080/20961790.2019.1588933

189. Katselou M, Papoutsis I, Nikolaou P, et al. AH-7921: the list of new psychoactive opioids is expanded. *Forensic Toxicol* 2015;**33**:195–201. https://doi.org/10.1007/s11419-015-0271-z

190. Kjellgren A, Jacobsson K, Soussan C. The quest for well-being and pleasure: experiences of the novel synthetic opioids AH-7921 and MT-45, as reported by anonymous users online. *J Addict Res Ther* 2016;**7**:287. https://doi.org/10.4172/2155-6105.1000287

191. Kjellgren A, Jacobsson K, Soussan C. The quest for well-being and pleasure: experiences of the novel synthetic opioids AH-7921 and MT-45, as reported by anonymous users online. *J Addict Res Ther* 2016;**7**:287. https://doi.org/10.4172/2155-6105.1000287

192. Mohr ALA, Friscia M, Papsun D, et al. Analysis of novel synthetic opioids U-47700, U-50488 and furanyl fentanyl by LC–MS/MS in post-mortem casework. *J Anal Toxicol* 2016;**40**:709–717. https://doi.org/10.1093/jat/bkw086

193. Elliott SP, Brandt SD, Smith C. The first reported fatality associated with the synthetic opioid 3,4-dichloro-N-[2-(dimethylamino)cyclohexyl]-Nmethylbenzamide (U-47700) and implications for forensic analysis. *Drug Test Anal* 2016;**8**:875–879. https://doi.org/10.1002/dta .1984

194. Kronstrand R, Thelander G, Lindstedt D, Roman M, Kugelberg FC. Fatal intoxications associated with the designer opioid AH-7921. *J Anal Toxicol* 2014;**38**(8):599–604.

195. European Monitoring Centre for Drugs and Drug Addiction (EMCDDA). Technical report on 3,4-dichloro-N-{[1-(dimethylamino)cyclohexyl]methyl}benzamide (AH-7921). Lisbon, EMCDDA, April 2014.

196. Hayes AG, Tyers MB. Determination of receptors that mediate opiate side effects in the mouse. *Br J Pharmacol* ;**79**:731–736.

197. Elliott S, Brandt S, Smith C. The first reported fatality associated with the synthetic opioid 3,4-dichloro-N-[2-(dimethylamino)cyclohexyl]-Nmethylbenzamide (U-47700) and implications for forensic analysis. *Drug Test Anal* 16- 0092–R1. https://doi.org/10.1002/dta.1984

198. Coppola M, Mondola R. AH-7921: from potential analgesic medicine to recreational drug. *Int J High Risk Behav Addict* 2017;**6**(2):e22593. https://doi.org/10.5812/ijhrba.22593

199. Tabarra I, Soares S, Rosado T, et al. Novel synthetic opioids – toxicological aspects and analysis. *Forensic Sci Res* 2019;**4** (2):111–140. https://doi.org/10.1080/20961790.2019.1588933

200. Hayes AG, Tyers MB. Determination of receptors that mediate opiate side effects in the mouse. *Br J Pharmacol* 1983;**79**:731–736.

201. Coppola M, Mondola R. AH-7921: a new synthetic opioid of abuse. *Drug Alcohol Rev* 2015;**34**:109–110.

202. Coppola M, Mondola R. MT-45: a new, dangerous legal high. *J Opioid Management* 2014;**10**:301–302.

203. Nakamura H, Shimizu M. Comparative study of 1-cyclohexyl-4-(1,2-diphenylethyl)-piperazine and its enantiomorphs on analgesic and other pharmacological activities in experimental animals. *Arch Int Pharmacodyn Thér* 1976;**221**:105–121.

204. Armenian P, Vo KT, Barr-Walker J, Lynch KL. Fentanyl, fentanyl analogs and novel synthetic opioids: a comprehensive review. *Neuropharmacology* 2017;**134**:121–132. https://doi.org/10.1016/j.neuropharm.2017.10.016

205. Prekupec MP, Mansky PA, Baumann MH. Misuse of novel synthetic opioids: a deadly new trend. *J Addict Med* 2017;**11**:256–265. https://doi.org/10.1097/ADM.0000000000000324

206. Ventura L, Carvalho F, Dinis-Oliveira RJ. Opioids in the frame of new psychoactive substances network: a complex pharmacological and toxicological issue. *Curr Mol Pharmacol* 2018;**11**:97–108. https://doi.org/10.2174/1874467210666170704110146

207. Solimini R, Pichini S, Pacifici R, Busardò FP, Giorgetti R. Pharmatoxicology of non-fentanyl derived new synthetic opioids. *Front Pharmacol* 2018;**9**:654. https://doi.org/10.3389/fphar.2018.00654

208. Helander A, Bradley M, Hasselblad A, et al. Acute skin and hair symptoms followed by severe, delayed eye complications in subjects using the synthetic opioid MT-45. *Br J Dermatol* 2017;**176**:1021–1027.

209. Tabarra I, Soares S, Rosado T, et al. Novel synthetic opioids – toxicological aspects and analysis. *Forensic Sci Res* 2019;**4** (2):111–140. https://doi.org/10.1080/20961790.2019.1588933

210. Vorce SP, Knittel JL, Holler JM, et al. A fatality involving AH-7921. *J Analyt Toxicol* 2014;**38**:226–230. https://doi.org/10.1093/jat/bku011

211. European Monitoring Centre for Drugs and Drug Addiction (EMCDDA). Drugs in Focus 2011.

212. Advisory Council on the Misuse of Drugs (ACMD). *ACMD's Recommendation on the Synthetic Opiate AH-7921*. London, ACMD, 2014.

213. Elliott S, Evans J. A 3-year review of new psychoactive substances in casework. *Forensic Sci Int* 2014;**243**:55–60. https://doi.org/10.1016/j.forsciint.2014.04.017

214. Soh YNA, Elliott S. An investigation of the stability of emerging new psychoactive substances. *Drug Test Anal* 2014;**6** (7–8):696–704. https://doi.org/10.1002/dta.1576

215. Kronstrand R, Thelander G, Lindstedt D, et al. Fatal intoxications associated with the designer opioid AH-7921. *J Anal Toxicol* 2014;**38**:599–604. https://doi.org/10.1093/jat/bku057

216. Fels H, Lottner-Nau S, Sax T, Roider G, Graw M. Postmortem concentrations of the synthetic opioid U-47700 in 26 fatalities associated with the drug. *Forensic Sci Int* 2019;**301**:e20–e28. https://doi.org/10.1016/j.forsciint.2019.04.010

217. Kriikku P, Pelander A, Rasanen I, Ojanperä I. Toxic lifespan of the synthetic opioid U-47700 in Finland verified by re-analysis of UPLC-TOF-MS data. *Forensic Sci Int* 2019;**300**:85–88. https://doi.org/10.1016/j.forsciint.2019.04.030

218. European Monitoring Centre for Drugs and Drug Addiction (EMCDDA). *Report on the Risk Assessment of MT-45 in the Framework of the Council Decision on New Psychoactive Substances*. Luxembourg, Publications Office of the European Union, 2015. Available at: www.emcdda.europa.eu/system/files/publications/1865/TDAK14006ENN.pdf [last accessed 23 April 2022].

219. European Monitoring Centre for Drugs and Drug Addiction (EMCDDA). *EMCDDA–Europol Joint Report on a New Psychoactive Substance: 1-cyclohexyl-4-(1,2- diphenylethyl) piperazine ('MT-45')*. Luxembourg, Publications Office of the European Union, 2014. Available at: www.emcdda.europa.eu/publications/joint-reports/MT-45_en [last accessed 23 April 2022].

220. Ruan X, Chiravuri S, Kaye AD. Comparing fatal cases involving U-47700. *Forensic Sci Med Pathol* 2016;**12**:369–371.

221. Jones MJ, Hernandez BS, Janis GC, et al. A case of U-47700 overdose with laboratory confirmation and metabolite identification. *Clin Toxicol (Phila)* 2017;**55**:55–59.

222. Coopman V, Blanckaert P, Van Parys G, Van Calenbergh S, Cordonnier J. A case of acute intoxication due to combined use of fentanyl and 3,4-dichloro-N-[2-(dimethylamino) cyclohexyl]-N-methylbenzamide (U-47700). *Forensic Sci Int* 2016;**266**:68–72. https://doi.org/10.1016/j.forsciint.2016.05.001

223. Papsun D, Krywanczyk A, Vose JC, Bundock EA, Logan BK. Analysis of MT-45, a novel synthetic opioid, in human whole blood by LC–MS–MS and its identification in a drug-related death. *J Anal Toxicol* 2016;**40**:313–317. https://doi.org/10.1093/jat/bkw012

224. Lucyk SN, Nelson LS. Novel synthetic opioids: an opioid epidemic within an opioid epidemic. *Ann Emerg Med* 2017;**69**:91–93. https://doi.org/10.1016/j.annemergmed.2016.08.445

225. Armenian P, Olson A, Anaya A, Kurtz A, Ruegner R, Gerona RR. Fentanyl and a novel synthetic opioid U-47700 masquerading as street 'Norco' in Central California: a case report. *Ann Emerg Med* 2017;**69**:87–90. https://doi.org/10.1016/j.annemergme d.2016.06.014

226. Brittain RT, Kellett DN, Neat ML, et al. Anti-nociceptive effects in N-substituted cyclohexylmethylbenzamides. *Br J Pharmacol* 1973;**49**:158–159.

227. Tabarra I, Soares S, Rosado T, et al. Novel synthetic opioids – toxicological aspects and analysis. *Forensic Sci Res* 2019;**4** (2):111–140. https://doi.org/10.1080/20961790.2019.1588933

Ketamine and Other Novel Psychoactive Substances with Dissociative Effects

6.1 'Dissociative' Drugs

Dissociative drugs distort perceptions of sight and sound and produce feelings of detachment (or dissociation) from the environment and self. Among the dissociative drugs, ketamine and phencyclidine (PCP) are the drugs most commonly used for recreational purposes.

In the last decade, a new generation of synthetic dissociative drugs appeared on the market, including methoxethamine (MXE), methoxphenidine, diphenidine and phencyclidine derivatives (e.g. 4-MeOPCP), which have rapidly spread, initially as legal replacements for the banned ketamine and PCP.

Ketamine is widely used in human and veterinary medicine and there is now increasing interest in its role in treatment-resistant depression, as discussed in this chapter. However, ketamine and then its novel analogues have also been used for recreational purposes and have been regarded as novel psychoactive substances, in order to differentiate it from controlled substances.[1] This document discusses the non-medical use of ketamine and its analogues and not its therapeutic role used in a controlled clinical setting.

Ketamine is a derivative of phencyclidine (PCP). Both these substances and their analogues are dissociative drugs and have been placed in this present text in the 'depressant' category for convenience and because they are predominantly sedative drugs. Ketamine, however, has a complex neuro-chemical profile, reflecting its actions as a psycho-stimulant, dissociative, anaesthetic and analgesic substance, with amnestic properties.

Ketamine can also distort perceptions of sight and sound and create feelings of detachment from the self and the environment. It can also be associated with hallucinogenic effects.

Drugs with dissociative effects act primarily as non-competitive antagonists at glutamate receptors of the N-methyl-D-aspartate (NMDA). One of their prominent effects is depersonalisation, or an 'alteration in one's experience and awareness of the self, leading to feelings of being unreal or detached from one's own body', and de-realisation, where individuals 'feel that the world around them has suddenly become unreal'.[2,3]

Ketamine hydrochloride is one of the dissociative drugs most commonly used for recreational purposes. At a global level, 96% of all ketamine quantities seized worldwide between 2013 and 2017 were reported by authorities in Asia, mostly in East and South-East Asia. However, ketamine trafficking appears to be spreading to other regions, including Europe, the Americas and Oceania.[4] In 2017, a total of 17 European countries reported police seizures of the drug. In the same year, last year prevalence of ketamine use among young adults (16–34 years) was estimated at 0.6 % in Denmark and 1.7 % in the UK.[5]

In addition to the recreational use of ketamine, the use of the novel psychoactive substance (NPS) analogues of ketamine and PCP has also been reported. As with other NPS, the control of one substance leads to the development of others. For example, methoxetamine ((RS)-2-(ethylamino)-2-(3- methoxyphenyl) cyclohexanone) 2-(3-methoxyphenyl)-2-(ethylamino) cyclohexanone (methoxetamine) was one of the first to be detected, but this gave rise to methoxphenidine (MXP) which was one of several NMDA antagonists marketed to replace methoxetamine (MXE) when this was controlled.[6]

As with other NPS, new compounds have been developed to replace those which become controlled. For example, methoxetamine was introduced as an alternative to ketamine, to be followed by methoxphenidine (MXP), which was one of several NMDA antagonists marketed in 2013 to replace the compound methoxetamine (MXE) which became a controlled substance.

Similarly, substituted analogues to ketamine, dextromethorphan (DXM), and phencyclidine (PCP) 3-methoxy-PCP (3-MeO-PCP), 4-MeO-PCP (also known as 'methoxydine'), diphenidine, and methoxphenidine (MXP, 2-MeO-diphenidine) have emerged on the NPS market as legal alternatives to the classical banned dissociatives.[7,8,9,10,11,12,13,14,15,16,17,18]

6.2 Street Names

Street names of illicit ketamine will differ between countries and languages. They include, but are not limited to: K, Ket, Special K, Kit-Kat, Cat Valium, Super K and Vitamin K.

Street names for methoxetamine include: M-ket, K-max, Mexxy, MXE powder, Special M and METH-O.

6.3 Legal Status

Ketamine has been widely used in human and veterinary medicine and is listed as an essential medicine by the World Health Organization (WHO).[19]

Because of the spread of its non-medical use and of counterfeit manufacturing, ketamine is a Schedule III substance.[20]

Methoxetamine (MXE) is controlled in Schedule II of the 1971 Convention, but derivatives such as 3-MeO-PCE and 4-MeO-PCP are not under international control.

6.4 Quality of the Research Evidence

In comparison with other club drugs and NPS, the international evidence on the management of the acute and chronic harms related to the use of ketamine in a clinical context is relatively wide and includes studies of healthy volunteers and animal studies. In contrast, the evidence on the harms associated with the misuse of ketamine and use in a recreational context is more limited and less robust.

The evidence regarding ketamine analogues is very limited.

6.5 Brief Summary of Pharmacology

Ketamine is a predominantly sedative drug, but its complex neurochemical profile reflects its actions as a dissociative, anaesthetic, psychostimulant and analgesic substance.[21]

Ketamine is a non-competitive N-methyl-D-aspartate (NMDA) receptor antagonist that acts as a dissociative anaesthetic with analgesic and amnestic properties. Ketamine is a derivative of phencyclidine (PCP) and is, as are its analogues, an arylcyclohexylamine. This is a miscellaneous group of dissociative anesthetic-type substances, acting by antagonism on

NMDA receptors.[14,15] Ketamine also acts at dopamine D2 and 5-HT2A receptors and the activation of 5-HT2A receptors is thought to be related to perceptual disorders and hallucinations. Ketamine also shows affinity for mu, delta, and sigma opioid receptors and affects monoamine transporters.[21]

Like phencyclidine (PCP), ketamine stimulates the vital functions of heartbeat and respiration, though it is less toxic and shorter acting than PCP.[22] The term 'dissociative' suggests that sensory loss and analgesia, as well as amnesia, are not accompanied by actual loss of consciousness.[23]

As a dissociative anaesthetic, ketamine has the capacity to induce narcosis and narcosis-like states in which consciousness appears to be separated from the body.[14] Its use can lead to a trance-like cataleptic state, unconsciousness, amnesia and deep analgesia, but with intact ocular, laryngeal and pharyngeal reflexes.[15] Ketamine impairs psychomotor performance in a dose-dependent fashion.

Ketamine has a plasma half-life of 2–4 hours.[24] Peak plasma concentrations are reached within a minute when ketamine is injected intravenously, 5–15 minutes when injected intramuscularly or snorted, and 4–6 hours when taken orally.[16,17]

Enzyme kinetic studies have shown that for ketamine the initial metabolic steps in humans (N-deethylation) are catalysed by CYP2B6 and CYP3A4. Therefore, caution should be addressed when co-administered orally with CYP3A4 and CYP2B6 inhibitors (such as ritonavir and cobicistat).[18,25]

Methoxetamine, which is 2-(3-methoxyphenyl)-2-(ethylamino)cyclohexanone, is an analogue of ketamine. It has and can be classified as a dissociative drug.[26] Its analogues are 1-[1-(3-methoxyphenyl)cyclohexyl]-piperidine (methoxyphencyclidine; 3-MeO-PCP) and N-ethyl-1- phenylcyclohexylamine (eticyclidine).

Methoxetamine was detected on drug markets in 2010 and was synthesised as a close structural analogue of ketamine in order to elude the classification of ketamine while retaining its psychoactive properties.[27] Because of its structural similarities to PCP and ketamine, it has been assumed that the effects of methoxetamine are broadly similar.[28]

Methoxetamine is both a dopamine reuptake inhibitor and an NMDA receptor blocker; its affinity for the NMDA receptor is comparable to or higher than that of ketamine. In addition, methoxetamine (in addition to PCP and its analogues) has affinity for the serotonin transporters.[29]

Methoxetamine has more potency and higher opioid receptor affinity than phencyclidine and weaker analgesic and anaesthetic effects, but longer duration of action, than ketamine.[30,31,32,33]

Methoxetamine has been marketed to drug users as much more powerful and as having longer-lasting effects than ketamine. The psychoactive effects should be anticipated to last longer than would be expected for ketamine.[28]

It was originally claimed that methoxetamine is a 'bladder-friendly' alternative to ketamine, and some users believed that methoxetamine was less damaging to their kidneys as well as their bladder than ketamine.[34,35,36,37] However, there is now evidence that this is not the case. Studies indicate that high-dose, chronic administration of methoxetamine induces urinary toxicity that is comparable to that induced by ketamine.[38]

6.6 Medical Uses of Ketamine

Ketamine is used as an anaesthetic and a powerful analgesic, particularly in paediatric, emergency medicine and veterinary medicine, and is considered as a safe battlefield anaesthetic due to its pharmacological profile. It also has a medical role in the management of pain in both humans and animals, including as an analgesic in chronic cancer pain (palliative care) and non-cancer pain.[39,40]

Ketamine has also been used for the treatment of substance misuse disorders, including alcohol, cocaine, cannabis, and opioid use and there is limited evidence that that ketamine may facilitate abstinence across multiple substances.[41] More recently, a number of studies have investigated the role of ketamine in treatment-resistant depression and major depressive disorders, whereby positive and encouraging outcomes have been reported.[42,43,44,45,46,47,48,49,50,51,52,53,54,55,56,57,58]

Nonetheless, concerns have been voiced over the medical use of ketamine for chronic conditions because of its toxic effects, especially associated with very high doses for prolonged periods of time. Recommendations for adequate monitoring of patients have been made.[59,60]

There are currently no clinical or non-clinical legitimate uses of methoxetamine. Some have argued however that because of its similarity to ketamine, methoxetamine may have some analgesic or anti-nociceptive properties, with enhanced potency and

duration of action.[61] It has also been argued that as an analogue of ketamine, it could be of pharmaceutical interest for treatment-resistant depression if it were to show rapid antidepressant properties similar to those of ketamine.[62,63,64] There is limited evidence that methamphetamine analogues (N-ethylnorketamine hydrochloride (NENK), 2-MeO-N-ethylketamine hydrochloride (2-MeO-NEK), and 4-MeO-N-ethylketamine hydrochloride (4-MeO-NEK)) elicit rapid antidepressant effects via activation of AMPA and 5-HT2 receptors.[65]

6.7 Prevalence and Patterns of Use

The recreational use of ketamine has been characterised by the EMCDDA as having 'potential for more widespread diffusion'.[66] The Global Drug Survey 2019 reported that darknet purchases of ketamine have increased over the last 5 years.[67]

The recreational use of ketamine has been reported among subgroups of drug users in Europe for the last two decades. However, national estimates, where they exist, show that the prevalence of its use in adult and school populations remains low. In 2017, last year prevalence of ketamine use among young adults (16–34) was estimated at 0.6% in Denmark and 1.7% in the UK.[68]

There is some evidence that initiation in ketamine use may take place at a slightly older age than for other substances, and that it is possible more experienced users add ketamine to their poly-use repertoire.[69] Research carried out in the US, England and Australia suggests that ketamine users tend to be white, male, urban and under 30 years old.[70,71,72,73]

Ketamine used for recreational purposes is typically made in clandestine laboratories, but can also be diverted from licit channels.[74,75] It is usually sold as ketamine, but in countries such as Indonesia and Thailand, ketamine may also be sold to unwitting users as 'ecstasy' or methamphetamine tablets.[76]

Ketamine is typically used intra-nasally, by insufflation. It is rarely injected. A study conducted in Scotland, for example, found that ketamine was injected by only 0.9% of users.[77]

6.8 Ketamine Use and High-Risk Sexual and Injecting Behaviours

Like other club drugs, ketamine is used as part of a socially active lifestyle and is associated with elevated, even pronounced, sexual health risks.[78]

Ketamine is associated with an increased incidence of unsafe sex among gay men.[79,80,81,82] A US study of gay and bisexual men attending 'circuit parties' in three cities found that over 60% had used ketamine at parties in the past year and unsafe sexual behaviour was associated with frequent ketamine use.[81]

There have also been reported cases of sexual dysfunction associated with ketamine abuse.[83,84]

As mentioned above, ketamine is rarely injected (typically being taken intra-nasally) but some use by injection has been reported. Laukenau et al. studied young ketamine injectors in US cities and described two types of ketamine injectors with different demographic profiles: experienced injecting drug users (IDUs), who injected a number of drugs and who tended to be homeless youth and homeless travellers;[85,86] and new IDUs, who initiated injecting with ketamine and tended to have stable housing and who associated with others who used ketamine.[86]

There is also some anecdotal evidence which suggests that it is possible that a minority of older injecting opiate drug users also inject ketamine[86,87] and that ketamine is sometimes injected.[88,89]

In interviews with ketamine injectors, subjects reported the advantages of injecting over snorting: sniffing aggravated the nasal passage and injecting produced what was referred to as a 'cleaner' high. Those who developed tolerance from sniffing found that injecting was a more potent and reliable mode of ingestion.[86] Most reported that the main reason for injecting was to achieve the 'k-hole' (where the user experiences feelings of detachment and perceptions appear divorced from reality), which was more reliably achieved and intensely experienced by injecting.[86]

Among those who injected ketamine only, a study has shown intramuscular injecting was more common than intravenous injecting. Injecting ketamine was shown to be associated with high-risk behaviours. Multiple injections were typical, for example eight to ten injections over several hours.[86]

6.9 Routes of Ingestion, Dosing and Frequency of Dosing

6.9.1 Ketamine

Illicit ketamine is mainly in powder form, typically sold in gram doses. It is less frequently available as a liquid, in which form it is possibly diverted from pharmaceutical supplies.

Illicit ketamine for recreational use is often sold as a powder of fine crystal and is crushed for insufflation. It is usually white or transparent but can also be off-white or brown. In some countries such as the UK for example, doses for recreational use are often measured as the quantity of powder that fits on the tip of a domestic key, a method therefore known as 'keying'.

Ketamine is sometimes sold in tablet form (in which form it is on occasion falsely sold to users as ecstasy). Ketamine is sometimes dissolved for injecting and then has a faster and more potent effect.

Ketamine is rarely taken orally, as it will then be metabolised into norketamine, which produces a sedative effect rather than the desired effect. It can also be smoked, used rectally[90,91] or swallowed in a wrap of paper.

The onset of the effects of ketamine is likely to occur approximately 5 minutes (but up to 30 minutes) after insufflation, the most common form of use. Effects occur in a matter of seconds or minutes after injection, smoking and smoke inhalation. This rapid onset of effect is thought to increase its potential for misuse. The effects themselves are generally short-lived, typically lasting 1–4 hours,[92] depending on dose, tolerance, individual factors and other drugs ingested. This short duration of effect may promote bingeing; ketamine users in a session will typically self-administer several doses in order to maintain psychotropic effects over time,[93] until supplies are exhausted.[94,95] On the other hand, the short duration of effects may also increase its appeal over longer-lasting hallucinogens.[69]

A typical recreational dose is approximately 10–25% of the effective general anaesthetic dose.[15] Single doses for intranasal use vary widely.[15,95,96] The small number of specialist treatment services offering specific treatment to ketamine users report that most of their patients use ketamine most days or every day and use up to several grams per day.[40] The highest dose noted in a series of 60 patients attending three clinical urology centres for a ketamine-related urological syndrome was 20 grams per day.[97]

6.9.2 Methoxetamine

Methoxetamine is generally sold as a white crystal powder, but can be found in tablet form. It is generally used by insufflation, but can be used rectally, by sublingual application and by injection (intramuscular mainly, but also intravenous).[28,98] It is also used orally, usually swallowed in a cigarette paper, or as tablets. The range of doses reported is 20–100 mg for oral administration and 10–50 mg for intramuscular injection.[23,28,98]

The onset of the effects of methoxetamine have been described to start 10–20 minutes after ingestion,[98] but can be delayed by 30–90 minutes after insufflation.[23]

One of the most significant differences between ketamine and methoxetamine appears to be the much slower onset of action of the latter (up to 90 minutes).[99,100,101] It is suspected to sometimes lead to repeated dosing and to inadvertent excessive dosing by people who think that their drug has had no effect.[102] This may lead to unintentional overdose[103] as users may ingest a second dose thinking that the first dose was inadequate. Compulsive re-dosing has also been described.[92] The effects after intramuscular injection are faster, with onset after approximately 5 minutes.[92]

The effects of methoxetamine last for approximately 1–7 hours, depending on the route of administration.[104] Drug user websites investigated by Corazza et al. stated that the duration of action of methoxetamine ranges from 5 to 7 hours when insufflated, less (approximately 1 hour) when administered by intramuscular injection.[64]

Powders and tablets sold as methoxetamine have been found typically to include a range of other compounds and adulterants, including mephedrone, caffeine and cocaine.[105]

Newer analogues of ketamine and PCP, such as dextromethorphan (DXM), 3-methoxy-PCP (3-MeO-PCP), 4-MeO-PCP, the methoxylated analogues of PCP 3- and 4-MeO-PCP, 1,2-diarylethylamines, have also been sold as 'legal highs' in a number of different forms including powders and tablets.[106]

6.10 Desired Effects for Recreational Use

6.10.1 Ketamine

The mind-altering effects of ketamine make it attractive to some drug users, along with its lack of hangover, short duration and relatively low cost. One of the earliest studies on the recreational use of ketamine found that users perceived it as a safe and potent hallucinogen with short duration of action and an equal balance of positive and negative effects.[107]

It has been argued by Benschop et al. (2000), that the expansion and coping motives were also associated with the use of dissociative drugs, as well as a higher endorsement of the coping motive.[108]

According to Teltzrow et al., ketamine has characteristic subjective effects which differ according to individual and setting of use.[109]

Overall, however, it can produce a range of experiences, depending on dose[110]:

- At low doses, ketamine produces distortion of time and space, visual and auditory hallucinations and mild dissociative effects.[111] It also has stimulant-type properties.[112]

- At high doses, it produces more severe dissociation, known by some users as the 'K-hole', where the user experiences feelings of intense detachment and perceptions appear completely divorced from reality.[111] With higher doses of ketamine, dissociative and hallucinogenic effects become the primary experience and the effect of the environment diminishes. Auditory hallucinations are fairly rare following ketamine use and have been reported much less consistently.[113]

Ketamine has been described as able to induce a 'raft' of intense experiences, including some that can be characterised as positive and negative psychotic-like features.[114] It is dissociative inasmuch as it causes users to feel both sedated and separate from their bodies.[86]

The combination of effects of ketamine has been described by some as 'alcohol-like intoxication, cocaine-like stimulation, opiate-like calming, and cannabis-like imagery'.[115] Moore et al. referred to the 'playful' effect of ketamine, in that it leads to improved moods and a child-like state. The intensity of ketamine was also emphasised.[69] Its effects include euphoria, depersonalisation and derealisation, feelings of universal empathy and experiencing synaesthesia (combinations of sense experiences such as sound and colour).[116]

Ketamine users also report that it enhances creativity and that it is used to manage the 'come-down' from other drugs, such as stimulants.

Ketamine users often experience floating sensations, sensory distortions and transcendental phenomena, such as mystical insight, spiritual trips, revelations or alternative realities.[111] Ketamine is sought by some because it induces a 'separate reality', 'near death', 'lack of fear of death' and out-of-body experiences.[117] States similar to those reported as near-death experiences have been described and include altered perceptions of time, a strong sense of detachment from the physical body and a sense of peace and joy.[118]

There are individual variations in motivations to use ketamine, as well as in what constitutes desired or unwanted effects. These have been described by a study as revolving around axes of sociability and intensity, with control over effect being an important concept. The voluntary versus involuntary entry into the K-hole[69] is a salient example: for some it is too intense; for others it is a desired journey or place. Interviews with users suggest that the dose is a key point of control, which users associate with the possibility of negative or positive consequences of ketamine use.

It has been reported that some users 'test' doses of ketamine to assess the strength of batches[69] and then adjust doses for desired effects. Self-administration of titrated ketamine is attempted by users to achieve the desired amount of dissociative sensation, hallucination and transcendental experience.[107]

In addition to dose used, the frequency of use and past exposure have been self-reported as influencing the experience. In a study of recreational users, 58% interviewed said they had experienced the K-hole and that this was related to increased exposure to the drug (more than 20 times).[71]

Ketamine is also used for self-medication for depression and studies are currently being conducted to examine its antidepressant action. There is also anecdotal evidence that it is also used as self-medication for sleep and anxiety. Anecdotal evidence also suggests that it is commonly used by men who have sex with men for some forms of anal sex because of its anaesthetic and muscle-relaxing effects.

6.10.2 Methoxetamine

Reports from users suggest that methoxetamine produces ketamine-like effects, but is more powerful and longer-lasting than ketamine (but less so than PCP).[23,28,119,120] Methoxetamine is linked to increased psychological effects (both desired and adverse) and increased toxicity compared with ketamine.[121]

Methoxetamine produced dissociative and stimulant wave outcome often lasting for days.[122] Effects described by users include euphoria, enhanced empathy and social interaction, pleasant intensification of sensory experiences (especially music),

distorted sense of reality, vivid hallucinations, derealisation, introspection, brief antidepressant effects, feelings of peacefulness and calmness, and spiritual and transcendental experiences.[123] Other desired effects include euphoria, feelings of peacefulness, increased empathy and social interaction and a sense of going deeper inside the self.[124] It is also associated with sensory deprivation and dissociation from the physical body, which are all features of a 'near-death experience' and part of the desired effects of methoxetamine.[125,126] It has been reported that a sense of empowerment occurs in the afterglow experience.[127]

The effects of methoxetamine are linked to mode of ingestion. Typically, it works as a short-acting mood enhancer, with powerful visual hallucinogenic and dissociative properties. The desired effects include euphoria, empathy, 'cosiness', intensification of sensory experiences, especially while listening to music, a mild to strong sense of dissociation, distortion of the sense of reality, vivid hallucinations, introspection and brief antidepressant effects.[23] An 'M-hole' has been described by users, typically referring to a subjective state of dissociation, which mimics the out-of-body experiences of near-death experiences,[118,128] and is often accompanied by feelings of derealisation, depersonalisation and disorientation, as well as vivid hallucinations.

There are also user reports that at high doses (>40 mg), methoxetamine can produce a wide range of unwanted effects including out-of-body or near-death experience, reduced ability to concentrate and focus, psychomotor agitation, intense dissociative and hallucinogenic experiences, paranoia, anxiety and distortions in the perception of time, distance, proportion and body image.[129,130,131]

6.11 Acute Ketamine Toxicity

In comparison with other drugs, ketamine in itself has a wide margin of safety,[132] but the use of illicit ketamine is not risk-free and ketamine is often co-ingested with other substances, which increases both its associated harms and those of other substances. It also gives rise to a greater risk of accidents (see Section 6.11.3) and chronic use can lead to urological problems, which can be severe (see Section 6.14.4).

Nevertheless, ketamine is characterised by its ability to cause unconsciousness, amnesia and analgesia, while sparing airway reflexes and maintaining haemodynamic stability.[15] Coughing and swallowing reflexes are maintained with minor suppression of the gag reflex, even when a user is very intoxicated, thus reducing the potential risk for users, if ketamine is used on its own.[132]

The Morgan and Curran review suggests a lack of severe acute physical health consequences, with no adverse outcome reported from large overdose, where no other substances are co-ingested.[132]

The main features of acute intoxication associated with ketamine are related to its psychoactive, dissociative and hallucinogenic properties. In humans, a single dose of ketamine induces dose-dependent impairments in working and episodic memory, which can have a profound effect on the user's ability to function.[133] Ketamine is associated with direct neurotoxicity and can cause acute neuropsychiatric effects, such as agitation or ketamine-related psychotic states. Often clinical features when people present to hospital are related to physical harm (e.g. agitation or accidents), and behaviours resulting from dissociative effects.

However, systemic toxicity with cardiovascular effects can occur and can be severe. Ketamine is a mild respiratory depressant, but its effects with clinical dose on the cardiovascular system are minimal and unusual for respiratory effects to occur. However, with recreational doses, especially higher doses, ketamine may increase heart rate, cardiac output, and blood pressure,[132,134] with a study reporting that tachycardia is the most common reason for presentation to emergency departments by recreational ketamine users.[135] It has been suggested that the stimulating effects of ketamine on the cardiovascular system may have implications for recreational users with pre-existing cardiac issues or hypertension.[136]

This will present a risk for people with hypertension or severe cardiac disease, and people at risk of stroke and raised intracranial pressure. Risks are increased with co-ingestion of stimulants[132] and should be emphasised in harm reduction messages (Section 6.16).

6.11.1 Features of Acute Ketamine Toxicity[137]

The reported acute effects of ketamine use are summarised in Box 6.1.

Case reports provide some insight into how common these ketamine-related effects are. In a study by Ng et al.[138] which reviewed 233 cases of presentations to an emergency department, the most common presenting symptoms were: impaired consciousness

> **Box 6.1** Analogues and Derivatives of Ketamine and Phencyclidine
>
> Ketamine is the most commonly used drug with dissociative effects, followed to some extent by methoxetamine.
>
> There are nonetheless a number of other NPS arylcyclohexylamine substances that have been notified to the Early Warning System in Europe. Like ketamine and its analogues, they are NMDA receptor antagonists. NPS with dissociative effects include:
>
> - 2-methoxyketamine
> - N-ethylnorketamine
> - 3-MeO-PCE (N-ethyl-1-(3-methoxyphenyl)
> - 4-MeO-PCP
> - cyclohexanamine
> - 1-[1-(3-methoxyphenyl) cyclohexyl]piperidine
> - 4-methoxyphencyclidine (4-MeO-PCP)
> - 1-[1-(4-methoxyphenyl)cyclohexyl]piperidine -N-ethyl norketamine
> - N-ethylketamine
> - tiletamine
> - dextromethorphan
> - N-ethyl norketamine
> - diphenidine (1-(1,2-diphenylethyl)piperidine)
> - methoxphenidine (MXP, 2-MeO-diphenidine)
> - 2-oxo-PCE
> - 2-(3-methoxyphenyl)-2-(propylamino) cyclohexan-1-one (methoxpropamine)

(45%), abdominal pain (21%), lower urinary tract symptoms (12%) and dizziness (12%). The most common physical symptoms included high blood pressure (40%), tachycardia (39%), abdominal tenderness (18%) and chest discomfort and palpitations (11%). However, no patient had serious cardiovascular complications (e.g. myocardial infarction or significant arrhythmias).

In that study, 46% of patients had a period of altered consciousness at some point after ketamine ingestion. This effect of ketamine was short-live; however, only 14% of the patients had a score on the Glasgow Coma Scale of less than 15 when examined in hospital. Among patients who had blood tests performed, leukocytosis (in 36%) and a raised creatinine kinase level (in 32%) were the most common abnormalities, whereas 16% had abnormal liver function test results and 3% had abnormal renal function test results. Most of the patients were

Box 6.2 The Reported Acute Effects of Ketamine Use

Dermatological

Transient rash, predominantly in face and neck

Gastrointestinal

Nausea

Vomiting

Neurobehavioural Effects/Psychiatric Effects[107,133,139]

Hallucinations (visual and auditory)

Slurred speech

Dizziness

Numbness

Confusion

Blurred vision

Insomnia

Decreased sexual motivation

Cognitive impairment

Aggression

Paranoia and display of dissociative-type symptoms

Ataxia

Dystonia

Agitation (agitated patients are at risk of other effects including hyperthermia, rhabdomyolysis, self-injury, enhanced perception, depersonalisation, movement disorders and confusion)

Paralysis and muscle rigidity

Ketamine-related psychotic states (typically short-lived with complete resolution).[114,140] Among patients with schizophrenia stabilised on an antipsychotic, however, ketamine can cause a relapse of psychotic symptoms,[141] which are idiosyncratic to those each individual exhibited during the acute phase of their illness[142,143]

Delirium

Polyneuropathy

Seizures

Convulsions

Cardiovascular and Respiratory[144,145,146]

Self-resolving sinus tachycardia (most commonly reported)

Hypertension (common)

Chest pain

Palpitation

Transient major Brugada ECG patterns (one case report)

Raised intracranial pressure

Pulmonary oedema

Respiratory depression

Cardiac and respiratory arrest

Increased muscle tone and activity may produce hyperpyrexia

managed solely in the emergency department (72%) and 85% had no or only minor complaints.[138]

6.11.2 Methoxetamine

The effects of methoxetamine are dose dependent and include mild euphoria, depersonalisation, de-realisation hallucinations, disorientation, confusion, vertigo, drowsiness, incoordination/falls, slurred speech, anxiety, reduced ability to focus and concentrate, analgesia, numbness, anxiety, impaired motor coordination, agitation, aggression, loss of consciousness, amnesia and catatonia.

Unwanted effects include vomiting, diarrhoea, insomnia, agitation, sweating, catatonia and hypertonia. They also include dysphoria, psychomotor agitation, vertical nystagmus, labile mood and dissociative confusion, including partial amnesia to the preceding events.[147]

Methoxetamine seems to have more severe side-effects than ketamine.[92] It has been argued that the acute methoxetamine toxidrome can be roughly divided into three types of symptoms: dissociative/delirious, sympathomimetic and cerebellar.[148]

Initial presentations to hospital generally involve loss of consciousness, incoordination with falls, agitation and aggression, and audio-visual hallucinations and delusions. It has been suggested that it was common at initial presentation for mental status to fluctuate between comatose, confusion, and agitation and aggression.[148] People have presented at hospital with methoxetamine intoxication with impaired consciousness and coma.[149]

Methoxetamine can cause rapid onset of neurological impairment, characterised by acute cerebellar toxicity.[149] Reversible cerebellar impairment has also been reported,[150] but recovery could extend over several days.[149] Cerebellar ataxia, incoordination, dysarthria and tremor have been reported.[28,149,151,152] There are also cases reporting truncal ataxia, dysarthria and nystagmus (horizontal, vertical and rotary).[153]

Although there is limited research, cognitive impairment has also been reported,[105] and there are a small number of cases of acute methoxetamine causing cerebellar toxicity[154] and cases of dissociation and catatonia.[155]

Methoxetamine has greater effects than ketamine in terms of hypertension and other stimulant-like effects, including agitation, tachycardia, hypertension and cerebellar features, such as ataxia.[105,153,156] It has

also been associated with pyrexia, tachypnea, elevated creatine kinase, tremor, as well as depressive thoughts and suicide attempts.[28,157,158,159]

6.11.3 Acute Withdrawal

For withdrawal see Section 6.13.2.

6.11.4 Poly-drug Use: Complicating Factors for Acute Toxicity

Acute ketamine toxicity, or toxicity associated with all arylcyclohexylamines, is often complicated by poly-drug use, which is common. In one study of attenders at an emergency department, 89% of self-reported ketamine users stated that they had used another drug and/or alcohol.[144] It is therefore recommended that when people present with acute toxicity after ketamine use, clinicians consider the possible impact of other drugs ingested.[15] Poly-drug use has also been implicated in death (see Section 6.10).

Box 6.3 3- and/or 4-MeO-PCP

It has been reported by the STRIDA Project that the adverse effects noted in acute intoxications involving 3- and/or 4-MeOPCP resembled those of classical dissociatives such as PCP, ketamine and methoxetamine.[160]

3-MeO-PCP is expected to elicit effects similar to other NMDA antagonists,[161,162,163] but half-life was approximately 11 hours.[164] Activity is reported to begin at doses as low as 5 mg.[165,166,167]

As with PCP, low doses are associated with anxiety, muscle tremors, drowsiness and hallucinations and higher doses have the potential to cause violent behaviour, tachycardia, hyperthermia, suicidal impulses, seizure or coma. At higher doses, individuals may also experience pulmonary aspiration or cardiovascular collapse, as with PCP.[168,169,170]

The most common features of acute toxicity have been reported to be tachycardia and hypertension followed by an altered mental status.[171,172] Delayed verbal responses to questions and ataxia have also been reported.[173]

A study presents two cases of intoxication due to consumption of 3-MeO-PCP and alcohol, respiratory acidosis, right anisocoria with mydriatic pupils and hypothermia. The patients were intubated for 7–8 hours. Almost 24 hours after hospitalisation, they were still in a delirious and agitated status.[174]

Box 6.4 Methoxphenidine and Diphenidine

Methoxphenidine (2-MXP; (±)-1-[1-(2-methoxyphenyl)-2-phnylethyl] piperidine; 2-Meo-diphenidine) 2-MXP, is a structural analogue of diephenidine and was introduced in the market as the replacement to methoxetamine (MXE). Anecdotal reports suggest 2-MXP has greater oral potency and effects reported online by users suggest that it may have a dopamine reuptake inhibitor action.[175]

The Swedish STRIDA study investigated cases of diphenidine (n=14) and methoxphenidine[176] (n=3) toxicity, which were reported to involve high levels of polyuse. The adverse effects noted in analytically confirmed cases were similar to those reported for other dissociative substances such as ketamine and methoxetamine, a fact also noted by other studies.[177,178]

Symptoms of toxicity reported commonly include hypertension (76%), tachycardia (47%), anxiety (65%), and altered mental state (65%) including confusion, disorientation, dissociation, and/or hallucinations. Just under half of cases (n=8) displayed severe intoxication. However, the high proportion of polysubstance use might have played a role in the intoxication and clinical features in some cases.[179] Other studies and case reports have mentioned the same symptoms[180,181,182,183]

Other features of methoxphenidine described in case reports also include symptoms such as, echolalia, confusion, agitation, opisthotonus, nystagmus and amnesia were consistent with phencyclidine-induced adverse effects.[184] A case of severe rhabdomyolysis and acute kidney injury associated with methoxphenidine has also been published.[185] According to online drug users, it can induce dissociation, visual effects and seems to be associated with seizures at heavy dosages.[186]

Box 6.5 2-oxo-PCE

2-oxo-PCE is another ketamine analogue. Its adverse effects are similar to those of ketamine, but are potentially more toxic, which led to it being described as 'a dangerous emerging arylcyclohexylamine analogue'.[187] A report of a cluster of 56 cases of 2-oxo-PCE-associated acute poisoning between October and November 2017 showed that the main clinical symptoms associated with sole 2-oxo-PCE use include impaired consciousness (84%), confusion (60%), abnormal behaviour (44%), hypertension (80%) and tachycardia (40%). Convulsion (16%) was also observed relatively frequently.[188]

6.11.5 Mortality

In terms of recreational use, fatalities solely linked to ketamine toxicity are relatively uncommon, but can happen. Ketamine-related deaths have been reported in adults using high doses[189] after intravenous doses of 500–1,000 mg.[74,75]

Deaths where ketamine is implicated, typically – but not always – involve the co-consumption of another additional substance, suggesting the particular risk is posed by poly-drug use and drug interaction. For example, the use of ketamine with other CNS depressants (e.g. alcohol) can potentiate CNS depression and/or increase the risk of developing respiratory depression. Concurrent use of diazepam or other benzodiazepines will increase plasma levels and reduce the clearance rate of ketamine.[190]

A retrospective study of all Australian cases in which self-administered ketamine was a mechanism contributory to death in 2000–2019 reported that other drugs were detected in 95.5% of cases. The study reported that pulmonary oedema was present in 82.2% of cases that underwent autopsy and pneumonia in 26.7%.[191]

It has also been noted that deaths from ketamine alone could have been associated with the increased likelihood of accidents caused by the drug's dissociative effects.[128] The effects of ketamine, notably a reduced awareness of risk, a reduced perception of pain, a lack of coordination, a temporary paralysis and an inability to speak, would put users at significant risk of injury or accidents. Although some argued that the highest risk of mortality from ketamine is through accidental death when intoxicated,[91,192] but evidence to support this is limited at present and more research is needed.[82]

6.11.5.1 Methoxetamine and Other Dissociative Novel Psychoactive Substances

Fatal and non-fatal intoxication associated with methoxetamine has been reported.[193] This was often associated with hyperthermia and/or the presence of other drugs.[92,194]

There are also reported deaths associated with 2-Methoxydiphenidine (2-MXP)[195,196] and 2-Methoxy diphenidine.[197,198] There are also reports of fatal and non-fatal acute intoxication associated with 3-MeO-PCP.[199,200,201] Also, case reports[202] associated with 4-methoxyphencyclidine (4-MeO-PCP).[203,204,205,206]

6.12 Management of Acute Harms

6.12.1 Identification and Assessment of Acute Toxicity

Diagnosis of acute ketamine, or other arylcyclohexylamine intoxication in an emergency department setting should be made on clinical assessment and the recognition of the clinical effects of ketamine, also taking into account the common co-ingestion of a number of substances, including alcohol.

A case series of US emergency department presentations suggested that the diagnosis of ketamine should be considered when people (especially young people) present with agitation, tachycardia and either visual hallucinations or nystagmus, although the absence of the latter two findings does not rule out the possibility of ketamine misuse. The authors also recommend that if symptoms are not improving, they should investigate other drugs co-ingested or another differential diagnosis.[145]

Because the onset of the effects of ketamine is rapid and effects are generally short-lived, people will typically develop adverse effects in the setting where the drug was ingested, and symptoms may resolve before they reach hospital. Indeed, some night clubs provide a room or area where unwell users of club drugs are initially assessed and managed prior to transfer to hospital, if required.[207]

This is not the case for all arylcyclohexylamine. The effects of other ketamine and PCP NPS analogues can last longer, as mentioned previously.

6.12.2 Clinical Management of Acute Toxicity

No antidote exists for ketamine overdose. The effects of ketamine are not reversed by naloxone and no other agents are available to reverse the effect in humans.[24] Activated charcoal is not necessary after ketamine acute intoxication, unless there is evidence that a co-ingestant may be contributing to the patient's symptoms or, in the case of a large ingestion, if the patient presents very early. Most patients will improve rapidly following acute ketamine toxicity.[15]

Even in the case of more toxic drugs, such as 2-oxo-PCE, most patients will not require intensive care. For example, in a cluster of 56 cases, only three patients required intensive care.[208]

Although randomised controlled trials and other robust studies are not available, there is consistency in case reports and series that patients are best managed with:

- Standard supportive care, with special attention to cardiac and respiratory functions, as the effects of the drug are usually short-lived;[15,145,209]
- Benzodiazepines may be required;
- Consideration of other causes for clinical presentation, for example co-ingestion of other psychoactive drugs, head injury, hypoglycaemia etc.
- Removal of the person from auditory and visual stimulation until symptoms resolve has been recommended. A quiet environment, with minimal external stimuli, may prevent excessive agitation.[15]

Observation of the patient until vital signs and mental state have normalised is also recommended. If symptoms fail to improve within an hour of presentation, the diagnosis and the management should be reviewed.[15,145] Profoundly obtunded (altered level of consciousness) patients may require airway support, intravenous fluids and titrated benzodiazepine therapy if they are agitated, hyperthermic or show overt sympathomimetic signs.[138]

A study of presentations at a Hong Kong emergency department[138] reported that most of the patients (197/233; 85%) developed no or only minor complications. The majority (168/233; 72%) were safely managed in the emergency department with supportive measures, including intravenous fluid and benzodiazepines for agitation. The five patients requiring management in an intensive care setting had all co-ingested other drugs that could have contributed to their clinical status.[138]

As for ketamine, in the management of acute methoxetamine intoxication, observation and symptom-directed supportive care[28] are recommended; cardiovascular and respiratory support is sometimes needed. In case reports, spontaneous recovery was observed, but the duration of recovery may extend to several days, as for example in a case whereby the patient's features of cerebellar toxicity persisted for 3–4 days before gradual recovery.[210]

As there are at present no specific management recommendations for acute methoxetamine toxicity and in light of the similarities with PCP and ketamine both in terms of pharmacology and clinical presentation, Craig et al. (2014) suggested that it would be reasonable to treat methoxetamine toxicity similarly to ketamine.[211]

Case reports show that oral benzodiazepines are commonly prescribed. Other symptomatic prescribing has also been described, such as antiemetics for nausea and vomiting, and intravenous fluids to prevent or manage rhabdomyolysis, for example.[212,213]

Low-dose benzodiazepines appear to have been sufficient in many cases of methoxetamine acute intoxication, depending on presentation. For example, in addition to observation in hospital, one report described patients being prescribed a dose of 5 mg of oral diazepam, but another needing 5 mg intramuscular of midazolam, to manage agitation, confusion and physiological features.[214]

Spontaneous recovery was reported, and many patients will recover quickly within 24 hours. However, not all will do so. The duration of recovery may extend to several days, as shown for example in a case report describing a patient with features of cerebellar toxicity which persisted for 3–4 days before gradual recovery.[215]

Based on the analysis of cases of suspected NPS intoxication originating from the emergency department or intensive care unit from July 2013 to March 2015, the STRIA project in Sweden identified nine patients who tested positive for 3-MeO-PCP, 4-MeO-PCP or both. It reported that the adverse effects noted in acute intoxications involving 3- and/or 4-MeOPCP resembled those of classical dissociatives such as PCP and ketamine. Management of toxicity was based on observation and standard supportive therapy. In addition, pharmacological treatment with sedatives was reported in 29 (49%) cases. Medical records showed benzodiazepine (primarily diazepam and/or midazolam) in 26 (44%), propofol in 13 (22%) and haloperidol in 5 (8%) medical records. Length of stay in hospital ranged between 1 and 9 days (mean and median of 2) days, but most patients (85%) stayed for 1 or 2 days.[216]

Similarly, a report of a cluster of 56 cases of 2-oxo-PCE-associated acute poisoning reported that the management of acute toxicity was mainly supportive,

whilst three patients required intensive care. All patients were described as having recovered uneventfully.[217] For all these substances, there are however some cases of fatalities associated with acute toxicity as discussed previously.

> For up-to-date guidance on the management of acute toxicity induced by ketamine, its analogues and other dissociatives, readers must consult their local or national guidelines and treatment protocols.
>
> Information should also be sought from the local or regional National Poisons Information Services. It is recommended that relevant clinicians and departments are registered to receive these facilities.

6.13 Harms Associated with Chronic Ketamine Use

The frequent and long-term recreational use of ketamine and its analogues has been shown to be associated with a number of adverse effects including:

6.13.1 Ketamine Dependence

There is evidence that the administration of NMDA receptor agonists, such as ketamine, increases the release of dopamine in the nucleus accumbens, which is typically associated with addiction liability.[218] There are case reports of ketamine dependence,[110,219,220,221] but a lack of large studies, so the incidence is not known.

Frequent ketamine use has been associated with tolerance. Animal studies[222,223] and human studies (children undergoing anaesthesia[224]) have shown a rapid development of tolerance with repeated ketamine dosing. A study of Australian recreational ketamine users found that 22% reported physical tolerance to ketamine.[71] Frequent users of recreational ketamine report escalating dose, with one case report of a 600% increase from dose at first use[95] and another reported a 760% increase from the initiation dose.[225] Also of concern among frequent users are the compulsive patterns of behaviour: bingeing or using without stopping until supplies run out.[227]

Ketamine is associated with craving and a study has shown a high prevalence of depression in patients with ketamine dependence, particularly those with higher levels of cravings. The authors suggest that clients presenting with greater cravings and more depression might require a longer duration of withdrawal treatment.[226]

6.13.1.1 Methoxetamine

Although this has not been thoroughly investigated, there are suggestions that methoxetamine has an abuse liability and addictive effects.[227,228]

Corazza et al. investigated through their analysis of drug user websites the effects of chronic methoxetamine use. Withdrawal symptoms were described and included low mood and depressive thoughts, cognitive impairment for many hours, as well as insomnia and suicide attempts.[23]

6.13.2 Ketamine Withdrawal

There is conflicting evidence on the existence of a specific ketamine withdrawal syndrome following cessation of ketamine use, but a specific ketamine withdrawal syndrome has not yet been described.[132]

In a study of 30 daily users, 28 reported having tried to stop taking ketamine but failing; all reported ketamine cravings as the reason for failure. The study also found that 12 of the 30 daily users reported withdrawal symptoms – anxiety, shaking, sweating and palpitations.[95] Other studies also reported craving and somatic and psychological symptoms (e.g. anxiety) of ketamine withdrawal.[116,229,230]

Clinical experience suggests that ketamine withdrawal does exist. Although ketamine rarely produces serious withdrawal symptoms, the marked drug tolerance and psychological dependence might contribute to difficulty in abstaining.[231] It has been argued that in cases of sustained and heavy use, the existence of a ketamine withdrawal syndrome must be considered.[116]

Although ketamine has a short half-life, metabolites are present for some hours and may be responsible for continuing symptoms.[116] In addition, it has also been argued the symptoms of acute withdrawal may be short-lived and therefore not identified.[232]

Nonetheless, case reports have described somatic and psychological aspects of anxiety as withdrawal symptoms.[116,231,232] One case report mentioned withdrawal symptoms such as 'chills', autonomic arousal, lacrimation, restlessness, nightmares and psychological craving, with further ketamine use to relieve these symptoms.[232] Another described in detail the effects of discontinuation of use on one patient, which included craving and drug hunting, anxiety,

shaking, sweating, palpitations, tiredness, low appetite and low mood.[116]

Even less is known about dependence to methoxetamine and other dissociatives. There are nonetheless reports from people who use it that symptoms following intoxication include low mood, cognitive impairment and insomnia. Craving and tolerance are reported.[233]

6.13.3 Other Harms of Chronic Use of Ketamine

6.13.3.1 Ketamine-Induced Damage to the Urinary Tract

Ketamine use is associated with damage to the urinary system, which can be in the form of severe and in some cases irreversible bladder damage. This has been referred to as ketamine-induced ulcerative cystitis,[132] although some have argued that it would be more appropriate and concise to describe it as ketamine-induced uropathy.[234] The mechanism of damage from ketamine is not yet clear but the effects, which are not specific to the bladder, are most likely to result from direct toxicity of ketamine or its metabolites. Damage can affect the entire urinary tract.[97]

The urological syndrome associated with ketamine use can lead to severe clinical symptoms:[97] a small, very painful bladder, dysuria, painful haematuria, urge incontinence, frequent and urgent urination, nocturia, obstruction of the upper urinary tract, papillary necrosis and hepatic dysfunction.[97,236,235,236,237]

Auxiliary examination showed cases of patients with symptoms including the following: sterile pyuria, contracted bladder (involving chronic inflammation with ulceration), erythematous swelling, necrotic mucosa, thin epithelium with neutrophilic and lymphoplasma cell infiltration in bladder mucosa, collagen and adipose tissue and bladder wall fibrosis with or without vesico-ureteric reflux and involvement of the upper urinary tract.[236] It has also been reported that high dosage and prolonged exposure to ketamine and its metabolites results in inflammatory changes, with microvascular damage, ischaemia and fibrosis.[17,238] End-stage renal disease from upper tract obstruction is another potentially severe harm which can affect chronic ketamine users.[239]

Cystoscopic inspection of the bladder also often shows a denuded urothelium, which, in the most severe cases, may slough off as intact sheets of cells.

There are reports of young patients at an end-stage of the disease process who required cystectomy (bladder removal) and reconstruction,[97] with a serious impact on life expectancy.

An analysis of the experiences of people with ketamine bladder problems has shown that initial symptoms are normalised due to their progressive nature and because they are common amongst other ketamine users. It is argued that this results in delayed help seeking, exacerbates disease progression and further complicates patient management.[240]

It has been reported that 20–30% of ketamine users suffer from lower urinary tract symptoms.[227,237] A study assessing the prevalence of urinary symptoms in a large cohort of non-treatment-seeking ketamine users found that harms to the urinary tract are dose-related and are particularly common among regular and dependent users. Urinary symptoms are associated with an increased frequency of use and increased amount used per session.[40] However, the duration and/or amount of ketamine used to induce lower urinary tract symptoms is not known.

The time of onset of lower urinary tract symptoms following ketamine misuse varies from a few days to a few years following the onset of use, with the severity being in part determined by the chronicity of use. Up to 100% of those using more than 5 grams per day report urinary symptoms.[241] Because of the severe bladder pain, users frequently self-medicate for severe pain with ketamine, as the only effective means of pain relief they know, thus perpetuating the damage to their urinary tract.[97]

Studies of patients in chronic pain and palliative care receiving pharmacological ketamine suggest individual variations, with some individuals more susceptible than others to ketamine-related urological damage.[97] Some series have reported a slight male predominance, but this is statistically insignificant and not universally reported.[242] 'At the present time, it would seem that ketamine-induced vesicopathy does not exhibit any gender bias.[237]

There is also a link between chronic ketamine use and kidney dysfunction. Hydronephrosis secondary to stenosis of the ureter seems to be an emerging health problem associated with frequent and high-dose ketamine use.[132] Chu et al.[237] reported in their study of ketamine-induced ulcerative cystitis that 51% of patients presented with unilateral or bilateral hydronephrosis. Four patients also showed papillary necrosis and this led to renal failure in one. Patients presenting with a history of ketamine use

and urological symptoms need to have their kidneys imaged to rule out ureteric strictures.

A study has shown that ketamine bladder problems have a considerable impact on those affected. In addition to pain and physical effects more generally, it is common that ketamine bladder problems cause feelings such as embarrassment, uncertainty, anxiety, guilt, self-loathing and depression. It has also been suggested that the emotional impact is perhaps further compounded by participants' relatively young age and the perceived self-inflicted nature of their condition. The study also shows that advanced symptoms appear to result in behaviour modification, such as staying close to a toilet, and that this can contribute to social isolation.[243]

Methoxetamine was marketed as a more 'bladder friendly' drug than ketamine. However, there is emerging evidence from an animal study that exposure to methoxetamine can induce changes in the kidney and bladder after daily use, suggesting that chronic use of methoxetamine in humans may be associated with similar lower urinary tract symptoms, as those described for chronic ketamine use.[244]

A cross-sectional, anonymous online survey in the US and UK investigated the prevalence of urinary symptoms in a group of methoxetamine users who had also used ketamine at least once in their lifetime. Approximately one-quarter of methoxetamine users questioned reported urinary symptoms; however, previous ketamine use cannot be ruled out as the cause of the symptoms.[245]

6.13.3.2 Gastrointestinal Toxicity

The use of ketamine has also been linked to gastrointestinal toxicity.[246] The intense abdominal pain associated with ketamine use is referred to by users in some countries as 'K-cramps'.[227]

The Ng study of presentations to emergency departments reported that 21% of ketamine patients presented with abdominal pain and 15% had abnormal liver function.[138] More recently, a cross-sectional study of 611 consecutive patients who were seeking treatment for ketamine uropathy found that 27.5% (n=168) of these patients reported the presence of upper gastrointestinal symptoms. The mean duration of ketamine use before symptom presentation was 5.0 ± 3.1 years.

In this study, the presenting symptoms included epigastric pain (n=155, 25.4%), recurrent vomiting (n=48, 7.9%), anaemia (n=36, 5.9%) and gastrointestinal bleeding (n=20, 3.3%).[247] Interestingly, the study found that uropathy symptoms were preceded by upper gastrointestinal symptoms for 4.4 ± 3.0 years in the majority (n=41, 83.9%) of patients. Other independent factors associated with upper gastrointestinal toxicity were older age, current use and longer duration of ketamine use.[248]

Little is currently known about ketamine-induced abdominal pain. A small number of case reports[238,249,250] have described colic-like, upper gastric pain in young ketamine users who also presented with abnormal liver function. CT scans showed dilation of the common bile duct, mimicking cholecystitis.

It has been suggested that ketamine may adversely affect the liver by direct toxicity to parenchymal cells, resulting in bile duct damage.[251] Impairment of the smooth muscle of the sphincter of Oddi may also be responsible for bile duct dilation.[138,238,251,252] A study has shown that the degree of dilation of the common bile duct was positively correlated with duration of ketamine use.[253]

These symptoms appear to resolve once the patient stops using ketamine and cessation of ketamine use potentially reverses the bile duct and liver injury in these patients.[254,255] However, in one case study, a person had a dilated common bile duct that regressed with abstinence but recurred following a return to ketamine use.[251]

6.13.3.3 Diabetic Ketoacidosis

Ketamine can precipitate diabetic ketoacidosis (DKA) in type 1 diabetes. The metabolic acidosis can be severe and has, in some cases, been associated with rhabdomyolysis.[256–275]

6.13.3.4 Drug Interaction

The use of ketamine raises general issues of adherence to antiretroviral regimens. As a substrate of the CYP450 system (specifically 3A4), ketamine may interact with certain antiretroviral medications, particularly the protease inhibitors with CYP450 inhibitive properties.[276]

Also, its cardiovascular effects may be deleterious among any patients with underlying heart disease or lipid abnormalities.

6.13.3.5 Neurobehavioural, Psychiatric and Psychological Effects

Cognitive Impairment and Memory Impairment

Overall, studies have shown that infrequent ketamine users do not appear to experience long-term cognitive impairment. However, there is evidence that frequent ketamine users do have profound impairments of their short-term and long-term memory, although many studies have been cross-sectional and hence unable to address causation.[132]

Neuropsychological harms appear to be related to frequency and quantity of dosing. Cognitive impairment and long-term psychological effects can result from prolonged use.[277] Ketamine is associated with direct neurotoxicity and can cause acute neuropsychiatric effects. One longitudinal study showed that frequent ketamine use impaired visual recognition and spatial working memory; the degree of impairment was correlated with changes in the level of ketamine use over 12 months.[194] Acute and acute-on-chronic use has been associated with impaired information handling within working memory and episodic memory, as well as deficits in semantic processing,[133,278] with men more affected than women.[279]

A case control study found that frequent ketamine use is associated with impairment of working memory, episodic memory, executive function and psychological wellbeing.[280] One-year follow-up with the same group showed the frequent users on increasing doses were more likely to have cognitive deficits, especially with spatial working memory and pattern recognition memory tasks, with both short-term and long-term memory affected.[279]

One study has shown that delusional thinking was positively correlated with the amount used by frequent users and persisted despite abstinence.[282] A dose-dependent relationship was found at one-year follow-up, with frequent users more delusional than infrequent, abstinent and non-users.[279]

Taking ketamine regularly has detrimental effects on memory function which last beyond the acute effects of the drug. Research suggests frequent use of ketamine produces long-lasting impairments in episodic memory and aspects of retrieval from semantic memory, which goes beyond ingestion.[93]

A three-year longitudinal study of people who had ceased or reduced ketamine use reported that some may continue to experience drug-related symptoms three years later. This is particularly in relation to impairment of episodic memory which was still present three years later and possibly also attentional functioning. Schizotypal symptoms and perceptual distortion may also continue after ketamine cessation.[281]

Research on infrequent users (defined as taking ketamine more than once a month but less than three times per week) and daily ketamine users found that scores on measures for delusion, dissociation and schizotypy were higher in the daily users.[70,279] Morgan et al. found that daily ketamine users had patterns of symptoms similar to individuals in the prodromal phase of schizophrenia.[279] Long-term ketamine users have more pronounced and persistent neuropsychiatric symptoms, generally characterised as schizophrenia-like symptoms. However, there is no evidence of clinically significant positive or negative psychotic symptoms among infrequent users.[282] There is also little evidence of a link between chronic heavy use of ketamine and diagnosis of a psychotic disorder.[132]

Depression

There is some evidence that ketamine may be of therapeutic use for the management of treatment-resistant depression,[56,57,283] as well as post-traumatic stress disorder.[284–305] A large clinical trial testing the efficacy of intravenous ketamine in mood disorders reported that it was associated with a rapid and large antidepressant effect at 24 hours, significantly superior to midazolam. Ketamine appears to possess rapid antidepressant effects independent of its transient psychoactive effects.[306]

In contrast, the frequent use of recreational ketamine or ketamine used outside medical supervision is typified by increased dissociative and depressive symptoms,[279,307] as well as subtle visual anomalies.[223] Morgan et al.'s longitudinal study[279] found increased levels of depression in both daily users and ex-ketamine users over the course of one year, but not among infrequent users. However, the depression was not at clinical levels and the increase was not correlated with changes in ketamine use.[132]

It is possible that rates of depression are higher among people who are getting treatment for ketamine use disorders. A study of case records of 129 patients classified as dependent on ketamine and receiving treatment at three substance use clinics in Hong Kong between January 2008 and August 2012 found a high frequency of psychosis and/or depression in patients with chronic ketamine use. In this study, substance-induced psychotic disorder accounted for 31.8% followed by depressive disorder (27.9%). The authors reported that depressive symptoms can either be premorbid or secondary to substance use.[308]

Neurological Effects

Animal studies have shown that ketamine is directly neurotoxic. Abnormalities were also found in ketamine-dependent patients in bilateral frontal (including corpus callosum and anterior cingulate cortex) and left temporoparietal white matter. A recent human study of 41 ketamine-dependent users and 44 drug-free volunteers showed bilateral degeneration of frontal and left temporoparietal white matter in ketamine users.[309] The study also reported that fractional anisotropy values negatively correlated with the total lifetime ketamine consumption.[311]

A case report has also demonstrated a reduction of frontal grey matter volume in ketamine-dependent patients. This reduction was correlated with duration of ketamine use; reduction in the left superior frontal gyrus correlated with estimated total lifetime consumption.[310]

Social Harms

A study of 100 recreational users of ketamine found that while one in five stated that they had ever experienced severe side-effects, more than one third (38%) reported having to deal with someone else who had suffered badly following ketamine use. The most commonly reported problems were in the areas of employment (20%), relationships (5%), financial (5%) and legal (1%).[71] The authors suggest that the problems were likely linked to the neurochemical consequences of ketamine use and the toxicity that might result.[71]

6.14 Management of Harms Related to Chronic Ketamine Use

6.14.1 Identification and Assessment

The first step for the identification of ketamine use and harms by specialist treatment services is to include questions relating to ketamine in routine care.

The modification of existing assessment instruments and data collection tools is indicated.

Assessment of ketamine use is similar to assessment for other drug use, with the addition of screening questions on urological and gastrointestinal symptoms and questions on the direct consequences of dissociation (e.g. cognitive impairment, sexual behaviours).

6.14.2 Psychosocial and Pharmacological Support

6.14.2.1 Psychological Support

Information on psychosocial support is presented in Chapter 2 and is relevant for ketamine users.

A small number of ketamine-specific studies have also been conducted. Copeland et al. suggest that the harms that require further investigation are the association of ketamine use with unsafe sex and injecting behaviours and its neurotoxic effects. They also argue that effective brief and early interventions are needed for those who are at risk of harm because of ketamine intoxication and/or excessive and regular consumption. Interventions should address ketamine use in situations where there is a heightened risk of accidental death because cognition is impaired.[24]

Critchlow described the treatment of a person with dependence on ketamine that involved three motivational interviewing sessions in the first instance.[116] Maxwell suggests an abstinence-oriented approach be used for ketamine, similar to that used for psychostimulants.[311] They suggest following the model used for cocaine and amphetamine dependence, with abstinence from all drugs from day 1. This may require the therapist to avoid being confrontational to prevent treatment drop-out; relapse prevention is also indicated.[94]

6.14.2.2 Pharmacological Interventions for Dependence and Withdrawal

Ketamine withdrawal is described in Section 6.13.2.

A case report describes medically assisted detoxification carried out in conjunction with three sessions of motivational interviewing. Detoxification was carried out using a reducing regimen of diazepam over 3 days. The regimen was successful and eliminated the majority of withdrawal symptoms.[116]

Others have also suggested that, in cases of sustained heavy use and where acute withdrawal syndrome is a possibility, a benzodiazepine detoxification regimen modified from alcohol detoxification regimens may lessen the symptoms arising from discontinuation.[312]

It has been suggested that symptomatic management of withdrawal is indicated in some cases, with low-dose benzodiazepine as a starting point. There are no studies to support the use of other pharmaceutical agents, so any prescribing must be based on clinical assessment.

There is also a case report of withdrawal symptoms which responded well to naltrexone.[313] There are a very small number of case reports that mention anti-psychotics and anti-depressants. For example, one case report mentioned that Paliperidone Palmitate may be useful in drug dose-reduction and maintaining abstinence.[314] Another report described what is called a significant reduction in craving and ketamine use after taking lamotrigine.[315]

A case report has shown a patient with a history of alcohol and ketamine dependence experiencing ketamine-like dissociative symptoms after alcohol consumption in the context of ketamine abstinence. It has been suggested that high dose alcohol may directly produce 'K-hole experiences' or perhaps trigger conditioned ketamine-like experiences in a patient who had been abstinent from ketamine for at least 1 year and was admitted for alcohol withdrawal treatment.[316]

6.14.2.3 Aftercare and Support

Chapter 2 presents information on aftercare. A few ketamine-specific studies have been conducted, with some suggesting that ketamine users' ability and willingness to abstain from using the drug may be low, even when (and perhaps because) experiencing significant urological problems. Chu et al. showed that 9 out of 24 ketamine users with bladder problems were able to abstain from the drug and complete the Pelvic Pain and Urgency/Frequency questionnaire.[237] Another study found that only 3 out of 10 patients stayed ketamine free for more than one year.[233]

6.14.3 Management of Urinary Tract Problems

Within substance misuse treatment centres, it is recommended that patients with a ketamine use history and with recurrent urological problems, or patients with unexplained urinary symptoms, are assessed by a urologist to exclude other causes and evaluate any damage. Any other patients with unexplained symptoms should be screened for ketamine use.[97] Appropriate support to stop ketamine use must be available, as well as advice regarding appropriate medical pain relief.

It has been argued that many health care professionals, including psychiatrists, are still unaware of the 'devastating potential of ketamine' for the urinary tract[317] and should be alerted to this problem.[318] The authors also recommend that ketamine use should be considered by other clinicians. Specifically, gastro-enterologists should consider ketamine use in a setting of biliary ectasia without an obstructive cause. They also suggest that ketamine should be considered by urologists and nephrologists in patients with a history of drug abuse and lower urinary tract symptoms in the absence of another aetiology.[319]

The most effective treatment for ketamine-related urological problems is cessation of use and it is essential that use of ketamine is stopped upon recognition of symptoms. Strategies are limited when use continues.[320] If drug cessation is achieved, the syndrome may be partially or completely reversed, but if ketamine use persists, so do symptoms. In a few patients, however, symptoms persist despite stopping drug use.[321,322]

Patients should also be referred to specialist drug services.[97] A survey of UK urologists suggested that approximately one third of urological problems resolved after drug cessation, one-third remained static and one-third progressed.[322]

There is limited literature to support how to manage patients with ketamine-related uropathy. It is suggested that most patients are managed conservatively, or with minimally invasive surgical intervention.

Early stages of the urological syndrome may present in casual or weekend users as episodes of cystitis, which can be treated empirically[97] (based on practical experience and observation). More frequent users may have irreversible damage and scarring. The most affected patients may require major surgery, in the form of cystectomy and bladder reconstruction.[97] Urinary tract reconstruction is reserved for those with refractory symptoms, contracted bladders or upper tract compromise.[323]

Where ketamine is identified as a factor, it has been recommended that renal function be assessed; a CT urogram can also be an important investigation to reveal the extent of the disease. A urine culture is mandatory. A routine evaluation of the upper tracts with a CT urogram can rule out ureteric stricture and cystoscopy can be used to assess bladder capacity.[97] In patients with normal renal function and with an ultrasound that shows no hydronephrosis, a CT scan may not be necessary.[324]

Treatment for urinary tract symptoms is either symptomatic (analgesia, urinary diversion) or the treatment of complications (e.g. percutaneous nephrostomy insertion).[322] Surgical and pharmacological approaches have been tried in order to relieve some symptoms and include cystoplasty, distention, partial cystectomy, opiates, pregabalin, duloxetine, tricyclic antidepressants, anticholinergics and anti-inflammatory drugs.[325]

Urinary tract reconstruction in patients with severe morbidity has been described as a major undertaking with a high risk of perioperative morbidity.[326] A study suggests that people with a history of ketamine use appeared to have a significantly higher rate of postoperative complications when compared with patients who underwent reconstructive surgery for other benign disease (congenital anomalies, neurogenic disease, intractable incontinence and interstitial cystitis/bladder pain syndrome (IC/BPS)).[327]

A strategy for the treatment of ketamine-related urological problems has been suggested by Wood et al.[97] Central to this is the requirement for patients to stop their ketamine use. However, this may be complicated by a need for pain control in those with ulcerative cystitis. This will require the treating team to develop an alternative pain management plan with the patient. There may also be a lack of motivation to abstain and non-compliance with urological investigation and treatment appointments.[97]

Winstock et al. recommended a multidisciplinary approach promoting harm reduction, cessation and early referral, to avoid progression to severe and irreversible urological pathologies.[324] Similarly, Wood et al. suggested a need for liaison between specialist drug services and local urology services.[324] Some drug agencies have developed proactive models.[97] However, this is not always possible, as patients can see urology departments outside their residential area. In this case, support is best organised by the general medical practitioner.[97]

It has been suggested that healthcare professionals can successfully engage young people during their stay in hospital for ketamine-related urological problems to participate in a package of psychosocial interventions, motivational interviewing and lifestyle re-design.[328]

In all cases, appropriate support to stop ketamine use must be available, as well as advice regarding appropriate medical pain relief.

6.15 Public Health and Public Safety

6.15.1 Viral and Bacterial Infections

Studies have reported that ketamine injecting is associated with high-risk behaviours like the sharing of injecting equipment and paraphernalia,[329,330] poly-drug use[331,332] and multiple injections. Ketamine injecting puts the user at risk of viral and bacterial infections and hence the potential risk of their transmission to others.

6.15.2 Accidents and Assaults

Ketamine impairs psychomotor functioning dose-dependently and higher doses increase the risk of accidents.[332,333] Ketamine use has been associated with driving accidents in Hong Kong: 9% of fatal drug- and alcohol-related single-car collisions in Hong King during 1996–2000 involved ketamine.[334] Driving accidents associated with methoxetamine have been reported.[335]

Ketamine use can place the user at risk of sexual assault, although studies have suggested that ketamine is not implicated in drug-facilitated assault.[336,337]

6.16 Harm Reduction

It has been recommended that all ketamine users are given the standard harm reduction advice, which includes not using the drug when alone, avoiding poly-use and co-ingestion of other substances, including alcohol, and information on a safe environment and safer injecting techniques.[24,93]

The following more specific harm reduction advice should be given to ketamine users:

- Users should be advised to measure dose carefully and start with a small test dose. They should also be advised to measure intervals between doses accurately.
- People who use or suspect that they are using methoxetamine should be aware that it has much slower onset of action of the latter (up to 90 minutes). Repeated dosing and inadvertent excessive dosing may result in unintentional overdose.
- The use of ketamine with other drugs, including alcohol, should be avoided.[24]
- Users should minimise the risk of accidental injury by ensuring that intoxicated friends are always accompanied by others who are not.[132] The dissociative effect of ketamine puts users at risk: drowning in shallow waters, including a bath, and hypothermia from long walks have been highlighted as risks.
- Users should be made aware of the link to urological problems, and other ketamine-related harms.

- Users who develop tolerance and who find themselves needing to use increasingly higher doses, and who are using more frequently than intended, should be advised to monitor their intake. Diaries and electronic tools can be very useful.
- Advice should be given to users that those acutely intoxicated should not be left alone in case of accidents and should have someone with them who has not used the substance.[132]
- Users should be made aware of the potential neurological and cognitive changes following frequent use of ketamine, which can result in poor performance at school, college or work.[132]
- Ketamine users who feel depressed and anxious when stopping or reducing ketamine should be encouraged to seek professional help to manage their symptoms during a gradual reduction or detoxification.
- Users should be made aware that the anaesthetic topical effects of ketamine mean that they may not feel pain from tissue trauma and extra caution must be exercised with any sexual activity which risks tissue damage.
- Daily use of ketamine should be avoided, due to the urological risks.
- Ketamine users with urological problems should be strongly encouraged to cease using the drug.

Advice should be given to users with urological problems not to deliberately dehydrate and to seek medical help and referral to a specialist to reduce the risk of permanent harm. Corazza et al. in their analysis of Internet sites found that users themselves suggested that dosages should increase only gradually. Users recommended that doses of 50 mg should not be exceeded on the first occasion of use, or when the drug was taken orally. The websites also advised users not to use methoxetamine with alcohol, tetra-hydrocannabinol, selective serotonin reuptake inhibitors or monoamine oxidase inhibitors. Users were advised to try a test dose of a few milligrams and to wait 2 hours before re-dosing.

References

1. World Drug Report 2019 (United Nations publication, Sales No. E.19.XI.8).

2. Craig CL, Loeffler GH. The ketamine analog methoxetamine: a new designer drug to threaten military readiness. *Mil Med* 2014;**179**(10):1149.

3. Zukin SR, Sloboda ZJ, Daniel C. Phencyclidine (PCP). In: *Substance Abuse: A Comprehensive Textbook*, 4th ed., pp. 324–335. Edited by JH Lowinson, P Ruiz, B Millmann, et al. Philadelphia, PA, Lippincott Williams & Wilkins, 1994.

4. World Drug Report 2019 (United Nations publication, Sales No. E.19.XI.8).

5. European Monitoring Centre for Drugs and Drug Addiction (EMCDDA). European Drug Report 2019: Trends and Developments. Luxembourg, Publications Office of the European Union, 2019.

6. Van Hout MC, Hearne E. 'Word of mouse': indigenous harm reduction and online consumerism of the synthetic compound methoxphenidine. *J Psychoactive Drugs* 2015;**47**(1):30–41. https://doi.org/10.1080/02791072.2014.974002

7. Bäckberg M, Beck O, Helander A. Phencyclidine analog use in Sweden: intoxication cases involving 3-MeO-PCP and 4-MeO-PCP from the STRIDA project. *Clin Toxicol* 2015;**53**(9):856–864. https://doi.org/10.3109/15563650.2015.1079325

8. See also Wallach JB, Simon D. Phencyclidine-based new psychoactive substances. *Handb Exp Pharmacol* 2018;**252**:261–303.

9. Berger ML, Schweifer A, Rebernik P, Hammerschmidt F. NMDA receptor affinities of 1,2-diphenylethylamine and 1-(1,2-diphenylethyl) piperidine enantiomers and of related compounds. *Bioorg Med Chem* 2009;**17**:3456–3462.

10. Wallach J, De Paoli G, Adejare A, Brandt SD. Preparation and analytical characterization of 1-(1-phenylcyclohexyl) piperidine (PCP) and 1-(1-phenylcyclohexyl)pyrrolidine (PCPy) analogues. *Drug Test Anal* 2014;**6**:633–650.

11. Anis NA, Berry SC, Burton NR, Lodge D. The dissociative anaesthetics, ketamine and phencyclidine, selectively reduce excitation of central mammalian neurones by N-methyl-aspartate. *Br J Pharmacol* 1983;**79**:565–575.

12. Helander A, Beck O, Bäckberg M. Intoxications by the dissociative new psychoactive substances diphenidine and methoxphenidine. *Clin Toxicol (Phila)* 2015;**53**:446–453.

13. Morris H, Wallach J. From PCP to MXE: a comprehensive review of the non-medical use of dissociative drugs. *Drug Test Anal* 2014;**6**:614–632.

14. Domino EF, Chodoff P, Corssen G. Pharmacologic effects of Ci-581, a new dissociative anesthetic, in man. *Clin Pharmacol Ther* 1965;**6**:279–291.

15. Kalsi SS, Wood DM, Dargan PI. The epidemiology and patterns of acute and chronic toxicity associated with recreational ketamine use. *Emerg Health Threats J* 2011;**4**:7107. https://doi.org/10.3402/ehtj.v4i0.7107

16. Quibell R, Prummer EC, Mihalyo M, Twycross R, Wilcock A. Ketamine. *J Pain Symptom Mgt* 2011;**41**:640–649.

17. Rabiner EA. Imaging of striatal dopamine release elicited with NMDA antagonists: is there anything there to be seen? *J Psychopharmacol* 2007;**21**:253–258.

18. Yanagihara Y, Kariya S, Ohtani M, et al. Involvement of CYP2B6 in n-demethylation of ketamine in human liver microsomes. *Drug Metab Dispos* 2001;**29**:887–890.

19. World Health Organization. Model List of Essential Medicines: 19th List (April 2015) amended November 2015.

20. Liao Y, Tang Y-L, Hao W. Ketamine and international regulations. *Am J Drug Alcohol Abuse* 2017(online). https://doi.org/10.1080/00952990.2016.1278449

21. Advisory Council on the Misuse of Drugs (ACMD). Ketamine: A Review of Use and Harm. London, Home Office, 2013.

22. Weil A, Rosen W. *Chocolate to Morphine: Understanding Mind-Active Drugs*. Boston, MA, Houghton Mifflin, 1983.

23. Corazza O, Schifano F, Simonato P, et al. Phenomenon of new drugs on the Internet: the case of ketamine derivative methoxetamine. *Hum Psychopharmacol* 2012;**27**(2):145–149. https://doi.org/10.1002/hup.1242

24. Copeland J, Dillon P. The health and psycho-social consequences of ketamine use. *Int J Drug Policy* 2005;**16**:122–131.

25. Hijazi Y, Boulieu R. Contribution of CYP3A4, CYP2B6, and CYP2C9 isoforms to N-demethylation of ketamine in human liver microsomes. *Drug Metab Dispos* 2002;**30**:853–858.

26. Halberstadt AL, Slepak N, Hyun J, Buell MR, Powell SB. The novel ketamine analog methoxetamine produces dissociative-like behavioral effects in rodents. *Psychopharmacology* 2016;**233**:1215–1225. https://doi.org/10.1007/s00213-016-4203-3

27. Gibbons S, Zloh M. An analysis of the 'legal high' mephedrone. *Bioorg Med Chem Lett* 2010;**20**:4135–4139.

28. Hofer KE, Grager B, Müller DM, et al. Ketamine-like effects after recreational use of methoxetamine. *Ann Emerg Med* 2012;**60**(1):97–99. https://doi.org/10.1016/j.annemergmed.2011.11.018

29. Roth BL, Gibbons S, Arunotayanun W, et al. The ketamine analogue methoxetamine and 3- and 4-methoxy analogues of phencyclidine are high affinity and selective ligands for the glutamate NMDA receptor. *PLoS One* 2013;**8**(3):e59334. https://doi.org/10.1371/journal.pone.0059334

30. Zanda MT, Fadda P, Antinori S, et al. Methoxetamine affects brain processing involved in emotional response in rats. *Br J Pharmacol* 2017;**174**(19):3333–3345. https://doi.org/10.1111/bph.13952

31. Coppola M, Mondola R. Methoxetamine: from drug of abuse to rapid-acting antidepressant. *Med Hypotheses* 2012;**79**:504–507.

32. Corazza O, Assi S, Schifano F. From 'Special K' to 'Special M': the evolution of the recreational use of ketamine and methoxetamine. *CNS Neurosci Ther* 2013;**19**:454–460.

33. Corazza O, Schifano F, Simonato P, et al. Phenomenon of new drugs on the Internet: the case of ketamine derivative methoxetamine. *Hum Psychopharmacol Clin Exp* 2012;**27**:145–149.

34. Winstock AR, Lawn W, Deluca P, Borschmann R. Methoxetamine: an early report on the motivations for use, effect profile and prevalence of use in a UK clubbing sample. *Drug Alcohol Rev* 2016;**35**:212–217. https://doi.org/10.1111/dar.12259

35. Lawn W, Borschmann R, Cottrell A, Winstock A. Methoxetamine: prevalence of use in the USA and UK and associated urinary problems. *J Subst Use* 2016;**21**:115–120.

36. Dargan P, Tang H, Liang W, Wood D, Yew D. Three months of methoxetamine administration is associated with significant bladder and renal toxicity in mice. *Clin Toxicol* 2014;**52**:176–180.

37. Wang Q, Wu Q, Wang J, et al. Ketamine analog methoxetamine induced inflammation and dysfunction of bladder in rats. *Int J Mol Sci* 2017;**18**:117.

38. Botanasa CJ, Bryan de la Penaa J, Kima HJ, Sup Lee Y, Hoon J. Methoxetamine: a foe or friend? *Neurochem Int* 2019; **122**:1–7.

39. Karlow N, Schlaepfer C H, Stoll C RT, et al. A systematic review and meta-analysis of ketamine as an alternative to opioids for acute pain in the emergency department. *Acad Emerg Med* 2018;**25**(10):1086–1097. https://doi.org/10.1111/acem.13502

40. National Poisons Information Service. Annual Report 2012/2013. London, Public Health England, 2013.

41. Jones JL, Mateus CF, Malcolm RJ, Brady KT, Back SE. Efficacy of ketamine in the treatment of substance use disorders: a systematic review. *Front Psychiatry* 2018;**9**:277. https://doi.org/10.3389/fpsyt.2018.00277

42. Malhi GS, Byrow Y, Cassidy F, et al. Ketamine: stimulating antidepressant treatment? *BJPsych Open* 2016;**2**:e5–e9. https://doi.org/10.1192/bjpo.bp.116.002923

43. Singh I, Morgan C, Curran V. Ketamine treatment for depression: opportunities for clinical innovation and ethical foresight. *Lancet Psychiatry* 2017;**4**(5):419–426.

44. Schoevers RA, Chaves TV, Balukova SM, van het Rot M, Kortekaas R. Oral ketamine for the treatment of pain and treatment-resistant depression *Br J Psychiatry* 2016;**208**:108–113. https://doi.org/1192/bjp.bp.115.165498

45. Swiatek KM, Jordan K, Coffman J. New use for an old drug: oral ketamine for treatment-resistant depression. *Br Med J Case Rep* 2016 (online). https://doi.org/10.1136/bcr-2016-216088

46. Zarate CA, Singh JB, Carlson PJ, et al. A randomized trial of an N-methyl-D-aspartate antagonist in treatment-resistant major depression. *Arch Gen Psychiatry* 2006;**63**(8):856–864.

47. Krystal JH. Ketamine and the potential role for rapid acting antidepressant medications. *Swiss Med Wkly* 2007;**137**:215–216.

48. Schwartz J, Murrough JW, Iosifescu DV. Ketamine for treatment-resistant depression: recent developments and clinical applications *Evid Based Mental Health* 2016;**19**(2):35–38.

49. Mathew SJ, Shah A, Lapidus K, et al. Ketamine for treatment-resistant unipolar depression. *CNS Drugs* 2012;**26**:189–204.

50. Murrough JW, Iosifescu DV, Chang LC, et al. An antidepressant efficacy of ketamine in treatment-resistant major depression: a two-site randomized controlled trial. *Am J Psychiatry* 2013;**170**:1134–1142.

51. Fond G, Loundou A, Rabu C, et al. Ketamine administration in depressive disorders: a systematic review and meta-analysis. *Psychopharmacology (Berl)* 2014;**231**:3663–3676.

52. McGirr A, Berlim MT, Bond DJ, et al. A systematic review and meta-analysis of randomized, double-blind, placebo-controlled trials of ketamine in the rapid treatment of major depressive episodes. *Psychol Med* 2015;**45**:693–704.

53. SchakJennifer KM, Van de Voort L, Johnson EK, et al. Potential risks of poorly monitored ketamine use in depression treatment. *Am J Psychiatry* 2016;**173**:3.

54. DeWilde KE, Levitch CF, Murrough JW, Mathew SJ, Iosifescu DV. The promise of ketamine for treatment-resistant depression: current evidence and future directions. *Ann N Y Acad Sci* 2015;**1345**:47–58. https://doi.org/10.1111/nyas.12646

55. Short B, Fong J, Galvez V, Shelker W, Loo CK. Side-effects associated with ketamine use in depression: a systematic review. *Lancet Psychiatry* 2018;**5**:65–78. https://doi.org/10.1016/S2215-0366(17)30272-9

56. Berman RM, Cappiello A, Anand A, et al. Antidepressant effects of ketamine in depressed patients. *Biol Psychiatry* 2000;**47**(4):351–354.

57. Zarate CA, Singh JB, Carlson PJ, et al. A randomized trial of an N-methyl-D-aspartate antagonist in treatment-resistant major depression. *Arch Gen Psychiatry* 2006;**63**(8):856–864.

58. Krystal JH. Ketamine and the potential role for rapid acting antidepressant medications. *Swiss Med Wkly* 2007;**137**:215–216.

59. Bell RF. Ketamine for chronic noncancer pain: concerns regarding toxicity. *Curr Opin Support Palliat Care* 2012;**6**(2):183–187. https://doi.org/10.1097/SPC.0b013e328352812c

60. Zhu W, Ding Z, Zhang Y, Shi J, Hashimoto K, Lu L. Risks associated with misuse of ketamine as a rapid-acting antidepressant. *Neurosci Bull* 2016;**32**(6):557–564. https://doi.org/10.1007/s12264-016-0081-2

61. Botanasa CJ, Bryan de la Penaa J, Kima HJ, Lee YS, Cheonga JH. Methoxetamine: a foe or friend? *Neurochem Int* 2019;**122**:1–7.

62. Coppola M, Mondola R. Methoxetamine: from drug of abuse to rapid-acting antidepressant. *Med Hypotheses* 2012;**79**:504–507.

63. Botanas CJ, de la Pena JB, Custodio RJ, de la PenKim HI, Cho MC, Lee YS. Methoxetamine produces rapid and sustained antidepressant effects probably via glutamatergic and serotonergic mechanisms. *Neuropharmacology* 2017;**126**:121–127.

64. Zanda M, Fadda P, Antinori S, et al. Methoxetamine affects brain processing involved in emotional response in rats. *Br J Pharmacol* 2017;**174**:3333–3345.

65. Sayson L V, Botanas C J, Custodio RJ et al. The novel methoxetamine analogs N-ethylnorketamine hydrochloride (NENK), 2-MeO-N-ethylketamine hydrochloride

(2-MeO-NEK), and 4-MeO-N-ethylketamine hydrochloride (4-MeO-NEK) elicit rapid antidepressant effects via activation of AMPA and 5-HT2 receptors. *Psychopharmacology* 2019;**236**(7):2201–2210. https://doi.org/10.1007/s00213-019-05219-x

66. European Monitoring Centre for Drugs and Drug Addiction (EMCDDA). 2012 Annual Report on the State of the Drug Problem in Europe.

67. Available at: www.globaldrugsurvey.com/wp-content/themes/globaldrugsurvey/results/GDS2019-Exec-Summary.pdf [last accessed 2 March 2022].

68. European Monitoring Centre for Drugs and Drug Addiction (EMCDDA). European Drug Report 2019: Trends and Developments. Luxembourg, Publications Office of the European Union, 2019.

69. Moore K, Measham F. 'It's the most fun you can have for twenty quid': motivations, consequences and meanings of British ketamine use. *Addict Res Theory* 2008;**16**(3):231–244.

70. Curran V, Morgan C. Cognitive, dissociative and psychotogenic effects of ketamine in recreational users on the night of drug use and 3 days later. *Addiction* 2000;**95**:575–590.

71. Dillon P, Copeland J, Jansen K. Patterns of use and harms associated with non-medical ketamine use. *Drug Alcohol Depend* 2003;**69**:23–28.

72. Clatts MC, Goldsamt L, Huso Y. Club drug use among young men who have sex with men in NYC: a preliminary epidemiological profile. *Subst Use Misuse* 2005;**40**:1317–1330.

73. Dalgarno PJ, Shewan D. Illicit use of ketamine in Scotland. *J Psychoactive Drugs* 1996;**28**:191–199.

74. Long H. Case report: ketamine medication error resulting in death. *Int J Med Toxicol* 2003;**6**:2.

75. Licata M, Pierini G, Popoli G. A fatal ketamine poisoning. *J Forensic Sci* 1994;**39**:1314–1320.

76. World Drug Report 2019 (United Nations publication, Sales No. E.19.XI.8).

77. Riley SC, James C, Gregory D, Dingle H, Cadger M. Patterns of recreational drug use at dance events in Edinburgh, Scotland. *Addiction* 2001;**96**(7):1035–1047.

78. Mitcheson L, McCambridge J, Byrne A, Hunt N, Winstock A. Sexual health risk among dance drug users: cross-sectional comparisons with nationally representative data. *Int J Drug Policy* 2008;**19**(4):304–310. https://doi.org/10.1016/j.drugpo.2007.02.002

79. Darrow WW, Biersteker S, Geiss T, et al. Risky sexual behaviors associated with recreational drug use among men who have sex with men in an international resort area: challenges and opportunities. *J Urban Health* 2005;**82**:601–609.

80. Lee SJ, Galanter M, Dermatis H, McDowell D. Circuit parties and patterns of drug use in a subset of gay men. *J Addictive Diseases* 2003;**22**(4):47–60.

81. Mattison AM, Ross MW, Wolfson T, Franklin D. Circuit party attendance, club drug use, and unsafe sex in gay men. *J Subst Abuse* 2001;**13**(1–2):119–126.

82. Ross MW, Mattison AM, Franklin D. Club drugs and sex on drugs are associated with different motivations for gay circuit party attendance in men. *Subst Use Misuse* 2003;**38**(8):1171–1179.

83. Jang MY, Long CY, Chuang SM, et al. Sexual dysfunction in women with ketamine cystitis: a case-control study. *BJU Int* 2012;**110**(3):427–431. https://doi.org/10.1111/j.1464-410X.2011.10780.x

84. Suppiah B, Vicknasingam B, Singh D, Narayanan S. Erectile dysfunction among people who use ketamine and poly-drugs. *J Psychoactive Drugs* 2016;**48**(2):86–92.

85. Lankenau SE, Bloom JJ, Shin C. Longitudinal trajectories of ketamine use among young injection drug users. *Int J Drug Policy* 2010;**21**(4):306–314. https://doi.org/10.1016/j.drugpo.2010.01.007

86. Lankenau SE, Clatts MC. Ketamine injection among high-risk youths: preliminary findings from New York City. *J Drug Issues* 2002;**32**(3):893–905.

87. Bristol Drug Project. Ketamine: just a harmless party drug? *Drink and Drug News*, **28** July 2008.

88. Darke S, Duflou J, Farrell M, Peacock A, Lappin J. Characteristics and circumstances of death related to the self-administration of ketamine. *Addiction* 2020 (online). https://doi.org/10.1111/add.15154

89. Han E, Kwon NJ, Feng L-Y, Li J-H, Chung H. Illegal use patterns, side effects, and analytical methods of ketamine. *Forensic Sci Int* 2016;**268**:25–34. https://doi.org/10.1016/j.forsciint.2016.09.001

90. Sinner B, Graf BM. Ketamine. *Handb Exp Pharmacol* 2008;**182**:313–333.

91. Jansen KL. A review of the nonmedical use of ketamine: use, users and consequences. *J Psychoactive Drugs* 2000;**32**:419–433.

92. Corazza O, Assi S, Schifano F. From 'Special K' to 'Special M': the evolution of the recreational use of ketamine and methoxetamine. *CNS Neurosci Ther* 2013;**19**(6):454–460. https://doi.org/10.1111/cns.12063

93. Curran HV, Monaghan L. In and out of the K-hole: a comparison of the acute and residual effects of ketamine in frequent and infrequent ketamine users. *Addiction* 2001;**96**(5):749–760.

94. Jansen KL, Darracot-Cankovic R. The nonmedical use of ketamine, part two: a review of problem use and dependence. *J Psychoactive Drugs* 2001;**33**:151–158.

95. Morgan CJ, Rees H, Curran HV. Attentional bias to incentive stimuli in frequent ketamine users. *Psychol Med* 2008;**38**:1331–1340.

96. Moreton JE, Meisch RA, Stark L, Thompson T. Ketamine self-administration by the rhesus monkey. *J Pharmacol Exp Ther* 1977;**203**:303–309.

97. Wood D, Cottrell A, Baker SC, et al. Recreational ketamine: from pleasure to pain. *BJU Int* 2011;**107**(12):1881–1884. https://doi.org/10.1111/j.1464-410X.2010.10031.x

98. Rosenbaum CD, Carreiro SP, Babu KM. Here today, gone tomorrow . . . and back again? A review of herbal marijuana alternatives (K2, Spice), synthetic cathinones (Bath Salts), Kratom, Salvia divinorum, methoxetamine, and piperazines. *J Med Toxicol* 2012;**8**(1):15–32. https://doi.org/10.1007/s13181-011-0202-2

99. Corazza O, Schifano F, Simonato P, et al. The phenomenon of new drugs on the Internet: a study on the diffusion of the ketamine derivative methoxetamine ('MXE'). *Hum Psychopharmacol* 2012;**27**:145–149.

100. Corazza O, Assi S, Schifano F. From 'Special K' to 'Special M': the evolution of the recreational use of ketamine and methoxetamine. *CNS Neurosci Ther* 2013;**19**:454e460. https://doi.org/10.1111/cns.12063

101. Hondebrink L, Kasteel EEJ, Tukker AM, et al. Neuropharmacological characterization of the new psychoactive substance methoxetamine. *Neuropharmacology* 2017;**123**:1–9.

102. Winstock AR, Lawn W, Deluca P, Borschmann R. Methoxetamine: an early report on the motivations for use, effect profile and prevalence of use in a UK clubbing sample. *Drug Alcohol Rev* 2016;**35**:212–217. https://doi.org/10.1111/dar.12259

103. Craig CL, Loeffler GH. The ketamine analog methoxetamine: a new designer drug to threaten military readiness. *Mil Med* 2014;**179**(10): 1149.

104. Botanasa CJ, Bryan de la Pena J, Kima HJ, Lee YS, Cheonga JH. Methoxetamine: a foe or friend? *Neurochem Int* 2019; **122**:1–7.

105. Advisory Council on the Misuse of Drugs (ACMD). Statement of Evidence on Methoxetamine. London, Home Office, 2012.

106. Gerace E, Bovetto E, Di Corcia D, Vincenti M, Salomone A. A case of nonfatal intoxication associated with the recreational use of diphenidine. *J Forensic Sci* 2017;**62**:1107–1111.

107. Siegel RK. Phencyclidine and ketamine intoxication: a study of four populations of recreational users. In: RC Peterson, RC Stillman, eds. *Phencyclidine Abuse: An Appraisal* (NIDA Research Monograph **21**), pp. 119–147. Bethesda, MD, National Institute on Drug Abuse, 1978.

108. Benschop A, Urbán R, Kapitány-Fövény M, et al. Why do people use new psychoactive substances? Development of a new measurement tool in six European countries. *J Psychopharmacol* 2020;**34**(6):600–611. https://doi.org/10.1177/0269881120904951

109. Teltzrow R, Bosch OG. Ecstatic anaesthesia: ketamine and GHB between medical use and self-experimentation. *Appl Cardiopulm Pathophysiol* 2012;**16**:309–321.

110. Hurt PH, Ritchie EC. A case of ketamine dependence. *Am J Psychiatry* 1994;**151**:779.

111. Teltzrow R, Bosch OG. Ecstatic anaesthesia: ketamine and GHB between medical use and self-experimentation. *Appl Cardiopulm Pathophysiol* 2012;**16**:309–321.

112. Ross S. Ketamine and addiction. *Prim Psychiatry* 2008;**15**(9):61–69.

113. Wolff K. Ketamine: the pharmacokinetics and pharmacodynamics in misusing populations. In: *The SAGE Handbook of Drug & Alcohol Studies*. London: Sage Publications, 2016.

114. Stirling J, McCoy L. Quantifying the psychological effects of ketamine: from euphoria to the K-hole. *Subst Use Misuse*. 2010;**45**(14):2428–2443. https://doi.org/10.3109/10826081003793912

115. Leary T, Sirius RU. *Design for Dying*. London: HarperCollins, 1998.

116. Critchlow DG. A case of ketamine dependence with discontinuation symptoms. *Addiction* 2006;**101**(8):1212–1213.

117. Gill JR, Stajíc M. Ketamine in non-hospital and hospital deaths in New York City. *J Forensic Sci* 2000;**45**(3):655–658.

118. Corazza O, Schifano F. Ketamine-induced near-death experience states in a sample of 50 misusers. *Subst Use Misuse* 2010;**45**(6):916–924.

119. Corazza O, Assi S, Schifano F. From 'Special K' to 'Special M': the evolution of the recreational use of ketamine and methoxetamine. *CNS Neurosci Ther* 2013;**19**:454e460. https://doi.org/10.1111/cns.12063

120. Corazza O, Schifano F, Simonato P, et al. Phenomenon of new drugs on the Internet: the case of ketamine derivative methoxetamine. *Hum Psychopharmacol* 2012;**27**:145e149. https://doi.org/10.1002/hup.1242

121. Horsley RR, Lhotkova E, Hajkova K, Jurasek B, Kuchar M, Palenicek T. Detailed pharmacological evaluation of methoxetamine (MXE), a novel psychoactive ketamine analogue: behavioural, pharmacokinetic and metabolic studies in the Wistar rat. *Brain Res Bull* 2016 (online). https://doi.org/10.1016/ j.brainresbull.2016.05.002

122. Van Hout MC, Hearne E. 'Word of Mouse': indigenous harm reduction and online consumerism of the synthetic compound methoxphenidine. *J Psychoactive Drugs* 2015;**47**(1):30–41. https://doi.org/10.1080/02791072.2014.974002

123. Botanasa CJ, Bryan de la Pena J, Kima HJ, Lee YS, Cheonga JH. Methoxetamine: a foe or friend? *Neurochem Int* 2019;**122**:1–7.

124. Zawilska JB. Methoxetamine: a novel recreational drug with potent hallucinogenic properties. *Toxicol Lett* 2014;**230**:402e407. https://doi.org/ 10.1016/j.toxlet.2014.08.011

125. Corazza O, Assi S, Schifano F. From 'Special K' to 'Special M': the evolution of the recreational use of ketamine and methoxetamine. *CNS Neurosci Ther* 2013;**19**:454e460. https://doi.org/10.1111/cns.12063

126. Corazza O, Schifano F, Simonato P, et al. Phenomenon of new drugs on the Internet: the case of ketamine derivative methoxetamine. *Hum Psychopharmacol* 2012;**27**:145e149. https://doi.org/10.1002/hup.1242

127. Van Hout MC, Hearne E. 'Word of Mouse': indigenous harm reduction and online consumerism of the synthetic compound methoxphenidine. *J Psychoactive Drugs* 2015;**47** (1):30–41. https://doi.org/10.1080/02791072.2014.974002

128. Schifano F, Corkery J, Oyefeso A, Tonia T, Ghodse AH. Trapped in the 'K-hole': overview of deaths associated with ketamine misuse in the UK (1993–2006). *J Clin Psychopharmacol* 2008;**28**:114–116.

129. Corazza O, Assi S, Schifano F. From 'Special K' to 'Special M': the evolution of the recreational use of ketamine and methoxetamine. *CNS Neurosci Ther* 2013;**19**:454e460. https://doi.org/10.1111/cns.12063

130. Craig CL, Loeffler GH. The ketamine analog methoxetamine: a new designer drug to threaten military readiness. *Mil Med* 2014;**179**:1149–1157.

131. Zanda MT, Fadda P, Chiamulera C, Fratta W, Fattore L. Methoxetamine: a novel psychoactive substance with serious adverse pharmacological effects: a review of case reports and preclinical findings. *Behav Pharmacol* 2016;**27**:489–496.

132. Morgan CJA, Curran HV. Ketamine use: a review. *Addiction* 2011;**107**:27–38.

133. Morgan CJ, Curran HV. Acute and chronic effects of ketamine upon human memory: a review. *Psychopharmacology* (Berl) 2006;**188**:408–424.

134. Haas DA, Harper DG. Ketamine: a review of its pharmacological properties and use in ambulatory anesthesia. *Anesth Prog* 1992;**39**:61–68.

135. Weiner AL, Vieira L, McKay CA, Bayer MJ. Ketamine abusers presenting to the emergency department: a case series. *J Emerg Med* 2000;**18**:447–451.

136. Sassano-Higgins S, Baron D, Juarez G, Esmaili N, Gold M. A review of ketamine abuse and diversion. *Depress Anxiety* 2016;**33**:718–727.

137. SPC data for ketamine hydrochloride for injection. SPC states that respiratory depression may occur with overdosage.

138. Ng SH, Tse ML, Ng HW, Lau FL. Emergency department presentation of ketamine abusers in Hong Kong: a review of 233 cases. *Hong Kong Med J* 2010;**16**(1):6–11.

139. Felser JM, Orban DJ. Dystonic reaction after ketamine abuse. *Ann Emerg Med* 1982;**11**(12):673–675.

140. Lahti AC, Weiler MA, Michaelidis T, Parwani A, Tammminga C. Effects of ketamine in normal and schizophrenic volunteers. *Neuropsychopharmacology* 2001;**25**:455–467.

141. Lahti AC, Koffel B, LaPorte D, Tamminga CA. Subanesthetic doses of ketamine stimulate psychosis in schizophrenia. *Neuropsychopharmacology* 1995;**13**:9–19.

142. Malhotra AK, Pinals DA, Adler CM, et al. Ketamine-induced exacerbation of psychotic symptoms and cognitive impairment in neuroleptic-free schizophrenics. *Neuropsychopharmacology* 1997;**17**:141–150.

143. Lahti AC, Holcomb HH, Medoff DR, Tamminga CA. Ketamine activates psychosis and alters limbic blood flow in schizophrenia. *Neuroreport* 1995;**6**:869–872.

144. Wood DM, Bishop CR, Greene SL, Dargan PI. Ketamine-related toxicology presentations to the ED. *Clin Toxicol* 2008;**46**:630.

145. Weiner AL, Vieira L, McKay CA, Bayer MJ. Ketamine abusers presenting to the emergency department: a case series. *J Emerg Med* 2000;**18**:447–451.

146. Rollin A, Maury P, Guilbeau-Frugier C, Brugada J. Transient ST elevation after ketamine intoxication: a new cause of acquired brugada ECG pattern. *J Cardiovasc Electrophysiol* 2011;**22**(1):91–94. https://doi.org/10.1111/j.1540-8167.2010.01766.x

147. Maskell SF, Bailey ML, Rutherfoord Rose S. Self-medication with methoxetamine as an analgesic resulting in significant toxicity. *Pain Med* **2016**;17:1773–1775. https://doi.org/10.10-93/pm/pnw041

148. Craig CL, Loeffler GH. The ketamine analog methoxetamine: a new designer drug to threaten military readiness. *Mil Med* 2014;**179**(10): 1149.

149. Shields JE, Dargan PI, Wood DM, Puchnarewicz M, Davies S, Waring WS. Methoxetamine associated reversible cerebellar toxicity: three cases with analytical confirmation. *Clin Toxicol* (Phila) 2012;**50**(5):438–440. https://doi.org/10.3109/15563650.2012.683437

150. Michelot D, Melendez-Howell LM. Amanita muscaria: chemistry, biology, toxicology, and ethnomycology. *Mycol Res* 2003;**107**:131–146.

151. Wood DM, Davies S, Puchnarewicz M, Johnston A, Dargan PI. Acute toxicity associated with the recreational use of the ketamine derivative methoxetamine. *Eur J Clin Pharmacol* 2012;**68**(5):853–856. https://doi.org/10.1007/s00228-011-1199-9

152. Ward J, Rhyee S, Plansky J, Boyer E. Methoxetamine: a novel ketamine analog and growing health-care concern. *Clin Toxicol* 2011;**49**:874–875.

153. Craig CL, Loeffler GH. The ketamine analog methoxetamine: a new designer drug to threaten military readiness. *Mil Med* 2014;**179**(10):1149.

154. Shields JE, Dargan PI, Wood DM, Puchnarewicz M, Davies S, Waring WS. Methoxetamine-associated reversible cerebellar toxicity: three cases with analytical confirmation. *Clin Toxicol* 2012;**50**:438–440.

155. Wood DM, Davies S, Puchnarewicz M, Johnston A, Dargan PI. Acute toxicity associated with the recreational use of the ketamine derivative methoxetamine. *Eur J Clin Pharmacol* 2012;**68**:853–856. https://doi.org/10.1007/s00228-011-1199-9

156. Sein Anand J, Wiergowski M, Barwina M, Kaletha K. Accidental intoxication with high dose of methoxetamine (MXE) – a case report. *Przegl Lek* 2012;**69**(8): 609–610.

157. Corazza O, Assi S, Schifano F. From 'Special K' to 'Special M': the evolution of the recreational use of ketamine and methoxetamine. *CNS Neurosci Ther* 2013;**19**:454e460. http://dx.doi.org/10.1111/cns.12063

158. Zawilska JB. Methoxetamine: a novel recreational drug with potent hallucinogenic properties. *Toxicol Lett* 2014;**230**:402e407. https://doi.org/ 10.1016/j .toxlet.2014.08.011

159. Shields JE, Dargan PI, Wood DM, Puchnarewicz M, Davies S, Waring WS. Methoxetamine-associated reversible cerebellar toxicity: three cases with analytical confirmation. *Clin Toxicol* 2012;**50**:438–440.

160. Bäckberg M, Beck O, Helander A. Phencyclidine analog use in Sweden: intoxication cases involving 3-MeO-PCP and 4-MeO-PCP from the STRIDA project. *Clin Toxicol* 2015;**53** (9):856–864. https://doi.org/10.3109/15563650.2015.1079325

161. Bakota E, Arndt C, Romoser AA, Wilson SK. Fatal intoxication involving 3-MeO-PCP: a case report and validated method. *J Anal Toxicol* 2016;**40**:504–510. https://doi.org/10.1093/jat/bkw056

162. Jacobs R, Nowell M. Phencyclidine hydrochloride: a challenge to medicine. *J Natl Med Assoc* 1981;**73**:170–172.

163. Bey T, Patel A. Phencyclidine intoxication and adverse effects: a clinical and pharmacological review of an illicit drug. *Calif J Emerg Med* 2007;**8**:9–14.

164. Johansson A, Lindsted D, Roman M, et al. A non-fatal intoxication and seven deaths involving the dissociative drug 3-MeO-PCP. *Forensic Sci Int* 2017;**275**:76–82.

165. Bakota E, Arndt C, Romoser AA, Wilson SK. Fatal intoxication involving 3-MeO-PCP: a case report and validated method. *J Anal Toxicol* 2016;**40**:504–510. https://doi.org/10.1093/jat/bkw056

166. Jacobs R, Nowell M. Phencyclidine hydrochloride: a challenge to medicine. *J Natl Med Assoc* 1981;**73**:170–172.

167. Bey T, Patel A. Phencyclidine intoxication and adverse effects: a clinical and pharmacological review of an illicit drug. *Calif J Emerg Med* 2007;**8**:9–14.

168. Bakota E, Arndt C, Romoser AA, Wilson SK. Fatal intoxication involving 3-MeO-PCP: a case report and validated method. *J Anal Toxicol* 2016;**40**:504–510. https://doi.org/10.1093/jat/bkw056

169. Jacobs R, Nowell M. Phencyclidine hydrochloride: a challenge to medicine. *J Natl Med Assoc* 1981;**73**:170–172.

170. Bey T, Patel A. Phencyclidine intoxication and adverse effects: a clinical and pharmacological review of an illicit drug. *Calif J Emerg Med* 2007;**8**:9–14.

171. Bäckberg M, Beck O, Helander A. Phencyclidine analog use in Sweden: intoxication cases involving 3-MeO-PCP and 4-MeO-PCP from the STRIDA project. *Clin Toxicol* 2015;**53** (9):856–864. https://doi.org/10.3109/15563650.2015.1079325

172. Thornton S, Lisbon D, Lin T, Gerona R. Beyond ketamine and phencyclidine: analytically confirmed use of multiple novel arylcyclohexylamines. *J Psychoactive Drugs* 2017;**49** (4):289–293. https://doi.org/10.1080/02791072.2017.1333660

173. Thornton S, Lisbon D, Lin T, Gerona R. Beyond ketamine and phencyclidine: analytically confirmed use of multiple novel arylcyclohexylamines. *J Psychoactive Drugs* 2017;**49** (4);289–293. https://doi.org/10.1080/02791072.2017.1333660

174. Bertol E, Pascali J, Palumbo D, et al. 3-MeO-PCP intoxication in two young men: first *in vivo* detection in Italy. *Forensic Sci Int* 2017;**274**:7–12.

175. Orsolin L, Papanti G, Schifano FR. Methoxphenidine (1-(1-(2-methoxyphenyl)-2-phenylethyl) Piperidine; 2-meo-diphenidine): preliminary data on chemical, pharmacological and clinical effects. *Eur Psychiatry* 2015;**30**(Suppl.1):1046.

176. Helander A, Beck O, Bäckberg M. Intoxications by the dissociative new psychoactive substances diphenidine and methoxphenidine. *Clin Toxicol* 2015;**53**(5):446–453. https://doi.org/10.3109/15563650.2015.1033630

177. Hofer KE, Degrandi C, Müller DM, et al. Acute toxicity associated with the recreational use of the novel dissociative psychoactive substance methoxphenidine. *Clin Toxicol* 2014;**52**(10):1288–1291. https://doi.org/10.3109/15563650 .2014.974264

178. Hofer KE, Degrandi C, Müller DM, et al. Acute toxicity associated with the recreational use of the novel dissociative psychoactive substance methoxphenidine. *Clin Toxicol* 2014;**52**(10):1288–1291. https://doi.org/10.3109/15563650 .2014.974264

179. Helander A, Beck O, Bäckberg M. Intoxications by the dissociative new psychoactive substances diphenidine and methoxphenidine. *Clin Toxicol* 2015;**53**(5):446–453. https://doi.org/10.3109/15563650.2015.1033630

180. Hofer KE, Degrandi C, Müller DM, et al. Acute toxicity associated with the recreational use of the novel dissociative psychoactive substance methoxphenidine. *Clin Toxicol* 2014;**52**(10):1288–1291. https://doi.org/10.3109/15563650 .2014.974264

181. Helander A, Beck O, Bäckberg M. Intoxications by the dissociative new psychoactive substances diphenidine and methoxphenidine. *Clin Toxicol* 2015;**53**:446–453.

182. Hofer EK, Degrandi C, Müller DM, et al. Acute toxicity associated with the recreational use of the novel dissociative psychoactive substance methoxphenidine. *Clin Toxicol* 2014;**52**:1288–1291.

183. Gerace E, Bovetto E, Di Corcia D, Vincenti M, Salomone A. A case of nonfatal intoxication associated with the recreational use of diphenidine. *J Forensic Sci* 2017;**62**:1107–1111.

184. Hofer EK, Degrandi C, Müller DM, et al. Acute toxicity associated with the recreational use of the novel dissociative psychoactive substance methoxphenidine. *Clin Toxicol* 2014;**52**:1288–1291.

185. Lam RPK, Yip WL, Tsui MSH, Ng SW, Ching CK, Mak TWL. Severe rhabdomyolysis and acute kidney injury associated with methoxphenidine. *Clin Toxicol* 2016;**54** (5):464–465. https://doi.org/10.3109/15563650 .2016.1157724

186. Orsolin L, Papanti G, Schifano FR. Methoxphenidine (1-(1-(2-methoxyphenyl)-2-phenylethyl) Piperidine;

2-meo-diphenidine): preliminary data on chemical, pharmacological and clinical effects. *Eur Psychiatry* 2015;**30** (Suppl. 1):1046.

187. Tang MHY, Chong YK, Chan CY, et al. Cluster of acute poisonings associated with an emerging ketamine analogue, 2-oxo-PCE. *Forensic Sci Int* 2018;**290**:238–243.

188. Tang MHY, Chong YK, Chan CY, et al. Cluster of acute poisonings associated with an emerging ketamine analogue, 2-oxo-PCE. *Forensic Sci Int* 2018;**290**:238–243.

189. Dobbs T. Report: after patient death, UVM medical center waited weeks to fix flawed systems. *VPR*, 7 July, 2015.

190. European Monitoring Centre for Drugs and Drug Addiction (EMCDDA). Technical report on 2-(3-methoxyphenyl)-2-(ethylamino)cyclohexanone (methoxetamine), Lisbon, EMCDDA, April 2014.

191. Darke S, Duflou J, Farrell M, Peacock A, Lappin J. Characteristics and circumstances of death related to the self-administration of ketamine. *Addiction* 2020 (online). https://doi.org/10.1111/add.15154

192. Stewart CE. Ketamine as a street drug. *Emerg Med Serv* 2001;**30** (11):30,32,34 passim.

193. Adamowicz P, Zuba D. Fatal intoxication with methoxetamine. *J Forensic Sci* 2015;**60**(S1). https://doi.org/10.1111/1556-4029.12594

194. European Monitoring Centre for Drugs and Drug Addiction (EMCDDA). Technical report on 2-(3-methoxyphenyl)-2-(ethylamino)cyclohexanone (methoxetamine), Lisbon, EMCDDA, April 2014.

195. Elliott SP, Brandt SD, Wallach J, Morris H, Kavanagh PV. First reported fatalities associated with the 'research chemical' 2-methoxydiphenidine. *J Anal Toxicol* 2015;**39**:287–293. https://doi.org/10.1093/jat/bkv006

196. Adamowicz P, Zuba D. Fatal intoxication with methoxetamine. *J Forensic Sci* 2015;**60**(S1). https://doi.org/10.1111/1556-4029.12594

197. Elliott SP, Brandt SD, Wallach J, Morris H, Kavanagh PV. First reported fatalities associated with the 'research chemical' 2-methoxydiphenidine. *J Anal Toxicol* 2015;**39**:287–293. https://doi.org/10.1093/jat/bkv006

198. Elliott S, Sedefov R, Evans-Brown M. Assessing the toxicological significance of new psychoactive substances in fatalities. *Drug Test Anal* 2018;**10**:120.

199. Bäckberg M, Beck O, Helander A. Phencyclidine analog use in Sweden: intoxication cases involving 3-MeO-PCP and 4-MeO-PCP from the STRIDA project. *Clin Toxicol* 2015;**53** (9):856–864. https://doi.org/10.3109/15563650.2015.1079325

200. Johansson A, Lindsted D, Roman M, et al. A non-fatal intoxication and seven deaths involving the dissociative drug 3-MeO-PCP. *Forensic Sci Int* 2017;**275**:76–82.

201. Bäckberg M, Beck O, Helander A. Phencyclidine analog use in Sweden: intoxication cases involving 3-MeO-PCP and 4-MeO-PCP from the STRIDA project. *Clin Toxicol* 2015;**53** (9):856–864. https://doi.org/10.3109/15563650.2015.1079325

202. Bakota E, Arndt C, Romoser AA, Wilson SK. Fatal intoxication involving 3-MeO-PCP: a case report and validated method. *J Anal Toxicol* 2016;**40**:504–510. https://doi.org/10.1093/jat/bkw056

203. McIntyre IM, Trochta A, Gary RD, Storey A, Corneal J, Schaber B. Hallucinogenic compounds: 4-methoxyphencyclidine and 4-hydroxy-*N*-methyl-*N*-ethyltryptamine. *J Anal Toxicol* 2015;**39** (9):751–755. https://doi.org/10.1093/jat/bkv089

204. de Jong LAA, Olyslager EJH, Duijst WLJM. The risk of emerging new psychoactive substances: the first fatal 3-MeO-PCP intoxication in the Netherlands. *J Forensic Leg Med* 2019;**65**:101–104.

205. Mitchell-Mata C, Thomas B, Peterson B, Couper F. Two fatal intoxications involving 3-methoxyphencyclidine. *J Anal Toxicol* 2017;**41**:503–507. https://doi.org/10.1093/jat/bkx048

206. Zidkova M, Hlozek T, Balik M, et al. Two cases of non-fatal intoxication with a novel street hallucinogen: 3-methoxy-phencyclidine. *J Anal Toxicol* 2017;**41**:350–354. https://doi.org/10.1093/jat/bkx009

207. Wood DM, Nicolaou M, Dargan PI. Epidemiology of recreational drug toxicity in a nightclub environment. *Subst Use Misuse* 2009;**44**:1495–1502.

208. Tang MHY, Chong YK, Chan CY, et al. Cluster of acute poisonings associated with an emerging ketamine analogue, 2-oxo-PCE. *Forensic Sci Int* 2018;**290**:238–243.

209. Smith KM, Larive LL, Romanelli F. Club drugs: methylene dioxymethamphetaine, flunitrazepam, ketamine hydrochloride, and gamma-hydroxybutyrate. *Am J Health Syst Pharm* 2002;**59**(11):1067–1076.

210. Shields JE, Dargan PI, Wood DM, Waring WS. Methoxetamine-associated reversible cerebellar toxicity: three cases with analytical confirmation. *Clin Toxicol* 2012;**50** (5):438–440. https://doi.org/10.3109/15563650.2012.683437

211. Craig CL, Loeffler GH. The ketamine analog methoxetamine: a new designer drug to threaten military readiness. *Mil Med* 2014;**179**(10): 1149.

212. Craig CL, Loeffler GH. The ketamine analog methoxetamine: a new designer drug to threaten military readiness. *Mil Med* 2014;**179**(10): 1149.

213. Wood DM, Dargan PI. Novel psychoactive substances: how to understand the acute toxicity associated with the use of these substances. *Ther Drug Monit* 2012;**34**(4):363–366.

214. Wood DM, Davies S, Puchnarewicz M, Johnston A, Dargan PI. Acute toxicity associated with the recreational use of the ketamine derivative methoxetamine. *Eur J Clin Pharmacol* 2012;**68**:853–856. https://doi.org/10.1007/s0022 8-011-1199-9

215. Shields JE, Dargan PI, Wood DM, Waring WS. Methoxetamine-associated reversible cerebellar toxicity: three cases with analytical confirmation. *Clin Toxicol* 2012;**50** (5):438–440. https://doi.org/10.3109/15563650.2012.683437

216. Bäckberg M, Beck O, Helander A. Phencyclidine analog use in Sweden: intoxication cases involving 3-MeO-PCP and

4-MeO-PCP from the STRIDA project. *Clin Toxicol* 2015;**53**(9):856–864. https://doi.org/10.3109/15563650.2015.1079325

217. Tang MHY, Chong YK, Chan CY, et al. Cluster of acute poisonings associated with an emerging ketamine analogue, 2-oxo-PCE. *Forensic Sci Int* 2018;**290**:238–243.

218. Matulewicz P, Kasicki S, Hunt MJ. The effect of dopamine receptor blockade in the rodent nucleus accumbens on local field potential oscillations and motor activity in response to ketamine. *Brain Res* 2010;**1366**:226–232.

219. Moore NN, Bostwick JM. Ketamine dependence in anesthesia providers. *Psychosomatics* 1999;**40**:356–359.

220. Pal HR, Berry N, Kumar R, Ray R. Ketamine dependence. *Anaesth Intensive Care* 2002;**30**:382–384.

221. Jansen KL. Ketamine – can chronic use impair memory? *Int J Addict* 1990;**25**:133–139.

222. Cumming JF. The development of an acute tolerance to ketamine. *Anesth Analg* 1976;**55**:788–791.

223. Bree MM, Feller I, Corssen G. Safety and tolerance of repeated anesthesia with CI 581 (ketamine) in monkeys. *Anesth Analg* 1967;**46**:596–600.

224. Byer DE, Gould AB Jr. Development of tolerance to ketamine in an infant undergoing repeated anesthesia. *Anesthesiology* 1981;**54**:255–256.

225. Muetzelfeldt L, Kamboj SK, Rees H, Taylor J, Morgan CJ, Curran HV. Journey through the K-hole: phenomenological aspects of ketamine use. *Drug Alcohol Depend* 2008;**95**(3):219–229. https://doi.org/10.1016/j.drugalcdep.2008.01.024

226. Chen L-Y, Chen C-K, Chen C-H, Chang H-M, Huang M-C, Xu K. Association of craving and depressive symptoms in ketamine-dependent patients undergoing withdrawal treatment. *Am J Addict* 2020;**29**(1):43–50. https://doi.org/10.1111/ajad.12978

227. Striebel JM, Nelson EE, Kalapatapu RK. 'Being with a Buddha': a case report of methoxetamine use in a United States veteran with PTSD. *Case Rep Psychiatry* 2017;**7**:2319094.

228. Botanasa CJ, Bryan de la Pena J, Kima HJ, Lee YS, Hoon J. Methoxetamine: a foe or friend? *Neurochem Int* 2019;**122**:1–7.

229. Blachut M, Solowiow K, Janus A, et al. A case of ketamine dependence. *Psychiatr Pol* 2009;**43**:593–599.

230. Lim DK. Ketamine-associated psychedelic effects and dependence. *Singapore Med J* 2003;**44**:31–34.

231. Wang YC, Chen SK, Lin CM. Breaking the drug addiction cycle is not easy in ketamine abusers. *Int J Urol* 2010;**17**(5):496. https://doi.org/10.1111/j.1442-2042.2010.02491.x

232. Monaghan DT, Bridges RJ, Cotman CW. The excitatory amino acid receptors: their classes, pharmacology and distinct properties in the function of the central nervous system. *Annu Rev Pharmacol Toxicol* 1989;**29**:365–402.

233. Craig CL, Loeffler GH. The ketamine analog methoxetamine: a new designer drug to threaten military readiness. *Mil Med* 2014;**179**(10):1149.

234. Wei YB, Yang JR. 'Ketamine-induced ulcerative cystitis' is perhaps better labelled 'ketamine-induced uropathy'. *Addiction* 2013;**108**(8):1515. https://doi.org/10.1111/add.12195

235. Chu PS, Ma WK, Wong SC, et al. The destruction of the lower urinary tract by ketamine abuse: a new syndrome? *BJU Int* 2008;**102**(11):1616–1622. https://doi.org/10.1111/j.1464-410X.2008.07920.x

236. Wong SW, Lee KF, Wong J, Ng WW, Cheung YS, Lai PB. Dilated common bile ducts mimicking choledochal cysts in ketamine abusers. *Hong Kong Med J* 2009;**15**(1):53–56.

237. Ramos SP, Zambonato TK, Graziott TM. Reduced functional bladder capacity associated with ketamine use. *Braz J Psychiatry* 2019;**41**(3):270–271. https://doi.org/10.1590/1516-4446-2018-0314

238. Sihra N, Ockrim J, Wood D. The effects of recreational ketamine cystitis on urinary tract reconstruction – a surgical challenge. *BJU Int* 2018;**121**:458–465.

239. Myers FA, Bluth MH, Cheung WW Ketamine : a cause of urinary tract dysfunction. *Clin Lab Med* 2016;**36**:721–744. https://doi.org/10.1016/j.cll.2016.07.008

240. Gill P, Logan K, John B, Reynolds F, Shaw C, Madden K. Participants' experiences of ketamine bladder syndrome: a qualitative study. *PhD Int J Urol Nurs* 2018;**12**:76–83.

241. Cottrell A, Warren K, Ayres R, Weinstock P, Gillatt DA. The relationship of chronic recreational ketamine use and severe bladder pathology: presentation, management of symptoms and public health concerns. *Eur Urol Suppl* 2009;**8**:170.

242. Middela S, Pearce I. Ketamine-induced vesicopathy: a literature review. *Int J Clin Pract* 2011;**65**(1):27–30. https://doi.org/10.1111/j.1742-1241.2010.02502.x

243. Gill P, Logan K, John B, Reynolds F, Shaw C, Madden K. Participants' experiences of ketamine bladder syndrome: a qualitative study. *PhD Int J Urol Nurs* 2018;**12**:76–83.

244. Yew DT, Wood DM, Liang W, Tang HC, Dargan PI. An animal model demonstrating significant bladder inflammation and fibrosis associated with chronic methoxetamine administration. *Clin Toxicol* 2013;**51**(4):278.

245. Lawn W, Borschmann R, Cottrell A, Winstock A. Methoxetamine: prevalence of use in the USA and UK and associated urinary problems. *J Subst Use* 2016;**21**(2):115–120. https://doi.org/10.3109/14659891.2014.966345

246. Liu SUQ, Ng SKK,Tam YH, et al. Clinical pattern and prevalence of upper gastrointestinal toxicity in patients abusing ketamine. *J Dig Dis* 2017;**18**(9):504–510.

247. Liu SUQ, Ng SKK,Tam YH, et al. Clinical pattern and prevalence of upper gastrointestinal toxicity in patients abusing ketamine. *J Dig Dis* 2017;**18**(9):504–510.

248. Liu SUQ, Ng SKK,Tam YH, et al. Clinical pattern and prevalence of upper gastrointestinal toxicity in patients abusing ketamine. *J Dig Dis* 2017;**18**(9):504–510.

249. Selby NM, Anderson J, Bungay P, Chesterton LJ, Kohle NV. Obstructive nephropathy and kidney injury associated with ketamine abuse. *Nephrol Dial Transplant Plus* 2008;**1**(2):310–312.

250. Ng SH, Lee HK, Chan YC, Lau FL. Dilated common bile ducts in ketamine abusers. *Hong Kong Med J* 2009;**15**:157.

251. Wong GL, Tam YH, Ng CF, et al. Liver injury is common among chronic abuses of ketamine. *Clin Gastroenterol Hepatol* 2014;**12**:1759–1762.

252. Wong GL, Tam YH, Ng CF, et al. Liver injury is common among chronic abuses of ketamine. *Clin Gastroenterol Hepatol* 2014;**12**:1759–1762.

253. Yu WL, Cho CC, Lung PF, et al. Ketamine-related cholangiopathy: a retrospective study on clinical and imaging findings. *Abdom Imaging* 2014;**39**:1241–1246.

254. Morgan CJ, Curran HV. Ketamine use: a review. *Addiction* 2011;**107**:27–38.

255. Liu SUQ, Ng SKK,Tam YH, et al. Clinical pattern and prevalence of upper gastrointestinal toxicity in patients abusing ketamine. *J Dig Dis* 2017;**18**(9):504–510.

256. Randall T. Ectasy-fuelled 'rave' parties become dances of death for English youths. *J Am Med Assoc* 1993;**269**:869–870.

257. Glasgow AM, Tynan D, Schwartz R, et al. Alcohol and drug use in teenagers with diabetes mellitus. *J Adolesc Health* 1997;**12**:11–14.

258. Gold MA, Gladstein J. Substance use among adolescents with diabetes mellitus: preliminary findings. *J Adolesc Health* 1993;**14**:80–84.

259. Martínez-Aguayo A, Araneda JC, Fernandez D, Gleisner A, Perez V, Codner E. Tobacco, alcohol, and illicit drug use in adolescents with diabetes mellitus. *Pediatr Diabetes* 2007;**8**:265–271.

260. Ng RS, Darko DA, Hillson RM. Street drug use among young patients with type 1 diabetes in the UK. *Diabet Med* 2004;**21**:295–296.

261. Lee P, Greenfield JR, Campbell LV. 'Mind the gap' when managing ketoacidosis in type 1 diabetes. *Diabetes Care* 2008;**31**:e58.

262. Rattray M. Ecstasy: towards an understanding of the biochemical basis of the action of MDMA. *Essays Biochem* 1991;**26**:77.

263. Britt GC, McCance-Katz EF. A brief overview of the clinical pharmacology of 'club drugs'. *Subst Use Misuse* 2005;**40**:1189–1201.

264. Seymour HR, Gilman D, Quin JD. Severe ketoacidosis complicated by 'ecstasy' ingestion and prolonged exercise. *Diabet Med* 1996;**13**:908–909.

265. Giorgi FS, Lazzeri G, Natale G, et al. MDMA and seizures: a dangerous liaison? *Ann NY Acad Sci* 2006;**1074**:357–364.

266. Rosenson J, Smollin C, Sporer KA, Blanc P, Olson KR. Patterns of ecstasy-associated hyponatremia in California. *Ann Emerg Med* 2007;**49**:164–171.

267. Kalantar-Zadeh K, Nguyen MK, Chang R, Kurtz I. Fatal hyponatremia in a young woman after ecstasy ingestion. *Nat Clin Pract Nephrol* 2006;**2**:283–288.

268. Ben-Abraham R, Szold O, Rudick V, Weinbroum AA. 'Ecstasy' intoxication: life-threatening manifestations and resuscitative measures in the intensive care setting. *Eur J Emerg Med* 2003;**10**:309–313.

269. Brvar M, Kozelj G, Osredkar J, Mozina M, Gricar M, Bunc M. Polydipsia as another mechanism of hyponatremia after 'ecstasy' (3,4 methyldioxymethamphetamine) ingestion. *Eur J Emerg Med* 2004;**11**:302–304.

270. Kwon C, Zaritsky A, Dharnidharka VR. Transient proximal tubular renal injury following ecstasy ingestion. *Pediatr Nephrol* 2003;**18**:820–822.

271. Lee P, Nicoll AJ, McDonough M, Colman PG. Substance abuse in young patients with type 1 diabetes: easily neglected in complex medical management. *Intern Med J* 2005;**35**:359–361.

272. Rome ES. It's a rave new world: rave culture and illicit drug use in the young. *Cleve Clin J Med* 2001;**68**:541–550.

273. Buchanan JF, Brown CR. 'Designer drugs'. A problem in clinical toxicology. *Med Toxicol Adverse Drug Exp* 1988;**3**:1.

274. Koesters SC, Rogers PD, Rajasingham CR. MDMA ('ecstasy') and other 'club drugs'. The new epidemic. *Paediatr Clin North Am* 2002;**49**:415.

275. Lee P, Campbell LV. Diabetic ketoacidosis: the usual villain or a scapegoat? A novel cause of severe metabolic acidosis in type 1 diabetes. *Diabetes Care* 2008;**31**:e13.

276. Romanelli F, Smith KM, Pomeroy C. Use of club drugs by HIV-seropositive and HIV-seronegative gay and bisexual men. *Top HIV Med* 2003;**11**(1):25–32.

277. Morgan CJ, Muetzelfeldt L, Curran HV. Consequences of chronic ketamine self-administration upon neurocognitive function and psychological wellbeing: a 1-year longitudinal study. *Addiction* 2010;**105**:121–133.

278. Morgan CJ, Rossell SL, Pepper F, et al. Semantic priming after ketamine acutely in healthy volunteers and following chronic self-administration in substance users. *Biol Psychiatry* 2006;**59**:265–272.

279. Morgan CJ, Perry EB, Cho HS, Krystal JH, D'Souza DC. Greater vulnerability to the amnestic effects of ketamine in males. *Psychopharmacology (Berl)* 2006;**187**:405–414.

280. Morgan CJ, Muetzelfeldt L, Curran HV. Ketamine use, cognition and psychological wellbeing: a comparison of frequent, infrequent and ex-users with polydrug and non-using controls. *Addiction* 2009;**104**:77–87.

281. Morgan CJ, Monaghan L, Curran HV. Beyond the K-hole: a 3-year longitudinal investigation of the cognitive and subjective effects of ketamine in recreational users who have substantially reduced their use of the drug. *Addiction* 2004;**99** (11):1450–1461.

282. Narendran R, Frankle WG, Keefe R, et al. Altered prefrontal dopaminergic function in chronic recreational ketamine users. *Am J Psychiatry* 2005;**162**:2352–2359.

283. Aan het Rot M, Collins KA, Murrough JW, et al. Safety and efficacy of repeated-dose intravenous ketamine for treatment-resistant depression. *Biol Psychiatry* 2010;**67**:139–145.

284. Womble AL. Effects of ketamine on major depressive disorder in a patient with posttraumatic stress disorder. *AANA J* 2013;**81**(2):118–119.

285. Berman RM, Cappiello A, Anand A, et al. Antidepressant effects of ketamine in depressed patients. *Biol Psychiatry* 2000;**47**(4):351–354.

286. Aan het Rot M, Collins KA, Murrough JW, et al. Safety and efficacy of repeated-dose intravenous ketamine for treatment resistant depression. *Biol Psychiatry* 2010;**67**:139–145.

287. Womble AL. Effects of ketamine on major depressive disorder in a patient with posttraumatic stress disorder. *AANA J* 2013;**81**(2):118–119.

288. Murrough JW. Antidepressant efficacy of ketamine in treatment-resistant major depression: a two-site, randomized, parallel-arm, midazolam-controlled, clinical trial. *Biol Psychiatry* 2013;**73**(9 Suppl. 1):142S.

289. Zarate CA, Singh JB, Carlson PJ, et al. A randomized trial of an N-methyl-D-aspartate antagonist in treatment-resistant major depression. *Arch Gen Psychiatry* 2006;**63**(8):856–864.

290. McGirr A, Berlim MT, Bond DJ, Fleck MP, Yatham LN, Lam RW. A systematic review and meta-analysis of randomized, double-blind, placebo-controlled trials of ketamine in the rapid treatment of major depressive episodes. *Psychol Med* 2015;**45**(4):693–704.

291. Iadarola ND, Niciu MJ, Richards EM, et al. Ketamine and other N-methyl-D-aspartate receptor antagonists in the treatment of depression: a perspective review. *Ther Adv Chronic Dis* 2015;**6**(3):97–114.

292. Mathew SJ, Zarate Jr. CA eds. *Ketamine for Treatment-Resistant Depression: The First Decade of Progress.* New York, Springer, 2016.

293. Singh JB, Fedgchin M, Daly EJ, et al. A double-blind, randomized, placebo-controlled, dose-frequency study of intravenous ketamine in patients with treatment-resistant depression. *Am J Psychiatry* 2016;**173**(8):816–826.

294. Albott C, Lim K. Forbes M, et al. 1001-Neurocognitive effects of repeated ketamine infusions in co-occurring posttraumatic stress disorder and treatment-resistant depression. *Biol Psychiatry* 2017;**81**(10):S405.

295. Al Shirawi MI, Kennedy SH, Ho KT, Byrne R, Downar J. Oral ketamine in treatment-resistant depression: a clinical effectiveness case series. *J Clin Psychopharmacol* 2017;**37**(4):464–467.

296. Singh I, Morgan C, Curran V, Nutt D, Schlag A, McShane R. Ketamine treatment for depression: opportunities for clinical innovation and ethical foresight. *Lancet Psychiatry* 2017;**4**(5):419–426.

297. Berman RM, Cappiello A, Anand A, et al. Antidepressant effects of ketamine in depressed patients. *Biol Psychiatry* 2000;**47**(4):351–354.

298. Zarate CA, Singh JB, Carlson PJ, et al. A randomized trial of an N-methyl-D-aspartate antagonist in treatment-resistant major depression. *Arch Gen Psychiatry* 2006;**63**(8):856–864.

299. Krystal JH. Ketamine and the potential role for rapid acting antidepressant medications. *Swiss Med Wkly* 2007;**137**:215–216.

300. Schwartz J, Murrough JW, Iosifescu DV. Ketamine for treatment-resistant depression: recent developments and clinical applications. *Evid Based Mental Health* 2016;**19**(2):35–38.

301. Mathew SJ, Shah A, Lapidus K, et al. Ketamine for treatment-resistant unipolar depression. *CNS Drugs* 2012;**26**:189–204.

302. Murrough JW, Iosifescu DV, Chang LC, et al. An antidepressant efficacy of ketamine in treatment-resistant major depression: a two-site randomized controlled trial. *Am J Psychiatry* 2013;**170**:1134–1142.

303. Fond G, Loundou A, Rabu C, et al. Ketamine administration in depressive disorders: a systematic review and meta-analysis. *Psychopharmacology (Berl)* 2014;**231**:3663–3676.

304. McGirr A, Berlim MT, Bond DJ, et al. A systematic review and meta-analysis of randomized, double-blind, placebo-controlled trials of ketamine in the rapid treatment of major depressive episodes. *Psychol Med* 2015;**45**:693–704.

305. SchakJennifer KM, Van de Voort L, Johnson EK, et al. Potential risks of poorly monitored ketamine use in depression treatment. *Am J Psychiatry* 2016;**173**:3.

306. Murrough JW. Antidepressant efficacy of ketamine in treatment-resistant major depression: a two-site, randomized, parallel-arm, midazolam-controlled, clinical trial. *Biol Psychiatry* 2013;**73**(9) Suppl. 1(142S).

307. Chang H, Huang MC, Chen LY. Major depressive disorder induced by chronic ketamine abuse: a case report. *Prim Care Companion CNS Disord* 2016;**18**(3):10. https://doi.org/10.4088/PCC.15l01881

308. Liang HJ, Tang KL, Chan F, Ungvari GS, Tang KW. Ketamine users have high rates of psychosis and/or depression. *J Addic Nurs* 2015;**26**(1):8–13.

309. Liao Y, Tang J, Ma M, et al. Frontal white matter abnormalities following chronic ketamine use: a diffusion tensor imaging study. *Brain* 2010;**133**:2115–2122.

310. Liao Y, Tang J, Corlett PR, et al. Reduced dorsal prefrontal gray matter after chronic ketamine use. *Biol Psychiatry* 2011;**69**(1):42–48. https://doi.org/10.1016/j.biopsych.2010.08.030

311. Maxwell JC. The response to club drug use. *Curr Opin Psychiatry* 2003;**16**:279–289.

312. Krystal J, Karper H, Bennett LP, et al. Interactive effects of sub anaesthetic ketamine and subhypnotic lorazepam in humans. *Psychopharmacology* 1998;**135**:213–229.

313. Bhad R, Dayal P, Kumar S, Ambekar A. The drug ketamine: a double-edged sword for mental health professionals. *J Subst Use* 2016;**21**(4):341–343. https://doi.org/10.3109/14659891.2015.1040092

314. Pérez Gómez L, González Martínez M, González Fernández A, et al. Possible use of paliperidone palmitate in ketamine addiction. *Eur Psychiatry* 2015;**30**(Suppl. 1):1085. https://doi.org/10.1016/S0924-9338(15)30856-7

315. Huang M-C, Chen L-Y, Chen C-K, Lin S-K. Potential benefit of lamotrigine in managing ketamine use disorder. *Med Hypotheses* 2016;**87**:97–100. https://doi.org/10.1016/j.mehy.2015.11.011

316. Chang F, Xu K, Huang M-C, Krystal J-H. Alcohol triggers re-emergence of ketamine-like experience in a ketamine ex-user. *J Clin Psychopharmacol* 2017;**37**(1):110–112. https://doi.org/10.1097/JCP.0000000000000635

317. de P. Ramos S, Zambonato TK, Graziottin TM. Reduced functional bladder capacity associated with ketamine use. *Braz J Psychiatry* 2019;**41**(3):270–271. https://doi:10.1590/1516-4446-2018-0314

318. de P. Ramos S, Zambonato TK, Graziottin TM. Reduced functional bladder capacity associated with ketamine use. *Braz J Psychiatry* 2019;**41**(3):270–271. https://doi:10.1590/1516-4446-2018-0314

319. de P. Ramos S, Zambonato TK, Graziottin TM. Reduced functional bladder capacity associated with ketamine use. *Braz J Psychiatry* 2019;**41**(3):270–271. https://doi:10.1590/1516-4446-2018-0314

320. Cottrell AM, Gillat DA. Ketamine-associated urinary pathology: the tip of the iceberg for urologists? *Br J Med Surg Urol* 2008;**1**:136–138.

321. Robles-Martínez M, Abad AC, Pérez-Rodríguez V, RosCucurull E, Esojo A, Roncero C. Delayed urinary symptoms induced by ketamine. *J Psychoactive Drugs* 2017 (online). https://doi.org/10.1080/02791072.2017.1371364

322. Winstock AR, Mitcheson L, Gillatt DA, Cottrell AM. The prevalence and natural history of urinary symptoms among recreational ketamine users. *BJU Int* 2012;**110**(11):1762–1766. https://doi.org/10.1111/j.1464-410X.2012.11028.x

323. Sihra N, Ockrim J, Wood D. The effects of recreational ketamine cystitis on urinary tract reconstruction – a surgical challenge. *BJU Int* 2018;**121**:458–465.

324. Wood D. Ketamine and damage to the urinary tract. *Addiction* 2013;**108**:1515–1519.

325. Robles-Martínez M, Abad AC, Pérez-Rodríguez V, Cucurull ER, Esojo A, Roncero C. Delayed urinary symptoms induced by ketamine. *J Psychoactive Drugs* 2017 (online). https://doi.org/10.1080/02791072.2017.1371364

326. Sihra N, Ockrim J, Wood D. The effects of recreational ketamine cystitis on urinary tract reconstruction – a surgical challenge. *BJU Int* 2018;**121**:458–465.

327. Sihra N, Ockrim J, Wood D. The effects of recreational ketamine cystitis on urinary tract reconstruction – a surgical challenge. *BJU Int* 2018;**121**:458–465.

328. Siu AMH, Ko FSL, Mak SK. Outcome evaluation of a short-term hospitalization and community support program for people who abuse ketamine. *Front Psychiatry* 2018;**9**:313.

329. Lankenau S, Clatts M. Drug injection practices among high-risk youth: the first shot of ketamine. *J Urban Health* 2004;**81**(2):232–248.

330. Lankenau S, Clatts M. Patterns of polydrug use among ketamine injectors in New York City. *Subst Use Misuse* 2005;**40**:1381–1397.

331. Lankenau S, Sanders B. Patterns and frequencies of ketamine injection in New York City. *J Psychoactive Drug* 2007;**39**(1):21–29.

332. Cheng WC, Ng KM, Chan KK, Mok VK, Cheung BK. Roadside detection of impairment under the influence of ketamine – evaluation of ketamine impairment symptoms with reference to its concentration in oral fluid and urine. *Forensic Sci Int* 2007;**170**:51–58.

333. Giorgetti R, Marcotulli D, Tagliabrac A, Schifano F. Effects of ketamine on psychomotor, sensory and cognitive functions relevant for driving ability. *Forensic Sci Int* 2015;**252**:127–142. https://doi.org/10.1016/j.forsciint.2015.04.024

334. Cheng JY, Chan DT, Mok VK. An epidemiological study on alcohol-/drugs-related fatal traffic crash cases of deceased drivers in Hong Kong between 1996 and 2000. *Forensic Sci Int* 2005;**153**:196–201.

335. Fassette T, Martinez A. An impaired driver found to be under the influence of methoxetamine. *J Anal Toxicol* 2016;**40**(8):700–702. https://doi.org/10.1093/jat/bkw054

336. Scott-Ham M, Burton FC. Toxicological findings in cases of alleged drug-facilitated sexual assault in the United Kingdom over a 3-year period. *J Clin Forensic Med* 2005;**12**:175–186.

337. Du Mont J, Macdonald S, Rotbard N, et al. Drug-facilitated sexual assault in Ontario, Canada: toxicological and DNA findings. *J Forensic Leg Med* 2010;**17**:333–338.

Nitrous Oxide (N₂O)

7.1 Quality of the Research Evidence

The evidence on the management of the acute and chronic harms associated with the recreational use of nitrous oxide (N_2O) is limited and consists mainly of case reports, with occasional experimental studies into acute effects. There are few findings on acute harms and interventions relating to the use of the drug, but consistent findings on the chronic effects of prolonged nitrous oxide use.

7.2 Brief Summary of Pharmacology

Nitrous oxide is a gas whose pharmacology is not well studied and existing evidence is not conclusive. It has been suggested, however, that opioid receptors may be responsible for its analgesic properties[1] and a study has shown that naloxone inhibits its analgesic effects.[2] Furthermore, nitrous oxide may act as an N-methyl-D-aspartate (NMDA) antagonist, similar in nature to ketamine, another anaesthetic (see Chapter 4).[3] Nitrous oxide works primarily via the opiate system, mediating the release of beta-endorphins and directly binding to mu, delta and kappa opiate receptors.[4] Nitrous oxide is used clinically as an anaesthetic gas with pain-relieving properties.

Nitrous oxide is a 'dissociative' drug. Although the effects of the drug on the brain are not fully understood, its dissociative effects are probably caused by preventing the normal action of the NMDA receptor.

When inhaled, nitrous oxide is rapidly absorbed via pulmonary circulation.[5] Due to high lipid solubility, it passes easily through the blood–brain barrier and has a rapid onset of action; it is cleared from the body within a few hours.[6] The use of nitrous oxide leads to vitamin B12 depletion, which is believed to be due to its effect on cobalt in vitamin B12, whereby the vitamin is converted from an active, monovalent form to an inactive, bivalent form.[7]

7.3 Clinical and Other Legitimate Uses of Nitrous Oxide

Nitrous oxide was first synthesised by the English chemist and philosopher Joseph Priestley in 1772. It has been used as a medical anaesthetic for over 150 years and continues to be widely used for medical, dental and veterinary purposes. It is also used for analgesia and can help relieve anxiety.[8] It is used in various settings, including ambulances, emergency departments, relief for women in labour and in dentistry, where its short duration of action is an advantage.[9,10] Nitrous oxide has been shown to ameliorate craving and withdrawal symptoms from alcohol, opioid, nicotine, cocaine and cannabis.[11,12,13,14,15,16]

Concerns have however been raised about use of nitrous oxide in anaesthesia, because of the potential adverse effects and hazards posed to both clinicians through unintended occupational exposure and patients, specifically by its haematological, neurological, myocardial and immunological effects, and because it can lead to postoperative nausea and vomiting and expansion of air-filled spaces.[17]

Outside of human and animal medical applications, nitrous oxide is used as a fuel additive, as an oxidising agent to increase the power of cars, as a component of rocket fuel, as an aerosol dispersant and in the catering industry in the dispensing of whipped cream.

The latter forms the basis of its sale for recreational use on websites, where users purchase it in the form of small canisters or larger tanks, which are labelled with 'approved for food use'.[18]

7.4 Prevalence and Patterns of Use

The use of nitrous oxide for recreational purposes is not new, as 'laughing gas parties' were popular in the UK in Victorian times, mostly in the context of variety performances in music halls, theatres and carnivals.

More recently, the Global Drug Survey 2018, which reported data from 123,814 people from more than 30 countries, showed that nitrous oxide was the tenth most used drug in the last 12 months (excluding tobacco and alcohol).[19] There are wide differences in the prevalence of use of nitrous oxide by country, with Germany being the country with lowest lifetime prevalence, (reported ≈11% lifetime nitrous oxide use, 3.5 times lower than in the UK, where over one third (≈38%) of participants reported lifetime).[20] Nonetheless, and despite varying rates of use, the recreational use of nitrous oxide has been reported in many parts of the world, including China.[21]

7.5 Routes of Ingestion and Frequency of Dosing

Nitrous oxide is a colourless gas that is slightly sweet smelling and tasting.

Nitrous oxide is typically inhaled, commonly via balloons, from small steel cartridges or cylinders (sometimes called 'bulbs' or 'chargers'). Cartridges contain highly pressurised nitrous oxide that are available from catering suppliers and used for whipped cream. They vary by brand, but are approximately 6 cm long, 1.8 cm wide and have a wall approximately 2 mm thick to withstand the pressure of the gas. Most contain approximately 8 g of nitrous oxide under pressure and are non-refillable.

These cartridges are supplied with a dispenser into which, when fitted, they release their compressed gas. If the dispenser is not filled with cream, the nozzle simply releases the gas only. A balloon can be placed over the nozzle to capture the nitrous oxide. Alternatively, the cartridges can be opened with the 'cracker' on the cream dispenser and the nitrous oxide again released into a balloon, from which it then can be inhaled. Both cartridges and crackers can be obtained from online suppliers. They are generally low cost.

The quality (purity) of the nitrous oxide depends on its source. Products intended for food use are of higher quality, especially if they originate from the EU. Products for industrial use may be adulterated or impure.

Nitrous oxide is also available in much larger gas cylinders intended for medical or industrial use. The use of these, for purposes other than those intended, can be dangerous. Unsafe methods include breathing directly from a cylinder using a face mask, opening a cylinder tank in a car or small room or filling a bag with the gas and putting it over the head. Cylinder tanks of nitrous oxide intended to boost horsepower of gasoline engines in cars can contain harmful contaminants like sulphur dioxide.

Nitrous oxide is rarely the only drug used by people who have taken it; instead it tends to be used as part of a wide repertoire of substances, or polydrug use.[22,23] It has been suggested that typically, the recreational use of nitrous oxide is moderate, with approximately 80% of users having less than 10 episodes per year.[24] It seems that people using nitrous oxide will usually take fewer than 10 balloons of nitrous oxide per episode,[25] with some case studies showing even smaller amounts, with an average number of fewer than five per session.[26] For example, a survey of students in Auckland found that recreational use typically amounted between two to five containers in a session.[27] However, not all use is 'moderate', as other studies report a range of 10–100 cylinders used in one session.[28,29,30,31,32,33,34,35,36,37,38,39]

Recreational users will typically inhale a number of small, imprecise doses from small containers and consequently it may be difficult to assess the quantity of nitrous oxide consumed. An experimental study testing the effects of nitrous oxide in 12 volunteers found that the primary effects were found only at the inhalation of 20% to 40% concentrations.[40] At the inhalation of 40% nitrous oxide (the highest concentration tested), subjects were confused, sedated, high, dysphoric and stimulated, but fatigue and depression were observed once the effects had worn off.

As nitrous oxide is used as an anaesthetic, official advice has been issued on the short-term occupational exposure limit, to avoid harms. The advice on this ranges from 25 parts per million (ppm) to 100 ppm,[41] and may provide an indication of the level at which harms can occur in recreational users. The harms resulting from nitrous oxide are largely determined by its mode of use rather than its direct physiological effects. Inhalation through balloons or canisters is relatively safe, whereas the use of airtight bags, masks or respirators carries a high risk of asphyxiation.[42]

7.6 Desired Effects of Nitrous Oxide for Recreational Use

Nitrous oxide is used recreationally because of its euphoric effect. The onset of the effects is immediate, with the peak around 1 minute after inhaling, lasting for approximately 2 minutes then fading.[43,44,45] Users may take many 'hits' over a few hours.

The short-lasting effects typically include a rush of dizziness, relaxation, reduction of anxiety, laughing fits, auditory distortions, feelings of dissociation and mild changes in perception and sometimes hallucinations.[46,47,48] It has been argued that these effects led to its use as a common recreational drug.[49] It is also reported that some people use it to self-manage pain and anxiety.[50] As an anaesthetic gas, it affects coordination and awareness[51] and reduces psychomotor performance.[52]

There is variability in the subjective effects of the drug. In one study, 12 individuals (under controlled, blinded conditions) were given a choice between oxygen and nitrous oxide after a sampling period for both. There was significant individual variability in the reported effects of the drug. Those who reported feelings of 'tingling', 'drunk', 'dreamy', 'coasting', 'floating' and 'having pleasant bodily sensations' during the nitrous oxide sampling period chose nitrous oxide more often during the choice period.[53] There is disagreement in the literature as to whether there are gender differences in the effects of nitrous oxide.[54,55]

The use of nitrous oxide is associated with unwanted effects. These include transient dizziness, dissociation, acute ataxia, disorientation, loss of balance, impaired memory and cognition, and weakness in the legs. Blurred vision, nausea and headache have been reported. When intoxicated, accidents like tripping and falling may occur.[56] There are a few cases reported from clinical practice in which patients experienced erotic hallucinations leading to accusations of molestation against dentists and other staff.[57,58,59]

7.7 Mortality

Nitrous oxide is generally considered to be safe as it produces minimal cardiorespiratory disturbance in fit patients and is rapidly and completely eliminated from the body after exposure.[60] However, recreational use can be associated with adverse effects and it may pose significant risks in some people, especially with particular methods of administration.[61]

A number of cases of death by asphyxiation are reported among individuals who were using nitrous oxide at the time. Although nitrous oxide does not depress the respiratory drive significantly, the normal physiological response to hypoxia is blunted when 50% nitrous oxide is given and deaths are often in relation to bags put over the head in order to facilitate inhalation[62] or inhalation in cars. There is also evidence that death is often linked to polydrug use.[63]

7.8 Acute Harms

7.8.1 Acute Toxicity

It has been argued that typically, the moderate recreational use of nitrous oxide is not associated with major side effects. It has been suggested that nitrous oxide typically has few short-term adverse effects, other than headache for some.[64]

Nonetheless, a systematic review of the case literature has shown an extensive number of case reports in the literature suggesting that nitrous oxide misuse and its sequelae occur more frequently than recognised. The vast majority of toxicities involve the neurological system, although there are psychiatric and other medical presentations as well. The authors also argue that the number of deaths related to nitrous oxide, which do not include cases where it was used to assist in suicide, suggest that the risks involved with abuse are more significant than previously recognised.[65]

Harms are likely to result from disorientation and unsteadiness caused by inhalation (e.g. falling down[66]). There are also isolated instances in the literature of hypothermic skin trauma resulting from contact with chilled canisters.[67]

However, heavy use of nitrous oxide can be associated with severe adverse effects. Acute exposure to nitrous oxide may irritate the respiratory tract and acute use of inhalants in general can result in sneezing, coughing, excess salivation and conjunctival erythema.[68] The use of nitrous oxide can also cause asphyxia, headache, nausea, vomiting, dizziness and excitement, and to the central nervous system (CNS) depression, convulsions and death. Hypertension and cardiac dysrhythmias are possible. Patients can present with altered mental state, paraesthesias, ataxia and weakness or spasticity of the legs.[69] Nausea, cyanosis and fainting have been reported as a result of nitrous oxide.[70]

When nitrous oxide is inhaled from a balloon it displaces the air in the lungs, thus temporarily preventing oxygen from entering the bloodstream and potentially causing tachycardia and transient peripheral neurological symptoms.[71] There have been reports of fatalities after acute exposure, due to asphyxiation.[72,73]

Nitrous oxide is insoluble in blood, and therefore rapidly clears into the alveoli from the blood once inhalation has ceased.[74] At the high concentrations (e.g. >70%) used in anaesthesia there is the potential for hypoxia if a high concentration of oxygen is not then provided. Nitrous oxide may have effects on immune function, but the evidence is unclear on this issue.[75]

There is a risk that users may confuse the much more toxic or potent gases or volatile substances, such as butane, with nitrous oxide. If a patient requires admission to an emergency department, there is a chance that he or she has used butane, which does not only have different effects but also different harms. The use of nitrous oxide is not as life-threatening as the use of butane, which can cause arrhythmia and increases the risk of sudden cardiac arrest. Life-threatening risks of nitrous oxide are linked to mode of use, which may lead to hypoxia or anoxia.

High concentrations of inhaled nitrous oxide constitute a hypoxic inspired mixture and the likelihood and severity of resultant hypoxaemia will depend on the effectiveness of nitrous oxide delivery, air entrainment, depth of respiration, and breath-holding to alter washout of nitrogen, oxygen, and carbon dioxide from the lungs. It is argued that such hypoxaemia should be well tolerated by a fit person, but could give rise to seizures, arrhythmias, or even respiratory or cardiac arrest in patients with epilepsy, cardiac disease, or other co-morbidities, especially if combined with other drugs that tend to produce cardiac arrhythmia.[76]

In a systematic review of the case literature, where 91 individual cases across 77 publications were included, a study found that the majority of cases (n=72) reported neurologic sequelae including myeloneuropathy and subacute combined degeneration, commonly (n=39) with neuroimaging changes. Psychiatric (n=11) effects included psychosis while other medical effects (n=8) included pneumomediastinum and frostbite. Across all cases, nitrous oxide misuse was correlated with low or low-normal Vitamin B12 (cyanocobalamin) levels (n=52) and occasionally elevated homocysteine and methylmalonic acid.[77]

The chronic use of nitrous oxide is associated with problems relating to the depletion of vitamin B12 and is discussed in Section 7.10.2.

The features are summarised in Box 7.1.[78]

Box 7.1 Features of Acute Toxicity Associated with Nitrous Oxide

Respiratory effects
Asphyxia
Hypoxia
Neurological and psychiatric effects
CNS depression
Convulsions
Psychiatric symptoms
Headache
Myeloneuropathy
Polyneuropathy
Dizziness
Excitement
Paraesthesias
Paralysis
Psychosis
Cardiovascular effects
Hypertension
Cardiac dysrhythmias
Megaloblastic anaemia
Leukopenia
Anoxia
Metabolic features
Thrombocytopenia
Gastrointestinal symptoms
Nausea and vomiting

Patients present to hospital with changes in gait or coordination, difficulty walking and falls.

7.8.2 Acute Withdrawal

For withdrawal see Section 7.10.1.1

7.8.3 Poly-drug Use and Drug Interactions

There may be some increase in the effects of nitrous oxide when it is combined with alcohol.[79] It is possible that nitrous oxide ingested at the same time as stimulants has a greater effect on blood pressure and heart rate. There is anecdotal evidence that nitrous oxide can briefly enhance the effects of psychedelics like LSD, or bring the effects back strongly when the drug is wearing off, which could be very frightening if unexpected.

Generally speaking, it has been suggested that the odds of nitrous-oxide-related disorders may be substantially higher in patients with comorbid substance use disorders.[80]

As it is not metabolised by the liver, the potential for drug interactions with other agents is low.

7.9 Clinical Management of Acute Toxicity

7.9.1 Identification and Assessment of Acute Toxicity

The diagnosis of acute nitrous oxide toxicity should be made by clinical assessment. There are no rapid urine or serum field tests, so analytical assessment should not be considered a component of routine diagnosis. Assessment should be based on the recognition of the clinical toxidrome associated with nitrous oxide and the potentially harmful modes of use.

7.9.2 Clinical Management of Acute Toxicity

The management of acute harms resulting from nitrous oxide must be based on local, national and international protocols and guidelines.

Management of acute nitrous oxide harms must include removal from exposure and providing symptomatic treatment for any resultant problems. It is recommended that patients are observed for at least 1 hour after exposure. A 12-lead ECG and a full blood count may be needed for symptomatic patients. Where there is chronic use of nitrous oxide, it is recommended that B12 concentration is checked in symptomatic patients (see Section 7.10.2). Guidance on diagnosis for psychiatrists has also been published.[81]

7.10 Harms Associated with Chronic Use and Dependence

7.10.1 Dependence

As the effects of nitrous oxide are short-lasting and pleasurable, people may use it frequently. There is no consensus on the dependence liability of nitrous oxide. Some argue that nitrous oxide use does not seem to result in dependence,[82] that its addictive

potential is low as it is only a partial opiate agonist, and its euphoric effects fade rapidly.[83] On the other hand, cases of tolerance and psychological dependence have been reported in chronic users[84,85] and it has been recommended that daily use of nitrous oxide should be avoided in particular by people with mental health problems or other psychological vulnerability.

7.10.1.1 Withdrawal

Nitrous oxide is sometimes used in a compulsive way by some individuals, possibly explaining one of its street names, 'hippie crack'. There are no significant withdrawal symptoms aside from the desire to use more nitrous oxide.

7.10.2 Other Harms – Mental Health – Vitamin B12 Deficiency

Although the evidence is limited, it is possible that nitrous oxide can worsen some mental health problems, and its use has been linked to manic relapse.[86] One case report describes a psychotic episode occurring in a patient with no history of psychosis who had been regularly using nitrous oxide.[87]

The chronic use of nitrous oxide has been linked to psychiatric symptoms which include cases of mild mood disorders, psychotic behaviour, fatigue, generalised weakness, and loss of memory. These symptoms often preceded the neurological impairments.[88]

The adverse effects of chronic nitrous oxide use are dominated by vitamin B12 deficiency. The vast majority of toxicity described in the literature and associated with nitrous oxide use involve the neurological system, although there are psychiatric and other medical presentations as well.[89] By inactivating vitamin B12, nitrous oxide can cause anaemia as well as neuropathy.

The harms caused by nitrous oxide tend to stem from heavy usage and the ensuing depletion of vitamin B12 leading to neurological problems.[90,91,92] Neurological deficits are more likely to occur when nitrous oxide is used at high doses and for prolonged durations.[93] Case reports describe vitamin B12 deficiency after repetitive use (e.g. 50–100 bulbs) of nitrous oxide within a few hours or heavy use over prolonged time, e.g. more than 10–20 'bulbs' (or canisters), daily for 10 days.[94,95,96,97]

Studies have shown that the most common complaints were 'numbness', 'paraesthesias' and 'weakness'.[98] A meta-analysis comprising of patients associated with adverse effects of nitrous oxide exposure in medical and recreational settings has shown that the most frequent clinical manifestations included paraesthesia (80%; 72.0–88.0%), unsteady gait (58%; 48.2–67.8%), and weakness (43%; 33.1–52.9%). At least one haematological abnormality was reported in 71.7% (59.9–83.4%) of patients.[99]

The most frequent outcomes were subacute combined degeneration (28%), myelopathy (26%), generalised demyelinating polyneuropathy (23%) or peripheral neuropathy.[100] Other common diagnoses include myeloneuropathy. An early sign of peripheral neuropathy is numbness in fingers[101] and heavy nitrous oxide use was associated with persistent numbness.

Studies and reports have described peripheral neuropathy[102] myelopathy[103–114] and polyneuropathy.[115] Severe myeloneuropathy[116,117,118] leukopenia and thrombocytopenia[119,120,121,122,123] have been reported. Nitrous oxide causes peripheral neuropathy in a dose-dependent manner.[124]

Less common neurological signs and symptoms at the time of presentation include changes in cognitive functioning, bowel and bladder dysfunction, sexual dysfunction, and Lhermitte's sign (an 'electric' sensation that travels down the limbs and back upon neck flexion).[125,126,127,128] In addition to neurological symptoms, functional vitamin B12 deficiency causes skin hyperpigmentation and vascular disease from hyperhomocysteinaemia, and is teratogenic.[129,130,131] A case report of cardiac arrest has been published.[132]

7.11 Management of Harms Related to Chronic Use

It has been suggested that there is a need to consider vitamin B12 deficiency in patients who arrive at a hospital with psychiatric manifestations who report a history of nitrous oxide exposure or misuse in the recent or remote past.[133]

The treatment for neuropathological effects of nitrous oxide toxicity is abstinence from nitrous oxide use, high doses of vitamin B12 therapy and physiotherapy.[134,135]

Suggested treatment for the chronic harms related to the use of nitrous oxide resulting from vitamin B deficiency include parenteral folic acid,[136,137] intramuscular vitamin B12 injection[138,139,140,141,142] and intravenous methylprednisolone.[143] A number of studies have shown that stopping exposure and introducing vitamin B supplementation[144] may result in either partial or complete recovery, although this can take months.[145] High-dose intramuscular B12 replacement is recommended.[146] Educating patients about the risks of nitrous oxide has also been recommended.[147,148]

A review of 18 published cases of nitrous oxide toxicity identified the most common neurological presentations as paraesthesiae and gait disturbance, improving over weeks to months with high-dose B12 replacement (although only 25% of cases regained their original level of function).[149]

It has been suggested that recovery is slow and long-term deficits can result.[150,151] Neurological recovery may be incomplete, particularly when patients continue to use nitrous oxide.[152] It has also been argued that B12 supplementation is not effective when nitrous oxide use persists.[153]

One case report suggests that where symptoms persist, methionine treatment has been successful where B12 treatment alone has failed.[154]

A review of 143 patients with B12 deficiency found that early diagnosis and treatment are crucial and that the severity of ataxia and paraesthesias after treatment was strongly related to the duration as well as the severity of symptoms prior to therapy.[155] It also similarly suggested that the extent of recovery under treatment was inversely related to the duration of symptoms.[156]

At a global level, it has been argued that population studies are needed to evaluate whether the correction of vitamin B12 deficiency prevents nitrous-oxide-related toxicity in the context of anaesthesia and recreational use, particularly in countries with a high prevalence of vitamin B12 deficiency.[157]

7.11.1 Psychosocial and Pharmacological Support

There is no relevant pharmacological support. For psychosocial support, see Chapter 2.

7.12 Harm Reduction and Public Health

It has been argued that health professionals should be aware of the toxic effects of nitrous oxide and be able to identify potential nitrous oxide abuse.[158]

The inhalation of nitrous oxide through the balloon method may carry less risk than other methods and minimises the risk of anoxia. Users will drop the balloon if they are getting too hypoxic or lose consciousness. Other methods may carry more risk, in that the user may become unconscious through anoxia and continue to have insufficient access to oxygen. The following harm reduction measures should be taken:

- Users should always inhale nitrous oxide from a balloon – never from a tube or mask, or directly from a dispenser or compressed air tank.
- Users must be careful not to confuse nitrous oxide with other gases and volatile substances, which have far greater risks.
- Users should avoid inhaling while standing up and should be aware of their immediate surroundings (e.g. steep drops, fires, rivers).
- The use of nitrous oxide should be avoided in particular by people with problems with low blood pressure or any mental health issues.
- Users should stop inhaling if they feel any physical discomfort, such as 'pins and needles' or numbness.

Regular and long-term users of nitrous oxide in particular should be aware of the purity of the products they use and of the impact of any impurities.

References

1. Savage S, Daqing MD. The neurotoxicity of nitrous oxide: the facts and 'putative' mechanisms. *Brain Sci* 2014;**4**:73–90. https://doi.org/10.3390/brainsci4010073

2. Berkowitz BA, Finck AD, Ngai SH. Nitrous oxide analgesia: reversal by naloxone and development of tolerance. *J Pharmacol Exp Ther* 1977;**203**:539–547.

3. Savage S, Daqing MD. The neurotoxicity of nitrous oxide: the facts and 'putative' mechanisms. *Brain Sci* 2014;**4**:73–90. https://doi.org/10.3390/brainsci4010073

4. Brouette T, Anton R. Clinical review of inhalants. *Am J Addict* 2001;**10**(1):79–94.

5. Brouette T, Anton R. Clinical review of inhalants. *Am J Addict* 2001;**10**(1):79–94.

6. Ghobrial GM, Dalyai R, Flanders AE, Harrop J. Nitrous oxide myelopathy posing as spinal cord injury. *J Neurosurg Spine* 2012;**16**(5):489–491. https:// doi.org/10.3171/2012.2 .SPINE11532

7. Nunn JF. Clinical aspects of the interaction between nitrous oxide and vitamin B12. *Br J Anaesthesia* 1987;**59**(1):3–13.

8. van Amsterdama J, den Brink W. Recreational nitrous oxide use: prevalence and risks. *Regul Toxicol Pharmacol* 2015;**73**(3):790–796.

9. Advisory Council on the Misuse of Drugs (ACMD). Consideration of the Novel Psychoactive Substances (Legal Highs). London, Home Office, October 2011.

10. Garakani A, Jaffe RJ, Savla D, et al. Neurologic, psychiatric, and other medical manifestations of nitrous oxide abuse: a systematic review of the case literature. *Am J Addict* 2016;**25**:358–369.

11. Gillman MA, Lichtigfeld FJ, Young TN. Psychotropic analgesic nitrous oxide for alcoholic withdrawal states. *Cochrane Database Syst Rev* 2007;**18**(2):CD005190.

12. Kripke BJ, Hechtman HB. Nitrous oxide for pentazocine addiction and for intractable pain: report of case. *Anesth Analg* 1972;**51**(4):520–527.

13. Lichtigfeld FJ, Gillman MA. The treatment of alcoholic withdrawal states with oxygen and nitrous oxide. *S Afr Med J* 1982;**61**(10):349–351.

14. Gillman MA, Lichtigfeld FJ. Analgesic nitrous oxide: adjunct to clonidine for opioid withdrawal. *Am J Psychiatry* 1985;**142**(6):784–785.

15. Carey C, Clark A, Saner A. Excellent results with analgesic nitrous oxide for addictive withdrawal states in general practice. *S Afr Med J* 1991;**79**(8):516.

16. Alho H, Methuen T, Paloheimo M, et al. Nitrous oxide has no effect in the treatment of alcohol withdrawal syndrome: a double-blind placebo-controlled randomized trial. *J Clin Psychopharmacol* 2003;**23**(2):211–214.

17. Sanders RD, Weimann J, Maze M. Biologic effects of nitrous oxide: a mechanistic and toxicologic review. *Anesthesiology* 2008;**109**(4):707–722.

18. Advisory Council on the Misuse of Drugs (ACMD). Consideration of the Novel Psychoactive Substances (Legal Highs). London, Home Office, October 2011.

19. Available at: www.globaldrugsurvey.com/wp-content/themes/ globaldrugsurvey/results/GDS2019-Exec-Summary.pdf [last accessed 4 March 2022].

20. Kaar SJ, Ferris J, Waldron J, Devaney M, Ramsey J, Winstock AR. Up: the rise of nitrous oxide abuse. An international survey of contemporary nitrous oxide use. *J Psychopharmacol* 2016(online). https://doi.org/10.1177 /0269881116632375

21. Chen R, Liao M, Ou J. Laughing gas inhalation in Chinese youth: a public health issue. *Lancet Public Health* 2018;**3**(10):e465. https://doi.org/10.1016/S2468-2667(18) 30134-8

22. Gillman M. Polydrug abuse associated with nitrous oxide causes death. *Oxf Med Case Reports* 2016;**6**:117.

23. Mancke F, Kaklauskaite G, Kollmer J, Weiler M. Psychiatric comorbidities in a young man with subacute myelopathy induced by abusive nitrous oxide consumption: a case report *Subst Abuse Rehab* 2016;**7**:155–159.

24. van Amsterdam J, den Brink W. Recreational nitrous oxide use: prevalence and risks. *Reg Toxicol Pharmacol* 2015;**73**(3):790–796.

25. van Amsterdam J, den Brink W. Recreational nitrous oxide use: prevalence and risks. *Reg Toxicol Pharmacol* 2015;**73**(3):790–796.

26. Cheng HM, Park JH, Hernstadt D. Subacute combined degeneration of the spinal cord following recreational nitrous oxide use. *BMJ Case Rep* 2013;**8**: bcr2012008509. https://doi.org/10.1136/ bcr-2012-008509

27. Ng J, O'Grady G, Pettit T, et al. Nitrous oxide use in first-year students at Auckland University. *Lancet* 2003;**361**:1349–1350.

28. Cheng HM, Park JH, Hernstadt D. Subacute combined degeneration of the spinal cord following recreational nitrous oxide use. *BMJ Case Rep* 2013;**8**: bcr2012008509. https://doi.org/10.1136/ bcr-2012-008509

29. Ng J, O'Grady G, Pettit T, et al. Nitrous oxide use in first-year students at Auckland University. *Lancet* 2003;**361**:1349–1350.

30. Wackawik A, Luzzio C, Juhasz-Poscine K, et al. Myelo-neuropathy from nitrous oxide abuse: unusually high methylmalonic acid and homocysteine level. *Wis Med J* 2003;**102**:43–45.

31. Gillman MA. Nitrous oxide abuse in perspective. *Clin Neuropharmacol* 1992;**15**:297–306.

32. Cartner M, Sinnott M, Silburn P. Paralysis caused by 'nagging'. *Med J Aust* 2007;**187**:366–367.

33. Alt RS, Morrissey RP, Gang MA, et al. Severe myeloneuropathy from acute high-dose nitrous oxide(N2O) abuse. *J Emerg Med* 2011;**41**:378–380.

34. Miller MA, Martinez V, McCarthy R, et al. Nitrous oxide 'whippit' abuse presenting as clinical B12 deficiency and ataxia. *Am J Emerg Med* 2004;**22**:124.

35. Shulman RM, Geraghty TJ, Tadros M. A case of unusual substance abuse causing myeloneuropathy. *Spinal Cord* 2007;**45**:314–317.

36. Ng J, Nanging FR. *Lancet* 2002;**360**(9330):384.

37. Tatum WO, Bui DD, Grant EG, et al. Pseudo-Guillain-Barre syndrome due to 'whippet'-induced myeloneuropathy. *J Neuroimaging* 2010;**20**:400–401.

38. Lin RJ, Chen HF, Chang YC, et al. Subacute combined degeneration caused by nitrous oxide intoxication: case reports. *Acta Neurol Taiwan* 2011;**20**:129–137.

39. Vasconcelos OM, Poehm EH, McCarter RJ, et al. Potential outcome factors in subacute combined degeneration: review of observational studies. *J Gen Intern Med* 2006;**21**:1063–1068.

40. Dohrn CS, Lichtor JL, Finn RS, et al. Subjective and psychomotor effects of nitrous oxide in healthy volunteers. *Behav Pharmacol* 1992;**3**(1):19–30.

41. Sanders RD, Weimann J, Maze M. Biologic effects of nitrous oxide: a mechanistic and toxicologic review. *Anesthesiology* 2008;**109**(4):707–722.

42. van Amsterdam J, Nabben T, van den Brink W. Recreational nitrous oxide use: prevalence and risks. *Regul Toxicol Pharmacol* 2015;**73**(3):790–796.

43. Advisory Council on the Misuse of Drugs (ACMD). Consideration of the Novel Psychoactive Substances (Legal Highs). London, Home Office, October 2011.

44. Lichtigfeld FJ, Gillman MA. The treatment of alcoholic withdrawal states with oxygen and nitrous oxide. *S Afr Med J* 1982;**61**(10):349–351.

45. Glijn NHP, van der Linde D, Ertekin E, van Burg PLM, Grimbergen YAM, Libourel EJ. Is nitrous oxide really that joyful? *Neth J Med* 2017;**75**(7):304–306.

46. Advisory Council on the Misuse of Drugs (ACMD). Consideration of the Novel Psychoactive Substances (Legal Highs). London, Home Office, October 2011.

47. Lichtigfeld FJ, Gillman MA. The treatment of alcoholic withdrawal states with oxygen and nitrous oxide. *S Afr Med J* 1982;**61**(10):349–351.

48. Glijn NHP, van der Linde D, Ertekin E, van Burg PLM, Grimbergen YAM, Libourel EJ. Is nitrous oxide really that joyful? *Neth J Med* 2017;**75**(7):304–306.

49. Kaar SJ, Ferris J, Waldron J, Devaney M, Ramsey J, Winstock AR. Up: the rise of nitrous oxide abuse. An international survey of contemporary nitrous oxide use. *J Psychopharmacol* 2016(online). https://doi.org/10.1177/0269881116632375

50. Lundin MS, Cherian J, Andrew MN, et al. One month of nitrous oxide abuse causing acute vitamin B$_{12}$ deficiency with severe neuropsychiatric symptoms *BMJ Case Reports CP* 2019;**12**:bcr-2018-228001.

51. Lundin MS, Cherian J, Andrew MN, et al. One month of nitrous oxide abuse causing acute vitamin B$_{12}$ deficiency with severe neuropsychiatric symptoms *BMJ Case Reports CP* 2019;**12**:bcr-2018-228001.

52. Walker DJ, Zacny JP. Within- and between-subject variability in the reinforcing and subjective effects of nitrous oxide in healthy volunteers. *Drug Alcohol Depend* 2001;**64**(1):85–96.

53. Walker DJ, Zacny JP. Within- and between-subject variability in the reinforcing and subjective effects of nitrous oxide in healthy volunteers. *Drug Alcohol Depend* 2001;**64**(1):85–96.

54. Dohrn CS, Lichtor JL, Finn RS, et al. Subjective and psychomotor effects of nitrous oxide in healthy volunteers. *Behav Pharmacol* 1992;**3**(1):19–30.

55. Zacny JP, Jun JM. Lack of sex differences to the subjective effects of nitrous oxide in healthy volunteers. *Drug Alcohol Depend* 2010;**112**(3):251–254.

56. van Amsterdam J, den Brink W. Recreational nitrous oxide use: prevalence and risks. *Reg Toxicol Pharmacol* 2015;**73**(3):790–796.

57. Bennett CR. Nitrous oxide hallucinations. *J Am Dent Assoc* 1980;**101**:595–597.

58. Jastak JT, Malamed SF. Nitrous oxide sedation and sexual phenomena. *J Am Dent Assoc* 1980;**101**:38–40.

59. Lambert C. Sexual phenomena hypnosis and nitrous oxide sedation. *J Am Dent Assoc* 1982;**105**:990–991.

60. Lichtigfeld FJ, Gillman MA. The treatment of alcoholic withdrawal states with oxygen and nitrous oxide. *S Afr Med J* 1982;**61**(10):349–351.

61. Randhawa G, Bodenham A. The increasing recreational use of nitrous oxide: history revisited. *Br J Anaesth* 2016;**116** (3):321–324. https://doi.org/10.1093/bja/aev297

62. Wagner SA, Clark MA, Wesche DL, Doedens DJ, Lloyd AW. Asphyxial deaths from the recreational use of nitrous oxide. *J Forensic Sci* 1992;**37**(4):1008–1015.

63. Gillman M. Polydrug abuse associated with nitrous oxide causes death. *Oxf Med Case Reports* 2016;**2016**(6):117.

64. Advisory Council on the Misuse of Drugs (ACMD). Consideration of the Novel Psychoactive Substances (Legal Highs). London, Home Office, October 2011.

65. Garakani A, Jaffe RJ, Savla D, et al. Neurologic, psychiatric, and other medical manifestations of nitrous oxide abuse: a systematic review of the case literature. *Am J Addict* 2016;**25**:358–369.

66. Dohrn CS, Lichtor JL, Finn RS, et al. Subjective and psychomotor effects of nitrous oxide in healthy volunteers. *Behav Pharmacol* 1992;**3**(1):19–30.

67. Hwang JC, Himel HN, Edlich RF. Frostbite of the face after recreational misuse of nitrous oxide. *Burns* 1996;**22** (2):152–153.

68. Brouette T, Anton R. Clinical review of inhalants. *Am J Addict* 2001;**10**(1):79–94.

69. Sanders RD, Weimann J, Maze M. Biologic effects of nitrous oxide: a mechanistic and toxicologic review. *Anesthesiology* 2008;**109**(4):707–722.

70. Rosenberg H, Orkin FK, Springstead J. Abuse of nitrous oxide. *Anesth Analg* 1979;**58**(2):104–106.

71. Ghobrial GM, Dalyai R, Flanders AE, Harrop J. Nitrous oxide myelopathy posing as spinal cord injury. *J Neurosurg Spine* 2012;**16**(5):489–491. https:// doi.org/10.3171/2012.2 .SPINE11532

72. Chadly A, Marc B, Barres D, Durigon M. Suicide by nitrous oxide poisoning. *Am J Forensic Med Pathol* 1989;**10** (4):330–331.

73. Suruda AJ, McGlothlin JD. Fatal abuse of nitrous oxide in the workplace. *J Occup Med* 1990;**32**(8):682–684.

74. Pasternak JJ, Lanier WL. Is nitrous oxide use appropriate in neurosurgical and neurologically at-risk patients? *Curr Opin Anaesthesiol* 2010;**23**(5):544–550.

75. Sanders RD, Weimann J, Maze M. Biologic effects of nitrous oxide: a mechanistic and toxicologic review. *Anesthesiology* 2008;**109**(4):707–722.

76. Randhawa G, Bodenham A. The increasing recreational use of nitrous oxide: history revisited. *Br J Anaesth* 2016;**116**(3):321–324. https:// doi.org/10.1093/bja/aev297

77. Garakani A, Jaffe RJ, Savla D, et al. Neurologic, psychiatric, and other medical manifestations of nitrous oxide abuse: a systematic review of the case literature. *Am J Addict* 2016;**25**:358–369.

78. Rosenberg H, Orkin FK, Springstead J. Abuse of nitrous oxide. *Anesth Analg* 1979;**58**(2):104–106.

79. Zacny JP, Walker DJ, Derus LM. Choice of nitrous oxide and its subjective effects in light and moderate drinkers. *Drug Alcohol Depend* 2008;**98**(1–2):163–168.

80. Mancke F, Kaklauskaite G, Kollmer J, Weiler M. Psychiatric comorbidities in a young man with subacute myelopathy induced by abusive nitrous oxide consumption: a case report. *Subst Abuse Rehab* 2016;**7**:155–159.

81. Sheldon R, Reid M, Schon F, Poole N. Just say N2O – nitrous oxide misuse: essential information for psychiatrists. *BJPsych Advances* 2020;**26**(2):72–81. https://doi.org/10.1192/bja .2019.57

82. van Amsterdam J, den Brink W. Recreational nitrous oxide use: prevalence and risks. *Regul Toxicol Pharmacol* 2015;**73** (3):790–796.

83. Gillman MA. Nitrous oxide abuse in perspective. *Clin Neuropharmacol* 1992;**15**:297–306.

84. Gilman MA. Nitrous oxide – an opioid agent: review of the evidence. *Am J Med* 1986; **81**:97–102.

85. Mancke F, Kaklauskaite G, Kollmer J, Weiler M. Psychiatric comorbidities in a young man with subacute myelopathy induced by abusive nitrous oxide consumption: a case report. *Subst Abuse Rehab* 2016;**7**:155–159.

86. Tym MK, Alexander J. Nitrous oxide induced manic relapse. *Aust NZ J Psychiatry* 2011;**45**(11):1002.

87. Sethi NK, Mullin P, Torgovnick J, Capasso G. Nitrous oxide 'whippit' abuse presenting with cobalamin responsive psychosis. *J Med Toxicol* 2006;**2**(2):71–74.

88. Cousaert C, Heylens G, Audenaert K. Laughing gas abuse is no joke: an overview of the implications for psychiatric practice. *Clin Neurol Neurosurg* 2013;**115**(7):859–862.

89. Garakani A, Jaffe RJ, Savla D, et al. Neurologic, psychiatric, and other medical manifestations of nitrous oxide abuse: a systematic review of the case literature. *Am J Addict* 2016;**25**:358–369.

90. Miller MA, Martinez V, McCarthy R, et al. Nitrous oxide 'whippit' abuse presenting as clinical B12 deficiency and ataxia. *Am J Emerg Med* 2004;**22**:124.

91. Stacy CB, Di Rocco A, Gould RJ. Methionine in the treatment of nitrous-oxide-induced neuropathy and myeloneuropathy. *J Neurol* 1992;**239**:401–403.

92. Luis-Ferdinand RT. Myelotoxic, neurotoxic and reproductive adverse effects of nitrous oxide. *Adverse Drug React Toxicol Rev* 1994;**13**:193–206.

93. Al-Sadawi M, Hidalgo C, Chinyere A, Apoorva J, Modupe O, McFarlane SI. Inhaled nitrous oxide 'whip-its!' causing subacute combined degeneration of spinal cord. *Am J Med Case Rep* 2018;**6**(12):237–240. https://doi.org/10.12691/ajmcr-6-12-3

94. Van Amsterdam J, Nabben T, van den Brink W. Recreational nitrous oxide use: prevalence and risks. *Regul Toxicol Pharmacol* 2015;**73**:790–796.

95. Stabler SP. Vitamin B12 deficiency. *N Engl J Med* 2013;**368**:2041–2042.

96. Massey TH, Pickersgill TT, Peal KJ. Nitrous oxide misuse and vitamin B12 deficiency. *BMJ Case Rep* 2016 (online). https://doi.org/10.1136/bcr-2016-215728

97. Cartner M, Sinnott M, Silburn P. Paralysis caused by 'nagging'. *Med J Aust* 2007;**187**:366–367.

98. Garakani A, Jaffe RJ, Savla D, et al. Neurologic, psychiatric, and other medical manifestations of nitrous oxide abuse: a systematic review of the case literature. *Am J Addict* 2016;**25**:358–369.

99. Oussalah A, Julien M, Levy J, et al. Global burden related to nitrous oxide exposure in medical and recreational settings: a systematic review and individual patient data meta-analysis. *J Clin Med* 2019;**8**:551.

100. Oussalah A, Julien M, Levy J, et al. Global burden related to nitrous oxide exposure in medical and recreational settings: a systematic review and individual patient data meta-analysis. *J Clin Med* 2019;**8**:551.

101. van Amsterdam J, van den Brink W. Recreational nitrous oxide use: prevalence and risks. *Regul Toxicol Pharmacol* 2015;**73**(3):790–796.

102. Richardson PG. Peripheral neuropathy following nitrous oxide abuse. *Emerg Med Australas* 2010;**22**(1):88–90.

103. Ghobrial GM, Dalyai R, Flanders AE, Harrop J. Nitrous oxide myelopathy posing as spinal cord injury. *J Neurosurg Spine* 2012;**16**(5):489–491. https://doi.org/10.3171/2012.2.SPINE11532

104. Cheng HM, Park JH, Hernstadt D. Subacute combined degeneration of the spinal cord following recreational nitrous oxide use. *BMJ Case Rep* 2013;**8**:bcr2012008509. https://doi.org/10.1136/bcr-2012-008509

105. Miller MA, Martinez V, McCarthy R, et al. Nitrous oxide 'whippit' abuse presenting as clinical B12 deficiency and ataxia. *Am J Emerg Med* 2004;**22**:124.

106. Shulman RM, Geraghty TJ, Tadros M. A case of unusual substance abuse causing myeloneuropathy. *Spinal Cord* 2007;**45**:314–317.

107. Tatum WO, Bui DD, Grant EG, et al. Pseudo-Guillain-Barre syndrome due to 'whippet'-induced myeloneuropathy. *J Neuroimaging* 2010;**20**:400–401.

108. Richardson PG. Peripheral neuropathy following nitrous oxide abuse. *Emerg Med Australas* 2010;**22**(1):88–90.

109. Diamond AL, Diamond R, Freedman SM, Thomas FP. 'Whippets'-induced cobalamin deficiency manifesting as cervical myelopathy. *J Neuroimaging* 2004;**14**(3):277–280.

110. Hsu CK, Chen YQ, Lung VZ, His SC, Lo HC, Shyu HY. Myelopathy and polyneuropathy caused by nitrous oxide toxicity: a case report. *Am J Emerg Med* 2012;**30**(6):1016.e3–6. https://doi.org/10.1016/j.ajem.2011.05.001

111. Probasco JC, Felling RJ, Carson JT, Dorsey ER, Niessen TM. Teaching neuroimages: myelopathy due to B12 deficiency in long-term colchicine treatment and nitrous oxide misuse. *Neurology* 2011;**77**(9):e51. https://doi.org/10.1212/WNL.0b013e31822c910f

112. Sotirchos ES, Saidha S, Becker D. Neurological picture: nitrous oxide-induced myelopathy with inverted V-sign on spinal MRI. *J Neurol Neurosurg Psychiatry* 2012;**83**(9):915–916.

113. Waters MF, Kang GA, Mazziotta JC, DeGiorgio CM. Nitrous oxide inhalation as a cause of cervical myelopathy. *Acta Neurol Scand* 2005;**12**(4):270–272.

114. Massey TH, Pickersgill TT, Peall JK. Nitrous oxide misuse and vitamin B₁₂ deficiency. *Case Rep* 2016;**2016**: bcr2016215728.

115. Richardson PG. Peripheral neuropathy following nitrous oxide abuse. *Emerg Med Australas* 2010;**22**(1):88–90.

116. Miller MA, Martinez V, McCarthy R, et al. Nitrous oxide 'whippit' abuse presenting as clinical B12 deficiency and ataxia. *Am J Emerg Med* 2004;**22**:124.

117. Dong X, Ba F, Wang R, Zheng D. Imaging appearance of myelopathy secondary to nitrous oxide abuse: a case report and review of the literature. *Int J Neurosci* 2019;**129**(3):225–229. https://doi.org/10.1080/00207454.2018.1526801

118. Williamson J, Huda S, Damodaran D. Nitrous oxide myelopathy with functional vitamin B ₁₂ deficiency. *BMJ Case Rep CP* 2019;**12**:e227439.

119. Miller MA, Martinez V, McCarthy R, et al. Nitrous oxide 'whippit' abuse presenting as clinical B12 deficiency and ataxia. *Am J Emerg Med* 2004;**22**:124.

120. Glijn NHP, van der Linde D, Ertekin E, van Burg PLM, Grimbergen YAM, Libourel EJ. Is nitrous oxide really that joyful? *Neth J Med* 2017;**75**(7):304–306.

121. Garriott J, Petty CS. Death from inhalant abuse: toxicological and pathological evaluation of 34 cases. *Clin Toxicol* 1980;**16**:305–315.

122. Bowen SE, Daniel J, Balster RL. Deaths associated with inhalant abuse in Virginia from 1987 to 1996. *Drug Alcohol Depend* 1999;**53**:239–245.

123. Suruda AJ, McGlothlin JD. Fatal abuse of nitrous oxide in the workplace. *J Occup Med* 1990;**32**:682–684.

124. Winstock AR. Ferris JA. Nitrous oxide causes peripheral neuropathy in a dose-dependent manner among recreational users. *J Psychopharmacol* 2020;**34**(2):229–236. https://doi.org/10.1177/0269881119882532

125. Garakani A, Jaffe RJ, Savla D, et al. Neurologic, psychiatric, and other medical manifestations of nitrous oxide abuse: a systematic review of the case literature. *Am J Addict* 2016;**25**:358–369.

126. Stabler SP. Vitamin B12 deficiency. *N Engl J Med* 2013;**368**:2041–2042.

127. Massey TH, Pickersgill TT, Peal KJ. Nitrous oxide misuse and Vitamin B12 deficiency. *BMJ Case Rep* 2016 (online). https://doi.org/10.1136/bcr-2016-215728

128. Mishra VA, Harbada R, Sharma A. Vitamin B12 and vitamin D deficiencies: an unusual cause of fever, severe hemolytic anemia and thrombocytopenia. *J Fam Med Prim Care* 2015;**4**:145–148.

129. Carey C, Clark A, Saner A. Excellent results with analgesic nitrous oxide for addictive withdrawal states in general practice. *S Afr Med J* 1991;**79**(8):516.

130. Cheng HM, Park JH, Hernstadt D. Subacute combined degeneration of the spinal cord following recreational nitrous oxide use. *BMJ Case Rep* 2013;**2013**:bcr2012008509. https://doi.org/10.1136/ bcr-2012-008509

131. Randhawa G, Bodenham A. The increasing recreational use of nitrous oxide: history revisited. *Br J Anaesthesia* 2016;**116** (3):321–324. https://doi.org/10.1093/bja/aev297

132. Cartner M, Sinnott M, Silburn P. Paralysis caused by 'nagging'. *Med J Aust* 2007;**187**:366–367.

133. Sethi NK, Mullin P, Torgovnick J, Capasso G. Nitrous oxide 'whippit' abuse presenting with cobalamin responsive psychosis. *J Med Toxicol* 2006;**2**(2):71–74.

134. Al-Sadawi M, Hidalgo C, Chinyere A, Apoorva J, Modupe O, McFarlane SI. Inhaled nitrous oxide 'whip-its!' causing subacute combined degeneration of spinal cord. *Am J Med Case Rep* 2018;**6**(12):237–240. https://doi.org/10.12691/ajmcr-6-12-3

135. Massey TH, Pickersgill TT, Peal KJ. Nitrous oxide misuse and Vitamin B12 deficiency. *BMJ Case Rep* 2016 (online). https:// doi.org/ 10.1136/bcr-2016-215728

136. Miller MA, Martinez V, McCarthy R, et al. Nitrous oxide 'whippit' abuse presenting as clinical B12 deficiency and ataxia. *Am J Emerg Med* 2004;**22**:124.

137. Butzkueven H, King JO. Nitrous oxide myelopathy in an abuser of whipped cream bulbs. *J Clin Neurosci* 2000;**7** (1):73–75.

138. Cheng HM, Park JH, Hernstadt D. Subacute combined degeneration of the spinal cord following recreational nitrous oxide use. *BMJ Case Rep* 2013;**2013**:bcr2012008509. https://doi.org/10.1136/ bcr-2012-008509

139. Miller MA, Martinez V, McCarthy R, et al. Nitrous oxide 'whippit' abuse presenting as clinical B12 deficiency and ataxia. *Am J Emerg Med* 2004;**22**:124.

140. Richardson PG. Peripheral neuropathy following nitrous oxide abuse. *Emerg Med Australas* 2010;**22**(1):88–90.

141. Diamond AL, Diamond R, Freedman SM, Thomas FP. 'Whippets'-induced cobalamin deficiency manifesting as cervical myelopathy. *J Neuroimaging* 2004;**14**(3):277–280.

142. Probasco JC, Felling RJ, Carson JT, Dorsey ER, Niessen TM. Teaching neuroimages: myelopathy due to B12 deficiency in long-term colchicine treatment and nitrous oxide misuse. *Neurology* 2011;**77**(9):e51. https://doi.org/10.1212/WNL .0b013e31822c910f

143. Ghobrial GM, Dalyai R, Flanders AE, Harrop J. Nitrous oxide myelopathy posing as spinal cord injury. *J Neurosurg Spine* 2012;**16**(5):489–491. https:// doi.org/10.3171/2012 .2.SPINE11532

144. Lundin MS, Cherian J, Andrew MN, et al. One month of nitrous oxide abuse causing acute vitamin B$_{12}$ deficiency with severe neuropsychiatric symptoms *BMJ Case Rep* 2019;**12**: bcr–2018–228001.

145. Diamond AL, Diamond R, Freedman SM, Thomas FP. 'Whippets'-induced cobalamin deficiency manifesting as cervical myelopathy. *J Neuroimaging* 2004;**14**(3):277–280.

146. Thompson AG, Leite MI, Lunn MP, Bennett DLH. Whippits, nitrous oxide and the dangers of legal highs. *Pract Neurol* 2015;**15**:207–209. https://doi.org/10.1136/practneurol-2014-001071

147. Keddie S, Adams A, Kelso ARC, et al. No laughing matter: subacute degeneration of the spinal cord due to nitrous oxide inhalation *J Neurol* 2018;**265**:1089–1095. https://doi.org/10 .1007/s00415-018-8801-3

148. Vasconcelos OM, Poehm EH, McCarter RJ, Campbell WW, Quezado ZMN. Potential outcome factors in subacute combined degeneration: review of observational studies. *J Gen Intern Med* 2006;**21**:1063–1068.

149. Massey TH, Pickersgill TT, Peal KJ. Nitrous oxide misuse and Vitamin B12 deficiency. *BMJ Case Rep* 2016 (online). https:// doi.org/ 10.1136/bcr-2016-215728

150. Shoults K. Case report: neurological complications of nitrous oxide abuse. *B C Med J* 2016;**58**(4):192–194.

151. Vasconcelos OM, Poehm EH, McCarter RJ, Campbell WW, Quezado ZMN. Potential outcome factors in subacute combined degeneration: review of observational studies. *J Gen Intern Med* 2006;**21**:1063–1068.

152. Keddie S, Adams A, Kelso ARC, et al. No laughing matter: subacute degeneration of the spinal cord due to nitrous oxide inhalation. *J Neurol* 2018; **265**:1089–1095. https://doi.org/10 .1007/s00415-018-8801-3

153. Blair C, Tremonti C, Edwards L, Haber PS, Halmagyi GM. Vitamin B12 supplementation futile for preventing demyelination in ongoing nitrous oxide misuse *Med J Aust* 2019;**211**(9):428. https://doi.org/10.5694/mja2.50371

154. Stacy C, DiRocco A, Gould R. Methionine in the treatment of nitrous oxide induced neuropathy and myeloneuroapthy. *J Neurol* 1992;**239**(7):401–403.

155. Ives R, Ghelani P. Polydrug use (the use of drugs in combination): a brief review. *Drugs Educ Prev Policy* 2006;**13** (3):225–232.

156. Mancke F, Kaklauskaite G, Kollmer J, Weiler M. Psychiatric comorbidities in a young man with subacute myelopathy induced by abusive nitrous oxide consumption: a case report. *Subst Abuse Rehab* 2016;7 155–159.

157. Garakani A, Jaffe RJ, Savla D, et al. Neurologic, psychiatric, and other medical manifestations of nitrous oxide abuse: a systematic review of the case literature. *Am J Addict* 2016;**25**:358–369.

158. Garakani A, Jaffe RJ, Savla D, et al. Neurologic, psychiatric, and other medical manifestations of nitrous oxide abuse: a systematic review of the case literature. *Am J Addict* 2016;**25**:358–369.

Introduction to Stimulant Club Drugs and Novel Psychoactive Substances

8A.1 An Introduction to Drugs with Stimulant Effects

Substances with a stimulant effect have been used by successive generations of people. A wide range of substances have been used, notably of course caffeine and nicotine. Psychostimulants can be plant-based substances or can also be of a synthetic nature.

Currently, the illicit market for stimulants includes cocaine and amphetamine-type stimulants (ATS), including new psychoactive substances with stimulant effect and ATS. The 2020 World Drug Report states that the manufacture of amphetamine-type stimulants continues to be dominated by methamphetamine.[1]

Stimulants constitute the main category of novel psychoactive substances (NPS) reported to the UNODC early warning advisory since 2009. The 2020 World Drug Report states that at this time, most of the NPS found on the drug markets of member states were stimulants, followed by synthetic opioid receptor agonists.[2] Simulant NPS include several synthetic cathinones, other phenethylamines, dimethoxyamphetamine and piperazines.

8A.2 Pharmacology in Brief

The patterns of effects of the various stimulant agents vary, but stimulant drugs overall stimulate the brain and central nervous system by increasing the activity of key neurotransmitters, such as noradrenaline, dopamine and serotonin. This takes place through a number of mechanisms, including increasing release of and/or inhibiting reuptake of these chemicals.

Different stimulants will work in different ways. Cocaine prevents dopamine reuptake while amphetamines increase its release. It is generally believed that dopamine reuptake blockade – in particular in the nucleus accumbens – is the most important action of cocaine.

On the other hand, enhancing the release of dopamine in the nucleus accumbens appears to be the mediating effect of amphetamines[3,4] and amphetamines increase the release of newly synthesised noradrenaline and dopamine.[3,5] The effects of amphetamines (and especially of methamphetamine, discussed in Chapter 10), also last longer than those of cocaine.[3]

The extent to which a specific drug elevates these levels will determine the effect. Drugs that elevate dopamine significantly will induce greater reward and pleasure or even euphoria, but are also more likely to increase a desire to re-dose. Those that elevate noradrenaline will be less euphoric, but may increase alertness and cause anxiety. They also increase strain on the heart and circulatory system.

Some stimulants act on serotoninergic receptors and exhibit monoamine reuptake as well. Stimulants that are linked with the release of serotonin are associated with feelings of empathy and compassion (sometimes referred to as empathogenic and entactogenic effects) and increased sociability and sex drive. Stimulants that act on the serotoninergic receptors exhibit hallucinogenic effects in addition to their stimulant effects.

Like other NPS, the toxic effects of NPS with stimulant effects have not been well studied, but are expected to be similar to those of better understood stimulants (see Box 8A.1).

8A.3 Stimulant Novel Psychoactive Substances in Europe

Recent data from Europe also suggest greater geographical diffusion and an overall increase in the consumption of all the commonly used classes of stimulant drugs.[12] As is the case world-wide, the main illicit stimulant drugs available in Europe are cocaine, amphetamine, methamphetamine and MDMA.

The extent of stimulant use and the types that are most common in Europe vary across countries, Overall, cocaine is the most frequently seized stimulant in many western and southern countries, while amphetamines and MDMA seizures are predominant in northern and eastern Europe.[12] There is also some evidence of a potential increase in stimulant injecting (see Box 8A.2).[12]

Box 8A.1 Novel Psychoactive Substance Stimulants

Over one third of all NPS identified at a global level since 2009 are stimulants. Up to December 2021 stimulant NPS have been the largest group of NPS identified and reported by Member States of the UN, followed by synthetic cannabinoids.[6]

The UNODC has reported that the number of stimulant NPS identified over the period 2009–2017 increased more than fourfold, from 48 new substances reported in 2009 to 206 reported in 2015. In 2017, 39% of all NPS identified that year were stimulants (26 out of 79), mostly cathinones or other phenethylamines.[7]

NPS with stimulant effects belong to the following groups:[8] phenethylamines, amphetamine, synthetic cathinones or beta-keto (bk) amphetamines, piperazines, pipradrols/piperidines, aminoidanes, benzofurans, tryptamines, 2C agents-substituted phenylethylamines, 2D agents-substituted phenylethylamines and NBome agents-substituted phenylethylamines.

Globally, the most widely seized NPS stimulants were synthetic cathinones[9] and cathinones form a significant part of the NPS drugs with stimulant effects that are used in Europe.[10]

There are others which are also used, including other amphetamine-type substances. These include a number that are novel derivatives of drugs such as 3,4-methylenedioxy-methamphetamine (MDMA), or 'ecstasy'. These amphetamine-type stimulants are discussed in Chapter 9.

Piperazines are also used because they have effects similar to MDMA/'ecstasy'. N-Benzylpiperazin (BZP) is one of the commonly used piperazines. It triggers the release of dopamine and norepinephrine and inhibits the uptake of dopamine, norepinephrine and serotonin. BZP has only one tenth of the potency of amphetamine, but at high doses can lead to hallucinations.[11]

Box 8A.2 Increase in Stimulant Injecting

There is increasing evidence of a potential rise in stimulant injecting in Europe.[12] A study examining the residue of syringes collected from the bins of street automatic injection kit dispensers and at harm reduction services in five sentinel EU cities in 2017 (Amsterdam, Budapest, Glasgow, Helsinki and Paris) reported that injected substances varied between and within cities but that traces of stimulants (cocaine, amphetamines and synthetic cathinones) were found in a high proportion of the syringes tested in each of the cities. The study also showed that half of the syringes tested contained two or more drugs; the most frequent combination being a mix of stimulant and opioid.[12]

The study findings may indicate a high prevalence of stimulant use among people who inject drugs. However, the high number of syringes containing residues of stimulants could reflect the higher frequency of injecting among stimulant users, rather than a high prevalence of stimulant use among people who inject drugs.

In some countries, there is increasing evidence of high levels of stimulant injection among people who inject drugs. A high prevalence of synthetic cathinones injection was reported in 2014 among clients of low-threshold programmes in Hungary (>50%).[13] In 2016, in Finland, 28% of treatment entrants reported injecting as a main route of administration of amphetamine. In Glasgow, a 2015 HIV outbreak among people who inject drugs has been strongly linked, among other factors, to injecting cocaine.[14,15]

The injecting of stimulants predominates in some countries,[16] as shown by data from drug services in Czechia, France, Hungary and Latvia.[21] Stimulants are reported as one of the main injected drugs in these four countries, where the substances used include synthetic cathinones (Hungary), cocaine (France), amphetamine (Latvia) and

Box 8A.2 (cont.)

methamphetamine (Czechia).[17] Synthetic cathinones were found in a majority of syringes from Budapest and in particular the synthetic cathinones pentedrone and MDPV[18] (see also Chapter 11).

Harms of Injecting Stimulant Drugs

Injecting drugs in general is associated with high levels of harms, including increased risk of overdose and likelihood of dependence. They are also associated with other harms. Simulants can be associated with compulsive and frequent injecting, making their users at particular risk of the acquisition and transmission of blood-borne viruses. To this are added the risks specifically linked to the injection of the various stimulants, which can include limb abscesses and vein clotting, damage and recession. This places injectors at risk of septicaemia, endocarditis, deep-vein thrombosis and other complications.

The injection of stimulants – including cocaine and synthetic cathinones – has been linked to increased risk of HIV and HCV transmission, through increased frequency of use and sharing of injecting paraphernalia.[19]

Despite overall decline in Europe, in recent years localised HIV outbreaks associated with stimulant injecting have been documented among marginalised populations of people who inject drugs in Bavaria[20] and Dublin 2014–2015 (synthetic cathinones, alpha-PVP), Luxembourg 2014–2017 (cocaine) and Glasgow 2015 (cocaine).[20,21] Information from low-threshold services in the area affected suggested that there might be an association between the increase in HIV cases and group consumption of stimulant new psychoactive substances, including synthetic cathinones.[22]

Regarding the risks associated with the injection of stimulants, high-HIV risk as a result of higher levels of unsafe sexual practices is discussed in Section 8.3.

Chapter 8B

Amphetamine-type Stimulants: An Overview

8B.1 Introduction

Amphetamine-type stimulants (ATS) are world-wide the second most popular group of drugs after cannabis (UNODC, 2019)[23] and a significant proportion of NPS with stimulant effects are ATS.

The World Health Organization (WHO) defines amphetamine-type stimulants (ATS) as a group of drugs whose principal members include amphetamine and methamphetamine. A range of other substances also fall into this group, such as methcathinone, ephedrine, pseudoephedrine, methylphenidate and 3,4-methylenedioxy-methamphetamine (MDMA).

Globally, seizures of ATS increased sharply from the second half of the 1990s until 2001 and over the period 2009–2017.[24] The largest number of seizures in the past few years have been methamphetamine, followed by amphetamine, 'ecstasy' type substances, other stimulants (MDPV, methcathinone, methylone, several other cathinones, dimethoxyamphetamine and several piperazines) and prescription stimulants.

8B.2 Pharmacology

Amphetamine itself, as well as the ATS, are derivatives of a beta-phenylethylamine core structure and are kinetically and dynamically characterised by easily crossing the blood–brain barrier; resistance to brain biotransformation; and the release of monoamine neurotransmitters from nerve endings. All the structural features that enable these physiological characteristics are present in the simplest derivative, amphetamine, as well as other ATS.[25]

Pharmacokinetically, amphetamines have a high oral bioavailability and low plasma protein binding (typically less than 20%). Their elimination half-lives range from 6 to 12 hours and renal and hepatic elimination occurs. Many amphetamines are extensively metabolised by the liver, but a significant proportion of several of these drugs is usually excreted without prior biotransformation.[36,26]

Chemically, amphetamines are weak basic drugs (with pKa value of approximately 9.9); they also have low molecular weight. This means that they can cross cellular membranes and lipidic layers easily, reaching high levels in tissues and biological fluids with a pH lower than blood, including saliva and sweat.[36,27]

ATS share common properties, but their effects must not be seen as homogeneous. There are significant variations between the various ATS.

Phenethylamines are a broad range of compounds that share a common phenylethan-2-amine structure. Studies have shown that phenethylamines have three different principal effects: central stimulant action; hallucinogenic action; and 'other' psychoactive action.[28] Some produce more than one of these effects.[29]

The subjective effects of these drugs range from stimulant effects (e.g. amphetamine, methamphetamine), empathogenic or entactogenic effects (e.g. MDMA, considered in Chapter 9), and hallucinogenic effects (e.g. the 2DC series such as 2CB, the 'D series', benzodifurans and others such as p-methoxymethamphetamine and PMMA).

It has been suggested that the predominant actions of a stimulant on serotonin versus dopamine transporters will determine its predominant effect. For example, among the NPS ATS, it is suggested that dimethylmethcathinones, 4-MA, and MMAI cause entactogenic/empathogenic effects similar to MDMA, whereas 3-MMC, 5-IT, and N-methyl-2-AI have more stimulant-type properties like amphetamine.[30,31]

8B.3 Medical and Other Legitimate Uses of Amphetamines

The clinical uses of amphetamines are currently limited. They have been utilised in the treatment of adults with attention deficit hyperactivity disorder (ADHD).[32] Dexedrine (dexamphetamine sulphate) is used in the treatment of narcolepsy and ADHD.

Methylphenidate has a similar chemical structure and effects to amphetamine and is also used for the treatment of ADHD. Methylphenidate is sometimes misused, including as a 'smart drug' or cognitive enhancer. In recent years, ethylphenidate, an NPS that mimics the effects of methylphenidate, has been manufactured in clandestine laboratories and sometimes sold on the illicit market or the Internet.

8B.4 Prevalence and Patterns of Use

The 2019 World Drug Report has confirmed that after cannabis, stimulants continue to constitute the second most widely used category of drugs globally. The type of stimulants used, however, varies considerably across the different sub-regions,[33] mainly cocaine, amphetamine, methamphetamine and 'ecstasy'; polydrug use is common.

The WHO suggested that there is no typical profile for ATS users and there is a wide range of desired effects from ATS. ATS are used by students and drivers to stay awake and concentrate, used by athletes to enhance performance, and used at parties and clubs to increase sociability.[34] ATS are also used to increase confidence and lift mood, lose weight and increase sex drive. A WHO 1997 report on ATS classified the patterns of use in the following way:[35]

1. Instrumental use. Amphetamines are exploited by users to achieve desired goals, such as improve concentration and ward off fatigue.
2. Sub-cultural/recreational use. Their stimulant properties are exploited to allow the user to remain active for longer periods in social and recreational settings, such as at music and dance events and all-night drinking venues.
3. Chronic use. For several reasons, including craving, tolerance and withdrawal, some amphetamine users develop chronic patterns of consumption to relieve unwanted effects of abstinence or in the context of dependence.

8B.5 Routes of Ingestion and Dosing

Depending on the substance, ATS can be taken orally, by insufflation, smoking or injected.

The association between route of administration and risks associated with use has been well documented. Smoked and injected ATS are more likely to lead to dependence than oral use,[36] while injecting also increases the risks of transmission of blood-borne viruses.[36]

The effects of ATS generally appear 30–40 minutes after ingestion and can last for 4–8 hours, but there are variations, depending on the ATS used, the dose, the potency and the length of the effects, as well as tolerance.

Some new ATS, such as the 2 desoxy form (2-DPMP,) have particularly long-lasting effects and have longer half-lives.[37,38,39]

There are also wide differences in physiological effects, with paramethoxyamphetamine (PMA) for example, having a much steeper dose–response curve than MDMA.

8B.6 Desired and Unwanted Subjective Effects of Amphetamine-type Stimulants

Overall, ATS are used for their stimulant, euphoric, anorectic and, in the case of some substances, empathogenic/entactogenic and hallucinogenic properties. ATS produce feelings of euphoria and relief from fatigue; they may improve performance on simple tasks and increase activity levels.[3] It is thought that the misuse liability of amphetamines is related to their euphorigenic effects.[3,40] A systematic review of the qualitative research evidence showed the heterogeneous nature of ATS users and the complicated dynamic of individual, social and environmental factors that shape different consumption trajectories.[41]

Unwanted subjective effects of amphetamines include increased anxiety, insomnia, irritability, aggression, restlessness and paranoia, and in some cases violent behaviour. Psychotic symptoms can occur when using amphetamines and can last for days or weeks. The 'come-down' from ATS, which is distinct from the physiological withdrawal observed in many dependent users, can last up to a few days; users may feel tired, anxious, depressed and some instances may experience restlessness, insomnia, muscle ache and fasciculation. Its intensity will depend on the substance, the dose consumed and the individual. Serotonin syndrome or toxicity is a potential risk (see Section 8B.9.2 for details on the serotonin syndrome).

8B.7 High-risk Injecting and Sexual Behaviours

There is evidence that injection of ATS is associated with high levels of infection risk.[42]

- People who inject ATS do so more frequently than those who inject other substances such as heroin.[53]

- There is evidence that the injecting of ATS is associated with a high HIV and blood-borne virus (BBV) risk behaviour. In the UK for example, data from the Unlinked Anonymous Monitoring (UAM) survey of people who inject drugs (PWID) showed that people who injected amphetamine and ATS as their main drug were more likely to report the sharing of injecting equipment than those who reported using other main drugs.[53] Those who reported injecting ATS alone as their main drug were also significantly less likely to have ever had an HIV test or a hepatitis C test than those who reported other main drugs.

ATS have also been linked to high-risk sexual behaviours, and risks related to HIV/AIDS and other blood-borne infections and sexually transmitted diseases. Some have argued that ATS can impair judgement and inhibition, and lead people to engage in high-risk sexual behaviours.[43] Some ATS, such as methamphetamine, has been reported to have pro-sexual effects, as discussed in Chapter 10. These drugs are sometimes used by gay men and other men who have sex with men, among other groups of people, as they are reported to increase sexual desire and make sexual intercourse less painful and more pleasurable[44] (see Chapter 10).

8B.8 Mortality

Mortality among amphetamine users is relatively low in comparison with other 'problem drugs', such as opioids. It is associated with longer drug careers and with injecting.[45] Deaths are often caused by blood-borne viruses and infectious diseases or damage to the cardiovascular system. Non-fatal overdoses related to amphetamine use, on the other hand, are common.[47,46,47] Amphetamine overdoses constitute only a small proportion of fatal overdoses, and are mainly associated with co-ingestion of opioids.[48] Direct amphetamine-related mortality typically occurs as a result of heart attacks, seizures, arrhythmias or respiratory failures.[58] Deaths due to NPS with stimulant effects have been reported.[49]

8B.9 Acute Harms

Stimulants have actions on multiple receptor sites within the central nervous system, with patterns of effects varying between drugs.

- Predominantly stimulant drugs inhibit monoamine (especially dopamine) reuptake and

are associated with a sympathomimetic toxidrome.
- Serotonergic effects predominate in toxicity of stimulants that provoke central serotonin release, or serotonin receptor agonists and therefore.[50]

Our knowledge of new ATS remains limited, although effects are expected to be broadly similar to the drugs they mimic. However, within each of these classes of ATS, there are variations between the various compounds based on the intrinsic toxicity of the substance consumed, the severity of effects and also their duration. There are however differences, including differences between the various new ATS. For example:

- There are reports of symptoms of 2-DPMP toxicity still being manifested 5–7 days after ingestion.[51]
- Phenethylamines in the 'D series' are described as longer lasting, more potent and more liable to induce vasoconstriction than other members of the phenethylamine family.[61]
- PMA, PMMA and 4-methylthioamphetamine have been more often associated with incidental deaths than other phenethylamines. PMA and PMMA are known to have a particularly high toxicity.[52]

Other factors that have an effect on the severity of acute ATS-related harm include the following:[36]

- Dose and frequency of use;
- Route of administration;
- Environmental conditions (including temperature, stressful environment and overcrowding, intense physical activity, too much or too little fluid intake);
- Individual variations and characteristics (including age, ethnicity, gender, physical and mental health co-morbidities, co-ingestion of more than one substance/poly-use, by-products of chemical synthesis).

8B.9.1 Features of Acute Toxicity

Chapters 9–11 give detailed information on the features of acute toxicity of selected drugs. Overall, ATS increase heart rate, blood pressure and breathing rates, constrict blood vessels, dilate pupils and release glucose and lipids into the bloodstream.[53] The toxicity, neurotoxicity and cardiotoxicity of amphetamines has been well documented, as has its impact on mental health.[47]

The acute toxic effects of amphetamine-type substances are summarised in Box 8B.1.

Box 8B.1 The Acute Toxic Effects of Amphetamine-type Substances

Sweating
Dilated pupils
Agitation
Confusion
Headache
Vomiting
Abdominal pain
Tremor
Anxiety
Seizures
Hallucinations or delusions
Chest pain
Tachycardia
Narrow-complex tachycardias
Dyspnoea
Systemic hypotension
Hypertension
Ventricular tachycardia
Ventricular fibrillation
Hyperpyrexia
Metabolic acidosis
Serotonin syndrome

There is a risk that the use of amphetamine induces strokes and heart attacks because it raises blood pressure and constricts blood vessels. Overall, there is evidence that psychostimulant use is associated with increased stroke risk, including fatal strokes among young adults. It has been recommended that in cases of haemorrhagic stroke among young adults, psychostimulant use should be considered.[54]

People at risk of heart disease or strokes are more likely to experience such complications.[36,55] Hyperthermia is one of the most life-threatening acute physiological consequences of ATS intoxication, with case reports suggesting that its incidence and severity varies between drugs, with those most implicated being methamphetamine, MDMA, MDEA and PMA.[36,56,57]

Hyperthermia associated with these drugs appears to be responsible for fatal complications, including rhabdomyolysis, acute renal failure, disseminated intravascular coagulation, multiple organ failure and acidosis.[36,66,58,59] Hepatocellular injury caused by ATS is well established, although not yet completely understood;[36] it may arise from both acute and chronic use of amphetamine.[36,66] (For more information on hyperthermia and its management, see Chapter 10, Sections 10.11.2 and 10.11.2.1).

8B.9.2 Serotonin Syndrome

Serotonin syndrome is a clinical condition that occurs as a result of a drug-induced increase in intrasynaptic serotonin levels, primarily resulting in activation of serotonin 2A receptors in the central nervous system.[60] Serotonin syndrome classically presents as the triad of autonomic dysfunction, neuromuscular excitation, and altered mental status.[61]

It is argued by some that the term 'serotonin toxicity' is preferable to 'serotonin syndrome', especially in relation to more severe cases, because it describes the serotonin excess more accurately.[71,62] In this document, the term 'serotonin syndrome' and 'serotonin toxicity' are used interchangeably.

Serotonin syndrome is a potentially life-threatening adverse reaction to the use of particular drugs (illicit or prescribed) or the interaction between drugs. A number of ATS used for recreational purposes are associated with serotonin syndrome, including (but not limited to) MDMA, MDPV, PMA and mephedrone, as well as methamphetamine and cocaine. There is also a dose–effect relationship; high doses or repeated doses of MDMA, for example, intensify serotonin release.[63] In addition, the simultaneous use of multiple serotonergic substances (e.g. ecstasy and methamphetamine) increases the risk of serotonin syndrome.[64] Drugs used therapeutically are also associated with serotonin syndrome (see Table 8B.1).[65,66,67,68,69,70,71,72,73,74,75]

It has been reported that the syndrome occurs in approximately 14–16% of individuals who have overdosed on SSRIs,[76] but a single therapeutic dose of SSRI has also been associated with it.[77] The use of illicit substances with therapeutic drugs increases the risks of serotonin toxicity. There is evidence that some users deliberately use monoamine oxidase inhibitors (MAOIs) to enhance the effect of psychoactive substances and/or help during the recovery period. For example, in an Australian study of 'ecstasy' users, 1 in 25 reported deliberately combining ecstasy and moclobemide.[77,78]

Three features have been described as critical in understanding the disorder:

- Serotonin syndrome is a predictable consequence of excess serotonergic agonism of central nervous system receptors and peripheral serotonergic receptors;

- Excess serotonin produces a spectrum of clinical features;
- The clinical manifestations range from the barely perceptible to lethal. Signs of excess serotonin range in mild cases from tremor and diarrhoea to neuromuscular rigidity and hyperthermia in life-threatening cases.[79]

Serotonin syndrome has three classic features of:

- Mental state changes
- Autonomic hyperactivity
- Neuromuscular abnormalities

Not all patients with the syndrome manifest signs and symptoms of all three features.[90] In a study of 2,222 consecutive cases of self-poisoning with serotonergic drugs, the clinical findings that had a statistically significant association with serotonin syndrome were primarily neuromuscular (including hyperreflexia, inducible clonus, myoclonus, ocular clonus, spontaneous clonus, peripheral hypertonicity and shivering), as well as autonomic derangement (including tachycardia on admission, hyperpyrexia, mydriasis, diaphoresis and diarrhoea) and mental health/psychiatric symptoms (agitation and delirium).[80] There is also evidence that, in severe cases, stroke, myocardial infarction, severe hyponatraemia, rhabdomyolysis, disseminated intravascular coagulation (DIC) and renal failure may occur. Hepatocellular damage has also been reported.[71]

The clinical symptoms are on a spectrum of severity, from mild to life-threatening (Table 8B.1).[90]

There is a dose–effect relationship, with more severe cases involving a combination of serotonergic drugs, rather than a single one. The simultaneous use of multiple stimulants increases the risk of serotonin toxicity and problems relating to sympathomimetic over-stimulation, such as dehydration and hyperthermia,[81] and cardiovascular problems,[82] as well as increasing the chances of neurotoxicity.[83] The risk is not only increased when two serotonergic psychoactive substances are co-ingested, but also when one psychoactive substance is ingested with a range of serotonin-releasing illicit drugs as well as a range of medications (Box 8B.2).[84,85,86,87,88,89,90,91,92,93,94]

Monoamine oxidase inhibitors (MAOIs) are strongly associated with serotonin syndrome or toxicity, especially when these are used in combination with a number of other drugs,

Table 8B.1 Clinical symptoms of the serotonin syndrome: severity spectrum

Mild	Patients can be afebrile. Tachycardia possible, shivering, diaphoresis, mydriasis
Moderate	Tachycardia, hypertension, hyperthermia (40° C is common), mydriasis, hyperactive bowel sounds, diaphoresis, hyperreflexia and clonus (considerably greater in lower extremities than upper); patient may exhibit horizontal ocular clonus; mild agitation or hypervigilance, slightly pressured speech; repetitive rotation of the head with the neck held in moderate extension
Severe	Severe hypertension and tachycardia that might deteriorate abruptly into frank shock. Patient may have agitated delirium, muscle rigidity and hypertonicity and increase in muscle tone (considerably greater in lower extremities than upper). Muscle hyperactivity may produce a core temperature of more than 41.1°C in some cases. Metabolic acidosis, rhabdomyolysis, elevated levels of serum aminotransferase and creatinine, seizures, renal failure, disseminated intravascular coagulopathy.

Box 8B.2 Therapeutic Drugs Used that Are Associated with Serotonin Syndrome

Monoamine oxidase inhibitors (MAOIs); tricyclic antidepressants; selective serotonin reuptake inhibitors (SSRIs); opiate analgesics; tramadol; over-the-counter cough medicines; antibiotics; weight-reduction agents; antiemetics; antimigraine agents; herbal products

---

including mephedrone, methylenedioxypyrovalerone (MDPV),[78,95,96,97,98,99] butylone, methylone[110] and phenethylamines (2C-I).[100] The potentially life-threatening interaction may have serious implications for people on antidepressants who also use these recreational substances.[101]

Serotonin toxicity generally presents abruptly and can progress quickly, sometimes within minutes,[102] especially when a combination of serotonergic drugs has been used.[71] It has been suggested that patients with serotonin toxicity will develop clinical manifestations within 6 hours.[71] Where a combination of drugs has been used, signs and symptoms will start when the second drug reaches effective blood levels, usually after one or two doses.[71]

8B.10 Management of the Acute Harms Associated with the Use of Amphetamine-type Stimulants

8B.10.1 Identification and Assessment of Acute Toxicity

Chapters 9–11 provide detailed information on the identification and diagnosis of acute toxicity specific to each drug discussed. Overall, for ATS, clear airway management and adequate ventilation in the case of unconsciousness should be carried out. In the case of cardiac arrest, cardiopulmonary resuscitation (CPR) should be continued for at least 1 hour and stopped only after discussion with a senior clinician.

Prolonged resuscitation for cardiac arrest is recommended following poisoning, as recovery with good neurological outcome may occur. This should be the case for all overdoses of recreational drugs, particularly as most patients are young and fit.

The benefits of gastric decontamination are uncertain, but it is suggested that oral activated charcoal be used if any amount of an ATS has been ingested within 1 hour, provided the airway can be protected. It also recommends that asymptomatic patients are observed for at least 4 hours, or 8 hours for patients who have ingested sustained-release preparations.

8B.10.2 Management of Serotonin Syndrome

It has been suggested that people with serotonin syndrome related to the use of psychoactive substances such as ecstasy usually present to hospitals with advanced symptoms because some of the early, mild signs of the syndrome are often perceived as normal drug effects.[78,112]

There are no laboratory tests to confirm the diagnosis. The diagnosis of serotonin syndrome remains challenging since it can only be made on clinical grounds. There is no objective diagnostic test. Yet, it has been suggested that failure to diagnose signs of serotonergic toxicity can turn mild and relatively harmless drug interactions into life-threatening, catastrophic events.[103]

Serotonin syndrome is difficult to diagnose for a number of reasons, including the variability in clinical manifestations, lack of awareness of the syndrome and limitations of the diagnostic criteria, which in turn may contribute to the lack of recognition.[71]

It has been argued that when assessing a patient with serotonin syndrome, the key elements of the history include the quantity and type of drugs ingested and the evolution and rate of progression of symptoms.[104] Boyer et al. suggest that clinicians should consider serotonin syndrome for patients who present with tremor, clonus or akathisia with no additional extrapyramidal signs, after consideration of the patient history and physical examination.[90]

Three diagnostic classification systems are available, the Sternbach (SC), Radomski (RC) (see Box 8B.3) and Hunter (HC) criteria (see Box 8B.4).[105,106,107] These classification systems try to reflect symptoms and symptom constellations thought to be indicative of serotonin syndrome. Whereas SC and RC draw on neuromuscular, cognitive and autonomous symptoms, HC focuses on neuromuscular symptoms such as clonus in its various forms, hyperreflexia and tremor.[108]

Diagnostic criteria for serotonin syndrome have also been adapted from Radomski et al.[109] and identified the following (Box 8B.3):

Box 8B.3 Features of serotinin syndrome

1. Manifestation of at least four major symptoms or three major symptoms plus two minor ones

   Mental (Cognitive and Behavioural) Symptoms
   - Major symptoms: confusion, elevated mood, coma or semi-coma
   - Minor symptoms: agitation and nervousness, insomnia

   Autonomic Symptoms
   - Major symptoms: fever, hyperhidrosis
   - Minor symptoms: tachycardia, tachypnoea and dyspnoea, diarrhoea, low or high blood pressure

   Neurological Symptoms
   - Major symptoms: myoclonus, tremors, chills, rigidity, hyperreflexia
   - Minor symptoms: impaired co-ordination, mydriasis, akathisia

2. These symptoms must not correspond to a psychiatric disorder, or its aggravation, that occurred before the patient took the serotonergic agent.

3. Infectious, metabolic, endocrine or toxic causes must be excluded.

4. A neuroleptic treatment must not have been introduced, nor its dose increased, before the symptoms appeared.[110]

Box 8B.4 Hunter Serotonin Toxicity Criteria

The 'Hunter Serotonin Toxicity Criteria: decision rules'[111] is based on the presence or absence of the seven clinical features below (see Figure 8.1).

Of all the clinical features, clonus was considered the most important sign (spontaneous, inducible and ocular).

IF (spontaneous clonus = yes)
THEN serotonin toxicity = YES

ELSE IF (inducible clonus = yes)
AND [(agitation = yes) OR (diaphoresis = yes)]
THEN serotonin toxicity = YES

ELSE IF (ocular clonus = yes)
AND [(agitation = yes) OR (diaphoresis = yes)]
THEN serotonin toxicity = YES

ELSE IF (tremor = yes) AND (hyperreflexia = yes)
THEN serotonin toxicity = YES

ELSE IF (hypertonic = yes) AND (temperature >38˚C)
AND [(ocular clonus = yes) OR (inducible clonus =yes)]
THEN serotonin toxicity = YES

Figure 8.1 The 'Hunter Serotonin Toxicity Criteria: decision rules' (in the presence of a serotonergic agent)

Most cases of serotonin syndrome are mild and may be treated by withdrawal of the offending agent and supportive care. Most mild cases will resolve spontaneously within 24 hours. Patients with moderate or severe cases of serotonin syndrome require hospitalisation. Although many cases will resolve within 24 hours after cessation of the drugs involved and initiation of treatment, clinical symptoms may persist for longer in cases involving serotonergic drugs with long duration of action, active metabolites or long half-lives.[90] If serotonin syndrome is recognised and complications are managed appropriately, the prognosis is favourable.[112]

Benzodiazepines are the standard treatment for agitation and tremor. Some have advised admission to the hospital for cardiac monitoring.[113] It has been suggested that 5-HT2A antagonists (cyproheptadine and chlorpromazine) could be used in more severe cases,[71,114,115,116] as they have been successfully used to treat serotonin syndrome following overdose. However, there are no controlled trials to support

this, and there is a risk of convulsions as serotonin toxicity lowers the seizure threshold.

An important part of the clinical management is control of agitation, autonomic instability and hyperthermia.[90,117] In moderate cases of serotonin syndrome, patients may have cardiorespiratory abnormalities and pyrexia, which should be treated aggressively.[71] Death of patients with serotonin syndrome is normally due to hyperpyrexia-induced multi-organ failure and it is therefore essential to rapidly lower the patient's temperature if it exceeds 39°C (ice-baths and internal cooling devices are recommended wherever available). Critically ill patients may require neuromuscular paralysis, sedation and intubation.[123]

It has been suggested that for severe cases, esmolol or nitroprusside may be used along with sedation and paralysis with non-depolarising agents,[118] but more research is needed. Intubation and intensive care unit admission should be considered in severe cases.[4,61]

Life-threatening serotonin syndrome may occur in 50% of cases of combined ingestion of an MAOI and an SSRI recreational drug, such as ecstasy. Rapid deterioration generally occurs and it has been recommended that patients be transferred to intensive care; toxicology investigations are also strongly recommended.[71]

The long half-life of some MAOIs (e.g. phenelzine, tranylcypromine) means that users could still be susceptible to interactions with ATS such as ecstasy up to 2 weeks after they have stopped using the drug.[119,120]

The principal differential diagnosis is neuroleptic malignant syndrome,[121] however, their treatments are distinct.[122] Whereas serotonin syndrome is associated with the use of a serotonergic agent, neuroleptic malignant syndrome is associated with the use of dopamine antagonists, which include first- and second-generation antipsychotics, as well as antiemetics.

In contrast to neuroleptic malignant syndrome, the onset of serotonin syndrome is usually rapid, although differential diagnosis between serotonin syndrome and neuroleptic malignant syndrome is not always clear-cut.[123] Both serotonin syndrome and neuroleptic malignant syndrome can present with nonspecific laboratory abnormalities including metabolic acidosis, rhabdomyolysis, transaminitis, elevated creatinine, myoglobinuria, leukocytosis, and elevated creatine kinase.[124]

8B.11 Harms Associated with Chronic Use of Amphetamine-type Stimulants

8B.11.1 Dependence and Withdrawal

The WHO has estimated that 11% of ATS users become dependent and may require specialist interventions. However, even occasional users may experience physical, social or psychological harms and may progress to more harmful or dependent drug use.[125]

Dopamine dysfunction has been reported as the main neurobiological mechanism in amphetamine dependence.[64] Amphetamines in general have low protein binding, which gives high bioavailability and supports their easy diffusion from the plasma to the extravascular compartment.[38] It has been reported that people dependent on amphetamines may have a larger volume of distribution and longer plasma elimination half-life relative to drug-naïve individuals (6 versus 4 l/kg). This is probably due to tissue sequestration as a result of the development of pharmacokinetic tolerance to the drug.[36,38]

Dependence on ATS is characterised by increased tolerance and withdrawal symptoms on cessation, which include sleep and appetite disturbances, fatigue, depression, irritability, craving, depression, anxiety and agitation. It is also characterised by the inability to reduce drug use despite significant negative social, health and psychological problems associated with use.

Amphetamine withdrawal is extremely common in people who are dependent on amphetamine.[126] There are variations in the level of intensity as discussed in Chapters 9–11. For amphetamine withdrawal[127] (amphetamine, dextroamphetamine and methamphetamine), when heavy chronic users discontinue their use abruptly, many will report time-limited withdrawal symptoms that commence up to 24 hours after their last dose and can last for three weeks or more. These can be sufficiently severe to result in relapse to drug use.

Phases of withdrawal include the initial 'crash', which resolves within approximately 1 week.[128,129] Severe symptoms include increased sleep (but of poor quality), increased appetite and a cluster of depression-related symptoms. Phase 2 is a sub-acute protracted set of withdrawal symptoms which are not well defined but include continued sleep disturbances and increased appetite.[139,140] Some symptoms may continue for weeks or months.

The WHO Technical Brief 2 on ATS[136] outlines three phases of ATS withdrawal. These are set out in Table 8B.2.[136]

8B.11.2 Physical and Psychiatric/Psychological Harms from Chronic Use

It is clear that amphetamine has a cardiotoxic effect and has been associated with chronic cardiac pathology. The risks of coronary artery disease are probably compounded by the chronic effect of amphetamines (including methamphetamine) in the heart tissue, as well as the effects of amphetamine intoxication, and this may be a cause of premature mortality, although other factors – such as tobacco and alcohol use – are often additional factors.[130] Hepatocellular damage may also occur from the chronic use of amphetamine.[36,66]

Table 8B.2 Phases of amphetamine-type stimulant (ATS) withdrawal

Phase	Time since last stimulant use	Common signs and symptoms
'Crash'	Typically commences 12–24 hours after last amphetamine use and subsides by 2–4 days	Exhaustion, fatigue, agitation and irritability, depression, muscle ache, akathisia, sleep disturbances (typically increased sleep, although insomnia or restless sleep may occur)
'Withdrawal'	Typically commences 2–4 days after last use, peaks in severity over 7–10 days and then subsides over 2–4 weeks	Strong cravings, fluctuating mood and energy levels, alternating between irritability, restlessness, anxiety and agitation, fatigue, lack of energy, may mimic narcolepsy
'Extinction'	Weeks to months (requires integration between withdrawal and post-withdrawal services)	Gradual resumption of normal mood with episodic fluctuations in mood and energy levels, alternating between irritability, restlessness, anxiety, agitation, fatigue, lack of energy, episodic cravings, disturbed sleep

Amphetamine dependence has been associated with mood disorders, depression and anxiety.[131] The prolonged use of ATS results in a series of mental and physical symptoms that include anxiety, confusion, insomnia, mood disturbances, cognitive impairments, paranoia, hallucinations and delusion.[132]

ATS are also linked to psychotic disorders,[133] attention deficit hyperactivity disorder (ADHD)[134] and antisocial personality disorder.[135] It has also been associated with sexual risk behaviour and increased risk of HIV[57] and suicide.[136]

The use of sympathomimetic drugs like amphetamine, methamphetamine and cocaine can induce acute psychosis. Overall, a wide range in prevalence of drug-induced psychosis among regular drug users has been reported, ranging from 8–46% for amphetamine.[137]

A minority of people who use amphetamines will develop a psychotic episode that requires care from emergency departments or psychiatric units.[138] A Cochrane review of treatment for amphetamine psychosis noted that it is difficult to determine in any robust way the prevalence of amphetamine-induced psychosis at local or global levels. The epidemiology of the disorder indicates that patients with the symptoms of psychosis due to amphetamine present to emergency departments and psychiatric units at low rates compared with the census of all patients; it also reports that significant psychotic symptoms are common to users with more extensive and severe patterns of amphetamine use.[149] Psychosis seems to be particularly associated with methamphetamine use.

Common symptoms of amphetamine-induced psychosis include paranoid and/or persecutory delusions, as well as auditory and visual hallucinations, with extreme agitation. However, even among those who use amphetamine frequently, psychotic symptoms are more likely to be sub-clinical and not to require highly intensive interventions. The development of psychosis and sub-clinical symptoms is related to the cumulative quantity of amphetamine ingestion, or the individual's lifetime history of amphetamine use.[149]

A European case series investigating psychosis associated with acute recreational drug toxicity found that psychosis was present in 6.3% of presentations to emergency departments in acute recreational drug toxicity cases (or 348 of 5,529 cases). Psychosis

varied considerably between drugs, but was a significant problem in amphetamine and methamphetamine poisoning, where it was seen in a large proportion of presentations with acute amphetamine toxicity. The number of cases in this study of presentations linked to NPS use was small, but suggests that psychosis was rare in mephedrone and methedrone poisoning, but occurred frequently with tryptamines, MDPV and the synthetic cannabinoid receptor agonists; psychosis was also common in presentations involving methylphenidate.[139]

Studies have suggested that there are similarities in clinical presentation between amphetamine-induced psychosis and schizophrenia, but the psychotic symptoms may be due solely to the heavy use of amphetamine, or heavy use of amphetamines may underlie a vulnerability to schizophrenia.[149] There are some indications that the two disorders may be linked genetically, with a study suggesting that relatives of users of methamphetamine with a lifetime history of amphetamine psychosis are five times more likely to have schizophrenia than methamphetamine users without such a history.[140]

8B.12 Management of Harms Associated with Chronic Use

8B.12.1 Identification and Assessment of Amphetamine-type Stimulant Use and Dependence[141]

Chapters 9–11 will look in greater detail at dependence to various ATS. Overall, the diagnosis of amphetamine use and dependence is based on criteria listed in the International Classification of Diseases (ICD-11). See Box 8B.5.

Daily use of amphetamine is considered to be the most harmful pattern; it often has adverse outcomes for the health and psychosocial functioning of the user. However, the use of amphetamines on a weekly basis or more has been associated with adverse effects, and injecting and smoking are associated with higher risk. Typically, the threshold signalling a high risk of developing dependence starts after 6–12 months of weekly use, although there are reports of users experiencing problems even after relatively low levels of exposure.[47]

Box 8B.5 International Classification
of Diseases (ICD-11)

**Stimulant Dependence Including Amphetamines,
Methamphetamine or Methcathinone**
Stimulant dependence including amphetamines,
methamphetamine or methcathinone is a disorder
of regulation of stimulant use arising from repeated
or continuous use of stimulants.

The characteristic feature is a strong internal
drive to use stimulants, which is manifested by
impaired ability to control use, increasing priority
given to use over other activities and persistence of
use despite harm or negative consequences. These
experiences are often accompanied by a subjective
sensation of urge or craving to use stimulants.
Physiological features of dependence may also be
present, including tolerance to the effects of
stimulants, withdrawal symptoms following
cessation or reduction in use of stimulants, or
repeated use of stimulants or pharmacologically
similar substances to prevent or alleviate withdrawal
symptoms.

The features of dependence are usually evident
over a period of at least 12 months but the diagnosis
may be made if stimulant use is continuous (daily or
almost daily) for at least 1 month.[142]

8B.12.2 Stepped Care for Amphetamine-type Stimulant Users

The WHO Technical Brief on ATS90 recommends
that services for ATS users are provided at a series of
levels, as set out in Table 8B.3.

8B.12.3 Psychosocial and Pharmacological Support for the Management of Dependence

At the time of writing, psychosocial interventions
remain the best treatment option for the management
of amphetamine dependence.[64]

8B.12.3.1 Psychosocial Interventions

For details on psychosocial interventions see Chapter 2.

Data are available on psychosocial interventions
specific to stimulants and/or ATS. A Cochrane review
of the psychosocial interventions for cocaine and psychostimulant amphetamine-related disorders
reported little significant behavioural changes, with
reductions in rates of consumption after an

intervention. In addition, current evidence does not
support a single treatment approach that is able to
tackle the multi-dimensional facets of addiction and
to yield better outcomes to resolve the chronic relapsing nature of addiction and its consequences.[143,144]

Nonetheless, a comparison between different types of
behavioural interventions by the Cochrane review[154]
showed results in favour of treatment with some form
of contingency management in respect to reducing treatment drop-outs and decreasing use and increasing
abstinence.[154] The more comprehensive behavioural
treatment, in which a contingency management programme is provided in addition to a community
reinforcement approach, had significantly better results
when compared to groups of patients receiving drug
counselling or behavioural treatment only, without the
added incentive programme involving vouchers to be
exchanged for goods contingent on cocaine-negative
urine samples.[154]

The Cochrane review's conclusions in terms of
implication for practice were that, until further studies are available, clinicians may consider contingency
management techniques as a good treatment
approach, provided this can be replicated in
a particular therapeutic setting. However, desired outcomes will not be achieved if the patient's readiness
for treatment and change is not managed and
addressed. Treatment interventions need to be
adequate to the particular stage of recovery a patient
is in at the time she or he seeks treatment.[154]

The Cochrane review suggests that currently, the
best results for treating psychostimulant dependence
are those of behaviour treatment with contingency management, in association with community reinforcement
and workplace behaviour interventions, but these have
limitations. Reductions in the amount or frequency of
use is a benefit, but short-term reduction is of little
lasting value. A patient must make effective changes in
his/her life, including sustained abstinence and the ability to work and maintain successful relationships with
others. The nature and amount of treatment must be
based on the range of problems a given patient faces. The
review therefore concludes from the best available evidence, clinicians should take into account the fact that
the best treatment has to match the patient's needs.[154]

A review has recently looked at the contingency
management (CM) provided at the same time as
pharmacological interventions and shown that CM
and medication as treatment for stimulant misuse
disorder could act synergistically and enhance each

Table 8B.3 Stepped Care for Amphetamine-type Stimulant Users

Steps	Type of user suited to intervention	Activities/interventions
Step 1	Occasional ATS users believed to be at relatively low risk	Personal care activities: Self/family care in reducing/stopping drug use. Self-help groups, informal community-based care. Information about the risks of drug use, brief counselling, peer outreach and education, drop-in centres, skills and vocational training, rehabilitation and reintegration services
Step 2	Problem' ATS users	Drug services in primary healthcare settings: assessment, brief counselling, harm reduction information, needle and syringe programmes, referral to specialist services if required, assistance with basic symptomatic detoxification and withdrawal. Referral back to the community for support, rehabilitation and reintegration services or referral to expert care
Step 3	Heavy/dependent ATS users	Specialised drug dependence clinical care: Assessment of dependence, pharmacologically assisted withdrawal, harm reduction, needle and syringe programmes, outpatient and/or inpatient or residential treatment and specialised counselling, referral to rehabilitation and reintegration services, and back to the community for support
Activities to be undertaken at every step	All users of ATS	Case management and counselling are important at every stage – though the exact technique and intensity will depend on the profile of the ATS user Also important is the provision of opportunities for ATS users to undergo vocational training and assistance to gain employment, as well as improve family relations, deal with legal problems and assist in the development of new recreational activities and social networks in the community

other's effect. The study suggests that combining CM and medications may be a key strategy for effective treatment, but more research is needed.[145]

There is also some early evidence that CM, when given in addition to behavioural activation, is feasible and acceptable to people who use treatment services and may be an option to augment the sustained impact of CM for this population, but again more research is needed.[146]

A randomised controlled trial (RCT) of Mindfulness-Based Relapse Prevention for Stimulant Dependent adults provided in conjunction with contingency management as a primary intervention approach for stimulant dependence, found that this may be effective in reducing stimulant use among stimulant-dependent adults with mood and anxiety disorders.[147]

We know less about the efficacy of other treatment approaches. A review of cognitive behavioural treatment (CBT) for amphetamine-type stimulant disorders reported that there currently is not enough evidence to establish the efficacy of CBT for ATS-use disorders, because of a paucity of high-quality research in this area currently.[148]

The WHO Technical Brief 278 suggests that crisis interventions may be needed in some instances for psychiatric symptoms, such as persecutory delusions or perceptual disturbances. It also recommends brief interventions, targeting ATS users to engage them in a discussion about their substance use and steer the discussion to encourage a person to decide if they want to change their behaviour. Brief interventions on their own have been shown to be successful at promoting behaviour change and can often be used as the first stage of more intensive treatment if needed. Information and counselling may also be needed, and a variety of approaches have been used from client-centred to open-ended counselling.[136]

There has recently been interest in the role of exercise as a potential treatment for substance use disorder. An RCT comparing an exercise dose with a health education dose aimed at stimulant users in residential treatment services found significantly lower probability of relapse to stimulant use in the exercise group versus the health education group and significantly fewer days of stimulant use among those who reported positive effects for exercise. The authors call for further research, including research on exercise dose sufficient to produce a significant treatment effect.[149] Similarly, it was also shown that patients with methamphetamine use disorder in early recovery who participated in a structured exercise programme, compared to a structured health education programme, demonstrated a greater improvement in depressive symptoms.[150,151] More research is needed.

Gender differences have been described by a few studies. Some have argued that there is some evidence of sexual dimorphism in response to stimulants, with some preliminary evidence that suggests a potential biological mechanism involving brain derived neurotrophic factor that might contribute to these differences and that additional research is needed.[152] Clinical and pre-clinical studies have for example found that women amphetamine users reported higher frequency of amphetamine use than men.[162,153,154]

A human laboratory study suggested that women self-administer more frequently but a lower dose of amphetamine than men.[155] It can be argued that although more research is needed before any conclusions are made, clinicians may want to consider gender-specific issues as an important element in the management of amphetamines.

8B.12.3.2 Pharmacological Interventions

Pharmacological interventions specific to each drug will be discussed in detail in all relevant chapters that follow.

Overall, and at the current time, no pharmacological intervention has demonstrated sufficient, consistent evidence of effectiveness to support its use in routine treatment.

A systematic review on treatment for amphetamine/methamphetamine dependence showed that currently no pharmacotherapy has provided convincing results; mostly studies were underpowered and had low treatment completion rates.[156]

For example, a placebo-controlled trial investigating the effectiveness of extended-release injectable naltrexone (XR-NTX) with intensive psychosocial therapy for amphetamine-dependent persons showed that adding naltrexone to treatment as usual did not improve outcomes.[157]

A recent systematic review identified five medications subject to multiple RCTs. Four of these demonstrated some limited evidence of benefit for reducing amphetamine use: methylphenidate (three studies), bupropion (three studies), modafinil (two studies), and naltrexone (one study). Four RCTs of

dexamphetamine suggest its benefit on secondary outcomes such as treatment retention, but not for reducing amphetamine use. Six other medicines indicate the potential for efficacy, but the number of studies is too small to draw conclusions.[158]

The findings were similar to a Cochrane review of the efficacy of psychostimulant drugs for amphetamine abuse or dependence which concluded that it does not support the use of psychostimulant medications at the tested doses as a replacement for amphetamines. The review also added that these conclusions may change in the future, as the number of included studies and participants were limited and information on outcomes was missing.[64]

There are some recommendations for symptomatic treatment of withdrawal. The WHO Technical Brief 2 on ATS recommends that treatment for severe insomnia be provided with light sedatives and that hydration is maintained. Clinicians should be aware that depressive symptoms of varying severity may occur during or after withdrawal and there may be risk of suicide.[136]

In terms of future developments, some have argued that these should target the restoration of dopaminergic function as a goal for the treatment of stimulant addiction.[159]

8B.12.4 Management of Amphetamine Psychosis

The resolution of symptoms among those who experience amphetamine-induced psychosis usually occurs with abstinence, although it may be incomplete, thus increasing risks of relapse.[160] Symptoms usually resolve with medication, which,[161] include antipsychotics and benzodiazepines.[149]

The prescribing of antipsychotic medication should consider the fact that there is an increasing risk of seizures and cardiac arrhythmias in patients who have taken a stimulant NPS and/or established recreational drug and that antipsychotics should probably be avoided while prominent sympathomimetic features are present. Prescribers should also consider the differences of typical vs. atypical antipsychotics; atypical antipsychotics may include serotonergic properties (5HT1A-receptor agonism) which could be unfavourable in subjects intoxicated with serotonergic agents.

A study found short-term olanzapine and haloperidol treatments had equivalent efficacies in the treatment of acute symptoms of mental disorders due to ATS. However, in this study olanzapine administration resulted in relatively earlier remission of symptoms, with less adverse reactions.[162] Several different types of antipsychotic medication have been used for treating agitation and psychosis, but it has been recommended that drugs with high DRD2 blockade should be used with caution.[163]

A Cochrane review[149] of the pharmacological treatment for amphetamine psychosis identified only one study that met criteria for inclusion. This RCT with 58 participants showed that antipsychotic medication reduced symptoms of amphetamine psychosis effectively, with the newer-generation medication olanzapine showing significantly greater safety and tolerability than the more commonly used haloperidol controls, measured by the frequency and severity of extrapyramidal symptoms.[164] However, the review also added that although antipsychotic medications have shown their efficacy in providing short-term relief when a heavy user of amphetamines experiences psychosis, there is no evidence regarding the long-term use of these medications for preventing relapse into psychosis.[149]

Because of the similarities in the clinical presentations of amphetamine psychosis and schizophrenia, it has been suggested that distinguishing between them is often determined by the quick resolution of symptoms in amphetamine psychosis, which is not a likely outcome of schizophrenia.[149,165] It has also been argued that the management, treatment and response to acute amphetamine psychosis are much like those for schizophrenia and antipsychotics produce similar results.[149,166]

Methamphetamine in particular has been linked with psychosis (discussed in detail in Chapter 10).

8B.12.5 Aftercare and Support

See Chapter 2 on psychosocial interventions.

8B.13 Public Health and Safety and Harm Reduction

The WHO Technical Brief on ATS suggests that clinicians should advise users of ATS (including methamphetamine) to reduce harms by considering the following[136]:

- ATS can stimulate excessive physical activity, leading to overheating. Users should therefore ensure they drink enough fluids, while taking care not to drink too much (not more than one pint in

1 hour when dancing) as this can cause hyponatraemia (an electrolyte disturbance in which the sodium ion concentration in the plasma is lower than normal).

- Users should not combine ATS with other drugs, including alcohol. The simultaneous use of more than one drug can cause serotonin syndrome, which can be severe.

- Users should think about safe sex. Methamphetamine in particular can increase sexual desire and the ability to have sex for longer periods. Users should always protect themselves by using condoms.

- Straws used for snorting should not be shared, as they carry the risk of transmission of blood-borne viruses.

- Where ATS are injected, users should never share equipment. They should also rotate sites to avoid vein damage.

Users should avoid taking ATS too many days in a row, to avoid dependence and to give their bodies a rest.

References

1. World Drug Report 2020 (United Nations publication, Sales No. E.20.XI.6).

2. World Drug Report 2020 (United Nations publication, Sales No. E.20.XI.6).

3. Srisurapanont M, Jarusuraisin N, Kittirattanapaiboon P. Treatment for amphetamine dependence and abuse (review). *Cochrane Database Syst Rev* 2001;(4):CD003022. Review update in: *Cochrane Database Syst Rev* 2014;4:CD003022.

4. Altman J, Everitt BJ, Glautier S, et al. The biological, social and clinical bases of drug addiction: commentary and debate. *Psychopharmacology* 1996;**125**(4):285–345.

5. Ellinwood Jr EH, Petrie WM. *Dependence on amphetamine, cocaine, and other stimulants.* In: SN Pradhan, SN Dutta, eds. *Drug Abuse: Clinical and Basic Aspects*, pp. 248–262. St. Louis, MO, CV Mosby, 1977.

6. United Nations Office on Drugs and Crime. Early Warning Advisory on New Psychoactive Substances. Available at: www .unodc.org/LSS/Page/NPS [last accessed 25 April 2022].

7. World Drug Report 2019 (United Nations publication, Sales No. E.19.XI.9).

8. Miliano C, Serpelloni G, Rimondo C, Mereu M, Marti M, De Luca AM. Neuropharmacology of new psychoactive substances (NPS): focus on the rewarding and reinforcing properties of cannabimimetics and amphetamine-like stimulants. *Front Neurosci* 2016 (online). https://doi.org/10 .3389/fnins.2016.00153

9. World Drug Report 2019 (United Nations publication, Sales No. E.19.XI.9).

10. World Drug Report 2020 (United Nations publication, Sales No. E.20.XI.6).

11. Miliano C, Serpelloni G, Rimondo C, Mereu M, Marti M, De Luca AM. Neuropharmacology of new psychoactive substances (NPS): focus on the rewarding and reinforcing properties of cannabimimetics and amphetamine-like stimulants. *Front Neurosci* 2016 (online). https://doi.org/10.3389/fnins.2016.00153

12. European Monitoring Centre for Drugs and Drug Addiction. European Drug Report 2019: Trends and Developments. Luxembourg, Publications Office of the European Union, 2019.

13. Kapitány-Fövény M, Rácz J. Synthetic cannabinoid and synthetic cathinone use in Hungary: a literature review. *Dev Health Sci* 2018;**1**(3): 63–69. https://doi.org/10.1556/2066.2.2018.18

14. McAule A, Palmateer NE, Goldberg DJ, et al. Re-emergence of HIV related to injecting drug use despite a comprehensive harm reduction environment: a cross-sectional analysis. *Lancet HIV* 201;6(5):e315–e324.

15. European Monitoring Centre for Drugs and Drug Addiction. Drugs in *Syringes* from *Six* European *Cities: Results* from the ESCAPE *Project* 2017. Luxembourg, Publications Office of the European Union, 2019.

16. European Monitoring Centre for Drugs and Drug Addiction. Drug-related *Infectious Diseases* in Europe: *Update* from the EMCDDA expert network. Luxembourg, Publications Office of the European Union, 2019.

17. European Monitoring Centre for Drugs and Drug Addiction. European Drug Report 2019: Trends and Developments. Luxembourg, Publications Office of the European Union, 2019.

18. Tarján A, Dudás M, Gyarmathy VA, Rusvai E, Tresó B, Csohán Á. Emerging risks due to new injecting patterns in Hungary during austerity times. *Subst Use Misuse* 2015;**50**(7):848–858.

19. Giese C, Igoe D, Gibbons Z, et al. Injection of new psychoactive substance snow blow associated with recently acquired HIV infections among homeless people who inject drugs in Dublin, Ireland. *Eurosurveillance* 2015;**20**(40):30036. https://doi.org/10.2807/1560-7917.ES.2015.20.40.30036

20. European Monitoring Centre for Drugs and Drug Addiction. Drug-related *Infectious Diseases* in Europe: *Update* from the EMCDDA expert network. Luxembourg, Publications Office of the European Union, 2019.

21. European Monitoring Centre for Drugs and Drug Addiction. European Drug Report 2019: Trends and Developments. Luxembourg, Publications Office of the European Union, 2019.

22. European Monitoring Centre for Drugs and Drug Addiction. Drug-related *Infectious Diseases* in Europe: *Update* from the EMCDDA expert network. Luxembourg, Publications Office of the European Union, 2019.

23. United Nations Office on Drugs and Crime. World Drug Report 2019. Vienna, Austria, UNODC, 2019.

24. World Drug Report 2019 (United Nations publication, Sales No. E.19.XI.9).

25. Carvalho M, Carmo H, Costa VM, et al. Toxicity of amphetamines: an update. *Arch Toxicol* 2012;**86**(8):1167–1231. https://doi.org/10.1007/s00204-012-0815-5

26. Kraemer T, Maurer HH. Toxicokinetics of amphetamines: metabolism and toxicokinetic data of designer drugs, amphetamine, methamphetamine, and their N-alkyl derivatives. *Ther Drug Monit* 2002;**24**(2):277–279.

27. de la Torre R, Farre M, Navarro M, Pacifici R, Zuccaro P, Pichini S. Clinical pharmacokinetics of amphetamine and related substances: monitoring in conventional and non-conventional matrices. *Clin Pharmacokinet* 2004;**43**(3):157–185.

28. Glennon RA, Young R, Dukat M, Cheng Y. Initial characterization of PMMA as a discriminative stimulus. *Pharmacol Biochem Behav* 1997;**57**(1–2):151–158.

29. Carroll FI, Lewin AH, Mascarella SW, Seltzman HH, Reddy PA. Designer drugs: a medicinal chemistry perspective. *Ann N Y Acad Sci* 2012;**1248**:18–38. https://doi.org/10.1111/j.1749-6632.2011.06199.x

30. Luethia D, Kolaczynska KE, Doccia L, Krähenbühla S, Hoenerb MC, Liechtia ME. Pharmacological profile of mephedrone analogs and related new psychoactive substances. *Neuropharmacology* 2018;**134**(Part A):4–12 https://doi.org/10.1016/j.neuropharm.2017.07.026

31. Iversen LL. *Speed, Ecstasy, Ritalin: The Science of Amphetamines.* Oxford, Oxford University Press, 2006.

32. Castells X, Blanco-Silvente L, Cunill R. Amphetamines for attention deficit hyperactivity disorder (ADHD) in adults. *Cochrane Database Syst Rev* 2018;**8**:CD007813. https://doi.org/10.1002/14651858.CD007813.pub3

33. United Nations Office on Drugs and Crime. World Drug Report, Booklet 4, Stimulants. World Drug Report 2019 (United Nations publication, Sales No. E.19.XI.9).

34. World Health Organization, Western Pacific Region. Patterns and Consequences of the Use of Amphetamine-Type Stimulants (ATS) (Technical Brief 1 on Amphetamine-Type Stimulants).

35. World Health Organization. Amphetamine-Type Stimulants. Published 1997.

36. European Monitoring Centre for Drugs and Drug Addiction (EMCDDA). The Levels of Use of Opioids, Amphetamines and Cocaine and Associated Levels of Harm: Summary of Scientific Evidence. Published March 2014.

37. Corkery JM, Elliott S, Schifano F, Corazza O, Ghodse AH. DPMP (desoxypipradrol, 2-benzhydrylpiperidine, 2-phenylmethylpiperidine) and D2PM (diphenyl-2-pyrrolidin-2-yl-methanol, diphenylprolinol): a preliminary review. *Prog Neuropsychopharmacol Biol Psychiatry* 2012;**39**(2):253–258. https://doi.org/10.1016/j.pnpbp.2012.05.021

38. Davidson C, Ramsey J. Desoxypipradol is more potent than cocaine on evoked dopamine efflux in the nucleus accumbens. *J Psychopharmacol* 2012;**26**(7):1036–1041. https://doi.org/10.1177/0269881111430733

39. Murray DB, Potts S, Haxton C, et al. 'Ivory wave' toxicity in recreational drug users; integration of clinical and poisons information services to manage legal high poisoning. *Clin Toxicol* 2012;**50**(2):108–113. https://doi.org/10.3109/15563650.2011.647992

40. King GR, Ellinwood Jr EH. Amphetamines and other stimulants. In: JH Lowinson, P Ruiz, RB Millman, JG Langrod, eds. *Substance Abuse: A Comprehensive Textbook*, 3rd edn., pp. 207–223. Baltimore, MD, Williams and Wilkins, 1997.

41. O'Donnell A, Addison M, Spencer L, et al. Which individual, social and environmental influences shape key phases in the amphetamine-type stimulant use trajectory? A systematic narrative review and thematic synthesis of the qualitative literature. *Addiction* 2019;**114**:24–47.

42. Public Health England, Health Protection Scotland, Public Health Wales, Public Health Agency Northern Ireland. Shooting Up: Infections among People Who Inject Drugs in the United Kingdom 2012. Public Health England, November 2013.

43. Harada T, Tsutomi H, Mori R, Wilson DB. Cognitive-behavioural treatment for amphetamine-type stimulants (ATS)-use disorders. *Cochrane Database Syst Rev* 2018;**12**: CD011315. https://doi.org/10.1002/14651858.CD011315.pub2

44. Harada T, Tsutomi H, Mori R, Wilson DB. Cognitive-behavioural treatment for amphetamine-type stimulants (ATS)-use disorders. *Cochrane Database Syst Rev* 2018;**12**: CD011315. https://doi.org/10.1002/14651858.CD011315.pub2

45. Singleton J, Degenhardt L, Hall W, Zábranský T. Mortality among amphetamine users: a systematic review of cohort studies. *Drug Alcohol Depend* 2009;**105**(1–2):1–8. https://doi.org/10.1016/j.drugalcdep.2009.05.028

46. Colfax G, Santos G-M, Chu P, et al. Amphetamine-group substances and HIV. *Lancet* 2010;**376**(9739):458–474. https://doi.org/10.1016/S0140-6736(10)60753-2

47. Darke S, Kaye S, McKetin R, Duflou J. Major physical and psychological harms of methamphetamine use. *Drug Alcohol Rev* 2008;**27**(3):253–262. https://doi.org/10.1080/09595230801923702

48. Grund J-P, Coffin P, Jauffret-Roustide M, et al. The fast and the furious: cocaine, amphetamines and harm reduction. In: T Rhodes, D Hedrich, eds. *Harm Reduction: Evidence, Impacts and Challenges*, pp. 191–232. Luxembourg, Publications Office of the European Union, 2010.

49. See for example Lehmann S, Kieliba T, Thevis M, et al. Fatalities associated with NPS stimulants in the Greater Cologne area. *Int J Legal Med* 2020;**134**:229–241. https://doi.org/10.1007/s00414-019-02193-z

50. Hill S, Thomas SH. Clinical toxicology of newer recreational drugs. *Clin Toxicol* 2011;**49**(8):705–719. https://doi.org/10.3109/15563650.2011.615318

51. Advisory Council on the Misuse of Drugs (ACMD). Desoxypipradrol (2-DPMP) advice. London, 2011. Available at:
    https://assets.publishing.service.gov.uk/government/uploads/system/uploads/attachment_data/file/119114/desoxypipradrol-report.pdf [last accessed 25 April 2022].

52. United Nations Office on Drugs and Crime, Laboratory and Scientific Section. Details for phenethylamines. Available at: www.unodc.org/LSS/SubstanceGroup/Details/275dd468-75a3-4609-9e96-cc5a2f0da467 [last accessed 8 March 2022].

53. Pérez-Mañá C, Castells X, Torrens M, Capellà D, Farre M. Efficacy of psychostimulant drugs for amphetamine abuse or dependence (review). *Cochrane Database Syst Rev* 2013;**2**(9): CD009695. https://doi.org/10.1002/14651858.CD009695.pub2

54. Darke S, Duflou J, Kaye S, Farrell M, Lappin J. Psychostimulant use and fatal stroke in young adults. *J Forensic Sci* 2019;**64**(5):1421–1426. https://doi.org/10.1111/1556-4029.14056

55. Henry JA, Jeffreys KJ, Dawling S. Toxicity and deaths from 3,4-methylenedioxymethamphetamine ('ecstasy'). *Lancet* 1992;**340**:384–387.

56. Green AR, O'Shea E, Colado MI. A review of the mechanisms involved in the acute MDMA (ecstasy)-induced hyperthermic response. *Eur J Pharmacol* 2004;**500**(1–3):3–13.

57. Jaehne EJ, Salem A, Irvine RJ. Pharmacological and behavioural determinants of cocaine, methamphetamine, 3,4-methylenedioxymethamphetamine, and para-methoxyamphetamine-induced hyperthermia. *Psychopharmacology* 2007;**194**(1):41–52.

58. Kalant H, Kalant OJ. Death in amphetamine users: causes and rates. *Can Med Assoc J* 1975;**112**:299–304.

59. Kendrick WC, Hull AR, Knochel JP. Rhabdomyolysis and shock after intravenous amphetamine administration. *Ann Int Med* 1977;**86**:381–387.

60. Sun-Edelstein C, Tepper SJ, Shapiro RE. Drug-induced serotonin syndrome: a review. *Expert Opin Drug Saf* 2008;**7**(5):587–596. https://doi.org/10.1517/14740338.7.5.587

61. Wang RZ, Vashistha V, Kaur S, Houchens NW. Serotonin syndrome: preventing, recognizing, and treating it. *Cleve Clin J Med* 2016;**83**(11):810–817. https://doi.org/10.3949/ccjm.83a.15129

62. Gillman PK. Triptans, serotonin agonists, and serotonin syndrome (serotonin toxicity): a review. *Headache* 2010;**50**:264–272.

63. Huether G, Zhou D, Ruther E. Causes and consequences of the loss of serotonergic presynapses elicited by the consumption of 3,4-methylenedioxymethamphetamine (MDMA, 'ecstasy') and its congeners. *J Neural Transm* 1997;**104**:771–794.

64. Schifano F. A bitter pill. *Overview of ecstasy (MDMA, MDA)-related fatalities. Psychopharmacology* 2004;**173**:242–248.

65. Sternbach H. The serotonin syndrome. *Am J Psychiatry* 1991;**148**:705–713.

66. Gill M, LoVecchio F, Selden B. Serotonin syndrome in a child after a single dose of fluvoxamine. *Ann Emerg Med* 1999;**33**:457–459.

67. Parrott AC. Recreational ecstasy/MDMA, the serotonin syndrome, and serotonergic neurotoxicity. *Pharmacol Biochem Behav* 2002;**71**:837–844.

68. Lee DO, Lee CD. Serotonin syndrome in a child associated with erythromycin and sertraline. *Pharmacotherapy* 1999;**19**:894–896.

69. Gardner MD, Lynd LD. Sumatriptan contraindications and the serotonin syndrome. *Ann Pharmacother* 1998;**32**:33–38.

70. Giese SY, Neborsky R. Serotonin syndrome: potential consequences of Meridia combined with demerol or fentanyl. *Plast Reconstr Surg* 2001;**107**:293–294.

71. DeSilva KE, Le Flore DB, Marston BJ, Rimland D. Serotonin syndrome in HIV-infected individuals receiving antiretroviral therapy and fluoxetine. *AIDS* 2001;**15**:1281–1285.

72. Callaway JC, Grob CS. Ayahuasca preparations and serotonin reuptake inhibitors: a potential combination for severe adverse reactions. *J Psychoactive Drugs* 1998;**30**:367–369.

73. Izzo AA, Ernst E. Interactions between herbal medicines and prescribed drugs: a systematic review. *Drugs* 2001;**61**:2163–2175.

74. Lange-Asschenfeldt C, Weigmann H, Hiemke C, Mann K. Serotonin syndrome as a result of fluoxetine in a patient with tramadol abuse: plasma level-correlated symptomatology. *J Clin Psychopharmacol* 2002;**22**:440–441.

75. Turkel SB, Nadala JG, Wincor MZ. Possible serotonin syndrome in association with 5-HT(3) antagonist agents. *Psychosomatics* 2001;**42**:258–260.

76. Isbister GK, Bowe SJ, Dawson A, Whyte IM. Relative toxicity of selective serotonin reuptake inhibitors (SSRIs) in overdose. *J Toxicol Clin Toxicol* 2004;**42**:277–285.

77. Copeland J, Dillon P, Gascoigne M. Ecstasy and the concomitant use of pharmaceuticals (NDARC Technical Report 201). National Drug and Alcohol Research Centre, University of New South Wales, 2004.

78. Copeland J, Dillon P, Gascoigne M. Ecstasy and the concomitant use of pharmaceuticals. *Addict Behav* 2006;**31**:367–370.

79. Boyer EW, Shannon M. The serotonin syndrome. *N Engl J Med* 2005;**352**:1112–1120.

80. Dunkley EJ, Isbister GK, Sibbritt D, Dawson AH, Whyte IM. The Hunter serotonin toxicity criteria: simple and accurate diagnostic decision rules for serotonin toxicity. *QJM* 2003;**96**:635–642.

81. Williams H, Dratcu L, Taylor R, Roberts M, Oyefeso A. 'Saturday night fever': ecstasy related problems in a London accident and emergency department. *J Accid Emerg Med* 1998;**15**(5):322–326.

82. Milroy CM, Clark JC, Forrest AR. Pathology of deaths associated with 'ecstasy' and 'eve' misuse. *J Clin Pathol* 1996;**49**(2):149–153.

83. Winstock AR, Griffiths P, Stewart D. Drugs and the dance music scene: a survey of current drug use patterns among a sample of dance music enthusiasts in the UK. *Drug Alcohol Depend* 2001;**64**(1):9–17.

84. Sternbach H. The serotonin syndrome. *Am J Psychiatry* 1991;**148**:705–713.

85. Gill M, LoVecchio F, Selden B. Serotonin syndrome in a child after a single dose of fluvoxamine. *Ann Emerg Med* 1999;**33**:457–459.

86. Parrott AC. Recreational ecstasy/MDMA, the serotonin syndrome, and serotonergic neurotoxicity. *Pharmacol Biochem Behav* 2002;**71**:837–844.

87. Lee DO, Lee CD. Serotonin syndrome in a child associated with erythromycin and sertraline. *Pharmacotherapy* 1999;**19**:894–896.

88. Gardner MD, Lynd LD. Sumatriptan contraindications and the serotonin syndrome. *Ann Pharmacother* 1998;**32**:33–38.

89. Giese SY, Neborsky R. Serotonin syndrome: potential consequences of Meridia combined with demerol or fentanyl. *Plast Reconstr Surg* 2001;**107**:293–294.

90. DeSilva KE, Le Flore DB, Marston BJ, Rimland D. Serotonin syndrome in HIV-infected individuals receiving antiretroviral therapy and fluoxetine. *AIDS* 2001;**15**:1281–1285.

91. Callaway JC, Grob CS. Ayahuasca preparations and serotonin reuptake inhibitors: a potential combination for severe adverse reactions. *J Psychoactive Drugs* 1998;**30**:367–369.

92. Izzo AA, Ernst E. Interactions between herbal medicines and prescribed drugs: a systematic review. *Drugs* 2001;**61**:2163–2175.

93. Lange-Asschenfeldt C, Weigmann H, Hiemke C, Mann K. Serotonin syndrome as a result of fluoxetine in a patient with tramadol abuse: plasma level-correlated symptomatology. *J Clin Psychopharmacol* 2002;**22**:440–441.

94. Turkel SB, Nadala JG, Wincor MZ. Possible serotonin syndrome in association with 5-HT(3) antagonist agents. *Psychosomatics* 2001;**42**:258–260.

95. Demirkiran M, Jankivic J, Dean JM. Ecstasy intoxication: an overlap between serotonin syndrome and neuroleptic malignant syndrome. *Clin Neuropharmacol* 1996;**19**:157–164.

96. Gillman PK. Ecstasy, serotonin syndrome and the treatment of hyperpyrexia. *Med J Aust* 1997;**167**:109–111.

97. Parrott AC. MDMA, serotonergic neurotoxicity, and the diverse functional deficits of recreational 'ecstasy' users. *Neurosci Biobehav Rev* 2013;**37**(8):1466–1484. https://doi.org/10.1016/j. neubiorev.2013.04.016

98. Garrett G, Sweeney M. The serotonin syndrome as a result of mephedrone toxicity. *BMJ Case Rep* 2010;**2010**: bcr0420102925. https://doi.org/10.1136/bcr.04.2010.2925

99. Mugele J, Nañagas KA, Tormoehlen LM. Serotonin syndrome associated with MDPV use: a case report. *Ann Emerg Med* 2012;**60**(1):100–102. https://doi.org/10.1016/j.annemergmed.2011.11.033

100. Bosak A, LoVecchio F, Levine M. Recurrent seizures and serotonin syndrome following '2C-I' ingestion. *J Med Toxicol* 2013;**9**(2):196–198. https://doi.org/10.1007/s13181-013-0287-x

101. Silins E, Copeland J, Dillon P. Qualitative review of serotonin syndrome, ecstasy (MDMA) and the use of other serotonergic substances: hierarchy of risk. *Aust NZ J Psychiatry* 2007;**41**(8):649–655.

102. Mason PJ, Morris VA, Balcezak TJ. Serotonin syndrome: presentation of 2 cases and review of the literature. *Medicine* 2000;**79**:201–209.

103. Werneke U, Jamshidi F, Taylor DM, Ott M. Conundrums in neurology: diagnosing serotonin syndrome – a meta-analysis of cases. *BMC Neurology* 2016;**16**:97. https://doi.org/10.1186/s12883-016-0616-1

104. Sun-Edelstein C, Tepper SJ, Shapiro RE. Drug-induced serotonin syndrome: a review. *Exp Opin Drug Safety* 2008;**7**(5):587–596.

105. Sternbach H. The serotonin syndrome. *Am J Psychiatry* 1991;**148**:705–713.

106. Radomski JW, Dursun SM, Reveley MA, Kutcher SP. An exploratory approach to the serotonin syndrome: an update of clinical phenomenology and revised diagnostic criteria. *Med Hypotheses* 2000;**55**:218–224.

107. Dunkley EJ, Isbister GK, Sibbritt D, Dawson AH, Whyte IM. The hunter serotonin toxicity criteria: simple and accurate diagnostic decision rules for serotonin toxicity. *QJM* 2003;**96**:635–642.

108. Werneke U, Jamshidi F, Taylor DM, Ott M. Conundrums in neurology: diagnosing serotonin syndrome – a meta-analysis of cases. *BMC Neurology* 2016;**16**:97. https://doi.org/10.1186/s12883-016-0616-1

109. Radomski JW, Dursun SM, Revely MA, Kutcher SP. An exploratory approach to the serotonin syndrome; an update of clinical phenomenology and revised diagnostic criteria. *Med Hypotheses* 2000;**55**:218–224.

110. Birmes P, Coppin D, Schmitt L, Lauque D. Serotonin syndrome: a brief review. *CMAJ* 2003;**168**(11):1439.

111. Watson WA, Litovitz TL, Rodgers GC Jr, et al. Annual report of the American Association of Poison Control Centers Toxic Exposure Surveillance System. *Am J Emerg Med* 2003;**21**:353–421.

112. Ables AZ, Nagubilli R. Prevention, recognition, and management of serotonin syndrome. *Am Fam Physician* 2010;**81**(9):1139–1142.

113. Dinesh D, Patel K, Galarneau D. Serotonin syndrome with fluoxetine: two case reports. *Ochsner J* 2016;**16**:554–557.

114. Mason PJ, Morris VA, BalcezaK TJ. Serotonin syndrome. Presentation of 2 cases and review of the literature. *Medicine* 2000;**79**:201–209.

115. Dinesh D, Patel K, Galarneau D. Serotonin syndrome with fluoxetine: two case reports. *Ochsner J* 2016;**16**:554–557.

116. Jaunay E, Gaillac V, Guelfi JD. Syndrome sérotoninergique. Quel traitement et quand? *Presse Med* 2001;**30**:1695–1700.

117. Gillman PK. The serotonin syndrome and its treatment. *J Psychopharmacol* 1999;**13**(1):100–109.

118. Dinesh D, Patel K, Galarneau D. Serotonin syndrome with fluoxetine: two case reports. *Ochsner J* 2016;**16**:554–557.

119. Gillman PK. Monoamine oxidase inhibitors, opioid analgesics and serotonin toxicity. *Br J Anaesth* 2005;**95**:434–441.

120. Ener R, Meglathery S, Van Decker W, Gallagher R. Serotonin syndrome and other serotonergic disorders. *Pain Med* 2003;**4**:63–74.

121. Birmes P, Coppin D, Schmitt L, Lauque D. Serotonin syndrome: a brief review. *JAMC* 2003;**168**(11):1439–1442.

122. Turner AH, Kim JK, McCarron RM, Nguyen CT. Differentiating serotonin syndrome and neuroleptic malignant syndrome. *Curr Psychiatr* 2019;**18**:30–36.

123. Werneke U, Jamshidi F, Taylor DM, Ott M. Conundrums in neurology: diagnosing serotonin syndrome – a meta-analysis of cases. *BMC Neurology* 2016;**16**:97. https://doi.org/10.1186/s12883-016-0616-1

124. Katus LE, Frucht SJ. Management of serotonin syndrome and neuroleptic malignant syndrome. *Curr Treat Options Neurol* 2016;**18**:39. https://doi.org/10.1007/s11940-016-0423-4

125. World Health Organization, Western Pacific Region. Harm Reduction and Brief Interventions for ATS Users (Technical Brief on Amphetamine-Type Stimulants 2). Available at: www.who.int/hiv/pub/idu/ats_brief2.pdf [last accessed 8 March 2022].

126. Schuckit MA, Daeppen JB, Danko GP, et al. Clinical implications for four drugs of the DSM-IV distinction between substance dependence with and without a physiological component. *Am J Psychiatry* 1999;**156**(1):41–49.

127. Shoptaw SJ, Kao U,Heinzerling K, Ling W. Treatment for amphetamine withdrawal. *Cochrane Database Syst Rev* 2009;(**2**):CD003021. https://doi.org/10.1002/14651858.CD003021.pub2

128. McGregor C, Srisurapanont M, Jittiwutikarn J, Laobhripatr S, Wongtan T, White JM. The nature, time course and severity of methamphetamine withdrawal. *Addiction* 2005;**100**(9):1320–1329.

129. Gossop MR, Bradley BP, Brewis RK. Amphetamine withdrawal and sleep disturbance. *Drug Alcohol Depend* 1982;**10**(2–3):177–183.

130. Kaye S, McKetin R. Cardiotoxicity associated with methamphetamine use and signs of cardiovascular pathology among methamphetamine users. *National Drug and Alcohol Research Centre*, University of New South Wales, 2005.

131. MacLean R, Sofuoglu M. Stimulants and mood disorders. *Curr Addict Rep* 2018;**5**:323–329. https://doi.org/10.1007/s40429-018-0212-0

132. Harada T, Tsutomi H, Mori R, Wilson DB. Cognitive-behavioural treatment for amphetamine-type stimulant (ATS)-use disorders. *Cochrane Database Syst Rev* 2018;**12**:CD011315. https://doi.org/10.1002/14651858.CD011315.pub2

133. Salo R, Flower K, Kielstein A, Leamon MH, Nordahl TE, Galloway GP. Psychiatric comorbidity in methamphetamine dependence. *Psychiatry Res* 2011;**186**(2–3):356–361.

134. Wilens TE. Attention-deficit/hyperactivity disorder and the substance use disorders: the nature of the relationship, subtypes at risk, and treatment issues. *Psychiatr Clin North Am* 2004;**27**(2):283–301.

135. Glasner-Edwards S, Mooney LJ, Marinelli-Casey P, Hillhouse M, Ang A, Rawson RA, Methamphetamine Treatment Project Corporate Authors. *Psychopathology in methamphetamine-dependent adults 3 years after treatment. Drug Alcohol Rev* 2010;**29**:12–20.

136. McKetin R, Kelly E, McLaren J, Proudfoot H. Impaired physical health among methamphetamine users in comparison with the general population: the role of methamphetamine dependence and opioid use. *Drug Alcohol Rev* 2008;**27**:482–489.

137. Bramness JG, Gundersen OH, Guterstam J, et al. Amphetamine-induced psychosis–a separate diagnostic entity or primary psychosis triggered in the vulnerable? *BMC Psychiatry* 2012;**12**:221.

138. Shoptaw SJ, Kao U, Ling W. Treatment for amphetamine psychosis. *Cochrane Database Syst Rev* 2009;(**1**):CD003026. https://doi.org/10.1002/14651858.CD003026.pub3

139. Vallersnes OM, Dines AM, Wood DM, et al. Psychosis associated with acute recreational drug toxicity: a European case series. *BMC Psychiatry* 2016;**16**:293.

140. Chen CK, Lin SK, Pak CS, Ball D, Loh EW, Murray RM. Morbid risk for psychiatric disorder among the relatives of methamphetamine users with and without psychosis. *Am J Med Genet B Neuropsychiatr Genet* 2005;**136B**(1):87–91.

141. World Health Organization, Western Pacific Region. Therapeutic Interventions for Users of Amphetamine-Type Stimulants (ATS) (Technical Briefs on Amphetamine-Type Stimulants 4).

142. World Health Organization. ICD-11 6C46.2 Stimulant dependence including amphetamines, methamphetamine or methcathinone. Available at: https://icd.who.int/browse11/l-m/en#/http://id.who.int/icd/entity/2016549355 [last accessed 25 April 2022].

143. Knapp WP, Soares B, Farrell M, Silva de Lima M. *Psychosocial interventions for cocaine and psychostimulant amphetamine-related disorders. Cochrane Database Syst Rev* 2007;(**3**): CD003023.

144. European Monitoring Centre for Drugs and Drug Addiction (EMCDDA). Best practice portal: treatment options for amphetamines users. Available at: www.emcdda.europa.eu/best-practice/treatment/amphetamines-users [last accessed 9 March 2022].

145. Soares Tardelli V, Pimentel Pádua do Lago M, Mendez M, Bisaga A. Management with pharmacologic treatment for stimulant use disorders: a review. *Behav Res Ther* 2018;**111**:57–63.

146. Mimiaga MJ, Closson EF, Pantalone DW, Safren SA, Mitty JA. Applying behavioral activation to sustain and enhance the effects of contingency management for reducing stimulant use among individuals with HIV infection. *Psychol Health Med* 2019;**24**(3):374–381. https://doi.org/10.1080/13548506.2018.1515492

147. Glasner S, Mooney LJ, Ang A, et al. Mindfulness-based relapse prevention for stimulant dependent adults: a pilot randomized clinical trial. *Mindfulness* 2017;**8**:126–135. https://doi.org/10.1007/s12671-016-0586-9

148. Harada T, Tsutomi H, Mori R, Wilson DB. Cognitive-behavioural treatment for amphetamine-type stimulants (ATS)-use disorders. *Cochrane Database Syst Rev* 2018;**12**: CD011315. https://doi.org/10.1002/14651858.CD011315.pub2

149. Carmody T, Greer TL, Walker R, Rethorst CD, Trivedi MH. A complier average causal effect analysis of the Stimulant Reduction Intervention using dosed exercise study. *Contemp Clin Trials Commun* 2018;**10**:1–8.

150. Haglund M, Ang A, Mooney L, et al. Predictors of depression outcomes among abstinent methamphetamine-dependent individuals exposed to an exercise intervention. *Am J Addict* 2015;**24**(3):246–251. https://doi.org/10.1111/ajad.12175

151. Zhu D, Xu D, Dai G, Wang F, Xu X, Zhou D. Beneficial effects of Tai Chi for amphetamine-type stimulant dependence: a pilot study. *Am J Drug Alcohol Abuse* 2016;**42** (4):469–478. https://doi.org/10.3109/00952990.2016.1153646

152. Heinzerling KG, Shoptaw S. Gender, brain-derived neurotrophic factor Val66Met, and frequency of methamphetamine use. *Gend Med* 2012;**9**(2):112–120. https://doi.org/10.1016/j.genm.2012.02.005

153. Holdcraft LC, Iacono WG. Cross-generational effects on gender differences in psychoactive drug abuse and dependence. *Drug Alcohol Depend* 2004;**74**:147–158.

154. Roth ME, Carroll ME. Sex differences in the acquisition of IV methamphetamine self-administration and subsequent maintenance under a progressive ratio schedule in rats. *Psychopharmacology* 2004;**172**:443–449.

155. Vansickel AR, Stoops WW, Rush CR. Human sex differences in d-amphetamine self-administration. *Addiction* 2010;**105**:727–731.

156. Siefried KJ, Acheson LS, Lintzeris N, et al. Pharmacological treatment of methamphetamine/amphetamine dependence: a systematic review. *CNS Drugs* 2020;**34**:337–365. https://doi.org/10.1007/s40263-020-00711-x

157. Runarsdottir V, Hansdottir I, Tyrfingsson T, et al. Extended-release injectable naltrexone (xr-ntx) with intensive psychosocial therapy for amphetamine-dependent persons seeking treatment: a placebo-controlled trial. *J Addict Med* 2017;**11**(3):197–204. https://doi.org/10.1097/ADM.0000000000000297

158. Lee NK, Jenner L, Harney A, Cameron J. Pharmacotherapy for amphetamine dependence: a systematic review. *Drug Alcohol Depend* 2018;**191**:309–337. https://doi.org/10.1016/j.drugalcdep.2018.06.038

159. Ashok AH, Mizuno Y, Volkow ND, Howes OD. Association of stimulant use with dopaminergic alterations in users of

cocaine, amphetamine, or methamphetamine: a systematic review and meta-analysis. *JAMA Psychiatry* 2017;**74** (5):511–519. https://doi.org/10.1001/jamapsychiatry.2017.0135

160. Ujike H, Sato M. Clinical features of sensitization to methamphetamine observed in patients with methamphetamine dependence and psychosis. *Ann NY Acad Sci* 2004;**1025**:279–287.

161. Leucht S, Pitschel-Walz G, Abraham D, Kissling W. Efficacy and extrapyramidal side-effects of the new antipsychotics olanzapine, quetiapine, risperidone, and sertindole compared to conventional antipsychotics and placebo. *A meta-analysis of randomised controlled trials. Schizophr Res* 1999;**35**(1):51–68.

162. Xue X, Song Y, Yu X, Fan O, Tang J, Chen X. Olanzapine and haloperidol for the treatment of acute symptoms of mental disorders induced by amphetamine-type stimulants: a randomized controlled trial. *Medicine* 2018;**97**:8.

163. Bramness JG, Rognli EB. Psychosis induced by amphetamines. *Curr Opin Psychiatry* 2016;**29**(4):236–241. https://doi.org/10.1097/YCO.0000000000000254

164. Leelahanaj T, Kongsakon R, Netrakom P. A 4-week, double-blind comparison of olanzapine with haloperidol in the treatment of amphetamine psychosis. *J Med Assoc Thailand* 2005;**88**(Suppl.3):43–52.

165. McIver C, McGregor C, Baigent M, Spain D, Newcombe D, Ali R. Guidelines for the Medical Management of Patients with Methamphetamine-Induced Psychosis. Drug and Alcohol Services, South Australia, 2006.

166. Fujii D. Risk factors for treatment-resistive methamphetamine psychosis. *J Neuropsychiatry Clin Neurosci* 2002;**14**(2):239–240.

'Ecstasy': MDMA (3,4-Methylenedioxy-N-Methylamphetamine), MDMA Analogues and Drugs with Similar Effects

9.1 Introduction

MDMA (3,4-methylenedioxy-N-methylamphetamine) has been popular among recreational drug users for a number of decades. This chapter also addresses issues pertaining to the consumption of MDMA analogues and other novel psychoactive substances (NPS) with MDMA-like effects[1] (see Table 9.1).

MDMA is sometimes referred to as 'ecstasy', and this chapter will use the term interchangeably, especially when this has been used by research cited. The term is also used to allude to the fact that the substance used may be MDMA, or may be another NPS with similar effect.

As is the case with other drugs, products sold as MDMA continue to change in form, purity and the product's primary psychoactive molecule, including NPS substituted for MDMA.

In recent years in Europe there has been a resurgence in the use of MDMA, the emergence of high-strength products and a shift from subcultural towards more mainstream use of the drug. It is argued that MDMA on Europe's contemporary market is in some respects a third-generation product with a different user profile and that this reflects the need to review interventions.[2]

MDMA is structurally similar to both amphetamine-type stimulants and to mescaline-type hallucinogens, but is pharmacologically different from other substance classes.[3] In addition to their stimulant and hallucinogenic effects, MDMA and similar substances share properties that are sometimes referred to as 'entactogenic'[4,5] or empathogenic.[6,7] This has been defined as combining a psychostimulant effect with changes in consciousness, leading to euphoria and feelings of empathy and closeness to others.[7] It has been argued that MDMA is the prototypical entactogenic/empathogenic drug and induces fewer psychostimulant effects than amphetamine,[8] but retains some psychostimulant effects.[9,10]

9.2 MDMA Analogues and Other Novel Psychoactive Substances with Similar Effects

A number of analogues and NPS with similar effects have been developed in recent years and sold, either as an alternative to MDMA, or mis-sold as MDMA to unsuspecting users.[11,12]

It has been reported that the euphoric and empathogenic/entactogenic effects of MDMA have proven very difficult to replicate.[13] For example, cathinones, benzofurans and others can mimic the effects of MDMA (see Chapter 11), but there are subtle differences in their psychoactive effects.[1]

Overall, numerous NPS have been used as adulterants/substitutes in products sold as 'ecstasy', but most seem to produce less desirable effects.[14] Some are also associated with high levels of toxicity, as discussed in this chapter.

A range of substances can produce different levels of empathogenic effects. These can be chemically divided into phenethylamines, amphetamines, synthetic cathinones, piperazines, pipradrols/piperidines, aminoindanes and benzofurans. Some hallucinogenic tryptamines can also produce empathogenic effects.[15]

Table 9.1 below lists some of the MDMA analogues and other substances with empathogenic properties that have been reported in the literature, including some cathinones, as seen in Chapter 11 (particularly those which are also beta-keto analogues of methylenedioxyphenethylamines[16]).

Some benzofurans derivatives, indanylalkylamine derivatives and aminoindane derivatives are also used recreationally for similar effects. They are addressed briefly at the end of this chapter.

Table 9.1 MDMA and MDMA-like novel psychoactive substances with 'empathogenic' effects

Substituted methylenedioxyphenethylamines[17]
- 3,4-methylenedioxy-N-methylamphetamine MDMA
- 3,4-methylenedioxy-N-ethylamphetamine MDEA
- 1,3-benzodioxolyl-N-methylbutanamine (N-methyl-1,3-benzodioxolylbutanamine) MBDB[18]
- 3,4-methylenedioxyamphetamine MDA[12]

Other substituted amphetamines
- 4-methylthioamphetamine 4-MTA[18,19]
- para-methoxyamphetamine 4-methoxyamphetamine PMA, 4-MA para-methoxy-N-methylamphetamine 4-methoxy-N-methylamphetamine PMMA, 4-MMA

Other substances with empathogenic properties
- 3,4-methylenedioxy-N-methylcathinone, bk-3,4-methylenedioxymethamphetamine bk-MDMA (MDMC, methylone)
- β-keto-N-methylbenzodioxolylbutanamine B1 bk-MBDB (beta-ketone-MBDB) (butylone)

9.3 MDMA Alternatives and Variations Over Time

There are significant variations in the compounds found in products sold on the illicit market as MDMA or 'ecstasy'. Studies have shown variations in the purity of MDMA over time and location, and variations in the compounds found in tablets sold as ecstasy.[10,12,20,21,22]

The adulteration of MDMA was common in the late 2000s, which saw the virtual disappearance of MDMA as the active ingredient in 'ecstasy' products, to be replaced by other psychoactive substances. By 2009, police seizure data suggested that the majority of MDMA tablets on European markets contained no MDMA at all.[23] Over the years, the latter have included non-MDMA products such as MDA, benzofuran, methylone,[24] piperazines such as BZP,[25] PMA and PMMA or a synthetic cathinone.

This was not limited to Europe; for example, in a study in an Australian emergency department, none of the 22 people seen with PMA toxicity reported deliberately taking the drug; rather, they had all intended to take ecstasy or MDMA.[26] Similarly, a report showing that among 150 seizures by police in Brazil, of drugs labelled as 'ecstasy', MDMA was found in only 44.7% of samples.[27] In the US, a study found that half of MDMA users in the sample reported that they had found out the products they bought as MDMA contained a drug other than MDMA or reported suspecting that they contained another drug.[28]

The large-scale substitution of MDMA with other products sold as 'ecstasy' subsided to a great extent in 2010/2011. MDMA products gradually re-emerged on the market, often at higher levels of purity. The EMCDDA reported that the first powders that appeared after the MDMA shortage were reportedly very pure, although their quality declined over time. There was also a growing popularity of MDMA crystals, which were perceived to be less easy to adulterate, although this was not always the case. It has also been reported that in 2015/2016 batches of MDMA tablets contained discernible crystals, apparently as a strategy to increase user trust.[29]

Many people choose to use crystals, assuming that these will be of better purity in comparison to tablets; there was a user preference for these as a 'premium' product, a purer and more reliable product than tablets.[30]

However, this is not necessarily the case and powders and crystals were not necessarily less adulterated than tablets, with one study for example showing that 'MDMA' crystals analysed were in fact methylone.[31] Similarly, information from the Spanish drug checking services Energy Control for example, has shown that caffeine was an adulterant in both tablets and crystal samples tested; tablets also contained the piperazines mCCP and TFMPP, while crystals were more commonly adulterated with procaine and methamphetamine.[32]

More recently, this situation changed. The 2019 European Drug Report has shown that data on drug purity obtained from eight drug checking services during the first half of 2018 confirmed recent reports on the increased availability of high-purity MDMA observed in drug markets in western Europe.

In recent years, there has been some evidence of an increase in the purity of MDMA sold on the illicit market in European countries, but not in other parts of the world (US).[33]

In comparison to previous years, MDMA users in Europe at least were less likely to be unknowingly using products that did not contain MDMA or also contained other substances. The report shows that samples presented to drug checking services as MDMA were unlikely to contain any unexpected active component, with adulterated MDMA powder or tablets representing less than 10% of all MDMA samples tested. Caffeine was the most common adulterant in these samples.[34]

However, although it is now more likely that products sold as MDMA only contain MDMA as the active ingredient, products that also contain other NPS are still sold on the illicit market and services that test drugs across Europe have also reported finding alpha PVP, 2CB, ketamine, piperazines (TMFPP, mCPP, BZP), amphetamine, PMA and PMMA,[35] mCCP and TFMPP (both piperazines), procaine and methamphetamine in samples sold as MDMA.[36]

This chapter will discuss the potentially increased risk of toxicity posed by some of these NPS. Data from European countries that collect this information show the MDMA content of tablets has been increasing since 2010 and reached a 10-year high in 2017.[37]

9.4 The Increase of MDMA and Rise in Purity

As shown above, people who currently set out to use MDMA are significantly more likely than they were a decade ago to purchase an MDMA product that contains MDMA.

However, although there was more consistency in the purity of MDMA sold on the illicit market, as discussed previously, this did not mean the elimination of variability between the various products sold, nor risk of adverse effects associated with MDMA use.

Two issues have been identified: (1) the increase in the average dose of MDMA and the rise of high-strength MDMA products, and (2) the significant variations in the potency and the onset of effects of MDMA products.

A significant development in recent years was the high strength of MDMA sold on the illicit market in Europe. The average MDMA content of tablets more than doubled over the period 2006–2016 in the countries of the European Union, with some very large amounts of MDMA found in some batches of the drug, resulting in increased harm and even death.[38] Indeed, in the 2000s in Europe, the mean dose of MDMA in a product was estimated to be 50–80 mg. By 2016, the mean dose reported in Europe was approximately 125 mg and batches of very high potency tablets, for example containing up to 340 mg have been identified.[39,40,41,42]

Similarly, a study analysing samples in 2016–2018 also found that products tend to have higher MDMA content compared to earlier years and that in 2018, the median MDMA content exceeded 100 mg freebase for the first time.[43] Individual tablets containing more than 250 mg of MDMA were reported in a number of countries,[44] with 'super pills' found on the illicit market with a reported range of 270–340 mg.[45]

It has been suggested that the predominance of high-strength MDMA products on the illicit market encouraged some people to seek lower-strength substances with similar effects. In the Netherlands, 4fluoroamphetamine (4FA), known as 'ecstasy light', has gained popularity because its effects reportedly range between those of amphetamine and MDMA.[46]

The higher doses are likely to cause toxicity,[47,48] as will be discussed in detail in the following section. An additional risk to people who use MDMA is therefore the unpredictability of content and the wide variations that exist between the potency of the various MDMA products. Studies reported for example that the MDMA content of a single ecstasy tablet or capsule of powder has varied from no MDMA content at all to doses as high as 245 mg or 270 mg.[49,50]

Similarly, a study of 24 separate groups of tablets sold as 'ecstasy' in Scotland were analysed to quantify their MDMA content, to determine the common dose and to identify any other drugs in the tablets. There was a 5.7-fold difference in the lowest to the highest concentration found. Variations were even found between tablets that carried the same logo and looked identical.[51] A more recent analysis of MDMA tablets (2016–2018) in the UK also showed dramatic within-batch content variability (up to 136 mg difference).[52]

The variations in unpredictability of the MDMA dose in a tablet poses the risk of acute harms, especially at high doses. To this is added variations in the onset of the effects of the MDMA, which may encourage people to re-dose, assuming that the MDMA they had already consumed had no effect.

A study based on the statistical evaluation of dissolution profiles at 15-minutes allowed tablets to be categorised as fast-, intermediate-, or slow-releasing, but showed that no tablet characteristics correlated with dissolution classification. The authors argue that this means that there would be no way of users knowing before they take a tablet whether it is more likely to be fast- or slow-releasing. There is significant risk of users re-dosing if absorption is delayed and this can cause MDMA toxicity and have severe adverse health effects, especially for high-content, slow-releasing tablets.[53]

9.5 Legal Status

MDMA was placed on Schedule I of the 1971 United Nations Convention on Psychotropic Substances in 1986.

9.6 Quality of Research Evidence

Although much more is known about MDMA than other club drugs, the evidence is limited albeit growing. It remains particularly limited about the use of illicit MDMA and its association with acute and chronic harms, and on the management of those harms. Much of the clinical evidence is derived from individual case reports and case series and a small number of prospective observational studies, retrospective audits and analysis of patient records.

As with other NPS and club drugs, the reliability of case reports is inconsistent. Many lack toxicological confirmation. Some authors have suggested that such case studies fail to convince that MDMA use is, on balance, the most plausible explanation for the clinical observations.[54,55] However, despite these limitations, these sources have built up a consistent picture of common patterns of acute 'ecstasy' toxicity.

A number of reviews of the evidence have been carried out,[56,57,58] but there is still no consensus on some of the harms among leading researchers.[59,60] For example, Parrott emphasises the accumulation of literature detailing the harms of the drug, particularly chronic neurotoxic effects.[57,58] However, his conclusions are not universally accepted.[59] A review by Cole takes a more critical approach to the evidence base, emphasising the lack of certainty about many of the harms putatively attributed to MDMA . He suggests that the number of clinical presentations relating to MDMA is far smaller than would be expected, given the high prevalence of its use.[60]

There are some controlled studies using legally obtained MDMA for research purposes and although accurate comparisons with illicit MDMA use cannot be made, they nonetheless provide important findings.[61] The evidence relating to specific NPS analogues of MDMA is much more limited. However, reports of their effects and toxicity generally fall within the range described in the larger literature on MDMA,[17] and on amphetamine-type stimulants (ATS), so useful inferences can be made from the existing literature.

9.7 Brief Summary of Pharmacology

MDMA and other ecstasy-type drugs have phenethylamine-derived molecular structures, and can be thought of pharmacologically, as atypical ATS. MDMA has multiple actions at different targets: it is a releaser and reuptake inhibitor of the monoamines serotonin, dopamine and noradrenaline.[62,63] It also has an MAOI effect and acts directly as an agonist at receptors, including the 5HT2A receptor, the serotonin receptor responsible for the hallucinogenic effects.[62] Its action on the noradrenaline transporter appears to explain much of the euphoric psychostimulant effect,[64] with the powerful serotonergic action being chiefly responsible for its pharmacological divergence from typical psychostimulants.[65,66]

However, among the stimulant and hallucinogenic drugs, the risk–effect profile of MDMA is unique, and comparison with drug classes with divergent properties can misguide as much as inform, so they have been increasingly seen as neither classical hallucinogens nor classical stimulants.[4]

In addition to its stimulant effects (such as increased energy, euphoria) and cardiovascular effects common to ATS and cocaine, MDMA produces characteristic alterations of mood and perception, particularly increased empathy, feelings of emotional wellbeing, sociability and sensuality.[4,67] MDMA has been described as intermediate between (or combining some properties of) stimulants and hallucinogens.[4]

Drugs with shared MDMA-like emotional and behavioural effects are sometimes described as 'entactogens' or 'empathogens',[3,6,68] although this terminology has not gained universal use. These drugs have been described as capable of inducing a reversible controlled alteration of consciousness in humans characterised by emotional relaxation, feelings of happiness and empathy with other [persons4] that has been called the 'entactogenic syndrome'.[69] MDMA induces altered states of consciousness characterised by increased empathy with others[70] and an 'open mind' state, characterised by heightened self-acceptance and openness for communication, and a decrease of fear responses, without hallucinogenic-like effects.[4] Other typical effects, including subjective 'relaxation',[71] 'peacefulness',[68] 'closeness to others',[72] and 'empathy',[72] may diverge from the effects expected from ATS, and the prosocial effects of MDMA are unique to MDMA relative to another stimulant.[73]

There is uncertainty regarding the pharmacology specific to the 'entactogenic' effects of MDMA and related drugs. In addition to the direct serotonergic effects on mood, the serotonin transporter (SERT), upon which MDMA and its analogues act, appears to mediate the release of the neuropeptide hormones oxytocin and prolactin.[74] It is now believed that MDMA's effect on enhancing desire to socialise and feelings of empathy may be related to increased oxytocin levels.[75] The action of MDMA on SERT are hypothesised to contribute[76] to its pro-social, entactogenic or empathogenic effects.

Doses or serum concentrations of MDMA and related drugs are often not closely associated with the level of acute harm observed, and lifetime dosage may not be closely associated with the degree of chronic harm either. One suggested explanation is that genetic polymorphisms affecting the hepatic metabolism of MDMA play a mediating role in toxicity.[66] The metabolism of MDMA (via steps which include pharmacologically active and toxic metabolites) is affected by the pattern of dosing,[77] with the metabolism of subsequent doses being inhibited by the limited availability of the cytochrome P450 (CYP2D6) enzyme.[62,78]

MDMA is rapidly absorbed. It typically takes 20–60 minutes to take effect, reaching peak effects between 60 and 90 minutes, and lasting up to 5 hours.[79] The half-life of a typical dose of 100 mg is around 8–9 hours.[62] While actively partying on ecstasy, saliva levels of cortisol can rise to more than eight times baseline levels.[80]

Parametisoxyamphetamine (PMA) and paramethoxymethamphetamine (PMMA) have often been substituted for MDMA and are associated with a high level of harm. They are potent noradrenaline and serotonin transporter inhibitors and releasers of these monoamines. They are associated with higher morbidity and mortality, particularly attributable to hyperthermia.[81,82] They have a potential for causing greater serotonin toxicity.

PMA, PMMA and 4-MTA are often characterised by severe hyperthermia, probably resulting from severe serotonin toxicity arising from the combined effects of marked serotonin release and strong monoamine oxidase inhibition.[83,84,85,86,87,88] Their hyperthermic properties are stronger than those of MDMA.[89] In combination with MDMA and other serotonergic drugs, this risk is multiplied further.[90]

The onset of the effects of similar substances varies. The onset of the effects of MDMA is typically 30 minutes, but can range from 20 minutes to 1 hour. User reports suggest the effects of MDAI are felt within 10–12 minutes of oral consumption. The duration of its effects has also been reported by users as varying considerably between individuals, with effects peaking after 30–45 minutes, to up to 3 hours,[91] a variability that has been attributed partially to products containing substances other than MDAI.[92]

The onset of the effects of PMA and PMMA is significantly later. This has caused concern, especially when users take it thinking it is MDMA. Users may take another dose, thinking that the first one has had no effect. There is, therefore, the risk of overdose, including fatal overdose.

9.8 Clinical Uses

MDMA is a Schedule 1 drug with no licensed clinical uses. However, prior to being classified and scheduled, MDMA had been used to facilitate psychotherapy.[93] In recent years, some research into its psychotherapeutic use has continued, and there is increasing evidence of MDMA as an adjunct to psychotherapy for treatment-resistant post-traumatic stress disorder (PTSD).

MDMA is hypothesised to support and enhance psychotherapy by increasing the subject's access to emotionally upsetting material, modulating the associated level of arousal and strengthening the therapeutic alliance.[94] MDMA is known to have major effects on serotonergic neurotransmission, but a downstream consequence of its effects on serotonin is the release of oxytocin and vasopressin, which may have relevance to producing trust and may reduce the threat response of being asked to revisit traumatic memories.[95] Brain imaging studies show reduced amygdala activity after MDMA administration, plus changes in the response to angry and happy facial expressions.[6]

There are marked differences of opinion among experts, with some arguing that MDMA has a potentially important therapeutic role, while other scientists believe that the evidence of MDMA's toxicity is already sufficient to conclude that 'there are no safe clinical applications for MDMA'.[59,96,97]

In recent years, there has been an increase in the number of studies that look at the role and effectiveness of therapeutic effects of MDMA in controlled settings,[98] especially in the treatment of post-traumatic stress.[99,100,101,102,103,104] Studies have demonstrated good preliminary results with minimal adverse effects, but larger trials are needed.[105,106,107,108] and some critics continue to argue that the potential dangers remain.[109]

The use of MDMA in other therapeutic interventions has also been examined by a few small studies, including a study on MDMA-assisted psychotherapy for autistic adults which showed rapid and durable improvement in social anxiety symptoms.[110] There is also some research on the use of MDMA for alcohol use disorder.[111] More research is needed.

The role of MDMA for a range of other conditions has also been explored, but more research is needed. MDMA was found in one case to give temporary, dramatic relief from the symptoms of Parkinson's disease;[112] this discovery, corroborated in animal studies, has led to drug development.[113] Although not widespread, it has been reported that some individuals may use MDMA in an attempt to self-medicate, for example to manage current stresses and lifetime traumas,[114] including PTSD symptoms.[115] In the US, there appears to be some 'underground' use of MDMA for therapeutic purposes.[116]

9.9 Prevalence and Patterns of Use

The recreational use of 'ecstasy' and MDMA has been well established in Europe for a number of decades, having appeared in Europe in the 1980s. Prevalence has varied over time. Following many years of high popularity, there was a decline in the use of MDMA. This coincided with the decline in the purity of products sold on the illicit market, which was has been associated in part with a shortage of the precursor safrole in 2008 (3,4methylenedioxyallybenzene, a liquid extracted from sassafras plants) and later PMK (piperonyl methyl ketone, itself derived from safrole). It has been argued that this dip in the quality of MDMA in earlier decades may have helped drive the emergence of mephedrone as a club drug.[117]

However, following a decade of decreasing MDMA/ecstasy use, the reported consumption of this drug appears to be increasing in several European countries[118,119,120,121] A new MDMA precursor called PMK-glycidate became available around 2010, revitalising MDMA production. PMK-glycidate is not derived from safrole and is therefore not vulnerable to natural shortages.[122]

There were differences between countries in the prevalence of use of MDMA or 'ecstasy', but overall, the 2019 European drug report has estimated that 13.7 million adults aged 15 to 64 years in the European Union have tried MDMA/ecstasy during their lives. MDMA is used particularly by people in younger age groups. It is suggested that 2.1 million young adults (15–34 years) used MDMA in the last year (1.7% of this age group), with national estimates ranging from 0.2% in Portugal and Romania to 7.1% in the Netherlands. Among those aged 15–24 years prevalence of use is higher, with 2.3% (1.3 million) young people estimated to have used MDMA in the last year.[123]

Although there has been an increase in the use of MDMA reported in some countries, this increased use was not found in all countries. Among the countries where robust national surveys have been conducted since 2016, four reported higher estimates than in the previous comparable survey, six reported stable estimates, and two reported a lower estimate.[124] Rates of use appear to be decreasing in Spain, although recent data suggest that this may be stabilising. Rates continue to be high in the Netherlands and increasing in the UK, Ireland and Bulgaria.[125]

Differences between countries were also found in other data sources. A 2018 multi-city analysis of wastewater in cities found the highest mass loads of MDMA in the wastewater in cities in Belgium, Germany and the Netherlands. Of the 37 cities that have data for 2017 and 2018, 21 reported an increase, nine a stable situation and seven a decrease in MDMA. Nonetheless, analysis that investigated longer-term trends found that in most cities with data for both 2011 and 2018 (10 cities), wastewater MDMA loads were higher in 2018 than they were in 2011. In 2017, the sharp increases observed over the 2011–2016 period appeared to be stabilising. However, the most recent data in 2018 point to increases in most cities.[126]

In the early years of MDMA/ecstasy's emergence as a recreational drug, it was strongly associated with underground raves, 'acid house' and associated dance subcultures. Clubs, parties and festivals remain the key locations for use, accompanying music and dancing. Ecstasy/MDMA has been reported as the favourite drug of surveyed club-goers.[30] More recently, a US study also found that higher frequency of nightclub/festival attendance was associated with increased odds of reporting lifetime MDMA use. Attending once a month or more was associated with double the odds for reporting use as compared to those attending less than once per month.[127]

As MDMA use has become more widespread, settings of use and types of users have diversified.[128] Although the use of MDMA/ecstasy is linked to the use of the night-time economy, use in other settings, such as homes, is not unusual.[129,130]

In fact, there are some indications from studies carried out in higher-prevalence countries that MDMA is no longer a niche or subcultural drug limited to dance clubs and parties, but is used by a broad range of young people in mainstream night-life settings, including bars and house parties.[131] It has been argued that in comparison to the 1990s, ecstasy has a new consumer profile, with a shift having taken place from subcultural towards more mainstream use of the drug.[132]

9.10 Forms, Routes of Ingestion and Frequency of Dosing

MDMA is sold in the form of tablets or pills, as a powder or crystals. Sometimes, the term 'ecstasy' is most often used for pressed tablets or capsules containing a dose of MDMA and the term MDMA is used for the powder or crystals.

Users may also refer to such products by the variable 'branding' colour, shape or imprinted logo of a tablet, with which manufacturers make them distinguishable (e.g. 'White Doves', 'Yellow Superman', 'Apples', 'Pink Hexagons').

MDMA is typically taken orally,[17] including in its powder/crystal form, which can be 'bombed' (wrapped in a cigarette paper or tissue and swallowed).[57] Some users consume MDMA by dipping a finger into powder[133] and licking it or through 'dabbing' it on gums. Doses consumed by the 'bombing' method (powder, typically wrapped in cigarette paper and swallowed) may be higher than average tablet doses.[57] For example, there was an apparent increase in 2013 of the number of MDMA users who accessed emergency treatment, according to reports by the Global Drug Survey. Users linked this to the current dominance of high-purity MDMA powder over pills, with Winstock suggesting that users may lack awareness of how to dose with powder.[134]

When not consumed orally, it may be insufflated, (snorted)[134] which is particularly common among experienced users.[128] User forums report that the insufflation of MDMA is painful and gives a shorter high, but with a rapid onset. According to the Global Drug Survey, oral ingestion remains the preferred method of administering MDMA, with only 15% of users snorting it (by insufflation).[134] Insufflation may be used as an alternative to oral use,[17] or sometimes as an additional route of administration for a boost, following oral ingestion. Rectal[17] ('plugging' or 'booty bumping') and injecting are uncommon.[57,135] The latter has been described by one study as 'too intense to enjoy', leading to reversion to oral use.[136] Other NPS with effects similar to MDMA, such as 5-APB and 6-APB,[97] are also most often used orally.

As mentioned in Section 9.10, even tablets of the same 'brand', can vary between batches, or can be easily mimicked in an uncontrolled market. Tablets of the same appearance may not deliver a consistent dose, or even contain the same psychoactive substance. For example, when two 'Yellow Rockstar' tablets from Glasgow were analysed, one contained 82 mg of MDMA, lower than doses administered to healthy humans in a recent research study,[137] and the other contained PMA and PMMA, along with caffeine.[51]

MDMA is often used as part of a wider repertoire of drugs. MDMA/ecstasy users are highly likely to be poly-drug users,[138,139] and more likely to report use of other drugs, including alcohol and novel psychoactive substances for example.[140,141] Ecstasy users have higher levels of consumption of alcohol, cigarettes and cannabis than non-ecstasy users.[142]

Among people who use MDMA/ecstasy, heavy and frequent users are significantly more likely to use other stimulants and hallucinogens at higher intensities than lighter ecstasy users.[140] Studies suggest that the heavier an individual's ecstasy use, the heavier and more varied their poly-drug use will be.[140] This could reflect the fact that people with higher levels of use may also be more likely to use other drugs with stimulant and hallucinogenic properties. Scholey et al. also suggest that this may represent a greater need (on the part of people with high levels of use) to boost drug effects as they become tolerant to the effects of MDMA.[140]

9.11 Desired Effects for Recreational Use

The unique combination of desired effects elicited by MDMA has been roughly summarised as the '3 Es' – energy, euphoria and empathy.[143] A study in six European countries has shown that the use of stimulant empathogens, such as NDMA, is associated with higher levels of enhancement and social motives and that that empathogen-type psychostimulants – usually consumed within the 'recreational scene' – are expected to increase sociability, feelings of friendliness or playfulness.[144]

MDMA's continued presence has been ascribed to its singular properties, combining unique desired effects with relatively low adverse effects at optimal doses.[47] MDMA topped a novel 'net pleasure index' among a large self-selected sample (22,000 people). In this index, subjective ratings of adverse effects were subtracted from ratings of desired effects to give a mean score that could be used to rank a range of drugs.[145] MDMA was also considered the best value drug overall by its users.[147]

Questionnaire evidence from people on ecstasy in a naturalistic party setting allowed ter Bogt and Engels to identify a hierarchy of motives for taking ecstasy.[146] Energy and euphoria were the leading motivations for a majority of users (as captured by users endorsing statements like 'dance all night' and 'feel absolutely great'). These were followed by sociability and flirtatiousness (e.g. 'flirting easier'), sexiness (e.g. 'sex better') and coping (e.g. 'forget my problems'); conformity (e.g. 'be cool') was the least important motivating factor.[148] When they contain MDMA, 'ecstasy' tablets are a relatively reliable producer of subjective pleasure.[47] Commonly reported positive effects, such as 'calmness', however, contrast sharply with paradoxical adverse effects that clinicians may encounter, such as agitation and anxiety.[67]

Based on evidence from 30 published studies, Kamilar-Britt and Bedi (2015) concluded that MDMA has 'prosocial' effects and that it dampens reactivity to negative emotional stimuli.[147] MDMA enhances sociability and interpersonal closeness, which may contribute to its recreational use, but its potential therapeutic use is also argued.[148] MDMA has a pro-sexual effect[149] and has been associated with increased sensual awareness, love, feeling of connection, desire, sexual intensity and satisfaction.[148] Paradoxically this may be coupled with erectile dysfunction in men and delayed orgasm in both sexes.[150,151] It has been hypothesised that this is due to release of prolactin and oxytocin, such that MDMA mimics the emotionally close but sexually impaired features of the post-orgasmic refractory period.[152] Female heterosexual ecstasy users, interviewed in one study, did not generally think that ecstasy increases the likelihood of high-risk sexual activities, although noted that they sometimes chose to engage in behaviours, such as anal sex, while intoxicated, which they otherwise may not have engaged in.[153] Roger et al.'s systematic review, which includes a meta-analysis, shows that ecstasy use is linked to small-to-moderate increases in sexual risk.[56] However, ecstasy is not one of the drugs most linked to 'chemsex' and the associated risks.[153]

Although a comparison with illicit MDMA and those dispensed by research, a study that analysed pooled data from nine placebo-controlled MDMA studies in healthy subjects in controlled clinical settings reported that acute subjective effects were predominantly positive. The study however also found that bad subjective drug effects and other adverse effects were more common in women.[154] A Dutch study similarly suggested that females may suffer a greater incidence of adverse effects, such as nausea, headache, dizziness and feeling faint.[148] Similarly, there is some evidence that the acute MDMA effects discussed in Section 9.14 below are more pronounced in women than they are in men.[155]

The subjective effects of some NPS have been reported to be similar subjective effects to those reported by MDMA,[24,156] especially its empathogenic effects or an 'entactogenic syndrome',[4] but evidence is limited. In combination with animal research, some anecdotal evidence supports the existence of subtle[17] to significant differences, with some drugs producing the empathogenic effects associated with MDMA, but with less of the stimulant and euphoriant effect.[157]

It has been reported that many MDMA-like NPS induce wellbeing, empathy, and prosocial effects and have only moderate psychostimulant properties. These MDMA-like substances primarily act by inhibiting the serotonin (5-HT) transporter (SERT) and NET, also inducing 5-HT and NE release. Monoamine receptor interactions vary considerably among amphetamine and MDMA-like NPS. Clinically, amphetamine- and MDMA-like NPS can induce sympathomimetic toxicity.[158]

9.12 Unwanted Effects

The use of MDMA is also associated with a number of unwanted effects. For example, a study reported that typical side-effects as experienced by more than half of a sample of users included jaw clenching (trismus, 'gurning'), dry mouth, tachycardia and sweating, with a minority having experienced urinary retention, dizziness, nausea and vomiting, and decreased libido.[159]

It has been argued that common side-effects, such as nystagmus, trismus, mild confusion and feeling hot, are the low end of a spectrum of serotonergic overactivity that has at the higher end serotonin syndrome and death.[160] Other adverse reactions include feeling cold and shivering.[162]

Products containing MDMA (at widely varying doses) were reported to have been associated with adverse effects 8% of the time and desired effects 74% of the time. Adverse effects reported from tablets containing MDMA included nausea (most common), headache, hallucinations, dizziness, 'allergic reactions' (note, however, that this term may not have been used by users in its medical sense) and, more rarely, palpitations, hyperthermic seizures, agitation and abdominal cramps.[47] In addition to unwanted acute side-effects, MDMA may have long-lasting effects. Users have described some symptoms that persisted up to 4 days.[161]

Other unwanted effects include 'mid-week blues' appearing 3 to 5 days after the use of MDMA/ecstasy. These 'blues' appear to increase in intensity and incidence[162] as users persist with the drug.[161]

Novice users may suffer fatigue, depressed mood and decreased appetite in the days after use. The majority of experienced users have experienced additional symptoms, such as nightmares and difficulty with memory and concentration.[161] The subacute effects are associated with depleted serotonin, so the worsening effects in experienced users,[162] especially when not associated with higher doses,[161] may indicate chronic serotonergic dysfunction, with heightening sensitivity to depletion.[163] Serotonin syndrome, or serotonin poisoning is discussed later.

Depressed mood following use is not universally found after administration of MDMA and other drugs with empathogenic effects in a therapeutic or research setting, and a positive mood change may even occur, as seen in a study with MDEA,[5] suggesting that the combined effect of the drug and environmental and behavioural stressors in typical use is important.[164]

As mentioned earlier, various NPS have been used as adulterants/substitutes for MDMA, but most seem to produce less desirable effects.[165] There is no evidence that PMA and PMMA have any prominent desired effects,[47,166] although their serotonergic pharmacology suggests that they could have 'entactogenic' effects. Indeed, a study linking the pharmacological content of a tablet consumed and its subjective effects on users reported that desired effects were nearly absent with tablets containing MDMA adulterated with PMMA.[47] In this study, adverse drug effects were reported by 16% of 924 users who had handed in MDMA for testing by a Dutch recreational drug-testing service.[47] The testing revealed that where adulterated 'ecstasy' had been handed in, a much greater proportion of users had complained of adverse effects.[47]

PMA and PMMA are particularly associated with adverse effects. The Dutch testing service found that tablets containing MDMA adulterated with PMMA had caused adverse effects in the majority of users (56% vs. 8% for MDMA-only tablets).[47] There is limited evidence on the detail, but self-experimentation by Shulgin, Shulgin et al. found that PMA (called 4-MA in their book) produced a sudden robust rise in blood pressure at 60 mg, and a feeling of 'druggedness' rather than a 'high' at 70 mg.[167] PMMA also produced tachycardia, eye-muscle twitch and compulsive yawning, and no enjoyable subjective effects.[168] The relative lack of desired MDMA-like effects combined with a slow onset is thought to lead to users believing they have taken weaker MDMA, taking more PMMA and suffering greater resulting toxicity.[168]

9.13 Mortality

The most frequently reported causes of death include hyperthermia and hyponatremia and MDMA can be associated with fatal serotonin syndrome. While toxicity can be severe, review of the literature reveals deaths related to MDMA toxicity to be rare. Confounding factors in some reports are that other drugs were co-ingested thus making it difficult to find MDMA as the sole cause of death. Its effects on the cardiovascular, neurologic, renal and hepatic systems can be devastating.[169]

Recent data show that MDMA (related deaths (MRDs) are on the rise in several countries.[170,171] And there has been concerns about the recent availability of some 'super-strength' formulations.[172]

Deaths resulting from other MDMA-like NPS have been reported in recent years. PMA and PMMA have been associated with a number of deaths. Compared with MDMA, they appear to have a high potential to cause life-threatening toxicity.[84] The emergence of PMA[47] and PMMA[44] on the ecstasy market internationally dates as far back as 1973, when PMA appeared in Canada, leading to fatalities.[173] Studies have shown a number of PMA-associated deaths, including as the sole drug.[174]

Similarly, in a case of a fatality linked to consumption of two capsules thought to be 'ecstasy', a single capsule from the batch was found to contain 422 mg bk-MDMA (methylone) and 53 mg bk-MBDB (butylone), far higher than typical reported doses.[11]

9.14 Acute Harms

Overall, reports of health problems associated with MDMA are relatively uncommon.[175] These are most likely to be linked to:

- The use of high-purity and high dose tablets;
- Polysubstance use. This could be associated with using MDMA with another substance. It could also be due to the ecstasy product used, which included more than one compound, causing possible metabolic interaction.[176]
- Toxicity associated with the use of tablets adulterated with other substances such as PMMA. For example, an Australian study reported that a majority of patients presenting with severe symptoms following the use of what had been sold as 'ecstasy' had in fact consumed PMA.[26]

A minority of users of MDMA/ecstasy will present to hospitals, often directly from parties, 'raves' or nightclubs.[177,178] The majority of presentations for MDMA are managed in hospital emergency departments; they are mild or moderate in severity and self-limiting.[56,180] In an Australian study, the median duration of stay in the emergency department was 3 hours.[130]

Studies from accident and emergency units show that the most common presentations after consuming MDMA include collapse and/or loss of consciousness, as well as feeling 'unwell', 'strange', 'weak' or 'dizzy'; nausea, vomiting and tachycardia are also common.[56,180] In a series of presentations to a London emergency department, 67% had consumed other substances.[180,179,] Similar and higher rates of co-intoxication were found in more recent reviews internationally, with alcohol, amphetamines and cocaine being common cointoxicants.[56,181]

MDMA can cause severe acute harms in some cases. Clinically, amphetamine- and MDMA-like NPS can induce sympathomimetic toxicity.[180] Severe acute harm following use of MDMA usually falls into the categories described below,[145,181] although the clinical picture is often complicated by concomitant drug use,[181] and a single case may have symptoms from more than one category:

- Hyperthermia/hyperpyrexia and secondary manifestations;
- Serotonin syndrome (a cause of hyperthermia[145]);
- Dilutional hyponatraemia and hyponatraemic encephalopathy. Hyponatraemia in particular is a cause of fatalities associated with MDMA and similar drugs in women;[179]
- Acute psychiatric presentations, including symptoms of anxiety, panic or psychosis;
- Other isolated physiological syndromes, including cardiac events, liver damage[182] and failure and pneumomediastinum. It has been suggested that hypoglycaemia, hyperkalaemia[183] and QRS elongation[26] may be features specific to PMA poisoning. However, all these signs have been observed occasionally in cases of severe MDMA toxicity not linked to PMA.[184,185,186]

It has also been noted that the increase in MDMA-related deaths has been mirrored by an increase in 'high-dose' MDMA pills in circulation, and/or the presence of high-risk adulterants such as PMA (para-methoxyamphetamine) and PMMA (paramethoxy-methamphetamine) in pills mis-sold as MDMA.[187]

When acute toxicity has occurred following the use of other NPS with effects similar to MDMA, such as PMA or PMMA for example, patterns of harms are similar to the broad spectrum of acute harm associated with MDMA and are described in the following.[17,84,188] However, the severity of symptoms may tend towards the higher or lower end of the spectrum seen with MDMA. PMA and PMMA are particularly associated with severe and life-threatening symptoms, such as seizures and coma.[56,82] A study from Norway, for example, reported 12 fatalities and 22 recoveries from a series of PMMA intoxications.[81]

As with other club drugs, mixed intoxications (from deliberate poly-drug use, alcohol or from ecstasy adulteration) are typical in general use and in presentations to acute clinical settings.[180] Poly-drug use appears to be associated with life-threatening outcomes at lower blood concentrations, as shown by a study which reported a mean post-mortem MDMA blood concentration of 2.90 mg/l in 22 ecstasy poly-drug deaths, whereas it was 8.43 mg/l in 13 cases where only MDMA was found.[180]

There is evidence that some adverse side-effects may be gender-specific. A study reported that women experienced more intense psychological effects, while men showed a greater increase in physiological measures, particularly systolic blood pressure. Although body weight may play a part, it also appears that there are pharmacokinetic and/or pharmacodynamic differences between genders.[189]

Adverse effects may be dose-dependent as well as gender-specific. In the analysis of clinical studies by Liechti et al., increasing dose was correlated with greater self-reporting of hallucinogen-like perceptual effects, in women in particular, and with greater reported dysphoric states in women alone. However, increasing dose was not associated with increases in measures of desired effects.[191]

There is evidence from an animal study that age may be a risk factor, but more research is needed, especially human research. A study found important age differences in the toxic events promoted by 'ecstasy', in relevant doses to the human scenario of drug usage. The hippocampus of aged animals revealed 5-HT neurotoxicity following MDMA use, while no neurotransmitter changes were seen in their adolescent counterparts. The study also found that aged animals were more susceptible than adolescent rats to tissue damage in the heart and kidneys following MDMA, thus suggesting a direct relationship between the age of the 'ecstasy' user and MDMA-related toxic events.[190]

It has been argued that there are difficulties in disaggregating the harmful effects specific to MDMA toxicity from the confounding effects of analogues, co-intoxicants and environmental and individual factors.[191] It is not yet clear how much of the overall MDMA-related harm is attributable to the toxicity of MDMA in isolation.[56]

A study showed that the levels recorded at autopsy in 13 deaths by toxicity alone, overlapped considerably with MDMA levels recorded from 24 cases where the drug was detected post-mortem, but trauma was the cause of death.[192]

9.14.1 Features of Acute MDMA Toxicity

Table 9.2 provides information on acute MDMA toxicity.

9.14.2 Hyperpyrexia/Hyperthermia and Its Consequences

MDMA use can promote the development of hyperthermia in two principal ways[145]: by adding to heat load and by reducing heat dissipation. It promotes a hypermetabolic state pharmacologically,[187] and behaviourally, often leading to muscular exertion through hours of dancing.[181]

Moreover, hot, overcrowded dance floors are a typical setting for its use.[215,216] Heat dissipation can be impaired by peripheral vasoconstriction, at least in rats,[217] or by dehydration. Another animal study has suggested that high ambient temperature conditions potentiated the toxic and lethal effects of MDMA.[218]

Many ecstasy-using dancers who suffer adverse effects display typical symptoms of heat illness, such as feeling unwell and collapsing in an exhausted state.[180,181,218] Some will move to a 'chill-out' room to recover at the dance venue, or be treated on site. Some will present to hospital, mostly with self-limiting symptoms, requiring minimal intervention beyond correcting dehydration and allowing rest. However, patients with more severe acute toxicity will present and will require intensive interventions.

The overheating associated with MDMA and drugs with similar effects can produce harms across a spectrum of severity; a minority of patients present with a severe hyperpyrexia that will not resolve spontaneously with rest in a cooler environment. This has been attributed to an idiosyncratic drug reaction causing a pharmacologically mediated central and peripheral thermogenesis.[56,219]

Hyperpyrexia associated with MDMA can appear across a broad dosage range.[56] The hyperpyrexia and serotonin syndrome seen in association with MDMA and related serotonergic drugs are clinically distinct from malignant hyperthermia and neuroleptic malignant syndrome.[145,220,221]

Hyperpyrexia is one of the predominant life-threatening adverse reactions to MDMA and similar drugs and is the underlying cause of many acute MDMA-related deaths. It is also a cause of severe chronic harm resulting from secondary complications such as liver failure and brain damage.[56,221] A case

Table 9.2 Features of acute MDMA toxicity

Reported effects associated with MDMA and other NPS with similar reported effects

CNS, neurobehavioural and psychiatric effects
Dilated pupils, mydriasis[11,180,181,193,194]
Feeling unwell/weak/dizzy[181]
Restlessness[5,129,195]
Nystagmus[19,24,82]
Euphoria[11]
Anxiety[5,195,196]
Panic[5,181]
Agitation[129,179,181,195,197,198]
Disorientation/confusion[19,129,181,195]
Psychosis[5,195,199]
Paranoid ideation, delusions[5,195,199]
Delirium[199]
Sleepiness[201]
Collapse, loss of consciousness[81,129,181,197]
Self-injury[199]
Convulsions, seizures[11,86,179,195,197,201]
Amnesia[19,200]
Hallucinations[5,82,85,195,200]
Coma[11,129,201]
Trismus, bruxism,[201] increase in jaw/facial tension,[5,24,82]
Headache[129,181,195]
Brain oedema[129]

Cardiovascular effects
Tachycardia[5,11,82,179,180,181,196,198,202]
Hyperthermia[6,11,19,81,82,86,129,181,196,200]
QT prolongation[198,203,204]
Hypertension[11,129,181,196,198]
Disseminated intravascular coagulation (DIC)[11,181,190,197,200]
Arrhythmias[205] (atrial fibrillation[206])
Myocardial infarction[207]
Chest pain[181,208]

Gastrointestinal effects
Nausea, vomiting[5,24,19,86,181,197]
Stomach cramps[86]
Dry mouth[5]

Respiratory effects
Tachypnoea[11,180]
'Hyperventilation'[5]
Pneumomediastinum, causing subcutaneous crepitation,[210] emphysema with neck/chest swelling[209,210]
Shortness of breath, dyspnoea, breathing difficulty[86,181,200,210,212]
Respiratory failure, acute respiratory distress[5,81]

Musculoskeletal effects
Hyperreflexia[11]
Shivering[11,19,85,145,180,196], Shaking[6,85,86,129]
Tremor[11,181,195,196]
Muscle spasms[82]
Myoclonus[11,181]
Increased muscle tone, muscle rigidity[11,82]
Inability to stand[86,200] Collapse[86]
Hyperactivity ('thrashing around')[175,211,212]

Other effects
Metabolic acidosis[213]
Sweating, diaphoresis[19,85,86,200]
Foaming at the mouth,[86,200]
Acute kidney injury/acute kidney failure[214]
Rhabdomyolysis[24,129,197,200]

report of a patient with severe pyrexia associated with MDMA reported severe multi-organ failure and profound disseminated intravascular coagulopathy.[222]

There may be considerable overlap between serotonin syndrome and this form of acute MDMA - related toxicity. Serotonin syndrome can be a trigger for uncontrolled hyperpyrexia, but hyperpyrexia can also occur without serotonin syndrome.[145] Acute kidney injury occurs as a consequence of the myoglobinuria seen with rhabdomyolysis, but may be compounded by a number of factors, which include a direct toxic effect of the drug in the kidney and volume depletion from dehydration.[216]

9.14.3 Serotonin Syndrome/Serotonin Toxicity

MDMA is a powerful releaser of serotonin and as such is linked to serotonin syndrome. Further information on the features and management of serotonin toxicity can be found in Chapter 8 and Section 9.14.

MDMA and similar drugs can be a cause of serotonin syndrome alone, or in combination with other factors that increase serotonin to toxic levels, including many recreational and pharmaceutical drugs,[223] such as MAOIs, SSRIs, tricyclics, tramadol and linezolid. In one Australian study, some ecstasy users reported deliberately taking these and other pharmaceuticals to magnify the effects of MDMA.[224]

The risks of serotonin syndrome associated with MDMA are boosted by several classes of serotonergic drug.[90,225] A recent fatality was associated with 6-APB and mirtazapine.[226] Some NPS entactogens inhibit monoamine oxidase.

PMA/PMMA poses a particular threat of severe serotonin toxicity.[81] It has been suggested that it may simultaneously promote serotonin toxicity in several ways – by causing serotonin release, inhibiting reuptake and inhibiting CYP2D6 metabolism.[82] Symptoms commonly seen in reports of severe PMA and PMMA toxicity are consistent with serotonin syndrome and hyperthermia. Serotonergic and sympathomimetic features may include bruxism, agitation, confusion, convulsions, rhabdomyolysis, coagulopathy, organ failure, coma and death.[84,185,227]

9.14.4 Dilutional Hyponatraemia and Hyponatraemic Encephalopathy

MDMA has been described as causing a 'perfect storm' of effects that can precipitate dilutional

hyponatraemia and it is argued that hyponatraemia appears to be a significant risk when hypotonic fluids are consumed during MDMA use.[228]

Women make up more than 85% of symptomatic cases in the literature, despite more males being users of MDMA.[179,216,229] It seems that MDMA has the potential to directly affect water balance via a syndrome of inappropriate anti-diuretic hormone (SIADH) secretion, particularly in women.[231]

The drug and the typical contexts of use promote exertion and sweating (resulting in loss of sodium). Hyponatraemia can occur when these effects are combined with the consumption of excessive quantities of low-electrolyte fluids such as beer and water.[203] The psychoactive effects of MDMA and similar drugs may encourage this, perhaps promoting obsessional repetitive behaviour, and masking awareness of emerging symptoms of hyponatraemia, such as confusion.[56,230] Furthermore, mistaken, or misunderstood, harm-reduction information has allegedly led to excessive drinking of water to avoid dehydration and heatstroke.[232]

Mild, asymptomatic hyponatraemia has recently been shown to be a common effect of the use of MDMA and similar drugs in a typical electronic dance music context. Women are more vulnerable than men, as they are more likely to have lower serum sodium levels before MDMA use. They are more likely to become mildly hyponatraemic while using, more likely to develop symptomatic hyponatraemic encephalopathy, and more likely to die as a result.[56] Fatalities are mainly women under 21 years of age, although men have suffered hyponatraemia, so the possibility of male cases should not be ignored.[56]

In contrast to other acute syndromes caused by MDMA and similar drugs, dilutional hyponatraemia often follows a uniform course, with symptoms mostly resulting from the progression of cerebral swelling. Initial headache, vomiting and disturbed mental state are followed by seizures, drowsiness, disorientation and muteness, progressing to coma, hypoxia and death, often due to tentorial herniation.[56] Patients may already be comatose upon admission to hospital.[231]

Relatively low doses, including single tablets, are not unusual in cases of hyponatraemia.[56] Also, the excess water intake required to cause symptomatic hyponatraemia, in the context of MDMA intoxication, is not extreme; 1,700 ml and 1,200 ml have been cited in case reports;[216,233] 3,500 ml was drunk in a case related to bk-MDMA (methylone) and ethcathinone.[24] Genetic variation in the function of alleles coding for the CYP2D6 enzyme and the COMT enzyme may predispose some individuals to MDMA-induced hyponatraemia.

9.14.5 Acute Psychiatric Presentations

Anxiety and panic are common presentations among users seeking medical help.[56] MDMA is an ATS, and is widely used, yet evidence linking it to psychosis is limited to a relatively small number of case reports and case series.[56] Collectively, these suggest that MDMA and similar drugs occasionally act as a stressor that precipitates acute psychosis, but at a much lower rate than amphetamine, their molecular relative.[195]

Psychotic symptoms can result from poly-drug use involving MDMA or, on occasion, from MDMA alone, particularly in vulnerable individuals.[56,195] No single characteristic pattern emerges from the evidence base; putative cases include previously healthy people experiencing sudden onset of psychosis after taking a single pill,[232,233] as well as chronic poly-drug users with complex vulnerabilities taking up to four tablets of ecstasy daily before admission with acute symptoms.[234] As with psychosis linked to other drugs, the prognosis varies from rapid resolution within hours (perhaps in those with a low intrinsic propensity to psychosis) to months or years as an inpatient (perhaps in those with a high vulnerability).[56,235]

The evidence base includes several cases where there is no toxicological evidence of MDMA consumption[55,235] and, in most cases, deliberate or unintended co-intoxication with other drugs linked to psychosis cannot be excluded as a factor.[236] It remains unclear whether the tendency for ATS to precipitate psychosis is more a direct pharmacological action or toxicity, or more an indirect product of severe psychological stress, such as that caused by sleep deprivation and bingeing behaviour.[257,236] In either case, MDMA is an exception among ATS, with lesser effects on dopamine and use typically confined to weekends, rather than multi-day binges, as may occur with methamphetamine and cocaine. Two cases of MDMA-induced psychosis occurred in individuals who were 'spiked' with the drug without their knowledge and consent.[56,238] This may indicate a substantial influence of psychological 'set' in determining the response to intoxication.

A case control study in a subacute population of males undergoing treatment for their first-episode psychosis found that those who had a recent history of 'ecstasy' use showed significantly different symptoms from those who had not used 'ecstasy', including shorter hospitalisation, less blunting of affect but increased hostility.[237]

9.14.6 Suicidal Ideation and Suicide

MDMA users have an increased risk of suicide attempts,[238] but it is uncertain how much of this association is causal, how much may relate to acute use and how much to chronic effects. Recent 'ecstasy' use has been linked to suicidal thoughts and behaviour, in some case reports in the context of acute psychosis as described previously, or subacutely, possibly triggered by the 'ecstasy' 'come-down' (for example one case followed a three-day session of injecting 'ecstasy').[56] MDMA overdose has been employed as a mechanism of suicide or suicide attempt,[239,240,241] as has bk-MDMA (butylone).[242]

9.14.7 Acute and Subacute Cardiac Events

There is some evidence that MDMA has cardio-toxic effects.[243]

MDMA alone, and in mixed intoxication, has been associated with acute cardiac events, including myocardial ischaemia and infarction.[56,244] It can also unmask underlying cardiac dysfunction. Myocardial infarction probably results from coronary artery spasms, similar to those observed in cocaine users. A series of three cases of acute coronary syndrome and ST elevation myocardial infarction (STEMI) demonstrates that, as with cocaine-induced heart problems, they may emerge long after plasma drug concentrations have peaked.[246] Hyperkalaemia could also contribute to cardiac arrhythmias. There is a single case report of severe dilated cardiomyopathy accompanying hepatic damage in a regular user of MDMA.[245]

Cardiac arrests occasionally occur without being precipitated by hyperpyrexia or serotonin syndrome.[181] When patients present with chest pain and other symptoms, concomitant use of other drugs should be considered, especially cocaine, which is well known for provoking cardiac dysfunction.[56]

9.14.8 Pulmonary Harms: Pneumothorax, Pneumomediastinum

A case report described a patient with MDMA toxicity presenting with pulmonary haemorrhage.[246]

One study has reported that MDMA has been associated (through uncertain mechanisms) with at least 23 cases of pneumomediastinum,[211] and a smaller number of pneumothorax cases are also reported in the systematic review by Rogers et al.[56] Patients usually present with pain in the chest and neck and shortness of breath, but subcutaneous emphysema and resultant swelling may also be apparent.[211] Sometimes presentations may be delayed as long as days after consumption. It is hypothesised that the muscle tension caused by MDMA, combined with exertion from dancing, jumping or sex,[212,247] could lead to air pressure against a closed glottis, similar to the Valsalva manoeuvre, raising alveolar pressures and causing ruptures.[211] This can result in air being forced out into spaces in the mediastinum.[248] One case with an alternative mechanism featured a tear in the oesophagus, allowing air into the mediastinum.[145]

9.14.9   Intracranial Haemorrhage

MDMA use has been associated with intracranial haemorrhage, even in the apparent absence of co-intoxicants.[56,249] Pre-existing aneurysms, or arteriovenous malformations, may rupture as a result of the acute surge in blood pressure caused by MDMA, similar to the mechanisms seen with cocaine.

There are some reports of cases of spontaneous intracranial haemorrhage in patients who have taken MDMA. One case report describes spontaneous subarachnoid haemorrhage and small acute cerebellar infarction in an otherwise healthy patient after ingestion of MDMA and the authors argue it is important to consider subarachnoid haemorrhages and cerebrovascular accidents as complications of MDMA use.[250]

9.14.10   Liver Failure

MDMA may cause liver failure in two ways. According to a review of the evidence, one group develop acute liver failure secondary to a severe hyperthermic reaction to MDMA. The other group appear to suffer isolated hepatotoxicity without any hyperthermia. This is generally a subacute effect which may emerge over the days following use, in contrast to the rapid onset of organ failure in hyperthermic patients.[56] Despite its rarity, this constitutes one of the more common causes of liver failure in this young age group. Patients may present in a critical condition, with hepatic encephalopathy, and some will require transplantation.[251] It has been suggested that MDMA may cause a greater amount of 'silent' liver damage than is recognised.[56]

9.14.11   Diabetic Ketoacidosis

A small number of case reports demonstrate that people with diabetes can suffer ketoacidosis and associated symptoms following MDMA use combined with exertion.[252,253]

9.14.12   Poly-drug Use and Drug Interactions

As discussed above, MDMA is commonly used with other psychoactive drugs and this can increase harm. For example, cocaine co-ingested with MDMA seems to increase the risk of severe anxiety. In an audit of 52 acute 'ecstasy'-related admissions, 13 with co-use of cocaine, four of the seven patients who suffered panic reactions were among the 13 cocaine users.[181] When MDMA is co-ingested with stimulants in general, the potential for toxicity is likely to be raised.[254] Co-intoxication with caffeine increases the risk of hyperpyrexia in rats.[255] PMMA and PMA produce greater toxicity in combination with other stimulants.[82]

Poly-drug use commonly confuses the clinical picture of MDMA intoxication, and can lead to paradoxical features that are not those expected from intoxication with MDMA alone. In a Swiss emergency department audit, hypothermia was, paradoxically, one of the most commonly recorded features, and brachycardia, coma, pupil constriction and hypotension were also noted.[181] These were associated with the co-use of substances, including GHB and opiates.[56] Consuming alcohol with MDMA and similar drugs is associated with a higher rate of harm. Concomitant alcohol use was implicated in 75% of cases of MDMA-related presentations in an Australian emergency department.[130]

In terms of drug interactions, MDMA and related drugs are substrates and inhibitors of CYP2D6, so combining them with other drugs or pharmaceuticals which compete for, inhibit or block CYP2D6 may cause greater unwanted effects or toxicity. For example, people taking the HIV antiretroviral drug ritonavir are likely to be at particular danger from MDMA toxicity.[256] Similar reactions may be possible with any drug sharing ritonavir's capacity to compete with MDMA as a substrate of CYP2D6 and inhibit the enzyme. Other drugs linked to apparent cases of adverse interactions include dextromethorphan (DXM), fluoxetine, paroxetine and moclobemide.[17,78] Drugs which could theoretically cause similar problems include haloperidol, thioridazine and quinidine.[17] CYP3A4 is also involved in the metabolism of MDMA and its derivatives, and co-ingestion of ritonavir has been linked with several cases of toxicity.[17] There may be risks associated with many other substances which affect CYP3A4.[17,257]

Importantly, MDMA is metabolised by CYP2D6 and inhibitors of this metabolic pathway may therefore increase its level and consequently toxicity.

9.15 Clinical Management of Acute Toxicity

Because of its common use in nightlife leisure settings, admissions to emergency departments following MDMA use often occur at peak times and therefore put pressure on resources.[130] PMA and PMMA may account for many cases of severe 'ecstasy' toxicity encountered in an emergency department.[81,84]

Due to the number of symptoms and complications associated with MDMA, the management of acute toxicity varies from initial management and assessment to supportive management of severe symptoms.[258]

The most common interventions required are clinical monitoring, observation and reassurance, and symptomatic treatment, including fluids.[181] The average duration of hospital stay reported by the Australian study was 3 hours,[130] but others recommend observation of asymptomatic patients for at least 4 hours. In an Australian emergency department, 14% of people presenting to hospital after MDMA consumption required admission.[130]

Dehydration should be addressed. Following MDMA-related presentation to a hospital emergency department, intravenous fluids were administered to 31% of patients in a UK study,[180] and to 71% of cases in a Swiss study,[181] but it is important to note that symptoms following MDMA use range from severe dehydration to severe hyponatraemia; the latter patients require fluid restriction, so it is dangerous to give hypotonic fluids or normal saline to patients prior to proper assessment[203,216] (see Section 9.14.4 for more detail).

There is no evidence to support gastric decontamination with activated charcoal, but it may be appropriate for cases of presentation within 1 hour of ingestion. Gastric lavage was used in a case with a positive outcome following an attempted suicide with 30 tablets.[241]

9.15.1 Hyperpyrexia and Hyperthermia

Patients presenting with high body temperatures (above 39°C) need aggressive cooling measures, such as ice baths or internal cooling, and benzodiazepine sedation.

It has been suggested that dantrolene may be considered when hyperthermia persists. However, this has been contested by some. No clinical trials have been conducted but a review has reported better survival rates for patients with temperatures above 40°C who received dantrolene, with minimal adverse effects.[259] However, a 2011 evaluation of options in MDMA-induced hyperthermia recommended against the use of dantrolene and antipyretics.[260]

An animal study suggests that by acting directly on blood vessels, carvedilol is modestly effective in attenuating MDMA-induced brain and body hyperthermia. The study also suggests that clozapine induces much more rapid and powerful hypothermic effects by both decreasing MDMA-induced brain activation and diminishing the sympathetic outflow to peripheral vessels. A therapeutic agent such as clozapine that not only mitigates, but reverses, MDMA-induced hyperthermia could be indispensable for emergency situations and could save the lives of highly intoxicated individuals.[261] However, much more research is needed before this can be recommended for humans

9.15.2 Serotonin Syndrome

The assessment, diagnosis and management of serotonin syndrome is described in detail in Chapter 8.

A case report describes extracorporeal life support as part of the management of haemodynamic instability induced by serotonin syndrome.[262]

A case series showed that supportive treatments in addition to the early use of cyproheptadine might have some beneficial effects in reducing the severity and hospital stay in patients presenting with life-threatening serotonin syndrome related to MDMA. Cyproheptadine has anti-histamine and 5-HT antagonist properties which are reported to be an effective agent in managing serotonin syndrome of moderate severity. However, more research is needed as there is little information concerning whether it is useful in life-threatening situations.[263]

For up-to-date guidance on the management of ecstasy/MDMA acute toxicity, it is recommended that information be sought from National or Regional Poisons Information Services and local protocols and national guidance be followed.

9.15.3 Acute Psychiatric Presentation Clinical Management

Most of the common features observed in acute patients can be at least partially attributable to anxiety, agitation and panic (e.g. dizziness, palpitations, hyperthermia, hypertension). Some features (e.g. tachycardia) can act as internal stimuli to anxiety and panic attacks. It is suggested that controlling agitation with benzodiazepines may relieve hypertension.

Many cases are resolved in a preclinical setting, or upon reassurance during the initial assessment. Agitation, anxiety and panic can be managed as they would be in the absence of a drug trigger, but cardiac monitoring is a higher priority.[180] Reassuring patients that they are not likely to be in physical danger may be sufficient, but benzodiazepines are the first-line pharmacological treatment. One study reported that benzodiazepines were administered to a quarter of all patients presenting following MDMA use at a Swiss emergency department.[145,181] Some suggest that haloperidol is contraindicated as a second-line option, because of possible dangerous interactions with MDMA and related drugs.[17]

9.16 Harms Associated with Chronic Use

While the association between MDMA and similar drugs consumption and several types of acute harm is relatively clear, current understanding of the chronic harm caused by MDMA use is limited, due to incomplete and disputed evidence.

Chronic use of MDMA has been linked to serotonergic neurological damage and dysfunction, which some researchers have suggested may be responsible for a broad range of neuropsychiatric symptoms and cognitive impairments. A meta-analysis shows these to be predominantly small, subclinical effects.[56] Significant trends indicating impairment are typically not identified in samples of 'ecstasy' users who have taken the drug on fewer than 50 occasions.[264]

Other harmful chronic consequences that have been attributed to long term and frequent use of MDMA include cardiovascular damage, particularly serotonergic valvular heart disease.

Evidence of long-term effects of NPS similar to MDMA use is not available, and so the potential for each of these to cause harm remains unknown. Chronic use of an NPS product containing MDAI and 2-AI (the latter of which appears to be more amphetamine-like than MDMA-like) has been linked to one case of cyanosis caused by methemoglobinaemia. Such effects may also result from chronic use of the many NPS products containing benzocaine as a cutting agent.[265]

9.16.1 Neurotoxicity

Differences in the serotonergic function of MDMA users, compared with controls, have been observed in neuroimaging studies.[266,267,268,269,270,271] Observed differences in markers of serotonergic function have been interpreted as indicating the degeneration and loss of serotonergic neurons and their terminals, i.e. 'neurotoxicity'.[271] Correlations have been demonstrated between presumed markers of toxicity seen in users and functional deficits in memory.[272,273] This supports the hypothesis that serotonergic neurotoxicity is the cause of the cognitive deficits and worsened neuropsychiatric status of MDMA users.[58]

The idea that MDMA is neurotoxic in typical human users is supported by some animal research,[268] but some experts do not consider the evidence to be conclusive.[60,274] Some have argued that the observations in such studies may be consistent with changes and loss of serotonergic markers, without loss of the neurons themselves (i.e. serotonergic dysfunction occurs but this may or may not amount to 'neurotoxicity').[275,276] Other authors highlight limitations in the predominantly retrospective and non-randomised studies supposedly indicative of 'neurotoxicity', claiming that current evidence is insufficient to exclude non-causal explanations,[276] such as pre-existing lower levels of serotonergic markers in the brains of MDMA users.[60,277] While poly-drug use in virtually all MDMA users has been cited as a confounding factor, recent investigations comparing MDMA users with LSD users[278] and other poly-drug users[279] add weight to the evidence for MDMA-specific neurotoxicity.

High lifetime intake may not necessarily be required for neurotoxicity to occur. One prospective study found evidence indicative of some brain changes in new users with an average lifetime intake of only six tablets. These changes did not, though, include losses in serotonin transporter density, which is the marker of toxicity most commonly observed. The authors concluded that it is possible that MDMA is neurotoxic even in small quantities.[280]

Studies have found evidence consistent with some recovery[281] and adaptation of the altered serotonin system,[273] but, conversely, other results indicate the persistence of serotonergic dysfunction following cessation of MDMA use.[269]

The degree of any lasting dysfunction or neurotoxicity caused by MDMA is thought to be a function of the bioenergetic stress undergone during acute intoxication.[282] This theory has led to the hypothesis that there are mediating factors for the bioenergetic stress experienced, and thus the vulnerability or resilience an individual may have to neurotoxicity, beyond the MDMA dose per session and frequency of use. These factors include: ambient temperature and level of exertion (increases of each may promote neurotoxicity), poly-drug use (with stimulants likely to promote neurotoxicity[283,284]) and others ranging from users' genetics and nutritional status to how well rested they are.[57]

A study suggests that people's age when they first used MDMA may be strongly linked to brain changes brought about by the drug, with those first exposed while their brains were still developing showing greater apparent deficits. The authors suggest that these age-related differences may reflect differences in the maturation stage of the 5-HT projection fields at the time of first exposure and enhanced outgrowth of the 5-HT system due to 5-HT's neurotrophic effects.[285]

Some NPS with empathogenic effects, for example 4-MTA,[86] have been referred to in the literature as 'non-neurotoxic' analogues of MDMA,[286,287] and some were developed for this purpose.[288] However, these assessments were based on pre-clinical evidence, and evidence from long-term human use is not available to confirm that these drugs do not cause serotonergic neurotoxicity. Animal and *in vitro* evidence suggests that among MDMA-like drugs, some are likely to be more neurotoxic (e.g. MDA) and some less neurotoxic (e.g. MDEA) than MDMA.[17]

9.16.2 Cognitive Deficits

A number of studies have compared the performance of community samples of MDMA users (current or past) against that of matched controls on many standard tests of cognitive performance. Weaker performance in certain domains has been identified in the MDMA users, with the greatest and most consistent effects seen on aspects of memory and recall,[56] such as verbal memory[275] and visual paired associate learning.[289]

One explanation for the poorer performance of the MDMA users is typically considered to be serotonergic neurotoxicity associated with the drug.[59] However, there is no consensus on this,[59] with many findings open to alternative, non-causal, interpretations, such as confounding cannabis use, or tendencies towards impulsivity and boredom leading to both ecstasy use and poorer performance on tests.[290]

The weaker performance of ecstasy users remains limited, according to some,[292] and deficits appear to be specific to certain domains rather than general, with one meta-analysis finding general intelligence unaffected and no impairments seen in simple cognitive functions like basic attention and reaction times.[56]

Deficits in verbal memory have been identified, whereas deficits in executive function and visual memory have been identified in some studies but not others.[292] The performance of users typically overlaps substantially with the performance of controls, and uncertainty and controversy remain over the clinical significance and real-world impact of the apparent deficits identified in these samples.[58,60]

A relatively high intensity of use may be necessary to produce significant deficits. In one study, which excluded anyone with significant poly-drug or alcohol use from the ecstasy-user sample, and which used controls who also shared the 'rave' or partying lifestyle, no marked deficits were found. The authors argued that the confounding influences of poly-drug use and lifestyle may lead to overestimation of the harm associated with MDMA .[291] However, in response, it has been argued that this study was nonetheless consistent with the serotonergic neurotoxicity of MDMA causing cognitive deficits, since it was not highly powered enough (with fewer than 50 users) to show subtle deficits associated with an average lifetime history of use.[266]

9.16.3 Psychiatric Symptoms and Harms

Community samples of current or past MDMA users have been compared with matched controls on measures of psychiatric and psychological health. A study has shown poorer results among MDMA users on several of these indices.[292] MDMA acutely increases cortisol levels, especially when the bioenergetic stress is magnified by behaviour and environment, but recent studies have also associated MDMA use with more chronic increases in cortisol and related dysfunction of hypothalamic–pituitary–adrenal axis. This in turn has been linked in chronic users to symptoms of distress, anxiety, aggression[293] and impaired coping.[294,295]

A meta-analysis in 2005 of 25 studies found a small but significant link between ecstasy use and depressive symptoms. However, the authors noted several methodological limitations and showed that publication bias may have occurred. They concluded that any effect of ecstasy on depression is unlikely to be clinically significant.[296] More recently, in a sample of 3,880 disadvantaged Canadian adolescents, those who self-reported ecstasy use were more likely to have elevated depression symptoms 1 year later (odds ratio 1.5) and those who used MDMA with methamphetamine had even higher rates (odd ratio 1.9).[297] However, studies have shown that circumstances such as a deprived home environment can provide a partial or even complete explanation for the higher incidence of depressive symptoms in ecstasy users.[298,299]

A US study using a national sample reported that suicide risk appears to be elevated among adolescent users of ecstasy, almost twice that of users of other illicit drugs and nine times the risk among non-users.[240]

A number of factors may be associated with long-term harms. A study by Soar et al. found that the 57 people who reported their MDMA use as having caused them problems (such as increased depression, somatisation and anxiety) did not differ from those who reported no harm in the duration of their use of ecstasy. However, those who reported problems also reported higher doses, in a pattern the authors call 'binge consumption', without further defining this.[300]

Concomitant use of other drugs is a confounding factor[193] that may explain much of the apparent heightened prevalence of various markers of psychopathology, such as depression and anxiety experiences.[301] Cannabis use, for example, has been found to mediate this relationship.[302] Early onset of cannabis use,[301] and tobacco use, have been shown to correlate with greater anxiety among MDMA users, where neither lifetime nor recent ecstasy use did.[301] However, in one sample of 30 users, the users were not more likely than controls to report pre-existing depression or anxiety symptoms.[303]

The come-down period after MDMA use is characterised by low mood and serotonin depletion, and it is possible that, for people vulnerable to depressive symptoms, this could exacerbate symptoms or potentially cause suicidality.[56]

In an experimental set-up, 12 male MDMA users performed a laboratory task involving monetary rewards. They were more 'aggressive' and 'irritable' than controls towards fictional co-players. It is not possible to exclude personality factors that pre-existed ecstasy use, and it is uncertain how this 'aggression' would translate to real-world face-to-face interactions.[295]

In addition to this evidence of poorer mental health in samples of MDMA users, mostly relating to subtle, subclinical differences, there is evidence from case reports of more profound psychiatric disturbances and disorders in individual users. One paper detailed two case studies of severe obsessive-compulsive disorder developing in chronic heavy users of MDMA, leading, in one case, to depression with psychotic features, and, in the other, to psychosis.[304] The former patient (a 16-year-old female who took four or five tablets per week for 1 year) was judged to have vulnerabilities to mental disorder, but the second patient did not (a 23-year-old male who took one or two tablets a week for more than 2 years). Both cases resolved with treatment. The authors conclude that causation cannot be determined, but is suggested by the case histories.

9.16.4 Harmful and Dependent Use and Withdrawal

MDMA is typically used occasionally.[57] Most people who try ecstasy will not escalate to regular or sustained use.[57] For example, UK population-level data suggest that although use of MDMA is relatively high in comparison to other drugs (except cannabis), only small percentages of people report using 'ecstasy' frequently and that the proportion of 'frequent' users of ecstasy has declined in the past 10 years. The majority of ecstasy users aged 16 to 59 reported having taken the drugs once or twice a year rather than more frequently.[305]

Nevertheless, using MDMA on many or most weekends is not uncommon among people sampled at clubs and raves.[148] Use of ecstasy several times a week, or even daily,[306] has been recorded, although this is exceptional and very likely to be linked to comorbidities.[137,236,308] One case has been reported of a poly-drug user who self-reported the consumption of 40,000 tablets between the ages of 21 and 30 years, before ceasing use following several collapses.[307] Bingeing for up to 48 hours and using up to 25 tablets has been reported,[57] but there is a lack of recent evidence, and the number of tablets is an imprecise guide to the total dose taken.

The tendency is for tolerance to the positive effects of MDMA to build up with use,[308] leading to diminishing returns from consumption. This may be protective against sustained heavy use or addiction.[57] It has been suggested that regular users often follow a trajectory of discovering and strongly liking MDMA, using it most weekends, sometimes with escalating dosages, for a year or two, suffering increasing adverse effects with decreasing enjoyment ('losing the magic') and then reducing or ceasing use spontaneously.[309] This pattern of decline has been described as almost unique among recreational drugs.[311] Nonetheless, a minority of ecstasy users will develop problems and drug-using patterns associated with harmful use even when no other problem drugs were also involved.

According to the 2019 European Drug Report, MDMA use is rarely cited as a reason for entering specialised drug treatment. In 2017, MDMA was reported by less than 1% (around 1,700 cases) of treatment entrants in Europe, with France, Hungary, UK and Turkey accounting for 68% of these.[310]

While MDMA is generally considered to have some potential for dependence,[5] use is often self-limiting and focused around weekend activities.[5] Reasons suggested for the low dependence potential include the relatively long period of recovery after one dose.[57]

It has been argued that although the physiological basis of MDMA dependence is relatively weak in comparison with some other drugs, other factors related to the behavioural and psychological aspects of reward and dependence may have a relatively greater contribution to dependence for ecstasy than for other drugs.[311]

Users may fulfil dependence criteria,[312–317] develop problematic chronic use patterns, have concerns about their use and seek treatment.[313] Several studies have demonstrated some features of dependence among MDMA users, such as worrying about use, thinking use was out of control and finding it difficult to abstain.[313,315]

A number of studies have shown that approximately one in five users have been found to be potentially dependent,[317,318,319,320] although studies which carried out detailed investigation of withdrawal symptoms have shown higher rates, as much as 43% in a US study of adolescents and young adults,[316,318] and as high as 64% in a study using DSM-IV criteria for amphetamine dependence.[322]

Some studies have suggested that how ecstasy is used, rather than how often, may be of key importance in ecstasy dependence, with 'binge' use and higher doses being associated with dependence.[315] Users who 'binge', who use ecstasy more frequently, and who experience more social and physical harm are more likely to become dependent users.[138]

Ecstasy 'craving' does not tend to follow the pattern typical with other drugs, as a symptom of dependence, but instead resembles anticipation of an enjoyed activity, typically being low during the week, but rising in the hours before weekend use.[144]

A withdrawal syndrome associated with MDMA has been reported. However, it has been argued that the wide between-study variations in the incidence of withdrawal symptoms indicate the need for improved distinction between the short- and the long-term effects of MDMA in standardised assessment tools, despite recent advances. As with other stimulants, the period following acute use is marked by a number of phases: an initial dysphoric 'crash', followed, in chronic users, by an extended 'withdrawal' phase, marked by anhedonia and anergia.[321] It has been argued that the application by some studies of withdrawal criteria related to the ecstasy come-down may have led to inflation of estimates of rates of potential dependence and withdrawal.[322] While 'true' withdrawal symptoms lead to users taking more of the drug to relieve them, adverse effects following an episode of ecstasy use have been seen as one reason why heavy users sometimes spontaneously quit MDMA.[311]

Some animal studies have shown that chronic use can lead to MDMA acting increasingly like an addictive stimulant. If chronic use of MDMA causes significant serotonergic damage but little or no dopaminergic damage (as supported by brain imaging[274]), then the dopaminergic effects may become more prominent than the serotonergic ones, similar to amphetamines with greater addictive potential.[323] This is partially supported by user experiences; many report 'losing the magic'[311] of the serotonergic effects with overuse and, outside the academic literature, users of drugs online for a note how, after overuse, MDMA feels more typically amphetamine-like.

MDMA dependence presents unique features.[315] In an online survey promoted to users of a dance-music website, ecstasy users were more likely than users of cocaine, ketamine or mephedrone to endorse three or more DSM-IV criteria, yet reported less harm, more pleasure and less desire to seek help than users of these other club drugs.[314]

MDMA is rarely reported as an individual's principal problem drug.[315,324]

Although MDMA is rarely a primary problematic drug, users of ecstasy are more likely than other drug users to have experienced substance use disorders in the past year involving drugs other than MDMA.[325] This was the case for 7 out of 10 MDMA users in an American population sample.[328]

9.16.5 Sleep Problems

A history of MDMA use has been linked to poorer sleep in some studies but other studies have found no differences.[56,326,327] Dysfunctional sleep processes may be involved in the memory deficits associated with MDMA use.[328]

9.16.6 Vascular Problems

The typical surge in blood pressure that MDMA causes may, over time, damage the blood vessels, in particular the walls of aneurysms and arteriovenous malformations.[56] This could lead to haemorrhage.[329] Therefore, patients with aneurysms, or any other history of vascular disorders, should be strongly advised of the risks from any drug with a hypertensive effect.

9.16.7 Heart Disease

A link between heavy, chronic MDMA use and valvular heart disease has been proposed, due directly to its serotonergic effects.[330,331] Activation of the 5-HT2B receptor in heart valves by (now obsolete) serotonergic pharmaceuticals such as fenfluramine and ergotamine have been demonstrated to cause cell proliferation,

fibrotic thickening and valve dysfunction.[332] There is some limited evidence that MDMA may be capable of causing such reactions in chronic, heavy users. A blinded study using echocardiography to identify abnormalities reported that MDMA may lead to mild to moderate valvular heart disease and valvular strands.[334]

A 33-year-old male smoker with an exceptionally high level of lifetime 'ecstasy' use (several pills per week since the age of 17)[333] reported shortness of breath and chest pain. He had severe mitral valve disease, with fibrotic thickening of the leaflets and resulting severe regurgitation, necessitating a valve replacement. It was suggested that the lack of reports of similar cases may be explained by the typically short 'ecstasy career' of most users, and the potential reversibility of the valve damage.[333]

In addition to valvular heart disease, chronic MDMA use has been linked to cardiomyopathy more generally,[333] although the evidence remains inconclusive. A retrospective analysis of autopsy records shows that the hearts of people who had MDMA in their bodies at post-mortem were more likely to have enlarged hearts, consistent with myocardial hypertrophy, as seen in users of cocaine and methamphetamine. However, this study did not appear to be controlled in a way that could exclude the confounding factor of poly-drug use.[334] A single case study of dilated cardiomyopathy associated with MDMA has been reported.[247]

9.17 Management of Chronic Harms

9.17.1 Treatments for Harmful Use and Dependence

As with other ATS, the treatment of harmful MDMA use is primarily psychosocial. No specific guidelines for psychosocial intervention have been described and validated for chronic MDMA users, but for general guidance on treatment options see Chapter 2.

In most cases, chronic ecstasy users will be poly-drug users, and existing interventions would be unlikely to focus on MDMA in isolation. For example, an intervention in the form of 45–60 minutes of structured motivational discussion was trialled in young stimulant users, most of whom had recently used ecstasy and cocaine, and most of whom were also regular users of cannabis and alcohol.[335] This discussion included exploration of the individual's pattern of use, 'good' and 'bad' effects of use, plans for behaviour change, likely outcomes of this and, for users with no immediate plans to change behaviour, reflection on what future scenarios would lead to a change (boundary setting).[338] In this study, the majority (59%) of participants did report making efforts to reduce or cease their stimulant use following the intervention, but 41% of the control group did as well. Average number of days with MDMA use in the previous 90 days fell from around 18 at baseline to around 8 at 6-month follow-up, and average dose fell from more than 2 tablets per session to around 1.5, with no significant difference seen between intervention and control groups.[338] Both the intervention and the control groups participated in baseline self-assessment and read health information, so the authors speculate that while there was no additional benefit from the intervention, contact with personnel and actions that focus attention on substance use may be enough to change behaviour.[338]

Similar results were found in a trial aiming to reduce MDMA use among Australian university students. A 50% reduction in use and a 20% reduction in reported severity of harm were recorded 24 weeks after 'motivational enhancement therapy', but the same changes followed the control condition, a 15-minute information session.[336] Another brief intervention for regular users did not produce significant reductions in quantity or frequency of use compared with the control condition (assessment only), but did significantly reduce reported symptoms of dependence, and a greater proportion (16%) achieved abstinence, although the study was underpowered to show whether this was statistically significant.[337]

It has been noted that 'ecstasy' users may not always accurately assess the harm that their drug use may be causing. The degree of apparent subclinical cognitive impairment in users appears to correlate not with the users' own assessments of how problematic their use is, but with the cumulative dose.[338]

However, most 'ecstasy' users are aware that there are risks associated with the drug, and will have reflected upon, contextualised and rationalised that risk.[339,340] Reducing risk of harm by encouraging ecstasy users to cease use (especially early in their career[338]) may be difficult because acute harm may be perceived as rare, and chronic harm too subtle to motivate behavioural change.[341]

Consequently, it has been suggested that the best approach to reducing the risk of harm may be to encourage users to minimise their intake as much as

possible.[344] This can be attempted by exploring users' experiences of the common unpleasant side-effects during and following use, and the disruption to other areas of life.[344] This approach may be supported by sharing the evidence that lighter users tend to maintain the positive effects from ecstasy, without the negative effects increasing much over time, whereas heavy users tend to find that the positive effects reduce sharply and unpleasant effects rise over time, to the point where they outweigh the enjoyment.[311] Doses higher than one average pill, or equivalent, are more likely to decrease the positive effects, with adverse effects rising steeply above 120 mg.[47,342]

9.17.2 Treatment of Depression in the Context of MDMA Use

It is recommended that clinicians prescribing antidepressants ask about recreational drug use and discuss the risk of drug interactions with those who use MDMA.[90] One study has reported that citalopram strongly reduces the desired effects of MDMA, and other SSRIs would be likely to act similarly.[343] Despite this reduction in enjoyment, it is possible that SSRIs or SNRIs could increase the risks of MDMA toxicity.[90,225] In rats, some effects of MDMA, including hyperthermia, are not diminished by citalopram, suggesting that if human users attempt to compensate for diminished enjoyment with higher doses, the risk of acute harm could be increased.[344] Furthermore, the pharmacological effects of these drugs involve multiple actions on serotonin release and reuptake, and this complexity may allow for unexpected interactions, including serotonin syndrome. MAOIs are strictly contraindicated in those who are unlikely to be able to abstain from MDMA and other similar serotonergic drugs, because the combination has a high risk of causing serotonin syndrome.

9.18 Public Health and Harm Reduction

Taking precautions and limiting dose were not found to be associated with experiencing a lower rate of adverse effects in a sample of 159 ecstasy poly-drug users, although most of this sample did not associate their use with adverse effects.[345] Ecstasy users sometimes believe that MDMA itself is virtually risk-free when it is 'clean',[346] i.e. that adulteration is responsible for most or all of the adverse effects, minor and severe. It may be beneficial to tell patients that while adulteration certainly does contribute to the risks, pure MDMA can cause harm and death,[349] especially in high doses and in environments that contribute to overheating and overexertion.[50] The principles for the reduction of the harms of ecstasy are similar to those for the reduction of ATS harms in general.

In addition:

- Ecstasy users should be made aware that not all ecstasy pills contain the same dose, and that some tablets sold as ecstasy may contain other drugs, like PMA, which can be stronger, take longer to take effect and have higher risks.
- Users should be advised to start with a small dose (half or quarter of a tablet). They should be made aware that taking more than one pill at once might not increase the effect, but can make a come-down worse and increase the risk.
- Users should be advised to take regular breaks from dancing and be sensitive to the possibility of exhaustion or overheating.
- Users should be advised to stay hydrated, but not to over-drink. It is best to take regular small sips of water and to drink no more than one pint of water per hour if dancing in a hot environment and half a pint if not dancing.
- Users should be advised to avoid mixing ecstasy with alcohol and other drugs, as this increases the risks.
- Users should avoid mixing MDMA with other stimulants as this increases the risk of cardiovascular adverse effects.
- Users should be aware that serotonin syndrome is dangerous and that they should watch out for anyone who looks flushed, hot and rigid and call emergency services immediately.
- A person on antidepressants who also takes ecstasy pills will be at greater risk of serotonin syndrome.

9.19 Benzofurans

Other substances used for their 'emphathogenic', and well as their stimulant effects, include benzofurans, principally 6-(2-aminopropyl)benzofuran (6-APB) and 5-(2- aminopropyl)benzofuran (5-APB), but also the other substances listed in Table 9.3.

Benzofurans are structurally very similar to MDMA and its active metabolite 3,4-methylenedioxyamphetamine (MDA)[349] 5-(2-aminopropyl)-benzofuran

Table 9.3 Benzofuran derivatives[347] (often referred to as Benzofury)

5-(2-aminopropyl)benzofuran 5-APB[18]
6-(2-aminopropyl)benzofuran 6-APB[18]
5-(2-aminopropyl)-2,3-dihydrobenzofuran 5-APDB
6-(2-aminopropyl)-2,3-dihydrobenzofuran 6-APDB
1-(benzofuran-5-yl)-N-methylpropan-2-amine 5-MAPB
1-(benzofuran-6-yl)-N-methylpropan-2-amine 6-MAPB
1-(benzofuran-5-yl)-N-ethylpropan-2-amine 5-EAPB
Indanylalkylamine derivative[18]
5-(2-aminopropyl)-2,3-dihydro-1 H-indene 5-APDI IAP[18]
Aminoindane derivatives[348]
5,6-methylenedioxy-2-aminoindane MDAI[91]
5-iodo-2-aminoindan 5-IAI[158]

(5-APB) and 6-(2- aminopropyl)-benzofuran (6-APB) were the first appear on the European market.

Benzodifurans include a group also known as the 'fly' drugs (for example, bromo-dragon fly, 2 C-B-fly). They are hallucinogens and are discussed in Chapter 12.

Benzofurans are ring-substituted amphetamine derivatives. Similar compounds have also appeared on the market in recent years, including 5- and 6-APB and their N-methyl derivatives. It was found that when these two materials were subjected to standard analytical techniques, it was not possible to distinguish between them. It is therefore very unlikely that those selling these drugs will know which form they are selling.[350]

Benzofurans were initially sold as 'legal ecstasy'. They were also sold as psychoactive substances in their own right, as 'Benzofury'. A study of Internet sites showed that when mephedrone became controlled, the vendors aggressively promoted the sale of Benzofury, as well as other new compounds (e.g. NRG-1 and NRG-2).[351]

The term Benzofury was originally applied to 6-APB; however, the name was later used interchangeably for 5-APB and 6-APB, as differentiation of the two isomers, even in laboratory analysis, is difficult.

9.19.1 Pharmacology

Understanding of benzofurans remains limited. Both 5- and 6-APB are phenethylamine-type materials and are related to methylenedioxyphenethylamines, such as MDMA and MDA.[353] They are potent inhibitors of the reuptake of noradrenaline, dopamine and serotonin with a potency on monoamine transporters similar to that of MDMA.[352] An animal study has shown that 5-APB and 6-APB are potent full agonists at 5-HT2B receptors.[353]

9.19.2 Patterns of Use, Modes of Ingestion

As with other substances, benzofurans are used as part of a wider drug repertoire.[196] Benzofurans are typically sold as a white powder, or in the form of pellets.[354] Routes of administration of benzofurans include nasal insufflation of powder and ingestion.

9.19.3 Desired Effects

The desired effects of benzofuran include increased empathy, euphoria, visual stimulation, appreciation for music and dancing, and an increase in mood and self-acceptance.[355] Users report that the effects of 5-APB and 6-APB are comparable to those of MDMA but more intense.[356] and that they have mood-enhancing, empathogenic and stimulant effects; they suggest that 5-APB is stronger than 6-APB.[353]

9.19.4 Clinical Uses

A patent application has been made for benzofuran compounds and their use as antidepressants and anxiolytics. The compounds inhibit serotonin reuptake, exhibit serotonin agonistic and antagonistic properties and are claimed to be suitable as antidepressants, anxiolytics, antipsychotics, neuroleptics and/or antihypertonics.[357]

9.19.5 Acute Harms

The unwanted effects of benzofurans include nausea, bruxism, dry mouth and eyes, diaorrhea, sensitivity to light, palpitations, increased heart rate, blood pressure and temperature, hot flushes, headaches, drowsiness, and clonus of the hands and feet. Benzofurans are also linked to psychological symptoms like hallucinations, depression, anxiety, panic attacks, insomnia and severe paranoia. Psychosis has been reported.[358] Some users also described an unpleasant 'comedown' that could last for several days.[359]

Very little information has been published on the acute harms of benzofuran, but a body of research is emerging.[360] It is suggested that such compounds produce clinical features similar to those of amphetamine, MDMA and mephedrone. Acute toxicity is characterised by serotonergic and sympathomimetic toxidrome, with nausea, agitation, anxiety, dizziness and hyperthermia.[361]

A case reported that (5-MAPB) (N-methyl-5-(2 aminopropyl)benzofuran) seems to have an acute toxicity profile similar to that of 5-APB and MDMA, with marked vasoconstrictor effect. In this case, observed symptoms and signs included paleness, cold and clammy skin, hypertension, elevated high-sensitive troponin T level, tachycardia, ECG change, diaphoresis, mild hyperthermia, mydriasis, tremor, hyperreflexia, clonus, agitation, disorientation, hallucinations, convulsions, reduced level of consciousness, and creatine kinase level elevation.[362]

Other reports also mentioned adverse effects, which include nausea, sympathomimetic stimulation and agitation.[259] Stimulant features of acute intoxication with benzofurans are most common, followed by mental health disturbances.[196] A study of the UK's National Poisons Information Service patient-specific telephone enquiries and user sessions for TOXBASE® from March 2009 to August 2013 was conducted, focusing on (2-aminopropyl)-2,3-dihydrobenzofurans. These data were compared with those of mephedrone collected over the same period. Ingestion of benzofuran was associated with similar toxic effects to those of amphetamines and cathinones. However, mental health disturbances and stimulant features were reported more frequently following reported ingestion of benzofuran compounds than after ingestion of mephedrone. However, there are limitations to these findings, resulting from a number of factors, including lack of analytical confirmation.[196]

Comparing the 57 patients who reported ingesting benzofuran compounds alone with 315 patients ingesting mephedrone alone, benzofurans were more often associated with stimulant features, including tachycardia, hypertension, mydriasis, palpitation, fever, increased sweating and tremor (72% vs. 38%) and mental health disturbances (58% vs. 38%). Other features reported after benzofuran compound ingestion included gastrointestinal symptoms (16%), reduced level of consciousness (9%), chest pain (7%) and creatinine kinase elevation (5%).[196]

One case report describes agitation and paranoia, but as a number of other drugs were ingested it is possible that another substance – or all – contributed to acute psychosis.[199]

It has been argued that the serotonin agonism of benzofuran raises the possibility that chronic use of this compound could be associated with valvular heart disease similar to that caused by fenfluramine and ergoline derivatives.[363,364]

9.19.6 Management of Acute Harms

See Section 9.15 for MDMA and drugs with similar effects.

A case with severe psychotic symptoms after use of 6-APB was successfully managed with benzodiazepines alone.[199]

9.19.7 Management of Chronic Harms

See Section 9.17 for MDMA and drugs with similar effects.

9.19.8 Harm Reduction

The harm reduction advice given for ATS and for MDMA is applicable here (see Chapter 8 and Section 9.18 in this chapter).

References

1. Iversen L, White M, Treble R. Designer psychostimulants: pharmacology and differences. *Neuropharmacology* 2014;**87**:59–65. https://doi.org/10.1016/j.neuropharm.2014.01.015

2. Mounteney J, Griffiths P, Bo A, Cunningham A, Matias J, Pirona A. Nine reasons why ecstasy is not quite what it used to be. *Int JDrug Policy* 2018;**51**:36–41.

3. Nichols DE. Differences between the mechanism of action of MDMA, MBDB, and the classic hallucinogens. Identification of a new therapeutic class: entactogens. *J Psychoactive Drugs* 1986;**18**:305–313.

4. Sáez-Briones P, Hernández A. MDMA (3,4-methylenedioxymethamphetamine) analogues as tools to characterize MDMA-like effects: an approach to understand entactogen pharmacology. *Curr Neuropharmacol* 2013;**11**(5):521.

5. Hermle L, Spitzer M, Borchardt D, Kovar KA, Gouzoulis E. Psychological effects of MDE in normal subjects. Are entactogens a new class of psychoactive agents? *Neuropsychopharmacology* 1993;**8**(2):171–176.

6. Bedi GD. Is ecstasy an 'empathogen'? Effects of MDMA on prosocial feelings and identification of emotional states in others. *Biol Psychiatry* 2010;**68**(12):1134–1140.

7. Iversen LL. *Speed, Ecstasy, Ritalin: The Science of Amphetamines*. Oxford, Oxford University Press, 2006.

8. Bershad AK, Miller MA, Baggott MJ, de Wit H. The effects of MDMA on socioemotional processing: does MDMA differ from other stimulants? *J Psychopharmacol* 2016;**30**:1248–1258. https://doi.org/10.1177/0269881116663120

9. Simmler LD, Liechti ME. Pharmacology of MDMA- and amphetamine-like new psychoactive substances. In: H Maurer, S Brandt (eds.), *New Psychoactive Substances. Handbook of Experimental Pharmacology*, vol. **252**. Cham, Springer, 2018.

10. Parrott AC. Is ecstasy MDMA? A review of the proportion of ecstasy tablets containing MDMA, their dosage levels, and the changing perceptions of purity. *Psychopharmacology* 2004;**173**:234–241.

11. Warrick BJ, Wilson J, Hedge M, Freeman S, Leonard K, Aaron C. Lethal serotonin syndrome after methylone and butylone ingestion. *J Med Toxicol* 2012;**8**(1):65–68. https://doi.org/10.1007/s13181-011-0199-6

12. Kalasinsky KS, Hugel J, Kish SJ. Use of MDA (the 'love drug') and methamphetamine in Toronto by unsuspecting users of ecstasy (MDMA). *J Forensic Sci* 2004;**49**(5):1106–1112.

13. European Monitoring Centre for Drugs and Drug Addiction. Recent changes in Europe's MDMA/ecstasy market, EMCDDA Rapid Communication. Luxembourg, Publications Office of the European Union, 2016.

14. European Monitoring Centre for Drugs and Drug Addiction. Recent changes in Europe's MDMA/ecstasy market, EMCDDA Rapid Communication. Luxembourg, Publications Office of the European Union, 2016.

15. Miliano M, Serpelloni G, Rimondo C, Mereu M, Marti M, De Luca MA. Neuropharmacology of new psychoactive substances (NPS): focus on the rewarding and reinforcing properties of cannabimimetics and amphetamine-like stimulants. *Front Neurosci* 2016 (online). https://doi.org/10.3389/fnins.2016.00153

16. Zaitsu K, Katagi M, Tatsuno M, Sato T, Tsuchihashi H, Suzuki K. Recently abused β-keto derivatives of 3,4-methylenedioxyphenylalkylamines: a review of their metabolisms and toxicological analysis. *Forensic Toxicol* 2011;**29**(2):73–84.

17. Freudenmann RW, Spitzer M. The neuropsychopharmacology and toxicology of 3,4-methylenedioxy-N-ethyl-amphetamine (MDEA). *CNS Drug Rev* 2004;**10**(2):89–116.

18. King LA. New phenethylamines in Europe. *Drug Test Anal* 2014;**6**:808–818.

19. Winstock AR, Wolff K, Ramsey J. 4-MTA: a new synthetic drug on the dance scene. *Drug Alcohol Depend* 2002;**67**(2):111–115.

20. Cole JC, Bailey M, Sumnall HR, Wagstaff GF, King LA. The content of ecstasy tablets: implications for the study of their long-term effects. *Addiction* 2002;**97**:1531–1536.

21. Cheng WC, Poon NL, Chan MF. Chemical profiling of 3,4-methylenedioxymethamphetamine (MDMA) tablets seized in Hong Kong. *J Forensic Sci* 2003;**48**:1249–1259.

22. Tanner-Smith EE. Pharmacological content of tablets sold as 'ecstasy': results from an online testing service. *Drug Alcohol Depend* 2006;**83**(3):247–254.

23. European Monitoring Centre for Drugs and Drug Addiction. Recent changes in Europe's MDMA/ecstasy market, EMCDDA Rapid Communication. Luxembourg, Publications Office of the European Union, 2016.

24. Boulanger-Gobeil C, St-Onge M, Laliberté M, Auger PL. Seizures and hyponatremia related to ethcathinone and methylone poisoning. *J Med Toxicol* 2012;**8**(1):59–61.

25. Elliott S, Smith C. Investigation of the first deaths in the United Kingdom involving the detection and quantitation of the piperazines BZP and 3-TFMPP. *J Analytic Toxicol* 2008;**32**(2):172–177.

26. Ling LH, Marchant C, Buckley NA, Prior M, Irvine RJ. Poisoning with the recreational drug paramethoxyamphetamine ('death'). *Med J Australia* 2001;**174**:453–455.

27. Togni LR, Lanaro R, Resende RR, et al. The variability of ecstasy tablets composition in Brazil. *J Forensic Sci* 2015;**60**:147–151.

28. Palamara JJ, Acosta P, Ompad DC, Cleland CM. Self-reported ecstasy/MDMA/'Molly' use in a sample of nightclub and dance festival attendees in New York City. *Subst Use Misuse* 2017;**52**(1):82–91. https://doi.org/10.1080/10826084.2016.1219373

29. European Monitoring Centre for Drugs and Drug Addiction. Recent changes in Europe's MDMA/ecstasy market, EMCDDA Rapid Communication. Luxembourg, Publications Office of the European Union, 2016.

30. Smith ZK, Moore K, Measham F. MDMA powder, pills and crystal: the persistence of ecstasy and the poverty of policy. *Drugs Alcohol Today* 2009;**9**(1):13–19.

31. Personal communication, John Ramsey.

32. European Monitoring Centre for Drugs and Drug Addiction. Recent changes in Europe's MDMA/ecstasy market, EMCDDA Rapid Communication. Luxembourg, Publications Office of the European Union, 2016.

33. Palamara JJ, Acosta P, Ompad DC, Cleland CM. Self-reported ecstasy/MDMA/'Molly' use in a sample of nightclub and dance festival attendees in New York City. *Subst Use Misuse* 2017;**52**(1):82–91. https://doi.org/10.1080/10826084.2016.1219373

34. European Monitoring Centre for Drugs and Drug Addiction. European Drug Report 2019: Trends and Developments. Luxembourg, Publications Office of the European Union, 2019.

35. European Monitoring Centre for Drugs and Drug Addiction. Recent changes in Europe's MDMA/ecstasy market, EMCDDA Rapid Communication. Luxembourg, Publications Office of the European Union, 2016. Available at: www.emcdda.europa.eu/system/files/publications/2473/TD0116348ENN.pdf [last accessed 23 April 2022].

36. European Monitoring Centre for Drugs and Drug Addiction. Recent changes in Europe's MDMA/ecstasy market, EMCDDA Rapid Communication. Luxembourg, Publications Office of the European Union, 2016.

37. European Monitoring Centre for Drugs and Drug Addiction. European Drug Report 2019: Trends and Developments. Luxembourg, Publications Office of the European Union, 2019.

38. World Drug Report 2019 (United Nations publication, Sales No. E.19.XI.9).

39. Home Office. Drug Misuse: Findings from the 2017/18 Crime Survey for England and Wales Statistical Bulletin 14/18 July 2018.

40. UK Focal Point on Drugs: United Kingdom Drug Situation 2017. Available at: https://assets.publishing.service.gov.uk/government/uploads/system/uploads/attachment_data/file/713101/Focal_Point_Annual_Report.pdf [last accessed 10 March 2022].

41. National Advisory Committee on Drugs and Alcohol, & Department of Health Northern Ireland. Prevalence of Drug Use and Gambling in Ireland and Drug Use in Northern Ireland 2014/15. Published 2016.

42. Scottish Government. Scottish Crime and Justice Survey 2014/15: Drug Use. Published 2016.

43. Couchman L, Frinculescu A, Sobreira C, et al. Variability in content and dissolution profiles of MDMA tablets collected in the UK between 2001 and 2018 – A potential risk to users? *Drug Test Anal* 2019;**8**: 1172–1182.

44. European Monitoring Centre for Drugs and Drug Addiction. European Drug Report 2019: Trends and Developments. Luxembourg, Publications Office of the European Union, 2019.

45. European Monitoring Centre for Drugs and Drug Addiction. Recent changes in Europe's MDMA/ecstasy market, EMCDDA Rapid Communication. Luxembourg, Publications Office of the European Union, 2016.

46. European Monitoring Centre for Drugs and Drug Addiction. Recent changes in Europe's MDMA/ecstasy market, EMCDDA Rapid Communication. Luxembourg, Publications Office of the European Union, 2016.

47. Brunt TM, Koeter MW, Niesink RJ, van den Brink W. Linking the pharmacological content of ecstasy tablets to the subjective experiences of drug users. *Psychopharmacology* 2012;**220**(4):751–762. https://doi.org/10.1007/s00213-011-2529-4

48. Sherlock K, Wolff K, Hay AW, Conner M. Analysis of illicit ecstasy tablets: implications for clinical management in the accident and emergency department. *J Accid Emerg Med* 1999;**16**(3):194–197.

49. Morefield KM. Pill content, dose and resulting plasma concentrations of 3,4-methylendioxymethamphetamine (MDMA) in recreational 'ecstasy' users. *Addiction* 2011;**106**(7):1293–1300.

50. Armenian PT. Multiple MDMA (ecstasy) overdoses at a rave event: a case series. *J Intensive Care Med* 2013;**28**(4):252–258.

51. O'Connor LC, Torrance HJ, McKeown DA, Simpson K. Analysis of 'ecstasy' tablets from Police Scotland in the Glasgow area – November 2013 to July 2014.

52. Couchman L, Frinculescu A, Sobreira C, et al. Variability in content and dissolution profiles of MDMA tablets collected in the UK between 2001 and 2018 – A potential risk to users? *Drug Test Anal* 2019;**11**(8):1172–1182.

53. Couchman L, Frinculescu A, Sobreira C, et al. Variability in content and dissolution profiles of MDMA tablets collected in the UK between 2001 and 2018 – A potential risk to users? *Drug Test Anal* 2019;**11**(8):1172–1182.

54. Bombe A, Dave-Momin N, Shah N, Sonavane S, Desousa A. MDMA dependence: a case report from urban India. *History* 2013;**3**(9):32–33.

55. Potash MN. Persistent psychosis and medical complications after a single ingestion of MDMA 'ecstasy': a case report and review of the literature. *Psychiatry* 2009;**6**(7):40.

56. Rogers G, Elston J, Garside R, et al. The harmful health effects of recreational ecstasy: a systematic review of observational evidence. *Health Technol Assess* 2009;**13**(6):iii–v. https://doi.org/10.3310/hta13050

57. Parrott AC. Human psychobiology of MDMA or 'ecstasy': an overview of 25 years of empirical research. *Hum Psychopharmacol* 2013;**28**(4):289–307. https://doi.org/10.1002/hup.2318

58. Parrott AC. MDMA, serotonergic neurotoxicity, and the diverse functional deficits of recreational 'ecstasy' users. *Neurosci Biobehav Rev* 2013;**37**(8):1466–1484. https://doi.org/10.1016/j. neubiorev.2013.04.016

59. Doblin R, Greer G, Holland J, Jerome L, Mithoefer MC, Sessa B. A reconsideration and response to Parrott AC (2013) 'Human psychobiology of MDMA or "ecstasy": an overview of 25 years of empirical research'. *Hum Psychopharmacol Clin Exp* 2014;**29**:105–108. https://doi.org/10.1002/hup.2389

60. Cole JC. MDMA and the 'ecstasy' paradigm. *J Psychoactive Drugs* 2014;**46**(1):44–56.

61. See for example: Vizeli P, Liechti ME. Safety pharmacology of acute MDMA administration in healthy subjects. *J Psychopharmacol* 2017;**31**(5):576–588. https://doi.org/10.1177/0269881117691569

62. De la Torre RM. Human pharmacology of MDMA: pharmacokinetics, metabolism, and disposition. *Ther Drug Monit* 2004;**26**(2):137–144.

63. Docherty JR, Green AR. The role of monoamines in the changes in body temperature induced by 3,4-methylenedioxymethamphetamine (MDMA, ecstasy) and its derivatives. *Br J Pharmacol* 2010;**160**(5):1029–1044. https://doi.org/10.1111/j.1476-5381.2010.00722.x

64. Hysek CM, Simmler LD, Ineichen M, et al. The norepinephrine transporter inhibitor reboxetine reduces stimulant effects of MDMA ('ecstasy') in humans. *Clin Pharmacol Ther* 2011;**90**(2):246–255. https://doi.org/10.1038/clpt.2011.78

65. Roiser JP. Association of a functional polymorphism in the serotonin transporter gene with abnormal emotional processing in ecstasy users. *Am J Psychiatry* 2005;**162**(3):609–612.

66. Pardo-Lozano R, Farré M, Yubero-Lahoz S, et al. Clinical pharmacology of 3,4-methylenedioxymethamphetamine (MDMA, 'ecstasy'): the influence of gender and genetics (CYP2D6, COMT, 5-HTT). *PLoS ONE* 2012;**7**(10):e47599.

67. Baylen CA. A review of the acute subjective effects of MDMA/ecstasy. *Addiction* 2006;**101**(7):933–947.

68. Gouzoulis-Mayfrank E. Differential actions of an entactogen compared to a stimulant and a hallucinogen in healthy humans. *Heffter Rev Psychedelic Res* 2001;**2**:64–72.

69. Shulgin AT. History of MDMA. In: SJ Peroutka, ed., *Ecstasy: The Clinical, Pharmacological and Neurotoxicological Effects of the Drug MDMA*, pp. 1–20. Norwell, MA, Kluwer Academic, 1990.

70. Greer GR, Tolbert R. The therapeutic use of MDMA. In: SJ Peroutka, ed., *Ecstasy: The Clinical, Pharmacological and Neurotoxicological Effects of the Drug MDMA*, pp. 21–36. Norwell, MA, Kluwer Academic, 1990.

71. Sessa B. Is there a case for MDMA-assisted psychotherapy in the UK? *J Psychopharmacol* 2007;**21**(2):220–224.

72. Harris DS, Baggott M, Mendelson JH, Mendelson JE, Jones RT. Subjective and hormonal effects of 3,4-methylenedioxymethamphetamine (MDMA) in humans. *Psychopharmacology* 2002;**162**(4):396–405.

73. Bershad AK, Mayo LM, Van Hedger K, et al. Effects of MDMA on attention to positive social cues and pleasantness of affective touch. *Neuropsychopharmacol* 2019;**44**:1698–1705. https://doi.org/10.1038/s41386-019-0402-z

74. Dumont GJ. Increased oxytocin concentrations and prosocial feelings in humans after ecstasy (3,4-methylenedioxymethamphetamine) administration. *Social Neurosci* 2009;**4**(4):359–366.

75. Bershada AK, Weafer JJ, Kirkpatrick MG, Wardle MC, Miller MA, de Wita Soc H. Oxytocin receptor gene variation predicts subjective responses to MDMA. *Neuroscience* 2016;**11**(6):592–599. https://doi.org/10.1080/17470919.2016.1143026

76. Bershada AK, Weafer JJ, Kirkpatrick MG, Wardle MC, Miller MA, de Wita Soc H. Oxytocin receptor gene variation predicts subjective responses to MDMA. *Neuroscience* 2016;**11**(6):592–599. https://doi.org/10.1080/17470919.2016.1143026

77. Peiró AM. Human pharmacology of 3,4-methylenedioxymethamphetamine (MDMA, ecstasy) after repeated doses taken 2 h apart. *Psychopharmacology* 2013;**225**(4):883–893.

78. Yubero-Lahoz SRM. Sex differences in 3,4-methylenedioxymethamphetamine (MDMA; ecstasy)-induced cytochrome P450 2D6 inhibition in humans. *Clin Pharmacokinet* 2011;**50**(5):319–329.

79. Green AR, Mechan AO, Elliott JM, O'Shea E, Colado MI. The pharmacology and clinical pharmacology of 3,4-methylenedioxymethamphetamine (MDMA, 'ecstasy'). *Pharmacol Rev* 2003;**55**(3):463–508.

80. Parrott AC, Lock J, Adnum L, Thome J. MDMA can increase cortisol levels by 800% in dance clubbers. *J Psychopharmacology* 2013;**27**(1):113–114.

81. Vevelstad M, Oiestad EL, Middelkoop G, et al. The PMMA epidemic in Norway: comparison of fatal and non-fatal intoxications. *Forensic Sci Int* 2012;**219**:151–157.

82. Lurie Y, Gopher A, Lavon O, Almog S, Sulimani L, Bentur Y. Severe paramethoxymethamphetamine (PMMA) and paramethoxyamphetamine (PMA) outbreak in Israel. *Clin Toxicol* 2012;**50**:39–43.

83. Hill SL, Thomas SHL. Clinical toxicology of newer recreational drugs. *Clin Toxicol* 2011;**49**:705–719.

84. Ling LH, Marchant C, Buckley NA, Prior M, Irvine RJ. Poisoning with the recreational drug

paramethoxyamphetamine ('death'). *Med J Australia* 2001;**174**:453–455.

85. De Letter EA, Coopman VAE, Cordonnier JACM, Piette MHA. One fatal and seven non-fatal cases of 4-methylthioamphetamine (4-MTA) intoxication: clinico-pathological findings. *Int J Legal Med* 2001;**114**:352–356.

86. Elliot SP. Fatal poisoning with a new phenethylamine: 4-methylthioamphetamine (4-MTA). *J Anal Toxicol* 2000;**24**:85–89.

87. Felgate HE, Felgate PD, James RA, Sims DN, Vozzo DC. Recent paramethoxyamphetamine deaths. *J Anal Toxicol* 1998;**22**:169–172.

88. Lamberth PG, Ding GK, Nurmi LA. Fatal paramethoxy-amphetamine (PMA) poisoning in the Australian Capital Territory. *Med J Australia* 2008;**188**:426.

89. Daws LC, Irvine RJ, Callaghan PD, Toop NP, White JM, Bochner F. Differential behavioural and neurochemical effects of para-methoxyamphetamine and 3,4-methylenedioxymethamphetamine in the rat. *Prog Neuropsychopharmacol Biol Psychiatry* 2000;**24**:955–977.

90. Silins E, Copeland J, Dillon P. Qualitative review of serotonin syndrome, ecstasy (MDMA) and the use of other serotonergic substances: hierarchy of risk. *Aust NZ J Psychiatry* 2007;**41**(8):649–655.

91. Corkery JM, Elliott S, Schifano F, Corazza O, Ghodse AH. MDAI (5,6-methylenedioxy-2-aminoindane; 6,7-dihydro-5Hcyclopenta[f][1,3]benzodioxol-6-amine; 'sparkle'; 'mindy') toxicity: a brief overview and update. *Hum Psychopharmacol Clin Exp* 2013;**28**:345–355.

92. Brandt SD, Sumnall HR, Measham F, Cole J. Analyses of second generation 'legal highs' in the UK: initial findings. *Drug Test Anal* 2010;**2**(8):377–382.

93. Greer GR, Tolbert R. A method of conducting therapeutic sessions with MDMA. *J Psychoactive Drugs* 1998;**30**(4):371–379.

94. Mithoefer MC, Wagner MT, Mithoefer AT, et al. Durability of improvement in post-traumatic stress disorder symptoms and absence of harmful effects or drug dependency after 3,4-methylenedioxymethamphetamine-assisted psychotherapy: a prospective long-term follow-up study. *J Psychopharmacol* 2013;**27**(1):28–39. https://doi.org/10.1177/0269881112456611

95. Johansen PØ, Krebs TS. How could MDMA (ecstasy) help anxiety disorders? A neurobiological rationale. *J Psychopharmacol* 2009;**23**(4):389–391. https://doi.org/10.1177/0269881109102787

96. Parrott AC. The potential dangers of using MDMA for psychotherapy. *J Psychoactive Drugs* 2014;**46**(1):37–43.

97. Capela JP. Molecular and cellular mechanisms of ecstasy-induced neurotoxicity: an overview. *Mol Neurobiol* 2009;**39**(3):210–271.

98. Sessa B, Higbed L, Nutt D. A review of 3,4-methylenedioxymethamphetamine (MDMA)-assisted psychotherapy. *Front Psychiatry* 2019 (online). https://doi.org/10.3389/fpsyt.2019.00138

99. Feduccia AA, Holland J, Mithoefer MC. Progress and promise for the MDMA drug development program. *Psychopharmacology* 2018;**235**(2):561–571. https://doi.org/10.1007/s00213-017-4779-2

100. Mithoefer MC, Mithoefe AT, Feduccia AA, et al.3,4-methylenedioxymethamphetamine (MDMA)-assisted psychotherapy for post-traumatic stress disorder in military veterans, firefighters, and police officers: a randomised, double-blind, dose-response, phase 2 clinical trial. *Lancet Psychiatry* 2018;**5**(6):486–497.

101. Sessa B. MDMA and PTSD treatment: 'PTSD: from novel pathophysiology to innovative therapeutics'. *Neurosci Lett* 2017;**649**:176–180.

102. Ot'alora MG, Grigsby J, Poulter B, et al.3,4-Methylenedioxymethamphetamine-assisted psychotherapy for treatment of chronic post-traumatic stress disorder: a randomized phase 2 controlled trial. *J Psychopharmacol* 2018;**32**(12):1295–1307.

103. Bouso JC, Doblin R, Farre M, et al. MDMA-assisted psychotherapy using low doses in a small sample of women with chronic post-traumatic stress disorder. *J Psychoactive Drugs* 2008;**40**:225–236.

104. Greer GR, Tolbert R. A method of conducting therapeutic sessions with MDMA. *J Psychoactive Drugs* 1998;**30**:371–379.

105. Thal SB, Lommen MJJ. Current perspective on MDMA-assisted psychotherapy for posttraumatic stress disorder. *J Contemp Psychother* 2018;**48**:99–108. https://doi.org/10.1007/s10879-017-9379-2

106. Oehen PR. A randomized, controlled pilot study of MDMA (±3,4-methylenedioxymethamphetamine)-assisted psychotherapy for treatment of resistant, chronic post-traumatic stress disorder (PTSD). *J Psychopharmacol* 2013;**27**(1):40–52.

107. Barone W, Beck J, Mitsunaga-Whitten M, Perl P. Perceived benefits of MDMA-assisted psychotherapy beyond symptom reduction: qualitative follow-up study of a clinical trial for individuals with treatment-resistant PTSD. *J Psychoactive Drugs* 2019;**51**(2):199–208. https://doi.org/10.1080/02791072.2019.1580805

108. Bahji A, , Forsyth A, Groll D, Hawken ER. Efficacy of 3,4-methylenedioxymethamphetamine (MDMA)-assisted psychotherapy for post-traumatic stress disorder: a systematic review and meta-analysis. *Prog Neuropsychopharmacol Biol Psychiatry* 2020;**96**:109735.

109. Schenk S, Newcombe D. Methylenedioxymethamphetamine (MDMA) in psychiatry: pros, cons, and suggestions. *J Clin Psychopharmacol* 2018;**38**(6):632–638. https://doi.org/10.1097/JCP.0000000000000962

110. Danforth AL, Grob CS, Struble C, et al. Reduction in social anxiety after MDMA-assisted psychotherapy with autistic adults: a randomized, double-blind, placebo-controlled pilot study *Psychopharmacology* 2018;**235**(11):3137–3148. https://doi.org/10.1007/s00213-018-5010-9

111. Sessa B. Why MDMA therapy for alcohol use disorder? *Neuropharmacology* 2018;**142**:83–88. https://doi.org/10.1016/j .neuropharm.2017.11.004

112. Concar D. Ecstasy has dramatic effect on Parkinson's symptoms. *New Scientist* 2002;**17**(2368):14.

113. Johnston TH, Millar Z, Huot P, et al. A novel MDMA analogue, UWA-101, that lacks psychoactivity and cytotoxicity, enhances l-DOPA benefit in parkinsonian primates. *FASEB J* 2012;**26**(5):2154–2163. https://doi.org/10 .1096/fj.11-195016

114. Moonzwe LS, Schensul JJ, Kostick KM. The role of MDMA (ecstasy) in coping with negative life situations among urban young adults. *J Psychoactive Drugs* 2011;**43**(3):199–210.

115. Jansen KLR. Ecstasy (MDMA) dependence. *Drug Alcohol Depend* 1999;**53**(2):121–124.

116. Sessa B. Can psychedelics have a role in psychiatry once again? *Br J Psychiatry* 2005;**186**(6):457–458.

117. McElrath K, Van Hout MC. A preference for mephedrone: drug markets, drugs of choice, and the emerging 'legal high' scene. *J Drug Issues* 2011;**41**(4):487–507.

118. European Monitoring Centre for Drugs and Drug Addiction (EMCDDA). European Drug Report. Trends and Developments 2015. Luxembourg, Publications Office of the European Union, 2015. Available at: www.emcdda.europa.eu/ system/files/publications/2637/TDAT16001ENN.pdf [last accessed 10 March 2022].

119. European Monitoring Centre for Drugs and Drug Addiction (EMCDDA). Recent changes in Europe's MDMA/ecstasy market. Results from an EMCDDA trendspotter study. Luxembourg, Publications Office of the European Union, 2016b. Available at: www.emcdda.europa.eu/system/files/pub lications/2473/TD0116348ENN.pdf [last accessed 10 March 2022].

120. Edland-Gryta M, Sandberg S, Pedersen W. From ecstasy to MDMA: recreational drug use, symbolic boundaries, and drug trends. *Int J Drug Policy* 2017;**50**:1–8.

121. Home Office. Drugs Misuse: Findings from the 2018/19 Crime Survey for England and Wales Statistical Bulletin. Published September 2019.

122. European Monitoring Centre for Drugs and Drug Addiction. Recent changes in Europe's MDMA/ecstasy market, EMCDDA Rapid Communication. Luxembourg, Publications Office of the European Union, 2016.

123. European Monitoring Centre for Drugs and Drug Addiction. European Drug Report 2019: Trends and Developments. Luxembourg, Publications Office of the European Union, 2019.

124. European Monitoring Centre for Drugs and Drug Addiction. European Drug Report 2019: Trends and Developments. Luxembourg, Publications Office of the European Union, 2019.

125. European Monitoring Centre for Drugs and Drug Addiction. European Drug Report 2019: Trends and Developments. Luxembourg, Publications Office of the European Union, 2019.

126. European Monitoring Centre for Drugs and Drug Addiction. European Drug Report 2019: Trends and Developments. Luxembourg, Publications Office of the European Union, 2019.

127. Palamar JJ, Acosta P, Omp DC, Cleland CM. Self-reported ecstasy/MDMA/'Molly' use in a sample of nightclub and dance festival attendees in New York City. *Subst Use Misuse* 2017;**52** (1):82–91. https://doi.org/10.1080/10826084.2016.1219373

128. Hansen DB. 'Weddings, parties, anything. . .': a qualitative analysis of ecstasy use in Perth, Western Australia. *Int J Drug Policy* 2001;**12**(2):181–199.

129. Halpern P, Moskovich J, Avrahami B, Bentur Y, Soffer D, Peleg K. Morbidity associated with MDMA (ecstasy) abuse – a survey of emergency department admissions. *Hum Exp Toxicol* 2011;**30**(4):259–266. https://doi.org/10.1177 /0960327110370984

130. Horyniak D, Degenhardt L, Smit de V, et al. Pattern and characteristics of ecstasy and related drug (ERD) presentations at two hospital emergency departments, Melbourne, Australia, 2008–2010. *Emerg Med J* 2014;**31**(4):317–322. https://doi.org /10.1136/emermed2012-202174

131. European Monitoring Centre for Drugs and Drug Addiction. European Drug Report 2019: Trends and Developments. Luxembourg, Publications Office of the European Union, 2019.

132. Mounteney J, Griffiths P, Bo A, Cunningham A, Matias J, Pirona A. Nine reasons why ecstasy is not quite what it used to be. *Int J Drug Policy* 2018;**51**:36–41.

133. Pearson G. Normal drug use: ethnographic fieldwork among an adult network of recreational drug users in inner London. *Subst Use Misuse* 2001;**36**(1–2):167–200.

134. Winstock A. The Global Drug Survey 2014 Findings. Global Drug Survey, April 2014. Available at: www .globaldrugsurvey.com/facts-figures/the-global-drug-survey-2 014-findings [last accessed 10 March 2022].

135. Jansen KLR. Ecstasy (MDMA) dependence. *Drug Alcohol Depend* 1999;**53**(2):121–124.

136. Topp L, Hando J, Dillon P, Roche A, Solowij N. Ecstasy use in Australia: patterns of use and associated harm. *Drug Alcohol Depend* 1999;**55**:105–115.

137. Carhart-Harris RL, Murphy K, Leech R, et al. The effects of acutely administered 3,4-methylenedioxymethamphetamine on spontaneous brain function in healthy volunteers measured with arterial spin labeling and blood oxygen level-dependent resting state functional connectivity. *Biol Psychiatry* 2014;**2014**:S0006-3223(14) 00005-5. https://doi.org/10.1016/j . biopsych.2013.12.015

138. Scholey AB, Parrott AC, Buchanan T, Heffernan TM, Ling J, Rodgers J. Increased intensity of ecstasy and polydrug usage in the more experienced recreational ecstasy/MDMA users: a WWW study. *Addict Behav* 2004;**29**(4):743–752.

139. Wu L-TA. The variety of ecstasy/MDMA users: results from the National Epidemiologic Survey on alcohol and related conditions. *Am J Addictions* 2009;**18**(6):452–461.

140. Palamar JJ, Acosta P, Omp DC, Cleland CM. Self-reported ecstasy/MDMA/'Molly' use in a sample of nightclub and dance festival attendees in New York City. *Subst Use Misuse* 2017;**52**(1):82–91. https://doi.org/10.1080/10826084.2016.1219373

141. Kinner SA, George J, Johnston J, Dunn M, Degenhardt L. Pills and pints: risky drinking and alcohol-related harms among regular ecstasy users in Australia. *Drug Alcohol Rev* 2012;**31**:273–280.

142. Hopper JW. Incidence and patterns of polydrug use and craving for ecstasy in regular ecstasy users: an ecological momentary assessment study. *Drug Alcohol Depend* 2006;**85**(3):221–235.

143. Hall AP, Henry JA. Acute toxic effects of 'ecstasy' (MDMA) and related compounds: overview of pathophysiology and clinical management. *Br J Anaesthesia* 2006;**96**(6):678–685.

144. Benschop A, Urbán R, Kapitány-Fövény M, et al. Why do people use new psychoactive substances? Development of a new measurement tool in six European countries. *J Psychopharmacol* 2020;**34**(6):600–611. https://doi.org/10.1177/0269881120904951

145. Winstock A. Drug Pleasure Ratings. Global Drug Survey, April 2014. Available at: www.globaldrugsurvey.com/facts-figures/the-net-pleasure-index-results [last accessed 10 March 2022].

146. ter Bogt TF, Engels RC. 'Partying' hard: party style, motives for and effects of MDMA use at rave parties. *Subst Use Misuse* 2005;**40**(9–10):1479–1502.

147. Kamilar-Britt P, Bedi G. The prosocial effects of 3,4-methylenedioxymethamphetamine (MDMA): controlled studies in humans and laboratory animals. *Neurosci Biobehav Rev* 2015;**57**:433–446.

148. Bershad AK, Miller MA, Baggott MJ, de Wit H. The effects of MDMA on socio-emotional processing: does MDMA differ from other stimulants? *J Psychopharmacol* 2016;**30**(12):1–11. https://doi.org/10.1177/0269881116663120

149. Dolder PC, Müller F, Schmid Y, Borgwardt SJ, Liecht ME. Direct comparison of the acute subjective, emotional, autonomic, and endocrine effects of MDMA, methylphenidate, and modafinil in healthy subjects. *Psychopharmacology* 2018;**235**:467–479. https://dooi.org/10.1007/s00213-017-4650-5

150. Zemishlany ZD. Subjective effects of MDMA ('ecstasy') on human sexual function. *Eur Psychiatry* 2001;**16**(2):127–130.

151. Kennedy KE. Ecstasy and sex among young heterosexual women: a qualitative analysis of sensuality, sexual effects, and sexual risk taking. *Int J Sex Health* 2010;**22**(3):155–166.

152. Passie T, Hartmann U, Schneider U, Emrich HM, Krüger TH. Ecstasy (MDMA) mimics the postorgasmic state: impairment of sexual drive and function during acute MDMA-effects may be due to increased prolactin secretion. *Med Hypotheses* 2005;**64**(5):899–903.

153. Bourne ARD. The chemsex study: drug use in sexual settings among gay and bisexual men in Lambeth, Southwark and Lewisham, London. Sigma Research, London School of Hygiene and Tropical Medicine, 2014.

154. Vizeli P, Liechti M E. Safety pharmacology of acute MDMA administration in healthy subjects. *J Psychopharmacol* 2017;**31**(5):576–588. https://doi.org/10.1177/0269881117691569

155. Papaseit E, Torrens M, Pérez-Mañá C, Muga R, Farré M. Key interindividual determinants in MDMA pharmacodynamics. *Exp Opin Drug Metab Toxicol* 2018;**14**(2):183–195. https://doi.org/10.1080/17425255.2018.1424832

156. Coppola M, Mondola R. Is the 5-iodo-2-aminoindan (5-IAI) the new MDMA? *J Addict Res Ther* 2012;**3**:134.

157. Nichols DE, Oberlender R. Structure-activity relationships of MDMA and related compounds: a new class of psychoactive drugs? *Ann NY Acad Sci* 1990;**600**(1):613–623.

158. Simmler LD, Liechti ME. Pharmacology of MDMA- and amphetamine-like new psychoactive substances. In: H Maurer, S Brandt, (eds.), *New Psychoactive Substances. Handbook of Experimental Pharmacology*, vol. **252**. Cham, Springer, 2018.

159. Raznahan M, Hassanzadeh E, Houshmand A, Kashani L, Tabrizi M, Akhondzadeh S. Change in frequency of acute and subacute effects of ecstasy in a group of novice users after 6 months of regular use. *Psychiatr Danub* 2013;**25**(2):175–178.

160. Parrott AC. Recreational ecstasy/MDMA, the serotonin syndrome, and serotonergic neurotoxicity. *Pharmacol Biochem Behav* 2002;**71**(4):837–844.

161. Fuit S, Brookhuis A, Karel C et al. Physical, affective and somatic effects of ecstasy (MDMA): an observational study of recreational users. *Curr Psychopharmacol* 2017;**6**(1):51–58.

162. O'Sullivan A, Parrott AC. Deteriorating cost–benefit ratios for ecstasy/MDMA with repeated usage. *Open Addiction J* 2011;**4**:38–39.

163. Young SN, Regoli M, Leyton M, Pihl RO, Benkelfat C. The effect of acute tryptophan depletion on mood and impulsivity in polydrug ecstasy users. *Psychopharmacology* 2014;**231**(4):707–716. https://doi.org/10.1007/s00213-013-3287-2

164. Travers KR, Lyvers M. Mood and impulsivity of recreational ecstasy users in the week following a 'rave'. *Addict Res Theory* 2005;**13**(1):43–52.

165. European Monitoring Centre for Drugs and Drug Addiction. Recent changes in Europe's MDMA/ecstasy market, EMCDDA Rapid Communication. Luxembourg, Publications Office of the European Union, 2016.

166. Al-Samarraie MS, Vevelstad M, Nygaard IL, Bachs L, Mørland J. Intoxication with paramethoxymethamphetamine. [Article in Norwegian.] *Tidsskr Nor Laegeforen* 2013;**133**(9):966–999. https://doi.org/10.4045/tidsskr.12.0417

167. Shulgin AT, Shulgin A. 4-MA; PMA; 4-methoxyamphetamine. In: *PIHKAL: A Chemical Love Story* (Monograph 97), pp. 707–709. Liverpool, Transform Press, 1991.

168. Shulgin AT, Shulgin A. 4-MA; PMA; 4-methoxyamphetamine. In: *PIHKAL: A Chemical Love Story* (Monograph 97), pp. 707–709. Liverpool, Transform Press, 1991.

169. Figurasin R, Maguire NJ. 3,4-Methylenedioxy-Methamphetamine (MDMA, Ecstasy, Molly) Toxicity. [Updated 2019 May 11]. In: StatPearls [Internet]. Treasure Island (FL), StatPearls Publishing, 2019. Available at: www

.ncbi.nlm.nih.gov/books/NBK538482/ [last accessed 10 March 2022].

170. Rigg KK, Sharp A. Deaths related to MDMA (ecstasy/molly): prevalence, root causes, and harm reduction interventions. *J Subst Use* 2018;**23**(4):345–352. https://doi.org/10.1080/14659891.2018.1436607

171. Roxburgh A, Lappin J. MDMA-related deaths in Australia 2000 to 2018. *Int J Drug Policy* 2020;**76**:102630.

172. Drugscope. Business as Usual? A Status Report on New Psychoactive Substances (NPS) and Club Drugs in the UK. Published 2014.

173. Cimbura G. PMA deaths in Ontario. *Can Med Assoc J* 1974;**110**(11):1263.

174. Office for National Statistics. Deaths Related to Drug Poisoning in England and Wales, 2013. Published 2014. Available at: www.ons.gov.uk/ons/dcp171778_375498.pdf [last accessed 10 March 2022].

175. European Monitoring Centre for Drugs and Drug Addiction. Recent changes in Europe's MDMA/ecstasy market, EMCDDA Rapid Communication. Luxembourg, Publications Office of the European Union, 2016.

176. See for example: Darracq MA, Thornton SL, Minns AB, Gerona RR. A case of 3,4-dimethoxyamphetamine (3,4-DMA) and 3,4-methylenedioxymethamphetamine (MDMA) toxicity with possible metabolic interaction. *J Psychoactive Drugs* 2016;**48**(5):351–354. https://doi.org/10.1080/02791072.2016.1225324

177. Rosenson J, Smollin C, Sporer KA, Blanc P, Olson KR. Patterns of ecstasy-associated hyponatremia in California. *Ann Emerg Med* 2007;**49**(2):164–171.

178. Williams H, Dratcu L, Taylor R, Roberts M, Oyefeso A. 'Saturday night fever': ecstasy-related problems in a London accident and emergency department. *J Accid Emerg Med* 1998;**15**(5):322–326.

179. Liechti ME, Kunz I, Kupferschmidt H. Acute medical problems due to ecstasy use. *Swiss Med Wkly* 2005;**135**(43–44):652–657.

180. Simmler LD, Liechti ME. Pharmacology of MDMA- and amphetamine-like new psychoactive substances. In: H Maurer, S Brandt (eds.), *New Psychoactive Substances. Handbook of Experimental Pharmacology*, vol. 252. Cham, Springer, 2018.

181. Degenhardt L, Hall W. The Health and Psychological Effects of 'Ecstasy' (MDMA) Use. National Drug and Alcohol Research Centre, University of New South Wales, 2010.

182. Cajanding RJM. MDMA-associated liver toxicity: pathophysiology, management, and current state of knowledge. *AACN Adv Crit Care* 2019;**30**(3):232–248. https://doi.org/10.4037/aacnacc2019852

183. Refstad S. Paramethoxyamphetamine (PMA) poisoning: a 'party drug' with lethal effects. *Acta Anaesthesiologica Scand* 2003;**47**:1298–1299. https://doi.org/10.1046/j.1399-6576.2003.00245.x

184. Giannikopoulos G, Stamoulis I, Panagi G, et al. P0494 severe hypoglycaemia, acute renal failure and rhabdomyolysis associated with the use of

185. Raviña P, Quiroga JM, Raviña T. Hyperkalemia in fatal MDMA ('ecstasy') toxicity. *Int J Cardiol* 2004;**93**(2):307–308.

186. Greene SL, Dargan PI, O'Connor N, Jones AL, Kerins M. Multiple toxicity from 3,4-methylenedioxymethamphetamine ('ecstasy'). *Am J Emerg Med* 2003;**21**(2):121–124.

187. Moore K, Wells H, Feilding A. Roadmaps to regulation: MDMA. *Br J Sociol* 2002;**53**(1):89–105.

188. Fineschi V, Masti A. Fatal poisoning by MDMA (ecstasy) and MDEA: a case report. *Int J Legal Med* 1996;**108**(5):272–275.

189. Liechti ME, Gamma A, Vollenweider FX. Gender differences in the subjective effects of MDMA. *Psychopharmacology* 2001;**154**(2):161–168.

190. Feio-Azevedo R, Costa VM, Barbosa DJ, et al. Aged rats are more vulnerable than adolescents to 'ecstasy'-induced toxicity. *Arch Toxicol* 2018;**92**:2275–2295. https://doi.org/10.1007/s00204-018-2226-8

191. Gouzoulis-Mayfrank E. The confounding problem of polydrug use in recreational ecstasy/MDMA users: a brief overview. *J Psychopharmacol* 2006;**20**(2):188–193.

192. Milroy CM. 'Ecstasy'-associated deaths: what is a fatal concentration? Analysis of a case series. *Forensic Sci Med Pathol* 2011;**7**(3):248–252.

193. Vecellio M, Schopper C, Modestin J. Neuropsychiatric consequences (atypical psychosis and complex-partial seizures) of ecstasy use: possible evidence for toxicity-vulnerability predictors and implications for preventative and clinical care. *J Psychopharmacol* 2003;**17**(3):342–345.

194. Kamour A, James D, Lupton DJ, et al. Patterns of presentation and clinical features of toxicity after reported use of ([2-aminopropyl]-2,3-dihydrobenzofurans), the 'benzofuran' compounds. A report from the United Kingdom National Poisons Information Service. *Clin Toxicol* 2014;**52**(10):1025–1031. https://doi.org/10.3109/15563650.2014.973115

195. Lin DL, Liu HC, Yin HL. Recent paramethoxymethamphetamine (PMMA) deaths in Taiwan. *J Anal Toxicol* 2007;**31**(2):109–113.

196. Gimeno Clemente C, Chiappini S, Claridge H, et al. The unregulated psychoactive compound: 'benzo fury'. *Curr Drug Abuse Rev* 2013;**6**(4):285.

197. Chan WL, Wood DM, Hudson S, Dargan PI. Acute psychosis associated with recreational use of benzofuran 6-(2-aminopropyl) benzofuran (6-APB) and cannabis. *J Med Toxicol* 2013;**9**(3):278–281. https://doi.org/10.1007/s13181-013-0306-y

198. Weinmann W, Bohnert M. Lethal monointoxication by overdosage of MDEA. *Forensic Sci Int* 1998;**91**(2):91–101.

199. Chen WH, Chui C, Yin HL. The antemortem neurobehavior in fatal paramethoxymethamphetamine usage. *Subst Abus* 2012;**33**(4):366–372.

200. Spatt J, Glawar B, Mamoli B. A pure amnestic syndrome after MDMA ('ecstasy') ingestion. *J Neurol Neurosurg Psychiatry* 1997;**62**(4):418.

201. Meehan TJ, Bryant SM, Aks SE. Drugs of abuse: the highs and lows of altered mental states in the emergency department. *Emerg Med Clin North Am* 2010;**28**(3):663–682. https://doi.org/10.1016/j. emc.2010.03.012

202. TOXBASE®. MDMA. www.toxbase.org

203. Drake WM, Broadhurst PA. QT-interval prolongation with ecstasy. *South African Med J* 1996;**86**(2):180–181.

204. Hartung TK, Schofield E, Short AI, Parr MJA, Henry JA. Hyponatraemic states following 3,4-methylenedioxymethamphetamine (MDMA, 'ecstasy') ingestion. *Q J Med* 2002;**95**:431–437.

205. Dowling GP, McDonough ET, Bost RO. 'Eve' and 'ecstasy': a report of five deaths associated with the use of MDEA and MDMA. *JAMA* 1987;**257**(12):1615–1617.

206. Madhok A, Boxer R, Chowdhury D. Atrial fibrillation in an adolescent – the agony of ecstasy. *Pediatr Emerg Care* 2003;**19**(5):348–349.

207. Qasim A, Townend J, Davies MK. Ecstasy-induced acute myocardial infarction. *Heart* 2001;**85**(6):e10.

208. Mutlu H, Silit E, Pekkafali Z, Incedayi M, Basekim C, Kizilkaya E. 'Ecstasy' (MDMA)-induced pneumomediastinum and epidural pneumatosis. *Diagn Interv Radiol* 2005;**11**(3):150–151.

209. Gungadeen A, Moor J. Extensive subcutaneous emphysema and pneumomediastinum after ecstasy ingestion. *Case Rep Otolaryngol* 2013;**2013**:795867. https://doi.org/10.1155/2013/795867

210. Clause AL, Coche E, Hantson P, Jacquet LM. Spontaneous pneumomediastinum and epidural pneumatosis after oral ecstasy consumption. *Acta Clinica Belgica* 2014;**69**(2):146–148.

211. James RA, Dinan A. Hyperpyrexia associated with fatal paramethoxyamphetamine (PMA) abuse. *Med Sci Law* 1998;**38**(1):83–88.

212. Els A, Coopman VAE, Cordonnier JACM, Piette MHA, Chemiphar NV. One fatal and seven nonfatal cases of 4-methylthioamphetamine (4-MTA) intoxication: clinico-pathological findings. In: A Els, Investigation of Fatalities Related to the Use of 3,4-Methylenedioxymethamphetamine (MDMA, 'Ecstasy') and Analogues: Anatomo-Pathological and Thanato-Toxicological Approach. PhD thesis, University of Ghent, 2002. Available at: http://lib.ugent.be/fulltxt/RUG01/000/745/574/RUG01-000745574_2010_0001_AC.pdf [last accessed 11 March 2022].

213. Pearson JM, Hargraves TL, Hair LS, et al. Three fatal intoxications due to methylone. *J Anal Toxicol* 2012;**36**(6):444–451. https://doi.org/10.1093/jat/bks043

214. Campbell GA, Rosner MH. The agony of ecstasy: MDMA (3,4-methylenedioxymethamphetamine) and the kidney. *Clin J Am Soc Nephrol* 2008;**3**(6):1852–1860. https://doi.org/10.2215/CJN.02080508

215. Watson JD. Exertional heat stroke induced by amphetamine analogues. *Anaesthesia* 1993;**48**(12):1057–1060.

216. Parrott AC. MDMA (3,4-methylenedioxymethamphetamine) or ecstasy: the neuropsychobiological implications of taking it at dances and raves. *Neuropsychobiology* 2004;**50**(4):329–335.

217. Kiyatkin EA. Critical role of peripheral vasoconstriction in fatal brain hyperthermia induced by MDMA (ecstasy) under conditions that mimic human drug use. *J Neurosci* 2014;**34**(23):7754–7762.

218. Chen Y, Tran HTN, Saber YH, Hall FS. High ambient temperature increases the toxicity and lethality of 3,4-methylenedioxymethamphetamine and methcathinone. *Pharmacol Biochem Behav* 2020;**192**:172912. https://doi.org/10.1016/j.pbb.2020.172912

219. Green AR. A review of the mechanisms involved in the acute MDMA (ecstasy)-induced hyperthermic response. *Eur J Pharmacol* 2004;**500**(1):3–13.

220. Hunt PA. Heat illness. *J R Army Med Corps* 2005;**151**(4):234–242.

221. Schütte JK, Schäfer U, Becker S, et al. 3,4-methylenedioxymethamphetamine induces a hyperthermic and hypermetabolic crisis in pigs with and without genetic disposition for malignant hyperthermia. *Eur J Anaesthesiol* 2013;**30**(1):29–37. https://doi.org/10.1097/EJA.0b013e32835a1127

222. Fritz-Patrick J, Pineau Mitchell A, Auzinger G. Too hot to handle: a case report of extreme pyrexia after MDMA ingestion. *Ther Hypothermia Temp Manag* 2018;**8**(3):173–175. https://doi.org/10.1089/ther.2018.0002

223. Pilgrim JL. Deaths involving MDMA and the concomitant use of pharmaceutical drugs. *J Analytic Toxicol* 2011;**35**(4):219–226.

224. Copeland JP. Ecstasy and the concomitant use of pharmaceuticals. *Addict Behav* 2006;**31**(2):367–370.

225. Pilgrim JL. Serotonin toxicity involving MDMA (ecstasy) and moclobemide. *Forensic Sci Int* 2012;**215**(1):184–188.

226. Advisory Council on the Misuse of Drugs (ACMD). Benzofurans: A Review of the Evidence of Use and Harm. Published 2013. Available at: https://assets.publishing.service.gov.uk/government/uploads/system/uploads/attachment_data/file/261783/Benzofuran_compounds_report.pdf [last accessed 23 April 2022].

227. Kraner JC, McCoy DJ, Evans MA, Evans LE, Sweeney BJ. Fatalities caused by the MDMA-related drug paramethoxyamphetamine (PMA). *J Anal Toxicol* 2001;**25**(7):645–648.

228. Baggott MJ, Garrison KJ, Coyle JR, et al. MDMA impairs response to water intake in healthy volunteers. *Adv Pharmacol Sci* 2016;**2016**:2175896. https://doi.org/10.1155/2016/2175896

229. Simmler LD, Hysek CM, Liechti ME. Sex differences in the effects of MDMA (ecstasy) on plasma copeptin in healthy subjects. *J Clin Endocrinol Metab* 2011;**96**(9):2844–2850. https://doi.org/10.1210/jc.2011-1143

230. Finch EL. Cerebral oedema after MDMA ('ecstasy') and unrestricted water intake. *Drug workers emphasise that water is not an antidote to drug.Br Med J* 1996;313(7058):690.

231. Chang JCYC. Late diagnosis of MDMA-related severe hyponatremia. *Case Rep Intern Med* 2014;1(2):153.

232. Virani S, Daya GN, Brainch N, et al. Persistent psychosis due to single dose of ecstasy. *Cureus* 2018;10(7):e3058. https://doi.org/10.7759/cureus.3058

233. Van Kampen J. Persistent psychosis after a single ingestion of 'ecstasy'. *Psychosomatics* 2001;42(6):525–527.

234. McGuire P, Fahy T. Chronic paranoid psychosis after misuse of MDMA ('ecstasy'). *Br Med J* 1991;302(6778):697.

235. Bramness JGM. Amphetamine-induced psychosis – a separate diagnostic entity or primary psychosis triggered in the vulnerable? *BMC Psychiatry* 2012;12(1):221.

236. Vaiva GV. An 'accidental' acute psychosis with ecstasy use. *J Psychoactive Drugs* 2001;33(1):95–98.

237. Rugani FS. Symptomatological features of patients with and without ecstasy use during their first psychotic episode. *Int J Environ Res Public Health* 2012;9(7):2283–2292.

238. Kim J, Fan B, Liu X, Kerner N, Wu P. Ecstasy use and suicidal behavior among adolescents: findings from a national survey. *Suicide Life Threat Behav* 2011;41:435–444.

239. Hinkelbein J, Gabel A, Volz M, Ellinger K. Suicide attempt with high-dose ecstasy. [Article in German.] *Der Anaesthesist* 2003;52(1):51–54.

240. Karlovšek MZ, Alibegovic A, Balažic J. Our experiences with fatal ecstasy abuse (two case reports). *Forensic Sci Int* 2005;147:S77–80.

241. Fernando T, Gilbert JD, Carroll CM, Byard RW. Ecstasy and suicide. *J Forensic Sci* 2012;57:1137–1139.

242. Rojek S, Małgorzata K, Strona M, Maciów M, Kula K. 'Legal highs' – toxicity in the clinical and medico-legal aspect as exemplified by suicide with bk-MBDB administration. *Forensic Sci Int* 2012;222(1):e1–e6.

243. Bonsignore A, Barranco R, Morando A, et al. MDMA-induced cardio-toxicity and pathological myocardial effects: a systematic review of experimental data and autopsy findings. *Cardiovasc Toxicol* 2019;19:493–499. https://doi.org/10.1007/s12012-019-09526-9

244. Hoggett KD. Ecstasy-induced acute coronary syndrome: something to rave about. *Emerg Med Australasia* 2012;24(3):339–342.

245. Mizia-Stec K, Gasior Z, Wojnicz R, et al. Severe dilated cardiomyopathy as a consequence of ecstasy intake. *Cardiovasc Pathol* 2008;17(4):250–253. https://doi.org/10.1016/j.carpath.2007.07.006

246. Rehman S, Khalid F, Kowsika S, Ghobrial I. As molly takes the party toll: MDMA toxicity presenting with pulmonary hemorrhage. *Am J Resp Crit Care Med* 2020;201:A1616.

247. Stull BW. Spontaneous pneumomediastinum following ecstasy ingestion and sexual intercourse. *Emerg Med J* 2008;25(2):113–114.

248. Marasco SF. Ecstasy-associated pneumomediastinum. *Ann R Coll Surg Engl* 2007;89(4):389.

249. Kahn DE. 3 cases of primary intracranial hemorrhage associated with 'Molly', a purified form of 3,4-methylenedioxymethamphetamine (MDMA). *J Neurol Sci* 2012;323(1):257–260.

250. Wong S, Afshani M. Intracranial vascular complications of 'molly' usage: case report and review of the literature. *Conn Med* 2016;80(8):467–469.

251. Garbino JJ. Ecstasy ingestion and fulminant hepatic failure: liver transplantation to be considered as a last therapeutic option. *Vet Hum Toxicol* 2001;43(2):99–102.

252. Seymour HG. Severe ketoacidosis complicated by 'ecstasy' ingestion and prolonged exercise. *Diabet Med* 1996;13:908–909.

253. Gama MP. Diabetic ketoacidosis complicated by the use of ecstasy: a case report. *J Med Case Rep* 2010;4(1):240.

254. Johnson MP, Nichols DE. Combined administration of a non-neurotoxic 3,4-methylenedioxymethamphetamine analogue with amphetamine produces serotonin neurotoxicity in rats. *Neuropharmacology* 1991;30(7):819–822.

255. Vanattou-Saïfoudine NR. Caffeine promotes dopamine D1 receptor-mediated body temperature, heart rate and behavioural responses to MDMA ('ecstasy'). *Psychopharmacology* 2010;211(1):15–25.

256. Papaseit E, Vázquez A, Pérez-Mañá C, et al. Surviving life-threatening MDMA (3,4-methylenedioxymethamphetamine, ecstasy) toxicity caused by ritonavir (RTV). *Intensive Care Med* 2012;38(7):1239–1240. https://doi.org/10.1007/s00134-012-2537-9

257. Antolino-Lobo I, Meulenbelt J, Nijmeijer SM, et al. 3,4-methylenedioxymethamphetamine (MDMA) interacts with therapeutic drugs on CYP3A by inhibition of pregnane X receptor (PXR) activation and catalytic enzyme inhibition. *Toxicol Lett* 2011;203(1):82–91. https://doi.org/10.1016/j.toxlet.2011.03.007

258. Davies N, English W, Grundlingh J. MDMA toxicity: management of acute and life-threatening presentations. *Br J Nurs* 2018;27(11):616–622.

259. Grunau BE, Wiens MO, Brubacher JR. Dantrolene in the treatment of MDMA-related hyperpyrexia: a systematic review. *CJEM* 2010;12(5):435–442.

260. Banks ML, Sprague JE. From bench to bedside: understanding the science behind the pharmacologic management of MDMA and other sympathomimetic-mediated hyperthermia. *J Pharm Technology.* 2011;27(3):123–31.

261. Kiyatkin EA, Ren S, Wakabayashi KT, Baumann MH, Shaham Y. Clinically relevant pharmacological strategies that reverse MDMA-induced brain hyperthermia potentiated by social interaction. *Neuropsychopharmacology* 2016;41:549–559.

262. Voizeux P, Lewandowski R, Daily T, et al. Case of cardiac arrest treated with extra-corporeal life support after MDMA

intoxication. *Case Rep Crit Care* 2019;**2019**:7825915. https://doi.org/10.1155/2019/7825915

263. Chu FK, Ming Yim AK, Ng SW. A case series of life-threatening 3,4-methylenedioxyamphetamine (MDMA) poisoning in an electronic dance music party in Hong Kong. *Asia Pac J Med Toxicol* 2018;**7**:3. http://apjmt.mums.ac.ir

264. Parrott AC. Residual neurocognitive features of ecstasy use: a re-interpretation of Halpern et al. (2011) consistent with serotonergic neurotoxicity. *Addiction* 2011;**106** (7):1365–1368.

265. Green D, Barry P, Green HD. Central cyanosis on a psychiatric unit treated at the Salford Royal Hospital. *Thorax* 2014;**69** (12):1157–1158. https://doi.org/10.1136/thoraxjnl-2014-205769

266. Di Iorio CR, Watkins TJ, Dietrich MS, et al. Evidence for chronically altered serotonin function in the cerebral cortex of female 3,4-methylenedioxymethamphetamine polydrug users. *Arch Gen Psychiatry* 2012;**69**(4):399–409. https://doi.org/10.1001/archgenpsychiatry.2011.156

267. Benningfield MM, Cowan RL. Brain serotonin function in MDMA (ecstasy) users: evidence for persisting neurotoxicity. *Neuropsychopharmacology* 2013;**38**(1):253–255.

268. Kish SJ, Lerch J, Furukawa Y, et al. Decreased cerebral cortical serotonin transporter binding in ecstasy users: a positron emission tomography/[(11)C] DASB and structural brain imaging study. *Brain* 2010;**133**(Pt 6):1779–1997. https://doi.org10.1093/brain/ awq103

269. Bauernfeind AL, Dietrich MS, Blackford JU, et al. Human ecstasy use is associated with increased cortical excitability: an fMRI study. *Neuropsychopharmacology* 2011;**36** (6):1127–1141. https://doi.org/10.1038/npp.2010.244

270. Urban NB, Girgis RR, Talbot PS, et al. Sustained recreational use of ecstasy is associated with altered pre and postsynaptic markers of serotonin transmission in neocortical areas: a PET study with [^{11}C]DASB and [^{11}C]MDL 100907. *Neuropsychopharmacology* 2012;**37**(6):1465–1473. https://doi.org/10.1038/npp.2011.332

271. Booij L, Soucy JP, Young SN, et al. Brain serotonin synthesis in MDMA (ecstasy) polydrug users: an alpha-[11C] methyl-tryptophan study. *J Neurochem* 2014;**131**(5):634–644. https://doi.org/10.1111/jnc.12826

272. McCann UD, Szabo Z, Vranesic M, et al. Positron emission tomographic studies of brain dopamine and serotonin transporters in abstinent (±) 3,4-methylenedioxymethamphetamine ('ecstasy') users: relationship to cognitive performance. *Psychopharmacology* 2008;**200**(3):439–450. https://doi.org/10.1007/s00213-008-1218-4

273. Bosch OG, Wagner M, Jessen F, et al. Verbal memory deficits are correlated with prefrontal hypometabolism in 18FDG PET of recreational MDMA users. *PLoS ONE* 2013;**8**(4):e61234. https://doi.org/10.1371/journal.pone.0061234

274. Gouzoulis-Mayfrank E, Daumann J. Neurotoxicity of methylenedioxyamphetamines (MDMA; ecstasy) in humans: how strong is the evidence for persistent brain damage? *Addiction* 2006;**101**(3):348–361.

275. Clemens KJ, McGregor IS, Hunt GE, Cornish JL. MDMA, methamphetamine and their combination: possible lessons for party drug users from recent preclinical research. *Drug Alcohol Rev* 2007;**26**(1):9–15.

276. Biezonski DK, Meyer JS. The nature of 3,4-methylenedioxymethamphetamine (MDMA)-induced serotonergic dysfunction: evidence for and against the neurodegeneration hypothesis. *Curr Neuropharmacol* 2011;**9** (1):84.

277. Krebs TS, Pål-Ørjan J. Methodological weaknesses in non-randomized studies of ecstasy (MDMA) use: a cautionary note to readers and reviewers. *Neuropsychopharmacology* 2012;**37**(4):1070.

278. Erritzoe D, Frokjaer VG, Holst KK, et al. In vivo imaging of cerebral serotonin transporter and serotonin2a receptor binding in 3,4-methylenedioxymethamphetamine (MDMA or 'ecstasy') and hallucinogen users. *Arch Gen Psychiatry* 2011;**68** (6):562–576. https://doi.org/10.1001/archgenpsychiatry.2011.56

279. Adamaszek M, Khaw AV, Buck U, Andresen B, Thomasius R. Evidence of neurotoxicity of ecstasy: sustained effects on electroencephalographic activity in polydrug users. *PLoS ONE* 2010;**5**(11):e14097. https://doi.org/10.1371/journal.pone.0014097

280. de Win MM. Sustained effects of ecstasy on the human brain: a prospective neuroimaging study in novel users. *Brain* 2008;**131**(11):2936–2945.

281. Thomasius R, Zapletalova P, Petersen K, et al. Mood, cognition and serotonin transporter availability in current and former ecstasy (MDMA) users: the longitudinal perspective. *J Psychopharmacol* 2006;**20**(2):211–225.

282. Parrott AC. MDMA and 5-HT neurotoxicity: the empirical evidence for its adverse effects in humans – no need for translation. *Br J Pharmacol* 2012;**166**(5):1518–1520; discussion 1521–1522. https://doi.org/10.1111/j.1476-5381.2012.01941.x

283. Peraile I, Granado N, Torres E, et al. Cocaine potentiates MDMA-induced oxidative stress but not dopaminergic neurotoxicity in mice: implications for the pathogenesis of free radical-induced neurodegenerative disorders. *Psychopharmacology* 2013;**230**(1):125–135. https://doi.org/10.1007/s00213-013-3142-5

284. Angoa-Pérez M, Kane MJ, Briggs DI, et al. Mephedrone does not damage dopamine nerve endings of the striatum, but enhances the neurotoxicity of methamphetamine, amphetamine, and MDMA. *J Neurochem* 2013;**125** (1):102–110. https://doi.org/10.1111/jnc.12114

285. Klomp A, den Hollander B, de Bruin K, Booij J, Reneman L. The effects of ecstasy (MDMA) on brain serotonin transporters are dependent on age-of-first exposure in recreational users and animals. *PLoS ONE* 2012;**7**(10): e47524. https://doi.org/10.1371/journal.pone.0047524

286. Huang X, Marona-Lewicka D, Nichols DE. p-Methylthioamphetamine is a potent new non-neurotoxic serotonin-releasing agent. *Eur J Pharmacol* 1992;**229**(1):31–38.

287. Nichols DE, Johnson MP, Oberlender R. 5-iodo-2-aminoindan, a nonneurotoxic analogue of

piodoamphetamine. *Pharmacol Biochem Behav* 1991;**38** (1):135–139.

288. Nichols DE, Marona-Lewicka D, Huang X, Johnson MP. Novel serotonergic agents. *Drug Des Discov* 1993;**9**(3–4):299–312.

289. Wagner D, Becker B, Koester P, Gouzoulis-Mayfrank E, Daumann J. A prospective study of learning, memory, and executive function in new MDMA users. *Addiction* 2013;**108** (1):136–145.

290. Schilt T, de Win MM, Koeter M, et al. Cognition in novice ecstasy users with minimal exposure to other drugs: a prospective cohort study. *Arch Gen Psychiatry* 2007;**64** (6):728–736.

291. Halpern JH, Sherwood AR, Hudson JI, Gruber S, Kozin D, Pope Jr HG. Residual neurocognitive features of long-term ecstasy users with minimal exposure to other drugs. *Addiction* 2011;**106**:777–786.

292. Taurah L, Chandler C, Sanders G. Depression, impulsiveness, sleep, and memory in past and present polydrug users of 3,4-methylenedioxymethamphetamine (MDMA, ecstasy). *Psychopharmacology* 2014;**231**(4):737–751.

293. Gerra G, Zaimovic A, Ampollini R, et al. Experimentally induced aggressive behavior in subjects with 3,4-methylenedioxy-methamphetamine ('Ecstasy') use history: psychobiological correlates. *J Subst Abuse* 2001;**13** (4):471–491.

294. Wetherell MA, Montgomery C. Basal functioning of the hypothalamic-pituitary-adrenal (HPA) axis and psychological distress in recreational ecstasy polydrug users. *Psychopharmacology* 2014;**231**(7):1365–1375.

295. Parrott AC, Montgomery C, Wetherell MA, Downey LA, Stough C, Scholey AB. MDMA, cortisol, and heightened stress in recreational ecstasy users. *Behav Pharmacol* 2014;**25**(5–6):458–472. https://doi.org/10.1097/FBP.0000000000000060

296. Sumnall HR, Cole JC. Self-reported depressive symptomatology in community samples of polysubstance misusers who report ecstasy use: a meta-analysis. *J Psychopharmacol* 2005;**19**(1):84–92.

297. Brière FN, Fallu JS, Janosz M, Pagani LS. Prospective associations between meth/amphetamine (speed) and MDMA (ecstasy) use and depressive symptoms in secondary school students. *J Epidemiol Community Health* 2012;**66** (11):990–994. https://doi.org/10.1136/jech-2011-200706

298. McCann M, Higgins K, Perra O, McCartan C, McLaughlin A. Adolescent ecstasy use and depression: cause and effect, or two outcomes of home environment? *Eur J Public Health* 2014;**24** (5):845–850. https://doi.org/10.1093/eurpub/cku062

299. Scott RM, Hides L, Allen JS, Burke R, Lubman DI. Depressive and anxiety symptomatology in ecstasy users: the relative contribution of genes, trauma, life stress and drug use. *Psychopharmacology* 2010;**209**(1):25–36. https://doi.org/10 .1007/s00213-009-1763-5

300. Soar K, Turner JJD, Parrott AC. Psychiatric disorders in ecstasy (MDMA) users: a literature review focusing on

personal predisposition and drug history. *Hum Psychopharmacol* 2001;**16**(8):641–645.

301. Bedi G, Van Dam NT, Redman J. Ecstasy (MDMA) and high prevalence psychiatric symptomatology: somatic anxiety symptoms are associated with polydrug, not ecstasy, use. *J Psychopharmacol* 2010;**24**(2):233–240. https://doi.org/10 .1177/0269881108097631

302. Daumann J, Hensen G, Thimm B, Rezk M, Till B, Gouzoulis-Mayfrank E. Self-reported psychopathological symptoms in recreational ecstasy (MDMA) users are mainly associated with regular cannabis use: further evidence from a combined cross-sectional/longitudinal investigation. *Psychopharmacology* 2004;**173**(3–4):398–404.

303. Thomasius R, Petersen KU, Zapletalova P, Wartberg L, Zeichner D, Schmoldt A. Mental disorders in current and former heavy ecstasy (MDMA) users. *Addiction* 2005;**100**:1310–1319.

304. Marchesi C, Tonna M, Maggini C. Obsessive-compulsive disorder followed by psychotic episode in long-term ecstasy misuse. *World J Biol Psychiatry* 2009;**10**(4–2): 599–602.

305. Home Office. Drugs Misuse: Findings from the 2018/19 Crime Survey for England and Wales Statistical Bulletin: 21/19. Published September 2019.

306. Miller JM, Vorel SR, Tranguch AJ, et al. Anhedonia after a selective bilateral lesion of the globus pallidus. *Am J Psychiatry* 2006;**163**(5):786–788.

307. Kouimtsidis CF. Neurological and psychopathological sequelae associated with a lifetime intake of 40,000 ecstasy tablets. *Psychosomatics* 2006;**47**(1):86–87.

308. Kirkpatrick MG, Baggott MJ, Mendelson JE, et al. MDMA effects consistent across laboratories. *Psychopharmacology* 2014;**231**(19):3899–3905. https://doi.org/10.1007/s00213-014-3528-z

309. O'Sullivan A, Parrott AC. Deteriorating cost–benefit ratios for ecstasy/MDMA with repeated usage. *Open Addiction J* 2011;**4**:38–39.

310. European Monitoring Centre for Drugs and Drug Addiction. European Drug Report 2019: Trends and Developments. Luxembourg, Publications Office of the European Union, 2019.

311. Degenhardt L, Bruno R, Topp L. Is ecstasy a drug of dependence? *Drug Alcohol Depend* 2010;**107**:1–10.

312. Uosukainen H, Tacke U, Winstock AR. Self-reported prevalence of dependence of MDMA compared to cocaine, mephedrone and ketamine among a sample of recreational poly-drug users. *Int J Drug Policy* 2015;**26**(1):78–83. https://doi .org/10.1016/j.drugpo.2014.07.004

313. Bruno R, Matthews AJ, Topp L, Degenhardt L, Gomez R, Dunn M. Can the severity of dependence scale be usefully applied to 'ecstasy'? *Neuropsychobiology* 2009;**60**(3–4):137–147. https://doi.org/10.1159/ 000253550

314. Cottler LB, Womack SB, Compton WM, Ben-Abdallah A. Ecstasy abuse and dependence among adolescents and young adults: applicability and reliability of DSM-IV criteria. *Hum Psychopharmacol Clin Exp* 2001;**16**:599–606.

315. Yen C, Hsu S. Symptoms of ecstasy dependence and correlation with psychopathology in Taiwanese adolescents. *J Nerv Ment Dis* 2007;**195**:866–869.

316. Scheier L, Abdullah A, Inciardi J, Copeland J, Cottler L. Tri-city study of ecstasy use problems: a latent class analysis. *Drug Alcohol Depend* 2008;**98**:249–263.

317. Abdallah A, Scheier L, Inciardi J, Copeland J, Cottler L. A psycho-economic model of ecstasy consumption and related consequences: a multi-site study with community samples. *Subst Use Misuse* 2007;**42**:1651–1684.

318. Winstock AR. Drugs and the dance music scene: a survey of current drug use patterns among a sample of dance music enthusiasts in the UK. *Drug Alcohol Depend* 2001;**64**(1):9–17.

319. Milani RM, Turner J, Parrott AC. The contribution of ecstasy dependence and stress to ecstasy-/MDMA-related psychiatric symptoms. *Open Addict J* 2011;**4**:28–29.

320. Topp L, Hall W, Hando J. Is There a Dependence Syndrome for Ecstasy? (National Drug and Alcohol Research Centre Technical Report No. 51). NDARC, 1997.

321. Parrott AC. Chronic tolerance to recreational MDMA (3,4-methylenedioxymethamphetamine) or ecstasy. *J Psychopharmacol* 2005;**19**:71–83.

322. McKetin R, Copeland J, Norberg MM, Bruno R, Hides L, Khawar L. The effect of the ecstasy 'comedown' on the diagnosis of ecstasy dependence. *Drug Alcohol Depend* 2014;**139**:26–32. https://doi.org/10.1016/j.drugalcdep.2014.02.697

323. Schenk S. MDMA self-administration in laboratory animals: a summary of the literature and proposal for future research. *Neuropsychobiology* 2009;**60**(3–4):130.

324. Public Health England. Drug Statistics from the National Drug Treatment Monitoring System (NDTMS): 2012–2013. PHE, 2013.

325. Wu LT, Parrott AC, Ringwalt CL, Patkar AA, Mannelli P, Blazer DG. The high prevalence of substance use disorders among recent MDMA users compared with other drug users: implications for intervention. *Addict Behav* 2009;**34**(8):654–661. https://doi.org/10.1016/j.addbeh.2009.03.029

326. Carhart-Harris RL, Nutt DJ, Munafo MR, Christmas DM, Wilson SJ. Equivalent effects of acute tryptophan depletion on REM sleep in ecstasy users and controls. *Psychopharmacology* 2009;**206**(2):187–196.

327. McCann UD. Effects of (±) 3,4-methylenedioxymethamphetamine (MDMA) on sleep and circadian rhythms. *Scientific World J* 2007;**7**:231–238.

328. Smithies V, Broadbear J, Verdejo-Garcia A, Conduit R. Dysfunctional overnight memory consolidation in ecstasy users. *J Psychopharmacol* 2014;**28**(8):751–762.

329. Gledhill JA. Subarachnoid haemorrhage associated with MDMA abuse. *J Neurol Neurosurg Psychiatry* 1993;**56**(9):1036.

330. Karch SB. A historical review of MDMA. *Open Forensic Sci J* 2011;**4**:20–24.

331. Droogmans SB. Possible association between 3,4-methylenedioxymethamphetamine abuse and valvular heart disease. *Am J Cardiol* (2007);**100**(9):1442–1445.

332. Bhattacharyya SA. Drug-induced fibrotic valvular heart disease. *Lancet* 2009;**374**(9689):577–585.

333. Montastruc F, Montastruc G, Vigreux P, et al. Valvular heart disease in a patient taking 3,4-methylenedioxymethamphetamine (MDMA, 'ecstasy'). *Br J Clin Pharmacol* 2012;**74**(3):547–548. https://doi.org/10.1111/j.1365-2125.2012.04252.x

334. Patel MM, Belson MG, Wright D, Lu H, Heninger M, Miller MA. Methylenedioxymethamphetamine (ecstasy)-related myocardial hypertrophy: an autopsy study. *Resuscitation* 2005;**66**(2):197–202.

335. Marsden J, Stillwell G, Barlow H, et al. An evaluation of a brief motivational intervention among young ecstasy and cocaine users: no effect on substance and alcohol use outcomes. *Addiction* 2006;**101**(7):1014–1026.

336. Norberg MM, Hides L, Olivier J, Khawar L, McKetin R, Copeland J. Brief interventions to reduce ecstasy use: a multi-site randomized controlled trial. *Behav Ther* 2014;**45**(6):745–759. https://doi.org/10.1016/j.beth.2014.05.006

337. Martin G, Copeland J. Brief intervention for regular ecstasy (MDMA) users: pilot randomized trial of a check-up model. *J Subst Use* 2010;**15**(2):131–142.

338. Fox HC. Ecstasy use: cognitive deficits related to dosage rather than self-reported problematic use of the drug. *J Psychopharmacol* 2001;**15**(4):273–281.

339. Larkin M. Dangerous sports and recreational drug use: rationalizing and contextualizing risk. *J Community Applied Social Psychol* 2004;**14**(4):215–232.

340. Gamma AL. Is ecstasy perceived to be safe? A critical survey. *Drug Alcohol Depend* 2005;**77**(2):185–193.

341. Baggott MJ. Preventing problems in ecstasy users: reduce use to reduce harm. *J Psychoactive Drugs* 2002;**34**(2):145–162.

342. Davies C, Murray R, eds. United Kingdom Drug Situation: Annual Report to the European Monitoring Centre for Drugs and Drug Addiction (EMCDDA), 2013. United Kingdom Focal Point at Public Health England, 2013.

343. Liechti ME. Acute psychological effects of 3,4-methylenedioxymethamphetamine (MDMA, 'ecstasy') are attenuated by the serotonin uptake inhibitor citalopram. *Neuropsychopharmacology* 2000;**22**(5):513–521.

344. Piper BJ. Dissociation of the neurochemical and behavioral toxicology of MDMA ('ecstasy') by citalopram. *Neuropsychopharmacology* 2007;**33**(5):1192–1205.

345. Fisk JE, Murphy PN, Montgomery C, Hadjiefthyvoulou F. Modelling the adverse effects associated with ecstasy use. *Addiction* 2011;**106**(4):798–805. https://doi.org/10.1111/j.1360-0443.2010.03272.x

346. Vanden Eede H, Montenij LJ, Touw DJ, Norris EM. Rhabdomyolysis in MDMA intoxication: a rapid and underestimated killer. 'Clean' ecstasy, a safe party drug?

J Emerg Med 2012;**42**(6):655–658. https://doi.org/10.1016/j
.jemermed.2009.04.057

347. Advisory Council on the Misuse of Drugs (ACMD). 6-APB and 5-APB: A Review of the Evidence of Use and Harm. Published 2013. Available at: https://assets.publishing.service.gov.uk/gov ernment/uploads/system/uploads/attachment_data/file/261783 /Benzofuran_compounds_report.pdf [last accessed 23 April 2022].

348. Sainsbury PD, Kicman AT, Archer RP, King LA, Braithwaite RA. Aminoindanes – the next wave of 'legal highs'? *Drug Test Anal* 2011;**3**(7–8):479–482. https://doi.org/ 10.1002/dta.318

349. Barceló B, Gomila I, Rotolo MC, et al. Intoxication caused by new psychostimulants: analytical methods to disclose acute and chronic use of benzofurans and ethylphenidate. *Int J Legal Med* 2017;**131**:1543–1553. https://doi.org/10.1007/s00414-01 7-1648-9

350. Advisory Council on the Misuse of Drugs (ACMD). Benzofurans: A Review of the Evidence of Use and Harm. Published 2013. Available at: https://assets .publishing.service.gov.uk/government/uploads/system/uploads/ attachment_data/file/261783/Benzofuran_compounds_report .pdf [last accessed 23 April 2022].

351. Jebadurai J, Schifano F, Deluca P. Recreational use of 1-(2-naphthyl)-2-(1-pyrrolidinyl)-1-pentanone hydrochloride (NRG-1), 6-(2-aminopropyl) benzofuran (Benzofury/6-APB) and NRG-2 with review of available evidence-based literature. *Hum Psychopharmacol Clin Exp* 2013;**28**(4):356–364.

352. Iversen L, Gibbons S, Treble R, Setola V, Huang XP, Roth BL. Neurochemical profiles of some novel psychoactive substances. *Eur J Pharmacol* 2013; **700**(1–3): 147–151. https:// doi.org/10.1016/j. ejphar.2012.12.006

353. Dawson P, Opacka-Juffry J, Moffatt JD, et al. The effects of benzofury (5-APB) on the dopamine transporter and 5-HT2-dependent vasoconstriction in the rat. *Prog Neuropsychopharmacol Biol Psychiatry* 2014;**48**:57–63.

354. Baron M, Elie M, Elie L. An analysis of legal highs – do they contain what it says on the tin? *Drug Test Anal* 2011;**3** (9):576–581

355. Barceló B, Gomila I, Rotolo MC, et al.Intoxication caused by new psychostimulants: analytical methods to disclose acute and chronic use of benzofurans and ethylphenidate. *Int J Legal Med* 2017;**131**:1543–1553. https://doi.org/10.1007/s00414-01 7-1648-9

356. Greene SL. Benzofurans and benzodifurans. In: PIDargan, DM Wood, eds., *Novel Psychoactive Substances: Classification, Pharmacology and Toxicology.* Oxford, Elsevier, 2013.

357. Hölzemann G, Böttcher H, Schiemann K, et al. Benzofuran compounds and their use as antidepressants and anxiolytics. US Patent No. 7,262,216 (28 August 2007).

358. Chan WL, Wood DM, Hudson S, Dargan PI. Acute psychosis associated with recreational use of benzofuran 6-(2-aminopropyl)benzofuran (6-APB) and cannabis. *J Med Toxicol* 2013;**9**:278–281. https://doi.org/10.1007/s13181-013-0306-y

359. Barceló B, Gomila I, Rotolo MC, et al.Intoxication caused by new psychostimulants: analytical methods to disclose acute and chronic use of benzofurans and ethylphenidate. *Int J Legal Med* 2017;**131**:1543–1553. https://doi.org/10.1007/s00414-01 7-1648-9

360. Roque Bravo R, Carmo H, Carvalho F, Dias da Silva D. Benzo fury: a new trend in the drug misuse scene. *J Appl Toxicol* 2019;**39**(8):1083–1095.

361. Liechti M. Novel psychoactive substances (designer drugs): overview and pharmacology of modulators of monoamine signalling. *Swiss Med Wkly* 2015;**45**:w14043.

362. Hofer KE, Faber K, Müller DM, et al. Acute toxicity associated with the recreational use of the novel psychoactive benzofuran N-methyl-5-(2 aminopropyl)benzofuran. *Ann Emerg Med* 2017;**69**(1):79–82. https://doi.org/10.1016/j .annemergmed.2016.03.042

363. Rothman RB, Baumann MH, Savage JE, et al. Evidence for possible involvement of 5-HT(2B) receptors in the cardiac vulvulopathy associated with fenfluramine and other serotonergic medications. *Circulation* 2000;**102**:2836–2841.

364. Dawson PO, Moffott JD. Cardiovascular toxicity of novel psychoactive drugs: lessons from the past. *Prog Neuropsychopharm Biol Pschiatr* 2012;**39**:244–252.

Methamphetamine

10.1 Introduction

It has been argued that globally, methamphetamine use represents the greatest challenge from all synthetic drugs. Whereas the highest prevalence of its use continues to be the US, where some commentators are suggesting it is developing into an epidemic,[1] new markets are emerging in many parts of the world, with Southeast Asia currently emerging as the world's fastest-growing methamphetamine market.[2]

10.2 Street Names

Street names at the time of publication include Crystal Meth, Tina, Christine, Ice, Glass, Crank, Yaba and Crazy Medicine. Other street names may be used locally.

10.3 Legal Status

Methamphetamine is placed in Schedule II of the United Nations Convention on Psychotropic Substances.

10.4 Quality of the Research Evidence

There is a much larger and more robust body of evidence on methamphetamine harms and treatment than for other club drugs. This includes a number of well conducted randomised controlled trials (RCTs) and Cochrane reviews, especially in relation to dependence.

However, most of the research evidence on methamphetamine comes from the US, Australia and Southeast Asia. European research is much more limited, reflecting the currently low rates of use across most of Europe. Some of the findings of international studies may be less relevant in a European context, especially those relating to epidemiology and trends.

10.5 Brief Overview of Pharmacology

Methamphetamine is an N,α-dimethylphenethylamine and a member of the phenethylamine family. It is a synthetic stimulant and a derivative of amphetamine.[3] Methamphetamine is a potent psychomotor stimulant with strong physiological effects on the peripheral and central nervous systems, resulting in physical and psychological effects.[4] It is typically described as a more potent stimulant than non-methylated amphetamines. It is highly lipophilic, and in comparison to amphetamine at similar doses, crosses the blood–brain barrier more easily, is more potent and has a more pronounced and a longer-lasting stimulant effect.[5] Methamphetamine has short-term and long-term effects that are similar to those produced by cocaine, but they last longer and can be more severe.[6]

The action of methamphetamine and other amphetamines have been well described.[5,7,8,9] Methamphetamine increases the activity of the noradrenergic and dopamine neurotransmitter systems. It increases the release and blocks the reuptake of dopamine. It has an active metabolite, amphetamine, and two inactive metabolites, p-OH-amphetamine and noradrenaline. It is oxidised and metabolised in the liver through enzymatic degradation primarily involving cytochrome P450-2D6. Approximately 10% of Caucasians are deficient in this enzyme, and a study has suggested that this makes them particularly sensitive to the effects of methamphetamine, as they lack the ability to metabolise and excrete the drug efficiently.[10]

Chronic methamphetamine alters brain function. Brain imaging studies have shown changes in the activity of the dopamine system that are associated with reduced motor skills and impaired verbal learning.[11] Imaging studies of methamphetamine-dependent individuals have found structural abnormalities: severe grey-matter deficits in the cingulate, limbic and paralimbic cortices, smaller hippocampal volumes, significant white-matter hypertrophy, medial temporal lobe damage and striatal enlargement.[12,13]

Studies have also shown severe structural and functional changes in areas of the brain associated with emotion and memory,[14,14] as well as neurochemical and metabolite changes in the ventral striatum.[15,16] Prolonged use has been reported to lead to downregulation of dopamine D2 receptors and uptake sites.[17] A state of hypo-dopaminergic activity has been reported.[18,19]

The psychiatric consequences of methamphetamine use are theorised to be secondary to its mechanisms of action: methamphetamine enters the synaptic neurons via monoamine transporters and, once in the neurons, displaces the monoamines from vesicular and intracellular locations, pushing the monoamines into the extra-neuronal spaces. Long-term use is associated with alterations in the levels of monoamines implicated with stimulant use, which include noradrenaline, serotonin and dopamine.[20,21]

10.6 Clinical and Other Legitimate Uses of Methamphetamine

Methamphetamine has been used in the US for the treatment of narcolepsy and attention deficit hyperactivity disorder (ADHD) and short-term treatment for exogenous obesity.[22]

10.7 Prevalence and Patterns of Use

Methamphetamine is one of the most widely misused drugs in the world, with over 35 million users estimated. Whereas the drug has been established in countries, such as the US, for a number of years, more recently the use of methamphetamine has been rising in many regions.

The methamphetamine market has been expanding, in particular in the two largest 'demand regions': Southeast Asia and North America. Southeast Asia emerges as the world's fastest-growing methamphetamine market, with quantities seized in East and Southeast Asia rising more than eightfold between 2007 and 2017. Other areas where methamphetamine is one of the predominant stimulant drugs used include Southwest Asia, Africa, North America, Central Asia and Trans-Caucasia, Australia and New Zealand.[23] More recently, there have been signs of growth of the methamphetamine market in Iraq and in Afghanistan, where it is increasingly manufactured.[24]

At a European level, the use of methamphetamine has historically been low in comparison with other stimulant drugs, and mainly found in a few countries with long-standing problems, including the Czechia and more recently Slovakia. However, the availability of methamphetamine has been slowly increasing and spreading geographically in other European countries, but it is still much lower than that of amphetamine.[25,26,27] In wastewater analysis carried out in 2018 and 2019, of the 42 cities that have data on methamphetamine in wastewater, 17 reported an increase, 16 a stable situation and 9 a decrease.[28]

An analysis of syringes in six European cities found methamphetamine in combinations of two or more stimulants (cocaine, amphetamine, methamphetamine or synthetic cathinone) were not uncommon and overall appeared in 10% of syringes (4% in Budapest, 5% in Paris, and 6% in Glasgow). This was particularly so in Helsinki, where 32% of syringes contained the residues of a mixture of stimulants, mostly of amphetamine and methamphetamine. Interestingly, it was also found in Helsinki that in the Finnish capital, half of the syringes containing traces of benzodiazepines tested positive for methamphetamine.[29]

Treatment entrants reporting primary methamphetamine use in Europe are concentrated in the Czech Republic, Slovakia, Poland and Turkey, which together account for 92% of the 8,300 methamphetamine clients reported in 2018.[30]

Similar figures have been reported by the 2020 European Drug Report which states that in Czechia, high-risk methamphetamine use among adults (15–64) was estimated at 0.50% in 2018 (corresponding to 33,500 users). In Slovakia, the prevalence derived from a treatment multiplier was estimated at 0.15% in 2018. The estimate for Cyprus was 0.03% or 155 high-risk methamphetamine users in 2018.[31] In the Czech Republic the consumption of methamphetamine has been firmly established for many years. By 2013, there were approximately 44,900 problem drug users in the Czech Republic, the majority of whom were methamphetamine users (34,200 methamphetamine users, compared to an estimated 10,700 opiate/opioid users).[32,33]

In the Czech Republic, methamphetamine is mainly produced in small-scale domestic cooking laboratories. (so-called kitchen laboratories) by users for their own or local use.[34] Home-produced methamphetamine powder is based on ephedrine and pseudoephedrine extracted from over-the-counter pharmaceutical products or, more recently, medicines imported from neighbouring countries.[35]

10.7.1 Population Sub-groups Using Methamphetamine

In Europe at the current time, methamphetamine is used by varied population sub-groups, ranging from socially integrated users who snort or swallow the drug, to marginalised users who inject or smoke methamphetamine.[36]

The demographic profile of methamphetamine users may change over time. For example, US and other studies have shown a change over time in the sociodemographic characteristics of methamphetamine users. A study of treatment admissions from the California Alcohol and Drug Data System from 1992 to 2002 showed not only a fivefold increase of methamphetamine admission, but also a shift towards usage by minority ethnic groups and a more vulnerable population in terms of homelessness, chronic mental health problems and disability. There was also a substantial increase in people reporting a legal supervision status (criminal justice intervention).[37]

A recent report from the US on data from the 2015–2018 National Surveys on Drug Use and Health (NSDUHs) has reported concerns about high rates of co-occurring substance use and/or? mental illness among adults using methamphetamine.[38]

10.7.1.1   Problem Drug Users

In Europe and specifically the Czech Republic and Slovakia, data show that there has been a spread of 'pervitin' (methamphetamine street name) use among problem drug users, which is reflected in increases in problem drug use estimates and in the number of people entering treatment for the first time who report 'pervitin' problems.[39] Frequent methamphetamine use was associated with injecting, sharing injecting paraphernalia, criminal behaviour and depression symptoms.[40]

A number of other European countries have also reported methamphetamine use, including Germany and in Norway where methamphetamine use appears to be interlinked with the older, more established amphetamine market. However, this is not always the case. The smoking of methamphetamine by injecting opioid users has been noted in Greece, and to a lesser extent Cyprus and Turkey.[41]

The increase in the use of methamphetamines by people admitted to heroin treatment has also been reported in the US, whereby a study has shown an increase from 1 in 50 primary heroin treatment admissions in 2008 to 1 in 12 admissions in 2017.[42]

An Australian qualitative study of the motivations for methamphetamine and opioid co-injection/co-use has shown that the aim is to facilitate intoxication, sometimes as the result of ineffective opioid substitution therapy (OST) treatment and perceived lack of pleasure after stabilisation on OST treatment.[43]

10.7.1.2   Clubbers

In some countries, the prevalence of methamphetamine use is higher among people who frequent nightclubs and night-time economic venues, sometimes referred to as 'clubbers'. For example, UK sample from the Global Drug Survey in 201 showed that the percentage of methamphetamine users among those described as 'regular clubbers' was higher, with 1% reporting use in the last 12 months.

10.7.1.3   Gay Men and Other Men Who Have Sex with Men (MSM)

There is also some evidence that in some regions at least, methamphetamine use is more common among gay men and other MSM, than it is among the general population and in some regions, its use is mainly concentrated in this population, such as the UK.[44]

Data from the UK[45,46,47,48] and Australia show that bisexual men report higher rates of methamphetamine use compared to heterosexual men[49,50] a fact also reported in the US.[51,52,53,54,55] Amphetamine-type-stimulants and methamphetamine have also been reported to be popular among MSM in Asia, where the drug is also used in a sexual context.[56]

Methamphetamine can be used in a sexual context to enhance sexual performance and pleasure. Methamphetamine is sometimes combined with other stimulants such as mephedrone and other drugs including gamma-hydroxybutyric acid (GHB), 'poppers' and medicines used for erectile dysfunction (e.g., sildenafil, tadalafil and vardenafil).[57] There is evidence that methamphetamine is sometimes injected by gay men and MSM who are using it in a sexual context.[58]

Studies have reported that HIV-positive men are more likely to use methamphetamine than other MSM.[59,60,61,62,63] US studies have shown that the incidence of HIV among MSM who use methamphetamine is more than double that among MSM who do not use methamphetamine.[64] One study suggested that there is also evidence that initiation of methamphetamine use increases sexual risk behaviour among HIV-uninfected MSM.[65,66]

Among heterosexuals, a study has found that methamphetamine use also associated with an increase in being sexually active, having multiple sex partners and casual sex partners and having condomless sex with casual partners, but it is not associated with a change in condom use *per se*. The study also found a dose-related increase in the likelihood of people having multiple sex partners.[67]

10.8 Routes of Ingestion and Dosing

Overall, methamphetamine on the illicit market is sold in Europe in two forms: (1) methamphetamine hydrochloride, in the most prominent crystalline solid form often called 'ice' or 'crystal meth'; and (2) powdered methamphetamine, which is similar to powdered amphetamine in many ways. It can also come in tablets, which carry logos similar to those on ecstasy tablets.

The most common form of methamphetamine is a hydrochloride salt, which comes as a white or off-white bitter-tasting powder, or as purer crystals that are soluble in water. Methamphetamine hydrochloride is stable and volatises easily so can be smoked, unlike amphetamine sulphate.

Whereas all methamphetamine is associated with adverse effects, an Australian study has reported that the increased availability and use of crystalline methamphetamine has been associated with increased regular use and harms.[68]

The method by which methamphetamine is administered depends on the form of the drug available. Methamphetamine is usually administered in the same way as amphetamine powder, either inhaled intra-nasally (snorted), 'bombed' (wrapped in cigarette paper and swallowed) or dissolved and ingested or injected. Although smokable as a powder, it is the larger crystals of relatively pure d-methamphetamine hydrochloride that are normally smoked, often in small glass pipes, and these crystals may also be dissolved and injected or crushed and snorted.[69]

Methamphetamine can also be used anally or inserted into the urethra. It has been noted that if too much methamphetamine is inserted anally, it may not all be completely dissolved and there is a risk of abrasion of condoms resulting from friction with this undissolved methamphetamine, which can contribute to the condom breaking.[70]

There is some evidence that smoking methamphetamine has more harmful psychological effects and a higher addictive potential than snorting or swallowing the drug, and that smokers have levels of dependence approaching those seen among methamphetamine injectors.[71,72] Methamphetamine is rapidly absorbed after ingestion and its half-life is 8–13 hours depending on route ingested.[73]

The stimulant effects depend on a number of factors, including route of ingestion and dose; they may last between 6 and 12 hours, but longer durations have been reported.[74] Intravenous injection and smoking have a rapid onset of action. Following oral administration, peak concentrations are seen in 2.6–3.6 hours and the mean elimination half-life is 10.1 hours (range 6.4–15 hours). Following intravenous use, the mean half-life is slightly longer (12.2 hours).

10.9 Desired Effects for Recreational Use and Unwanted Effects

The effects of methamphetamine result from a surge in newly synthesised catecholamines and serotonin; these include excitation, wellbeing, increased alertness, energy and confidence, highly focused attention and decreased appetite. Methamphetamine use creates feelings of increased confidence, sociability and euphoria.[75] In methamphetamine-naïve individuals, acute doses can improve cognitive processing. Studies show that single low to moderate doses increase arousal and alertness, and improve attention and concentration, particularly among those who are sleep-deprived. Methamphetamine has an apparent aphrodisiac effect, with increased sexual drive, decreased fatigue and loss of sexual inhibition. It can delay ejaculation, assist longer intercourse and decrease humoral secretions.[76,77] Paradoxically, there is evidence that long-term use is associated with decreased sexual functioning in some men.[78]

Higher doses of methamphetamine can cause dysphoria, restlessness and anxiety, and are associated with tremors and dyskinesia. In binge use of methamphetamine, the euphoric effects decrease over time, while dysphoria and compulsive behaviour increase. Bingeing has also been reported to induce sleeplessness, hallucinations and paranoia.[79]

The negative psychological effects of methamphetamine use may include anxiety, restlessness, insomnia, grandiosity, paranoia, psychosis, hallucinations (including delusional parasitosis), depression, unprovoked aggressive or violent behaviour and irritability. Individuals can talk excessively, be agitated, aggressive and restless, and may be observed performing repetitive meaningless tasks.[11,80]

Unwanted effects of methamphetamines have been reported to be common. A US study of 350 individuals found that the majority reported problems associated with methamphetamine use, which included weight loss (84%), sleeplessness (78%), financial problems (73%), paranoia (67%), legal problems (63%), hallucinations (61%), work problems (60%), violent behaviour (57%), dental problems (55%), skin problems (36%) and high blood pressure (24%).[81] In a survey of gay men, 40.4% of men who had used methamphetamine in the past year reported concerns about this drug.[47]

The 'come-down' from methamphetamine is one of the most common unwanted effects reported by users.[82] Users may feel irritable, restless, anxious, depressed and lethargic, and there are reports of the use of benzodiazepines or heroin to soften the come-down. It has been reported in New Zealand that methamphetamine is often sold in a package with GHB/GBL so that the GHB/GBL can be used to help with methamphetamine come-down effects.[83]

10.10 Mortality

A study of cohorts of individuals in California hospitalised from 1990 to 2005 with a diagnosis of disorders relating to methamphetamine, cocaine, alcohol, opiates and cannabis and followed up for 16 years (74,139 individuals and 4,122 deaths) found that hospitalised methamphetamine users had a higher mortality risk than the users of all substances, except for opiates. The standardised mortality rate for methamphetamine found by the study was 4.67, which is similar to rates found by studies in inpatient or treatment settings in the Czech Republic,[84] Denmark[85] and Taiwan,[86] but slightly larger than those reported by a community-based sample of amphetamine users in Sweden.[87]

Deaths associated with methamphetamine have been attributed to homicide, suicide, motor vehicle accidents, manufacturing, distribution and sales of the drug as well as its direct toxic effects.[88] Biologically based causes include stroke, cardiovascular collapse, pulmonary oedema, myocardial infarction, hyperpyrexia and renal failure.[89,90]

For up-to-date guidance on the management of methamphetamine acute toxicity, it is recommended that information be sought from national and regional Poisons Information Services. Local or national guidelines should also be consulted.

10.11 Acute Harms

Methamphetamine use is associated with a range of health harms, including psychosis and other mental disorders, cardiovascular and renal dysfunction, infectious disease transmission and overdose.[91]

10.11.1 Acute Toxicity

The features of acute toxicity are summarised in Box 10.1.

10.11.2 Cardiovascular and Respiratory Harms

The link between the use of methamphetamine and cardiovascular disease is well established,[92] with a study reporting that cardiovascular disease represents the second leading cause of death among

---

Box 10.1 Features of Acute Methamphetamine Toxicity

Cardiovascular and Respiratory
  Narrow-complex tachycardias (common)
  Chest pain
  Tachycardia
  Systemic hypotension or hypertension
  Ventricular tachycardia or ventricular fibrillation
  Dyspnoea
Gastrointestinal and Urological
  Abdominal pain
  Vomiting
  Metabolic acidosis
Neurological and Psychiatric
  Sweating
  Dilated pupils
  Agitation
  Confusion
  Headache
  Anxiety
  Hallucinations or delusions
  Psychotic symptoms
  Seizures
  Tremor
  Hyperpyrexia (may be severe)
  Serotonin syndrome (especially if more than one stimulant drug has been used) (serotonin syndrome is discussed in depth in Chapter 8).

methamphetamine users following only accidental overdose.[93] The association between methamphetamine use and cardiomyopathy has been established for many decades.[94]

Methamphetamine exerts cardiovascular effects on people who use it by causing catecholamine excess, through excessive noradrenaline release and reuptake inhibition at the sympathetic synaptic receptors.

The acute (and chronic) use of methamphetamine can severely affect the cardiovascular system.[11] It causes an acceleration of heart and lung action through vasoconstriction and bronchodilation, while muscle activity is primed via transient hyperglycaemia and dilation of blood vessels in skeletal muscles.[95] Some non-essential physiological activity is inhibited (e.g. stomach and intestinal function); levels of stress hormones – including cortisol and adrenocorticotropic hormone – are increased by 200% in humans following ingestion[96] and remain elevated for hours.[5] Tachycardia and hypertension are common features of methamphetamine toxicity.[7]

Chest pain is a common complaint associated with methamphetamine use,[97] with one study reporting that they account for 38% of emergency department visits and 28% of admissions among patients using methamphetamine.[98] It has also been suggested that although in some patients chest pain is due to methamphetamine-induced hypertension, tachycardia or anxiety, acute coronary syndrome (ACS) is also common among methamphetamine users. One study recommended that patients with chest pain in the context of methamphetamine use should be evaluated for ACS.[99] The prevalence of ACS was found to be 25% in a small series of patients presenting to an emergency department with chest pain after methamphetamine use.[100]

Methamphetamine users have significantly higher rates of coronary artery disease than the general population.[101] Even those with normal coronary arteries are at risk of methamphetamine-induced myocardial infarction, because of coronary spasm, which may be refractory to intracoronary vasodilator therapy.[102] The putative mechanisms of myocardial infarction in the context of methamphetamine use include accelerated atherosclerosis, rupture of pre-existing atherosclerotic plaques, hypercoaguability and epicardial coronary artery spasm.[104,103,104] Acute myocardial infarction following methamphetamine use can be severe and can result in cardiogenic shock and death.[105]

A study in Hawaii (where the prevalence of methamphetamine use is high) reported that methamphetamine use accounts for 40% of all admissions of patients under the age of 45 years with cardiomyopathy. More than 20% of patients with heart failure were former or current methamphetamine users.[106] A US registry containing information on more than 11,000 patients with decompensated heart failure reported that more than 5% were stimulant users.[107]

One case series reported that more than a quarter (27.2%) of methamphetamine-intoxicated patients had a prolonged corrected QT interval (QTc>440ms), suggesting that methamphetamine-induced alterations in cardiac conduction may be partly responsible for the drug's dysrhythmogenic effects.[108]

Other conditions related to methamphetamine intoxication include premature ventricular contractions, premature supraventricular contractions, accelerated atrioventricular conduction, atrioventricular block, intraventricular conduction delay, bundle branch block, ventricular tachycardia, ventricular fibrillation, and supraventricular tachycardia.[102,110,109] Methamphetamine-induced dysrhythmias may also occur because of myocardial ischaemia or infarction.[99]

Methamphetamine use may also be associated with aortic dissection and carries a greater risk for that than cocaine; it may be second only to hypertension in its importance as a risk factor for aortic dissection.[110] Methamphetamine can cause cerebral infarct, haemorrhage and hypertension,[75,111] and is a risk factor for intracerebral haemorrhage.[112] The ingestion of large quantities of methamphetamine in particular has been associated with cerebrovascular haemorrhage.[113,114,115]

Haemorrhagic strokes have been associated with methamphetamine use and methamphetamine-related stroke linked with poor clinical outcomes.[116,117] Cardiac and systemic thrombus caused by methamphetamine has been reported.[118]

Like other drugs injected, the injection of methamphetamine has been associated with endocarditis.[99] Cardiovascular events are often involved in medical complications and death associated with methamphetamine.[119]

The risks associated with the long-term use of methamphetamine are discussed in Section 10.13.

10.11.3 Hyperthermia and Rhabdomyolysis

The ingestion of large quantities of methamphetamine has been associated with hyperthermiaby promoting heat generation and preventing heat dissipation and by its effects on increasing body metabolism and causing vasoconstriction.[115,116,117] and, Methamphetamine has also been associated with rhabdomyolysis.[120,121]

10.11.4 Urological/Liver

The ingestion of large quantities of methamphetamine has been associated with renal and liver failure.[115,116,117]

10.11.5 Mental Health Effects

Acute intoxication can cause panic, agitation and transient symptoms of hallucinations and paranoia. It can increase aggressive responses to threatening situations.[122,123,124] Amphetamines and methamphetamine have been consistently associated with elevated rates of suicide and evidence suggests a likely causal link.[125,126]

A recent systematic review and meta-analysis found compelling evidence for a causal association between the use of amphetamines and increased risk of psychosis. There also appeared to be some level of specificity in this effect, with elevated risk relative to other substance use.[127]

Methamphetamine can also exacerbate psychosis in people with schizophrenia.[128,129,130] It can also crease the severity of a range of psychiatric symptoms, and the need to distinguish these symptoms from underlying psychiatric disorders, to avoid misdiagnosis and sub-optimal care, has been recommended.[131]

10.11.6 Methamphetamine Use and High-risk Sexual Behaviours

There is evidence that methamphetamine in particular is associated with high-risk behaviours and chemsex,[132] especially by gay men and other men who have sex with men (MSM). There is also some evidence that initiation of methamphetamine use increases sexual risk behaviour among HIV-uninfected MSM.[133]

'Chemsex' is sometimes referred to as 'party and play' and is a term that is used to describe sex between men that occurs under the influence of drugs taken immediately before and/or during the sexual session in order to enhance and prolong the sexual experience.[61,134] Chemsex has been reported internationally and across a number of European countries.[135,136,137,138,139,140,141,142]

A number of drugs are typically used within the context of 'chemsex', with some differences by country. For example, in addition to methamphetamine, in the UK γ-hydroxybutyrate (GHB), γ-butyrolactone (GBL), and previously mephedrone, were used in chemsex.[143] In Spain in contrast, a retrospective study of the role of chemsex in episodes of acute street drug poisoning in HIV-infected patients in an emergency department over a period of 1 year suggest that cocaine had a significant role, with methamphetamine and GHB the next street drugs implicated.[144]

High-risk behaviours associated with methamphetamine have been reported,[145] Three patterns of behaviour are associated with methamphetamine use: high-risk sexual practices, sexualised injecting and the sharing of injecting equipment. For example, a study of gay and bisexual men found that methamphetamine and poly-drug use were independently predictive of reporting >20 recent partners, unprotected anal intercourse with a casual partner and a sexually transmitted infection.[146]

The use of club drugs in a sexual context has been described.[147,148] Methamphetamine is one of the drugs most commonly used in a sexual context (chemsex)[147] and elsewhere. In a US study of 60 MSM, 68% reported using methamphetamine during sex more than 50% of the time.[149]

A relatively large body of evidence shows heightened sexual risk-taking associated with methamphetamine use.[150,151,152,153,154,155,156] There is some evidence that compared with use of other drugs, methamphetamine use is a particularly strong predictor of unprotected anal sex among MSM.[157,158]

Methamphetamine use has also been associated with sexually transmitted infections (STIs), with increased rates of STIs,[66,159,160] including HIV infection.[149,161,162,163,164,165,166,167,168,169] There is also an association between methamphetamine use and rates of HIV and hepatitis C.[170,171,172,173,174,175,176,177] and a relationship has been observed between increased severity of methamphetamine use and HIV risk.[157]

Studies have shown that MSM who use methamphetamine, regardless of their HIV status, have a greater risk of STIs than those who do not.[63,178] Men who use methamphetamine are 1.5–2.9 times more likely to acquire HIV than those who do not.[156,179,180,181,182]

Studies also suggest that HIV-positive MSM who use methamphetamine are significantly more likely than MSM who do not use methamphetamine (regardless of their HIV status) to engage in unprotected anal sex[63,183,184,185] and group sex,[186] to have multiple sexual partners,[50,63 101 ,187,188] to find sexual partners on the Internet,[63] to have sex with an injecting drug user[185] and to be intoxicated during sex.[63,185] Among HIV-infected MSM men who have a sero-discordant partner (i.e. HIV negative, or status unknown), the use of methamphetamine is significantly associated with unprotected anal sex.[64,189,190]

It has been noted that HIV-positive men are more likely to inject psychoactive substances (including methamphetamine) than other MSM, with injecting increasingly common with older age, peaking among men in their 40s.[61] There are some reports from methamphetamine users of increased sexual desires with injecting methamphetamine, in comparison with other forms of methamphetamine use.[191,192]

Social media and mobile phone applications (Apps) have been described by Bourne et al. as a facilitator of drug use during sex among gay men in London, or 'chemsex'.[193] Location-based, social networking applications (mobile phone apps) are providing men with the opportunity to source both sexual partners and drugs in their local area. 'Apps' have been described as playing a major role in the organisation of sex parties and 'chemsex', typically linked with high-risk drug use and sexual behaviours.[194]

An outbreak of syphilis has also been linked to seeking sex partners through an online chatroom, as well as to the use of methamphetamine.[195]

A number of factors and sub-groups of methamphetamine users have been associated with particularly high-risk behaviours for transmission of HIV and STIs. These include methamphetamine users who use sildenafil (Viagra)[159,160,161,192,196] or other illicit drugs during sex,[197,198] those who exchange sex for methamphetamine,[199] those who report high levels of sexual compulsivity,[192,200] those who engage in sexual encounters in public spaces[65,201] and those who report methamphetamine binges.[202]

A recent review of outcomes among MSM who use methamphetamines has reported a low adherence to HIV medication by HIV-positive MSM who use methamphetamine. This, the authors believe, may contribute to the transmission of HIV virus resistant to medication which has been seen in newly infected MSM who use methamphetamine.[158]

However, it is important to note that a causal link between methamphetamine use and STIs, HIV and other blood-borne viruses (BBV) has not been established. There is some evidence that individuals who engage in high-risk sexual activity are more likely to use recreational drugs[203] and evidence that among MSM, recreational drug use in general (rather than methamphetamine use specifically) is associated with high-risk activity.[204,205]

The link between methamphetamine use and high-risk sexual activities is not unique to MSM, although most of the research has been carried out among MSM and less evidence is available for heterosexuals.[206] Studies of male and female heterosexual populations also suggest that methamphetamine users have a higher frequency of sexual activity, have more sexual partners and engage in higher-risk sexual behaviours (unprotected vaginal sex and anal sex) than the users of any other drugs.[207,208,209,210,211]

10.11.7 Injecting Risks

Methamphetamine injecting is a serious public health concern, as well as heightening risks and harms to the individual user.[212] The evidence on the elevated injecting-related risk behaviours among methamphetamine users in comparison with other injectors has been ambiguous.[153,213,214,215] Regardless, methamphetamine injecting has been identified as a significant risk factor and injectors often present with more complex needs. Studies have shown that methamphetamine injectors are more dependent than non-injectors,[216] are at increased risk of non-fatal overdose,[217] and are more likely to engage in HIV-risk behaviours;[215,218,219,220] a study has reported a higher prevalence of STIs than among non-injecting methamphetamine users.[221]

Methamphetamine injectors are more likely to have co-morbid psychiatric disorders than non-injecting methamphetamine users.[222,223] The use of methamphetamine by injecting in particular has been linked to suicide.[224]

There is evidence that methamphetamine injectors may be more likely to attempt suicide than those who smoke or snort the drug,[225,225] with a seven-year study reporting that people who injected methamphetamine had an 80% greater risk of attempting suicide than those who did not inject, even after taking into account a wide range of potential confounders. The study also showed a dose–response relationship between frequency of injecting methamphetamine and suicidal behaviour. The conclusion was that individuals who inject methamphetamine should be considered at high risk of suicide among populations of methamphetamine users, as well as the broader injecting population.[226]

10.11.8 Acute Harms of Poly-drug Use and Drug Interactions

The high level of poly-drug use among methamphetamine users has been well established.[227] Cross-sectional population surveys suggest that the concurrent use of alcohol and cocaine is particularly common.[228] This can cause harm as it increases blood pressure. Methamphetamine can also mask the effects of alcohol, which may increase the risk of alcohol poisoning and accidents due to false feelings of being sober. Concurrent use of amphetamine including methamphetamine and cannabis can increase psychotic symptoms in some users. The combination of methamphetamine and cocaine has been shown to increase substantially the cardiotoxic effects of both drugs.[229]

The co-ingestion of GHB and methamphetamine might increase the risk of GHB overdose, as methamphetamine can mask the signs of acute toxicity and can impair the accurate measurement of GHB doses, which increases the risk of GHB overdose. There are also risks associated with the use of methamphetamine with other serotonergic substances, leading to the risk of serotonin syndrome. The potential for drug interactions with CYP2D6 inhibitors is high and coadministration of these agents may increase the toxicity of methamphetamine. Well known CYP2D6 inhibitors include: amiodarone, citalopram, codeine, fluoxetine, haloperidol, methadone, paroxetine and valproic acid. Among the antiretrovirals, while low-dose ritonavir does not seem to affect CYP2D6 activity,[230] the newer booster cobicistat is included in the list of CYP2D6 inhibitors.

10.11.9 Acute Withdrawal

For withdrawal see Section 10.13.2.

10.11.10 Emergency Hospital Admissions

In countries where rates of methamphetamine use are high, admissions to emergency departments (EDs) are reportedly very common. US data demonstrate that regular users of methamphetamine have a high rate of presentation to ED[100,231,232] and there is some evidence that adult methamphetamine users use ED and other hospital resources more than the users of other substances.[100,233] A Canadian study of homeless and street-based youth reported that frequent injecting of methamphetamine was associated with increased risk of ED utilisation.[228]

Studies have also shown relatively high levels of methamphetamine-related hospital presentations for psychiatric problems. Psychiatric symptoms, including acute psychosis, depression and anxiety disorders, have been associated with both acute and chronic methamphetamine use.[227,234,235,236,237,238,239,240,241,242,243,244,245,246,247]

In methamphetamine-endemic areas, studies have shown that 1–2% of all ED visits are related to methamphetamine use, with psychiatric conditions being the most common complaints.[227,236–246]

Some studies have also suggested that more methamphetamine-related presentations to EDs were for psychiatric problems than for other problems. For example, a US study reported that methamphetamine-related psychiatric visits to EDs represented 7.6% of all psychiatric attendances, a percentage which the authors described as 'disproportionate'. In comparison, 1.8% of all trauma visits were methamphetamine-related and 2.1% of presentations with chest pain were methamphetamine-related.[249]

Other studies also showed that methamphetamine-related ED visits associated with psychiatric complaints or diagnosis represented the largest patient sub-group visiting EDs with psychiatric issues.[236,249] For example, a study of 378 presentations with methamphetamine toxicity to an Australian ED reported that the most common clinical effect was acute behavioural disturbance, occurring in 295 (78%) presentations. Other effects included tachycardia in 212 (56%), hypertension in 160 (42%) and hyperthermia in 17 (5%) presentations.[248]

A study of psychiatric admissions to EDs reported that there were no differences in heart rate, admission route or cost of care of methamphetamine-related visits and other visits. This, according to the study, suggests that methamphetamine users presenting for psychiatric problems are clinically similar to non-amphetamine users with psychiatric problems.[249]

However, in comparison with other patients presenting to EDs for toxicology-related issues, some studies have shown that those presenting with methamphetamine-related problems are more agitated, violent and aggressive and more likely to present on arrival with tachycardia and hypertension.[247,248] It has been argued that methamphetamine use presents a significant challenge to EDs and acute mental health services.[249]

10.12 Management of Acute Harms

Interventions required are clinical monitoring, observation and symptomatic treatment. It is recommended that where a patient has impaired consciousness, emergency clinicians should ensure clear airways and adequate ventilation. As with other amphetamines, in the event of cardiac arrest, resuscitation should be continued for at least 1 hour and only stopped after discussion with a senior clinician. Prolonged resuscitation for cardiac arrest is recommended following poisoning, as recovery with good neurological outcome may occur.

The benefit of gastric decontamination is uncertain. Clinicians should consider oral activated charcoal if methamphetamine has been ingested within 1 hour, provided the airway can be protected. Asymptomatic patients should be observed for at least 4 hours, or 8 hours for patients who have ingested sustained-release preparations. Agitated adults can be sedated with an initial dose of oral or intravenous diazepam.

A study of 378 methamphetamine-related presentations to EDs in Australia reported that acute behavioural disturbance, occurring in almost 80% of presentations, was successfully managed with oral sedation alone in 180 (61%) patients, with the remainder receiving parenteral sedation.[250]

10.12.1 Treatment of Methamphetamine-induced Psychosis

Any treatment for methamphetamine-induced psychosis must focus on abstinence from drugs and the prevention of relapse. It has been argued that in many patients, transient psychosis will subside after a few weeks to a month of abstaining from methamphetamine and prescribing antipsychotic to these patients may not be needed in light of the mental and physical side effects associated with the medications.[251] There is no standardised treatment for methamphetamine-induced psychosis and studies have shown the effectiveness of a range of antipsychotic medications.[252,253] However, even when

anti-psychotics are prescribed, it is recommended that treatment also includes psychosocial interventions and relapse prevention. It is also good practice to deliver treatment for other co-occurring psychiatric disorders including depression and anxiety.[254]

10.13 Harms of Chronic Use and Dependence

People who use methamphetamine regularly are at the risk of dependence. Regular or dependent use is associated with comorbidities including depression, anxiety, psychosis and cardiovascular disease. In addition, there are risks associated with contextual social factors related to the use of methamphetamine including sexually transmitted or blood-borne infections and legal issues.[255]

10.13.1 Dependence

Methamphetamine is a potent central nervous system stimulant and the risk of dependence is high.[256]

Dependence on methamphetamines follows the same principles discussed in Chapter 8.

Tolerance to methamphetamine takes place when the drug is taken frequently, leading to users taking higher doses or using more frequently or changing the route of administration in order to achieve the desired effect. There is some emerging evidence that craving to methamphetamine cues can be measured in dependent individuals[257,258,259] and that cue-elicited methamphetamine craving is a strong predictor of subsequent use.[260]

There is some evidence that methamphetamine-dependent users show a decrease in everyday functioning, disruption in everyday activities and increased errors in planning a daily schedule. Methamphetamine dependence has also been linked to impairments in the domains of communication, work and recreation.[261,262] There is also evidence that the chronic use of methamphetamine causes cognitive deficits after withdrawal.[263,264,265,266] Studies have also shown that this may be associated with disruptions of the dopaminergic and serotonergic systems.[266,267,268,269,270] Chronic use of methamphetamine causes neurochemical and neuroanatomical changes, which include memory impairment.

Dependence results in deficits in memory and in decision-making and verbal reasoning.[271] There is limited evidence that this functional deficit continues several months after abstinence.[264,272] One study has reported deteriorating cognitive performance during the first three months of abstinence from methamphetamine, with abstinent patients or abstinent patients with a recent lapse scoring worse on neuropsychological testing than patients with ongoing methamphetamine use. This reflects the difficulties in attention, understanding and memory often encountered in methamphetamine patients in treatment settings.[267] Although it needs to be substantiated by larger studies, Henry et al. suggest that this may have important implications for treatment interventions, as individuals with poor functional ability may have difficulty responding to cognitive-behavioural therapy (CBT) and the cognitive enhancement techniques commonly used in the treatment of methamphetamine misuse.[274]

A recent study of 108 participants has reported that methamphetamine dependence was associated with poorer performance in decision-making and disinhibition over and above other predictors and that duration of methamphetamine use was linked to disinhibition. The authors suggest the need to target disinhibition and impulsive decision-making as part of methamphetamine dependence treatment.[273]

10.13.2 Withdrawal

Methamphetamine is associated with a clear withdrawal syndrome. A time-limited withdrawal syndrome may occur within 24 hours of the last dose when heavy chronic users of methamphetamine cease to use the drug abruptly. The withdrawal syndrome is common and severe enough to cause relapse outside a contained environment.[274]

Chapter 8 (the overview of amphetamine-type stimulants) has discussed in greater detail the phases of amphetamine withdrawal and should be read in conjunction with this chapter. Phases of withdrawal symptoms have also been identified with methamphetamine users. For example, a study of 21 inpatients suggested that methamphetamine withdrawal has two phases: an acute phase lasting 7–10 days, in which overall symptom severity declines in a linear pattern from a high initial peak; and a sub-acute phase lasting at least a further 2 weeks, with some studies reporting much longer periods.[275] Withdrawal from methamphetamine has been described as more characterised by psychological and psychiatric symptoms than physical symptoms.[91]

Table 10.1 outlines the two phases of methamphetamine withdrawal, according to the reported symptoms.[83,91,116,225,276,277,278,279,280]

Table 10.1 The two phases of methamphetamine withdrawal

Acute withdrawal symptoms	Longer-term withdrawal symptoms (can last up to 12 months)
Severe dysphoria	Anhedonia
Irritability	Impaired social functioning
Melancholia	Intense craving
Anxiety	Hyper-arousal
Hypersomnia and marked fatigue	Vegetative symptoms
Paranoia	Severe dysphoria
Intensity of post-binge dysphoria can lead to suicide ideation and attempts have also been linked to withdrawal[91,282] (for more information on the withdrawal syndrome see Chapter 8	Mood volatility
Akathisia/restless legs	Irritability
	Sleep pattern disruption

Greater severity of withdrawal symptoms in methamphetamine-dependent individuals has been reported among those who are older, who have been using methamphetamine longer and who have more severe methamphetamine use disorder.[277,282]

10.13.3 Physiological, Psychological and Psychiatric Effects of Long-term Use and Dependence

Chronic use has been associated with malnourishment.[281]

10.13.3.1 Cardiovascular Effects

Long-term use of methamphetamine can result in severe cardiovascular complications related to chronic hypertension and cardiovascular disease, such as angina, arrhythmias, valvular disease, haemorrhagic/ischaemic strokes and a high incidence of myocardial infarction.[107,108,116,282,283,284,285,286] Chronic methamphetamine can be associated with the development of a dilated cardiomyopathy.[287]

A study on patients with methamphetamine-associated cardiomyopathy has shown that some present with an acute stress cardiomyopathy, which is often characterised by a shorter duration of methamphetamine use, a 'reverse Takotsubo' (RT) pattern, higher levels of cardiac enzymes and a greater scope for early recovery of ventricular function. Others, particularly with a longer history of use, have evidence of atrial and ventricular remodelling on initial echocardiography and/or fibrosis on cardiac magnetic resonance imaging (CMR) and present with a chronic dilated cardiomyopathy; they have limited scope for recovery.[288]

10.13.3.2 Neurological Effects

Chronic CNS hyper-stimulation can lead to frequent headaches, tremors, athetoid movements and seizures.[11] There is evidence that users of amphetamine-type substances, including methamphetamine, may have an above-normal risk of developing Parkinson's disease (PD) because of enduring damage to the brain's dopamine neurons. This was shown by a retrospective population-based cohort study of inpatient hospital episodes and death records from 1990 through to 2005 in California. Patients at least 30 years of age were followed for up to 16 years. The study found that methamphetamine users had a 76% increased risk of developing Parkinson's disease in comparison with the matched population proxy control group. The authors noted that this finding may be limited to high-dose, chronic methamphetamine users and only when they reach middle and older age, when they have suffered age-related loss of dopamine neurons.[289]

10.13.3.3 Pulmonary and Respiratory Harms

The smoking of methamphetamine can cause respiratory symptoms and disorders such as pulmonary oedema, bronchitis, pulmonary hypertension, haemoptysis and granuloma.[11] Methamphetamine is associated with pulmonary arterial hypertension (PAH),[290] although its precise role remains unclear.[99]

10.13.3.4 Blood-borne Infections and Haematological, Gastrointestinal and Urological effects

Methamphetamine has been reported to cause acute liver injury, with hepatic necrosis and centrilobular degeneration, even in the absence of hepatitis.[291] There are reports of mesenteric infarction,[292] segmental ischaemic colitis, vasculitis[293] or vasospasm with spontaneous resolution.[294] Severe acute necrotic haemorrhagic pancreatitis has been reported in cases of sudden death of chronic methamphetamine use.[99]

Because of the increased likelihood of high-risk sexual behaviours discussed in Section 10.10.2,

methamphetamine users are more likely to be diagnosed with a sexually transmitted infection than non-users.[209,212] Methamphetamine users are also at greater risk of viral hepatitis, especially where the drug is injected, but even among methamphetamine smokers and insufflators, hepatitis C is more common than it is in the general population.[295,296,297]

10.13.3.5 Dermatological

Methamphetamine users may suffer from skin lesions resulting from compulsive scratching (due to formication – a sense of having insects moving under the skin). These lesions can result in bacterial cellulitis and, in some cases, bacteraemia and sepsis. In a case series of methamphetamine users presenting to an emergency department, skin infection accounted for 6% of the initial presentations and 54% of subsequent admissions to hospital.[100]

10.13.3.6 Pott Puffy Tumour

There is a case report of Pott puffy tumour (PPT) associated with the intranasal use of methamphetamine. This is an anterior extension of a frontal sinus infection that results in frontal bone osteomyelitis and subperiosteal abscess.[298]

10.13.3.7 Ophthalmological Harms

Acute unilateral vision loss has been reported following a single dose of intranasal methamphetamine use and is believed to be due to ischaemic optic neuropathy secondary to methamphetamine-induced vasospasm and methamphetamine-associated vasculitis.[299,300]

10.13.3.8 Mental Health, Psychological and Psychiatric effects

The frequent and prolonged use of methamphetamine has a number of adverse effects. There is a well-established association between methamphetamine use and mental health problems.[116,301]

Studies have found elevated rates of mood disorders, anxiety disorders and antisocial personality behaviour and disorder, even after treatment.[302] A recent systematic review and meta-analysis found elevated levels of psychosis, depression, suicidality and violence amongst people who use amphetamines, including methamphetamine.[303] Depressive disorders and symptoms are frequently associated with methamphetamine use,[243,245,246,304,305,306,307,308] with depression being described as pervasive amongst heavy users.[309] The disorder is often associated with mood disturbances.[310]

A systematic review has found that people who use methamphetamine are at a significantly elevated risk of poor mental health when compared to people who do not use the drug. The review found that they around twice as likely to experience depression and psychosis and four times more likely to be suicidal.[311]

The state of catecholamine and serotonin depletion after several days of methamphetamine use can manifest itself as exhaustion, depression, lethargy and anhedonia. Psychological symptoms include persistent anxiety, paranoia, insomnia, auditory hallucinations, delusion, psychotic or violent behaviour and suicidal or homicidal thinking.[11,312] The link between psychotic symptoms and amphetamine-induced sleep deprivation has also been reported.[313]

Methamphetamine contributes significantly to the risk of psychosis, although the majority of people who use it experience only milder transient symptoms, which recede when they are no longer intoxicated.[314] Nonetheless some of the symptoms can resemble those of paranoid schizophrenia,[273] or symptoms almost indistinguishable from schizophrenia,[315] including persecutory delusions and auditory hallucinations.[316]

Methamphetamine-induced psychosis can occur in individuals with no history of psychosis.[74,240] Nevertheless, it has also been shown that methamphetamine users with a family history of schizophrenia may be five times more likely to develop psychosis than those without one. Nonetheless, it has also been shown that methamphetamine users with a family history of schizophrenia may be five times more likely to develop psychosis than those without one.[317,318]

It is well established that substance misuse can exacerbate mental health problems.[319] There is some evidence that serious psychiatric disorders may emerge or worsen as a result of methamphetamine use,[83,91,225,320,321] including increased risk of suicide.[322] It was also reported that a previous history of psychotic disorders relates to worse outcomes in methamphetamine-induced psychosis.[323,324] Methamphetamine use can increase the severity of a range of psychiatric symptoms.[325]

Risk of psychosis following methamphetamine use has also been shown to be higher in victims of sexual abuse.[326,327] Amphetamine and methamphetamine-induced psychosis are associated with environmental and genetic risk factors, but it has also been shown that higher frequency, severity, and length of use have been reported as the most robust risk factors.[328,329] Psychotic symptoms typically amplify over time with continued methamphetamine use.[330] Methamphetamine-induced psychotic disorder has been associated with the chronic, high-dose and continuous use of methamphetamine.[331] A systematic review of the literature has found that the most consistent correlates of psychotic symptoms were increased frequency of methamphetamine use and dependence on methamphetamine.[332]

A literature review looking at the prevalence of substance-induced psychosis that included 17 studies in the meta-analysis, resulted in a composite event rate of 36.5% in methamphetamine users. It was significantly higher when the period of assessment was lifetime use (42.7%) and when only individuals with methamphetamine use disorders (43.3%) were included.[333]

Symptoms may include auditory, visual and tactile hallucinations and paranoid delusions, persecutory delusions and other delusions. Research seems to suggest that delusions in methamphetamine psychosis are primarily persecutory in nature.[334,335,336,337,338] A wide spectrum of psychotic symptoms can occur in methamphetamine users, ranging from brief delusional experiences, to persistent psychosis characterised by first-rank symptoms and cognitive impairment.[339]

Methamphetamine-induced psychosis can be transient or persistent. Even if the psychotic symptoms produced by methamphetamine are transient, recurrent drug use can lead to a symptom course that appears chronic in nature.[340]

Symptoms usually remit after acute intoxication but some individuals may develop psychosis weeks or months after stopping methamphetamine,[312,341] and may prove to be refractory to antipsychotic medication.[342] Stress can precipitate spontaneous psychosis in former methamphetamine users who are abstinent.[343]

Much of the literature on persistent methamphetamine psychosis comes from Japan, where methamphetamine has been illicitly used for over 50 years, which suggests that persistent methamphetamine psychosis is not uncommon.[344] Japanese studies have also reported that psychotic symptoms may recur where there is new exposure to the drug.[344,344,345,346,347,348] Japanese research has also reported discouraging results with standard anti-psychotic drugs, as many patients remain clinically psychotic after many months of treatment.[343,349]

10.13.3.9 Cognitive Effects

There are direct physiological effects of methamphetamine intoxication, but the cognitive and behavioural changes associated with its use may be secondary to neurotoxicity.[350]

Neuroimaging in chronic methamphetamine users has shown significant neural damage in patients and evidence of cognitive impairment, but it is not established whether the link is causal.[75,351]

A study has shown that the effects of cocaine and methamphetamine on the neuropsychological profiles of people who use them are similar. However, there is some evidence that cocaine use is more associated with working memory impairments, which are typically frontally mediated, while methamphetamine appears to be more associated with memory impairments that are linked with temporal and parietal lobe dysfunction.[352]

10.13.4 Co-morbidities of Methamphetamine Use Disorders and HIV

Methamphetamine has been shown to interfere with the efficacy of HIV medication and treatment.[353] Its use has been linked to non-adherence to medication regimens[354] and there is a suggestion that it may be associated with increased viral loads, even among those taking antiretroviral medication.[355] Both methamphetamine use and HIV may be associated with impaired cognitive function, and in combination may result in greater impairment than each condition alone.[355] There is evidence that hepatitis C increases these cognitive deficits.[356]

10.14 Management of Harms of Chronic and Dependent Use of Methamphetamine

10.14.1 Identification and Assessment of Dependence

The identification and assessment of chronic use of methamphetamine and ensuing harms are similar to those for ATS in general (see Chapter 8).

10.14.2 Psychosocial Interventions for Dependence

Studies have shown that some people dependent on drugs may achieve abstinence, without the need for treatment.[357,358] It has also been shown that people in treatment can remit from methamphetamine dependence, reduce their frequency of use or cease entirely and maintain abstinence over long periods.[359] There is also some evidence that behavioural-based treatment for methamphetamine misuse can be effective in reducing HIV infections, by reducing high-risk injecting behaviours and unsafe sexual practices.[170,360]

An economic evaluation of the cost-effectiveness of counselling for methamphetamine dependence showed that greater investment in this cost-effective strategy will produce significant cost-savings and improve health outcomes as well as improve many externality issues associated with drug use.[361]

At present, the most effective treatments for methamphetamine addiction are psychosocial interventions and behavioural therapies. Historically, treatment for stimulant dependence has relied on cognitive-behavioural therapy (CBT), with efforts to integrate contingency management (CM) (for more information see Chapter 8).

Overall, the evidence suggests that psychosocial interventions, such as CBT and CM, are moderately effective in achieving methamphetamine abstinence.[362]

A number of US studies have reported the effectiveness of CM within specific research and drug treatment settings,[363] as well as outside those settings.[364] CM in combination with other interventions, such as CBT, has proved to be modestly effective at reducing methamphetamine dependence.[366,365,366,367]

CM was also shown to have superior efficacy to CBT during drug treatment.[365,368] A Cochrane review of psychosocial interventions for cocaine and psychostimulant amphetamine disorders reported that comparisons between different types of behavioural interventions showed results in favour of treatments with some form of contingency management with respect to both reducing drop-outs and lowering use. However, the review also reports there are few significant behavioural changes even after reductions in drug consumption and conclude that there are no data supporting a single-treatment approach that is able to tackle the multidimensional facets of addiction and to resolve the chronic, relapsing nature of addiction, with all its correlates and consequences.[369]

10.14.2.1 Implementation of Contingency Management

Some studies have looked in greater detail at the impact of CM and at variations in CM models used and which specific factors were most effective in producing positive treatment outcomes. Roll et al. found that there were significant differences in terms of a CM schedule's ability to initiate and maintain abstinence. The schedule based on an escalating programme of reinforcement with a reset contingency (developed by Higgings[370]) showed the best results for a successful treatment episode.[371]

Ling Murtaugh et al. found, in their study of 162 MSM methamphetamine-dependent users, that it was the act of voucher redemption, rather than the receipt or size of payment, that affected subsequent abstinence from methamphetamine. Participants who delayed spending the vouchers, and those who saved the vouchers, had worse outcomes once they did finally redeem them. The authors recommend that frequent purchases in incentive-based programmes should be promoted to improve abstinence outcomes.[372]

Overall, studies have shown some efficacy in psychological treatment for methamphetamine use, but retention in psychological therapies of methamphetamine-using patients has been an issue.[373] Some have argued that although psychosocial and behavioural interventions have been the most effective treatment for methamphetamine use, their role is still in question. It has been argued, for example, that CM interventions have shown benefit, but a key limitation includes its failure to address adequately mental health needs or develop relapse prevention plans for after the intervention.[158] There is also some evidence that CM is not likely to have a sustained and large effect on methamphetamine use.[374] One RCT of CM to reduce methamphetamine use and sexual risk studied 217 non-treatment-seekers over 12 weeks and found that CM was potentially associated with an increase in methamphetamine use and decreases in sexual risk, but these were not statistically significant.[376]

A systematic review and meta-analysis of mental health outcomes associated with methamphetamine use has argued that services that interact with people who use methamphetamine need to have the capacity to treat and manage co-occurring mental health conditions. The review also recommends that more work is needed to ensure that people who use this drug are provided with adequate mental health care and that generic responses are tailored to make sure they are acceptable, safe and effective for people who use methamphetamine.[375]

As relapse rates from methamphetamine are high,[376] there have been calls for more work in improving methamphetamine treatment. Further research into cognitive-behavioural and behavioural treatments for methamphetamine users is required, with a focus on increasing the duration of the effect of interventions and improving their effectiveness among patients with more complex presentations.[377]

The is also evidence that services that target specific groups and meet their specific needs provide effective treatment. For example, in an Australian LGBTI-specific treatment service, clients showed reductions in methamphetamine use and improved psychosocial functioning over time.[378]

10.14.2.2 Social Support and Other Interventions

Other support may also be required. Social interventions, such as securing stable housing, training and employment are often needed. For example, homelessness has been independently associated with the initiation of methamphetamine use among people who inject drugs,[379,380] and a recent study found that the loss of stable housing through residential eviction was associated with an increased hazard of crystal methamphetamine or relapse into methamphetamine use, even after adjusting for a range of potential confounders including homelessness.[381]

There is increasing interest in the role of exercise in the management of chronic harms associated with stimulant use. A systematic review was to evaluate the effectiveness of exercise for reducing anxiety and depression, and improving fitness and quality of life in adults who have previously used methamphetamine. The review suggests that overall recovery in methamphetamine-dependent users might be improved by including an effective exercise programme in the rehabilitation process; significant improvements were found for anxiety, depression, fitness and quality of life following exercise, as compared to all control groups.[382]

A small number of studies have looked at electroconvulsive therapy (ECT) with patients who were unresponsive to antipsychotic medications and reported improvement to psychotic symptoms, cravings, withdrawal, and mood.[383,384,385] There have also been a limited number of studies looking at electro-acupuncture and a RCT reported significant improvement to Positive and Negative Syndrome Scale (PANSS) scores after 1 week of treatment that continued to improve until the end of the 4-week trial.[386]

A RCT of people who are dependent on methamphetamine looked at the role of electro-acupuncture and found that it is effective in treating the methamphetamine withdrawal symptoms in methamphetamine, including anxiety, and depression.[387] More research is needed.

Mindfulness-based relapse prevention (MBRP) has shown some benefit, although more research is needed. It has been reported that MBRP can decrease craving and depressive symptoms for comorbid substance use in depressive disorders.[388] A RCT evaluating the efficacy of MBRP in conjunction with contingency management as a primary intervention approach for stimulant dependence found that MBRP reduces negative affect and psychiatric impairment and is particularly effective in reducing stimulant use among stimulant-dependent adults with mood and anxiety disorders.[389]

10.14.3 Pharmacological Interventions for Methamphetamine Dependence and Withdrawal

The need to develop safe and effective medication for methamphetamine dependence continues to be a global strategic aim.

According to the US National Institute on Drug Abuse (NIDA), one approach currently tried is to target the activity of glial cells with a drug called AV411 (ibudilast). This has been shown to inhibit methamphetamine self-administration in rats; it is now being studied in clinical trials to establish its safety and effectiveness in humans. Other approaches currently under study use the body's immune system to neutralise the drug in the bloodstream before it reaches the brain. These approaches involve injecting a user with (anti) methamphetamine antibodies or with vaccines that stimulate the body to produce its own antibodies.[390] A clinical study is currently being conducted to establish the safety of an anti-methamphetamine monoclonal antibody, known as mAb7F9, in human methamphetamine users.[392]

Methamphetamine vaccines, which recruit the body's immune system to keep the drug from entering the brain, are currently being tested in animals, and a human clinical trial is currently underway to test an immunologic agent called a monoclonal antibody, which binds to methamphetamine and neutralises it before it can exert its effects.[89,391]

Over the years, in addition to new compounds, a number of medications approved for other conditions have been tested for their efficacy and safety in treating methamphetamine dependence. These have included serotonergic agonists, dopaminergic agonists, monoamine agonists and mixed monoamine agonists/antagonists.[92,394,392,393,394,395,396,397,398,399,400,401,402,403,404,405,406,407]

As mentioned in Chapter 8, a recent systematic review reported that there is currently no pharmacotherapy that has shown convincing results for the treatment of amphetamine and methamphetamine dependence; this is mainly because most studies were underpowered and had low treatment completion rates. However, there were positive signals from several agents that warrant further investigation in larger scale studies.[408]

The systematic review that included 43 studies also found that there are a few pharmacotherapy candidates for the treatment of amphetamine and methamphetamine dependence/use disorder that demonstrate some weak positive signals, although more research is needed. The most consistent positive findings were shown with stimulant agonist treatment (dexamphetamine and methylphenidate), naltrexone and topiramate. Less consistent benefits were shown with bupropion, the glutamatergic agent, riluzole, and antidepressant mirtazapine. In general, antidepressant medications (e.g. SSRIs, TCAs) have not been effective in reducing amphetamine and methamphetamine use.[409]

Similarly, a study of pharmacotherapeutic agents in the treatment of methamphetamine dependence reported that no agent has demonstrated a broad and strong effect in achieving methamphetamine abstinence in Phase II trials. However, agents with novel therapeutic targets appear promising, with more research needed.[410]

Similarly, another review looked at 14 different drugs, including antidepressants, antipsychotics, psychostimulants, anticonvulsants, and opioid antagonists. Although there was no evidence of benefit for psychostimulants overall, there was low strength evidence from two RCTs that methylphenidate may reduce methamphetamine use. Antidepressants had no effect on abstinence or retention based on moderate to high strength evidence. Studies of anticonvulsants, antipsychotics (aripiprazole), and opioid antagonists (naltrexone) provided either low strength evidence of no effect on the outcomes of interest, or insufficient evidence to draw conclusions. Most pharmacotherapies were ineffective in treating methamphetamine use disorder.[411]

Another systematic review and meta-analysis also found that none of the drug classes studied in patients with methamphetamine disorder had strong or consistent evidence of benefit on methamphetamine abstinence, or treatment retention. The study suggests that methylphenidate and topiramate are promising drugs deserving more research.[412]

Similarly, another systematic review that has medications evaluated for methamphetamine/ amphetamine use disorder has reported that many of its findings were insufficient to form strong conclusions. However, there was moderate-strength evidence that antidepressants had no statistically significant effect on abstinence or retention, and low-strength evidence of no statistically significant effect on harms. The review also reported on low-strength evidence that psychostimulants had no statistically significant effect on abstinence and retention. However, methylphenidate may be more effective than placebo in reducing use. Similarly, although the evidence for anticonvulsants/muscle relaxants was insufficient, the review found low-strength evidence that topiramate may be more effective than placebo for reducing methamphetamine/amphetamine use.

In addition, there was low-strength evidence that methylphenidate may reduce amphetamine/methamphetamine use[413] and that naltrexone did not improve treatment retention.

A trial has shown the safety and effectiveness of buprenorphine and bupropion in the treatment of methamphetamine withdrawal craving, although buprenorphine was shown to be superior compared with bupropion.[414] More research is needed.

A Cochrane review[415] of the efficacy and safety of psychostimulant medications for amphetamine dependence (dexamphetamine, bupropion, methylphenidate and modafinil), in addition to psychosocial interventions, reported that no significant differences were found between psychostimulants and placebo for any of the studied outcomes. Overall retention in

studies was low (50.4%). Psychostimulants did not reduce amphetamine use, or amphetamine craving, and did not increase sustained abstinence. The proportion of drop-outs due to adverse events was similar for psychostimulants and placebo. The review concluded that the evidence does not support the prescribing of psychostimulants (at the tested doses) as replacement therapy, although further research may change this conclusion.[418]

A recent systematic review of 43 RCTs examined 23 pharmacotherapies for substance use disorder or drug dependence due to amphetamine/methamphetamine, with various outcomes pertaining to use and associated symptoms. The review found that while some drugs demonstrated results that were statistically significantly better than placebo outcomes, the studies were generally small and the samples biased and study protocol completion was low. The most consistent positive findings have been demonstrated with stimulant agonist treatment (dexamphetamine and methylphenidate), naltrexone and topiramate.[416] Another systematic review has shown there was low-strength evidence that methylphenidate may reduce amphetamine/methamphetamine use.[417]

The evidence on naltrexone is also not consistent.

One the one hand, a small double-blind placebo-controlled study on the use of N-acetyl cysteine plus naltrexone found no significant difference with placebo on treatment outcomes.[406] Similarly, another study has shown that in comparison with placebo, extended-release naltrexone does not appear to reduce methamphetamine use or sexual risk behaviours among methamphetamine-dependent men who have sex with men.[418]

A recent multisite, double-blind, two-stage, placebo-controlled trial to evaluate the efficacy and safety of extended-release injectable naltrexone (380 mg every 3 weeks) plus oral extended-release bupropion (450 mg per day) over a period of 12 weeks in adults with moderate or severe methamphetamine use disorder. The primary outcome found was that a reduction in amphetamine use (defined as at least three methamphetamine-negative urine samples out of four samples obtained in the last 2 weeks of each stage) was overall low, but was higher in those than received the bupropion/ naltrexone than those who received the placebo.[419] Another study has found that naltrexone may be especially effective in methamphetamine-dependent individuals with low executive function.[420]

Other trials conducted with methamphetamine users have tested selegeline, ondansetron, paroxetine,[397] fluoxetine[421,422] and sertraline,[367,399] usually accompanied by a psychosocial structured therapy. A placebo-controlled trial studying the selective serotonin reuptake inhibitor sertraline for the treatment of methamphetamine use showed that subjects receiving sertraline did not show improvements in depressive symptoms or craving compared with those who did not receive it.[399] It has been argued that, overall, results suggest that sertraline, and possibly all selective serotonin reuptake inhibitors, are ineffective and may even be contraindicated for methamphetamine dependence.[399]

A number of small studies have suggested that there may be a potential for the use of mirtazapine (a noradrenergic and specific serotonergic antidepressant).[11,151,423] Mirtazapine (in addition to counselling) was shown to reduce use among active methamphetamine users.[151] It was also shown to lessen the symptoms of methamphetamine withdrawal (including the subjective symptoms) over 10 days of abstinence, with reductions in agitation, anxiety, fatigue, irritability, paranoid ideation, anhedonia, vivid dreams and suicide ideation. It also increased the amount of sleep.[407]

The impact of mirtazapine, in addition to counselling, on sexual behaviours that were shown by one study is noteworthy. A 12-week double-blind trial of mirtazapine among 60 MSM found that most sexual risk behaviours decreased significantly in the mirtazapine arm of the study in comparison with the placebo arm, even though both arms received HIV risk-reduction counselling at baseline. The study also found that the reduction in sexual risks was associated with a reduction in negative test results for amphetamine use, perhaps suggesting a possible causal pathway between the two outcomes.[151]

Not all studies of mirtazapine have shown its effectiveness in the management of methamphetamine dependence.[408] One study which focused on patients with acute withdrawal symptoms showed that it does not facilitate retention or recruitment in outpatient methamphetamine withdrawal treatment.[408]

The use of anticonvulsants has also been investigated. A randomised controlled trial of 140 methamphetamine-dependent adults prescribed topiramate (at doses of up to 200 mg/day) suggested that this medication does not promote abstinence. However, there is some indication that it may reduce amounts ingested and can reduce relapse rates among those already abstinent.[395]

Similarly, a trial randomly assigning people to an active medication regimen – comprising flumazenil (2 mg infusions on days 1, 2, 3, 22, 23), gabapentin (1,200 mg to day 40) and hydroxyzine (50 mg to day 10) – or placebo showed that the regimen was no more effective than placebo in reducing methamphetamine use, retaining patients in treatment or reducing craving.[424] These results were different from those of another study using the same protocol that found fewer positive urine tests for methamphetamine throughout the trial and decreased cravings.[405] Differences may be due to study conditions and different demographic characteristics of participants in a private medical setting.[427]

A double-blind study of 60 subjects with bipolar or major depressive disorder and methamphetamine dependence randomised them to placebo or citicolin, an over-the-counter nutritional supplement (2,000 mg/day), for 12 weeks. A significant between-group difference in depressive symptoms was observed. The study also showed significantly higher completion rates among those on citicolin than those on placebo.[321]

For the moment, however, psychosocial therapies continue to be the cornerstone of treatment, with drug therapy regarded as an adjunct rather than a replacement for psychosocial approaches.[11] There is currently no approved pharmacotherapy for methamphetamine dependence[378] and no specific medication to counteract the effects of methamphetamine withdrawal, or prolong abstinence.[425,426]

10.14.4 Treatment Effectiveness, Impact, Retention and Completion

Some studies have shown that, when methamphetamine users seek treatment, there is a substantial likelihood of treatment drop-out and relapse,[427] although the treatment outcomes for methamphetamine users are not necessarily different from those of the users of other drugs.[428,429] There is, though, a lack of treatment provision.[430]

Although still limited in Europe, the treatment of methamphetamine use disorder can be effective in leading to improvements in substance misuse, injecting, health and criminal behaviour at 1 year after discharge from treatment.[431,432]

Treatment for methamphetamine use/dependence can have a positive impact on other high-risk behaviours. A study of CM and CBT interventions delivered to a group of MSM found that those who reported the greatest decrease in methamphetamine use also reported the greatest and quickest reduction in depressive symptoms and high-risk sexual behaviour.[433] The authors suggest that lowering methamphetamine use can have an effect on depression and sexual behaviour and that some users who respond well to treatment may show improvements in these co-occurring problems, without the need for more intensive targeted interventions.[436]

Similar findings were reported by other studies.[151] There is some evidence that interventions to reduce or eliminate methamphetamine use for MSM in drug treatment settings also produce reductions in high-risk sexual behaviours and resultant HIV transmission. Drug treatment may be an important part of an HIV/STI prevention strategy for MSM.[365] One study of methamphetamine users found that longer treatment retention and greater rates of treatment completion were significantly related to greater reductions in risky sexual and injecting behaviours and were associated with reductions in HIV risk three years after treatment.[434]

There is a growing body of evidence on the factors that help predict methamphetamine treatment success, and most particularly failure, including retention in treatment and treatment completion.[430] There is consistent evidence that poorer outcomes are associated with:

- Greater frequency of use previously
- More extensive history of previous treatment[435,436,437]
- Lower educational attainment,[430,438] although conflicting evidence on this has been reported.[438,439]
- Polydrug use[440]
- Residing in unstable accommodation[441]
- Engaging in criminal behaviours[442]

Conversely, there is some evidence that factors associated with remission from methamphetamine use including maintaining or gaining employment and increased levels of perceived social support were shown to be predictive of remission.[443]

Other factors have also been associated with success or failure, but the evidence is either limited or inconsistent. These include greater craving for methamphetamine,[262] legal coercion of treatment,[430]

residential versus outpatient treatment,[438] shorter treatment duration,[440] disability,[430] selling methamphetamine[440] and intravenous use.[430,439] Race, gender and ethnicity have also been associated with treatment success or failure, but the findings have differed between studies.

Similar factors were identified as affecting health-related quality of life (HRQOL) for those completing treatment. A study of the HRQOL trajectories of 723 people dependent on methamphetamine, resulting from treatment completion and continued care over one year, found greater improvements in mental health. It described 'fairly static' trajectories in physical health status, in comparison with those who did not complete treatment or who continued to use services. The study showed differential patterns of health improvement. Factors identified as negatively affecting HRQOL included unemployment, lifetime trauma, suicide history, interpersonal conflict, continued use of methamphetamine, poly-drug use and medical and psychiatric impairment.[444]

The study also found that higher education was associated with a poorer health outcome, a finding that is not supported by the literature. The authors speculated that this might be because drug use among highly educated subjects can lead to a lower perceived health status, with the subjects not being able to maintain previous health standards and not being able to fulfil goals they had set before drug use. The study also showed poorer health outcomes for women on methamphetamine.[447]

The frequency of use at entry to treatment and early treatment responsiveness have been identified as predictors of treatment success. One study of 60 individuals looked at whether cognitive performance can predict success in treating methamphetamine dependence, and considered whether cognitive performance is more or less predictive of treatment success than established factors, such as frequency of use.[445]

The study found that, although a few neurocognitive and psychiatric variables were associated with treatment outcome, the frequency of methamphetamine use at the study outset was a much stronger predictor of outcomes. Participants who had two or fewer urine tests positive for methamphetamine during the first two weeks were much more likely to complete treatment and achieve abstinence in the majority of the treatment weeks,[448] a finding that was consistent with several other studies.[430,400,438,439,439,441]

The authors suggest that it is possible that this finding was partially due to study design. Nonetheless, the study did show that patterns of methamphetamine use during the initial stages of treatment were able to predict the outcomes in terms of continued use and treatment attendance. A few cognitive measures were related to treatment outcome, but these did not allow for prediction after adjustment for methamphetamine use at the beginning of the study. The authors concluded that clinicians who want to identify patients at risk of treatment failure should use multiple urine tests. They also suggest that it is more plausible to predict treatment failure than treatment success.[448]

Similarly, a study of bupropion found that early treatment responsiveness may be important for positive outcomes, a finding consistent with smoking cessation[403] and with some research in cocaine treatment.[403,404] Data analysis showed that the inability of users to provide at least three methamphetamine-free samples in the first two weeks of treatment was associated with a likelihood of treatment failure exceeding 90%. The authors suggest that clinicians prescribing bupropion can predict treatment failures confidently within two weeks when they carry out drug testing three times a week, with weekly testing yielding acceptable predictive power within three weeks. The ability to predict treatment failure was substantially more precise than the prediction of treatment success, which the authors attributed partially to the overall treatment failure rates. The absence of an early response predicts treatment failure better than the presence of an early good response predicting treatment success. The authors therefore suggest that this prediction of treatment failure is relevant to clinicians, as it signals the need to change treatment modality and intensity.[402]

10.14.5 Access to Treatment

People dependent on methamphetamine may not access treatment services for many years and there is often a delay between first use, first recognising a problem with methamphetamine, and first treatment assessment. Different studies have shown a range for average length of time for the first treatment. An Australian study found that methamphetamine users can wait an average of 5 years from first experiencing problems to seeking treatment.[447] US studies have reported an average of 8[448] and 9 years.[83]

There are many reasons why this may be the case. A US study reported a common belief among methamphetamine users that it is a 'functional drug', which may encourage frequent and prolonged daily use.[83,449] Similarly, Kenny et al. reported common reasons for not seeking methamphetamine treatment: users did not believe that they were dependent (despite meeting DSM-IV criteria for dependence); they did not feel that regular use of methamphetamine warranted formal treatment; they discounted their dependence; and they recognised their dependence but were not ready to do anything about it.[450]

There is also some evidence that treatment services may not be, or be perceived to be, accessible to methamphetamine users. An Australian study[451,452] suggested that the reasons for under-representation of methamphetamine users in the treatment system include poor orientation of services for this group, lack of information about treatment options and little confidence in the effectiveness of programmes.

Barriers to treatment are not only constructed by service users but also by clinical staff. A study has also looked into barriers to methamphetamine treatment from the perspective of treatment providers, who saw barriers as extensive and wide-ranging. They included the particular personality characteristics of methamphetamine users, complexities associated with mental health co-morbidity, waiting periods resulting in loss to treatment, the binge nature of methamphetamine use, lack of pharmacological options and negative attitudes of staff towards this patient group.[453]

Improved understanding of the ways methamphetamine users access other treatment services could be used to facilitate effective referral pathways. Studies have looked at the factors, and user characteristics, that make individuals more likely to seek support.[454,455] GPs have been identified as a likely common starting point for patients seeking referral for all drug-related problems.[456]

Quinn et al.'s study suggests that service utilisation for other problems, such as mental health or other drug problems, increases the likelihood of accessing treatment for methamphetamine use.[458] They suggest that contact with other services may increase the opportunity for treatment of methamphetamine misuse and break down barriers to professional support, such as ignorance of the services available and stigma associated with service utilisation.[457] People who use services for other issues are more receptive to seeking treatment for methamphetamine misuse.[458] The authors also note that these findings suggest a need to facilitate professional support pathways for treating methamphetamine users who engage in harmful use patterns.[458]

The availability of appropriate and relevant services has been identified as enhancing service uptake. Australian studies have suggested that methamphetamine injectors are more likely than those who smoke or snort the drug to seek and receive treatment from specialist services.[458,458,459] It has been suggested that there is greater availability of services for people who inject and fewer barriers to treatment (such as needle exchanges).

In comparison with other substances such as opiates, it may be important to make the treatment settings specific to methamphetamine users, to accommodate the different nature of methamphetamine dependence and withdrawals. Although this may be beyond the means of many drug treatment systems and services, services can undertake some small changes that could have a large impact on user perception, such as allocating some time each day for methamphetamine clients or allocating specific staff or rooms with specific methamphetamine resources.[453]

The cultural competence of services has also been identified as enhancing treatment uptake and enhancing effective harm reduction.[460] A study of behavioural psychological interventions on depression, sexual risk behaviour and methamphetamine use among 162 MSM found that a gay-specific CBT intervention reported the greatest reduction in all three outcomes.[436]

Treatment readiness may also be key to accessing support for methamphetamine problems. Quinn et al. found that two key factors were associated with seeking help for methamphetamine problems: seeking help from family or peers in the year before entry into the study; and adoption of personal methods for the reduction or cessation of methamphetamine use.[458] It has been suggested that targeted interventions to identify and access individuals when they first experience readiness to change could be important. Motivational interviewing and stepped care could be beneficial.

One study found that only a small number of methamphetamine-using participants had reported access to more intensive drug treatment services (i.e. residential detoxification and/or rehabilitation), maybe suggesting a preference for low- rather than high-threshold treatment services,[458,461] or that many individuals feel that they are able to address harmful and/or dependent use without the need for intensive professional intervention.[360]

It has been suggested that elevated rates of violent behaviour amongst people who use amphetamines and methamphetamines indicate that health services need to be equipped to manage this risk.[462]

10.14.6 Interventions for Mental Health

In a summary of clinical and policy implications of a recent systematic review and meta-analysis of mental health problems associated with methamphetamine use, McKetin et al. (2019) have suggested that the current treatment responses, and the siloed arrangement of mental health and substance use services in many countries, hinder the provision of care for co-occurring disorders. The authors also argue that the provision of treatment for co-occurring mental health and substance use disorders is hindered by diagnostic issues, particularly whether psychosis or depression is considered to be amphetamine-related or whether it represents a 'primary' or 'independent' disorder. This can lead to suboptimal management of mental health conditions in cases where symptoms are thought to be amphetamine-related.[463]

10.14.7 Aftercare and Support

See Section 8B.12.5.

10.15 Harm Reduction

The implications of driving under the influence of methamphetamine has been discussed.[464] Harm reduction is covered in Chapter 8.

It is argued that there is a need to revisit harm reduction approaches when applied to stimulant use, as existing harm reduction approaches were developed largely for opioid injectors, and they have been metropolitan based.[465]

References

1. Ben-Yehuda O, Siecke N. Crystal methamphetamine: a drug and cardiovascular epidemic. *JACC Heart Fail* 2018;6:219–221. https://doi.org/10.1016/j.jchf.2018.01.004

2. World Drug Report 2019 (United Nations publication, Sales No. E.19.XI.9). Available at: https://wdr.unodc.org/wdr2019/

prelaunch/WDR19_Booklet_1_EXECUTIVE_SUMMARY .pdf [last accessed 13 March 2022].

3. World Health Organization, Western Pacific Region. Harm Reduction and Brief Interventions for ATS Users (Technical Brief on Amphetamine-Type Stimulants 2). Available at: www .who.int/hiv/pub/idu/ats_brief2.pdf [last accessed 13 March 2022].

4. Panenka WJ, Procyshyn RM, Lecomte T, et al. Methamphetamine use: a comprehensive review of molecular, preclinical and clinical findings. *Drug Alcohol Depend* 2013;**129**(3):167–179. https://doi.org/10.1016/j .drugalcdep.2012.11.016

5. Pérez-Mañá C, Castells X, Torrens M, Capellà D, Farre M. Efficacy of psychostimulant drugs for amphetamine abuse or dependence. *Cochrane Database Syst Rev* 2013; **2**(9):CD009695.

6. Newton TF, De La Garza R, Kalechstein AD, Nestor L. Cocaine and methamphetamine produce different patterns of subjective and cardiovascular effects. *Pharmacol Biochem Behav* 2005;**82**(1):90–97.

7. Weiland-Fiedler P, Erickson K, Waldeck T, et al. Evidence for continuing neuropsychological impairments in depression. *J Affect Disord* 2004;**82**(2):253–258.

8. Fleckenstein AE, Volz TJ, Hanson GR. Psychostimulant-induced alterations in vesicular monoamine transporter-2 function: neurotoxic and therapeutic implications. *Neuropharmacology* 2009;**56**(Suppl. 1_:133–138. https://doi .org/10.1016/j.neuropharm.2008.07.002

9. Sulzer D, Sonders MS, Poulsen NW, Galli A. Mechanisms of neurotransmitter release by amphetamines: a review. *Prog Neurobiol* 2005;**75**(6):406–433.

10. Rose ME, Grant JE. Pharmacotherapy for methamphetamine dependence: a review of the pathophysiology of methamphetamine addiction and the theoretical basis and efficacy of pharmacotherapeutic interventions. *Ann Clin Psychiatry* 2008;**20**:145–155.

11. Volkow ND, Chang L, Wang GJ, et al. Association of dopamine transporter reduction with psychomotor impairment in methamphetamine abusers. *Am J Psychiatry* 2001;**158**(3):377–382.

12. Chang L, Cloak C, Patterson K, et al. Enlarged striatum in abstinent methamphetamine abusers: a possible compensatory response. *Biol Psychiatry* 2005;**57**:967–974.

13. Thompson PM, Hayashi KM, Simon SL, et al. Structural abnormalities in the brains of human subjects who use methamphetamine. *J Neurosci* 2004;**24**:6028–6036.

14. London ED, Simon SL, Berman SM, et al. Mood disturbances and regional cerebral metabolic abnormalities in recently abstinent methamphetamine abusers. *Arch Gen Psychiatry* 2004;**61**(1):73–84.

15. Baicy K, London ED. Corticolimbic dysregulation and chronic methamphetamine abuse. *Addiction* 2007;**102**(Suppl. 1):5–15.

16. Aron JL, Paulus MP. Location, location: using functional magnetic resonance imaging to pinpoint brain differences relevant to stimulant use. *Addiction* 2007;**102**(Suppl. 1):33–43.

17. Volkow ND, Wang GJ, Fowler JS, et al Brain DA D2 receptors predict reinforcing effects of stimulants in humans: replication study. *Synapse* 2002;**46**:79–82.

18. Volkow ND, Li TK. Drug addiction: the neurobiology of behaviour gone awry. *Nat Rev Neurosci* 2004;**5**:963–970.

19. Goldstein RZ, Volkow ND. Drug addiction and its underlying neurobiological basis: neuroimaging evidence for the involvement of the frontal cortex. *Am J Psychiatry* 2002;**159**:1642–1652.

20. Brackins T, Brahm NC, Kissack JC. Treatments for methamphetamine abuse: a literature review for the clinician. *J Pharm Pract* 2011;**24**(6):541–550. https://doi.org/10.1177 /0897190011426557

21. Sora I, Li B, Fumushima S, et al. Monoamine transporter as a target molecule for psychostimulants. *Int Rev Neurobiol* 2009;**85**:29–33.

22. See www.accessdata.fda.gov/drugsatfda_docs/label/2013/0053 78s028lbl.pdf [last accessed 13 March 2022].

23. World Drug Report 2019 (United Nations publication, Sales No. E.19.XI.9).

24. World Drug Report 2020 (United Nations publication, Sales No. E.20.XI.6).

25. European Monitoring Centre for Drugs and Drug Addiction. European Drug Report 2019: Trends and Developments. Luxembourg, Publications Office of the European Union, 2019.

26. van Hout MC, Hearne E. Shake 'N Bake: the migration of 'Pervitin' to Ireland. *Int J Ment Health Addict* 2016;**15** (4):919–927.

27. European Monitoring Centre for Drugs and Drug Addiction. European Drug Report 2020: Trends and Developments. Luxembourg, Publications Office of the European Union, 2020.

28. European Monitoring Centre for Drugs and Drug Addiction. European Drug Report 2020: Trends and Developments. Luxembourg, Publications Office of the European Union, 2020.

29. European Monitoring Centre for Drugs and Drug Addiction. Drugs in Syringes from Six European Cities: Results from the ESCAPE Project 2017. Luxembourg, Publications Office of the European Union, 2019.

30. European Monitoring Centre for Drugs and Drug Addiction. European Drug Report 2020: Trends and Developments. Luxembourg, Publications Office of the European Union, 2020.

31. European Monitoring Centre for Drugs and Drug Addiction. European Drug Report 2020: Trends and Developments. Luxembourg, Publications Office of the European Union, 2020.

32. Mravčík V, Chomynová P, Grohmannová K, et al. National Report: The Czech Republic – 2013 Drug Situation. Praha, Úřad vlády České Republik.

33. Šefránek M, Miovský M. Treatment outcome evaluation in therapeutic communities in the Czech Republic: changes in

methamphetamine use and related problems one year after discharge. *J Groups Addict Recover* 2018 (online). https://doi.org/10.1080/1556035X.2017.1280718

34. European Monitoring Centre for Drugs and Drug Addiction. European Drug Report. Trends and Developments 2015. (EMCDDA Papers). Luxembourg, Publications Office of the European Union, 2015.

35. European Monitoring Centre for Drugs and Drug Addiction. Exploring Methamphetamine Trends in Europe. (EMCDDA Papers). Luxembourg, Publications Office of the European Union, 2014a.

36. European Monitoring Centre for Drugs and Drug Addiction and Europol. Methamphetamine in Europe, EMCDDA-Europol Threat Assessment. Luxembourg, Publications Office of the European Union, 2019.

37. Brecht ML, Greenwell L, Anglin MD. Methamphetamine treatment: trends and predictors of retention and completion in a large state treatment system (1992–2002). *J Subst Abuse Treat* 2005;**29**(4):295–306.

38. Jones CM, Compton WM, Mustaquim D. Centre for Disease Control and Prevention. Patterns and characteristics of methamphetamine use among adults – United States, 2015–2018. *Morb Mortal Wkly Rep* 2020;**69**(12):317.

39. European Monitoring Centre for Drugs and Drug Addiction. European Drug Report: Trends and Developments. Luxembourg, Publications Office of the European Union, 2014.

40. Šefránek M, Miovský M. Treatment outcome evaluation in therapeutic communities in the Czech Republic: changes in methamphetamine use and related problems one year after discharge. J Groups Addict Recover 2017 (online). https://doi.org/10.1080/1556035X.2017.1280718

41. European Monitoring Centre for Drugs and Drug Addiction. Perspectives on drugs. Health and social responses for methamphetamine users. Updated 27 June 2014. Accessed 5 September 2019.

42. Jones CM, Compton WM, Mustaquim D. Centre for Disease Control and Prevention. Patterns and characteristics of methamphetamine use among adults – United States, 2015–2018. *Morb Mortal Wkly Rep* 2020;**69**(12):317.

43. Palmer A, Scott N, Dietze P, et al. Motivations for crystal methamphetamine-opioid co-injection/co-use amongst community-recruited people who inject drugs: a qualitative study. *Harm Reduct J* 2020;**17**:31714. https://doi.org/10.1186/s12954-020-00360-9

44. Home Office. Drug Misuse: Findings from the 2013/14 Crime Survey for England and Wales. July 2001. Available at: https://assets.publishing.service.gov.uk/government/uploads/system/uploads/attachment_data/file/335989/drug_misuse_201314.pdf [last accessed 25 April 2022].

45. Keogh P, Reid D, Bourne A, et al. Wasted Opportunities. Problematic Alcohol and Drug Use Among Gay and Bisexual Men. Available at: www.sigmaresearch.org.uk/files/report2009c.pdf [last accessed 14 March 2022].

46. Stonewall's Gay and Bisexual Men's Health Survey. Available at: www.stonewall.org.uk/system/files/Gay_and_Bisexual_Men_s_Health_Survey__2013_.pdf [last accessed 14 March 2022].

47. Buffin J, Roy A, Williams H, Yorston C (National LGB Drug & Alcohol Database). Part of the Picture: Lesbian, Gay and Bisexual People's Alcohol and Drug Use in England. Substance Dependency and Help-Seeking Behaviour. UCLAN and Lesbian and Gay Foundation. Published 2012.

48. Bonell CP, Hickson FCI, Weatherburn P, et al. Methamphetamine use among gay men across the UK. *Int J Drug Policy* 2010;**21**:244–246.

49. Lea T, Kolstee J, Lambert S, Ness R, Hannan S, Holt M. Methamphetamine treatment outcomes among gay men attending a LGBTI-specific treatment service in Sydney, Australia. *PLOS ONE* 2017 (online). https://doi.org/10.1371/journal.pone.0172560

50. Lea T, Mao L, Hopwood M, et al.Methamphetamine use among gay and bisexual men in Australia: trends in recent and regular use from the Gay Community Periodic Surveys l. Int J Drug Policy 2016;**29**:66–72.

51. Buchacz K, McFarland W, Kellogg TA, et al. Amphetamine use is associated with increased HIV incidence among men who have sex with men in San Francisco. *AIDS* 2005;**19**:1423–1424. https://doi.org/00002030-200509020-00011

52. Plankey MW, Ostrow DG, Stall R, et al. The relationship between methamphetamine and popper use and risk of HIV seroconversion in the multicenter AIDS cohort study. *J Acquir Immune Defic Syndr* 2007;**45**:85–92. https://doi.org/10.1097/QAI.0b013e3180417c99

53. Thiede H, Jenkins RA, Carey JW, et al. Determinants of recent HIV infection among Seattle-area men who have sex with men. *Am J Public Health* 2009;**99**(Suppl. 1):S157–164. https://doi.org/10.2105/AJPH.2006.098582

54. Glick S, Burt R, Moreno C, Ketchum J, Thiede H. Highlights from the 2015 Seattle area National HIV Behavioral Surveillance survey of injection drug use. HIV/AIDS Epidemiology Unit, Public Health – Seattle & King County and the Infectious Disease Assessment Unit, Washington State Department of Health HIV/AIDS Epidemiology Report 2015;**85**:51–58.

55. Glick S, Burt R, Shiver C, Moreno C, Thiede H. Highlights from the 2014 Seattle area National HIV Behavioral Surveillance survey of men who have sex with men. HIV/AIDS Epidemiology Unit, Public Health – Seattle & King County and the Infectious Disease Assessment Unit, Washington State Department of Health HIV/AIDS Epidemiology Report 2015;**84**:55–68.

56. Lima SH, Akbarb M, Wickershamb JA, Kamarulzaman A, Frederick L. The management of methamphetamine use in sexual settings among men who have sex with men in Malaysia. *Int J Drug Policy* 2018;**55**:256–262. https://doi.org/10.1016/j.drugpo.2018.02.019

57. World Drug Report 2019 (United Nations publication, Sales No. E.19.XI.9).

58. Maxwell S, Shahmanesh M, Gafos M. Chemsex behaviours among men who have sex with men: a systematic review of the literature. *Int J Drug Policy* 2019;**63**: 74–89.

59. Bourne A, Reid D, Hickson F, Torres Rueda S, Weatherburn P. The chemsex study: drug use in sexual settings among gay and bisexual men in Lambeth, Southwark and Lewisham. London, Sigma Research, London School of Hygiene and Tropical Medicine. Published 2014. Available at:www .sigmaresearch.org.uk/chemsex[lastaccessed14March2022].

60. Bolding G, Hart G, Sherr L, Elford J. Use of crystal methamphetamine among gay men in London. *Addiction* 2006;**101**:1622–1630.

61. Forrest D, Metsch L, LaLota M, Cardenas G, Beck D, Jeanty Y. Crystal methamphetamine use and sexual risk behaviors among HIV-positive and HIV-negative men who have sex with men in South Florida. *J Urban Health* 2010;**87**:480–485.

62. Schwarcz S, Scheer S, McFarland W, et al. Prevalence of HIV infection and predictors of high transmission sexual risk behaviors among men who have sex with men. *Am J Public Health* 2007;**97**:1067–1075.

63. Whittington W, Collis T, Dithmer-Schreck D, et al. Sexually transmitted diseases and human immunodeficiency virus-discordant partnerships among men who have sex with men. *Clin Infect Dis* 2002;**35**:1010–1017.

64. Buchacz K, McFarland W, Kellogg T, et al. Amphetamine use is associated with increased HIV incidence among men who have sex with men in San Francisco. *AIDS* 2005;**19**:1423–1424.

65. Hoenigl M, Chaillon A, Moore DJ, Morris SR, Davey M, Smith S J. Little, clear links between starting methamphetamine and increasing sexual risk behavior: a cohort study among men who have sex with men. *J Acquir Immune Defic Syndr* 2016;**71**:551–557.

66. Nelson Glick S, Burt R, Kummer K, Tinsley J, Banta-Green CJ, Golden MR. Increasing methamphetamine injection among MSM who inject drugs in King County. *Washington Drug Alcohol Depend* 2018;**182**:86–92. https://doi.org/10.1016/j.drugalcdep .2017.10.011

67. McKetin R, Lubman DI, Baker A, et al.The relationship between methamphetamine use and heterosexual behaviour: evidence from a prospective longitudinal study. *Addiction* 2018;**113**:1276–1285.

68. Degenhardt L, Grant S, Mcketin R, et al. Crystalline methamphetamine use and methamphetamine-related harms in Australia. *Drug Alcohol Rev* 2016 (online). https://doi.org/ 10.1111/dar.12426

69. European Monitoring Centre for Drugs and Drug Addiction and Europol. Methamphetamine in Europe, EMCDDA-Europol Threat Assessment. Luxembourg, Publications Office of the European Union, 2019.

70. Schifano F, Corkery JM, Cuffolo G. Smokable ('ice', 'crystal meth') and non-smokable amphetamine-type stimulants: clinical pharmacological and epidemiological issues, with special reference to the UK. *Ann Ist Super Sanita* 2007;**43** (1):110–115.

71. McKetin R, Kelly E, McLaren J. The relationship between crystalline methamphetamine use and methamphetamine dependence. *Drug Alcohol Depend* 2006;**85**(3):198–204.

72. McKetin R, McLaren J, Lubman DI, Hides L. The prevalence of psychotic symptoms among methamphetamine users. *Addiction* 2006;**101**(10):1473–1478.

73. Barr AM, Panenka WJ, MacEwan GW, et al. The need for speed: an update on methamphetamine addiction. *J Psychiatry Neurosci* 2006;**31**:301–313.

74. Gawin FH, Ellinwood EH Jr. Cocaine and other stimulants. Actions, abuse, and treatment. *N Engl J Med* 1988;**318**:1173–1182.

75. De La Garza R, Zorick T, Heinzerling KG, et al. The cardiovascular and subjective effects of methamphetamine combined with gammavinylgamma-aminobutyric acid (GVG) in non-treatment seeking methamphetamine-dependent volunteers. *Pharmacol Biochem Behav* 2009;**94**:186–193.

76. Gay GR, Sheppard CW. Sex in the 'drug culture'. *Med Asp Hum Sex* 1972;**6**:28–50.

77. Bell DS, Trethowan WH. Amphetamine addiction and disturbed sexuality. *Arch Gen Psychiatry* 1961;**4**:74–78.

78. National Institute on Drug Abuse (NIDA). Are methamphetamine abusers at risk for contracting HIV/AIDS and hepatitis B and C? (Research Report Series: Methamphetamine Abuse and Addiction). Bethesda, MD, Department of Health and Human Services, National Institutes of Health. Revised September 2006. Available at: www.nida.nih.gov/researchreports/methamph/methamph5 .html#hiv [last accessed 14 March 2022].

79. Leamon MH, Flower K, Salo RE, Nordahl TE, Kranzler HR, Galloway GP. Methamphetamine and paranoia: the methamphetamine experience questionnaire. *Am J Addict* 2010;**19**:155–168.

80. Leslie EM, Smirnov A, Cherney A, et al. Predictors of aggressive behavior while under the influence of illicit drugs among young adult methamphetamine users. *Subst Use Misuse* 2018;**53** (14):2439–2443. doi.org/10.1080/10826084.2018.1473434

81. Brecht ML, O'Brien A, von Mayrhauser C, Anglin MD. Methamphetamine use behaviors and gender differences. *Addict Behav* 2004;**29**(1):89–106.

82. Degenhardt L, Topp L. Crystal methamphetamine use among polydrug users in Sydney's dance party subculture: characteristics, use patterns and associated harms. *Int J Drug Policy* 2003;**14**(1):17–24.

83. United Nations Office on Drugs and Crime (UNODC). World Drug Report 2013 (United Nations Publication, Sales No. E.13. XI.6). UNODC, 2013.

84. Lejckova P, Mravcik V. Mortality of hospitalized drug users in the Czech Republic. *J Drug Issues* 2007;**37**:103–118.

85. Arendt M, Munk-Jorgensen P, Sher L, Jensen SO. Mortality among individuals with cannabis, cocaine, amphetamine, MDMA, and opioid use disorders: a nationwide follow-up study of Danish substance users in treatment. *Drug Alcohol Depend* 2010;**114**:134–139.

86. Kuo CJ, Liao YT, Chen WJ, Tsai SY, Lin SK, Chen CC. Causes of death of patients with methamphetamine dependence: a record-linkage study. *Drug Alcohol Rev* 2010;**30**:621–628.

87. Stenbacka M, Leifman A, Romelsjo A. Mortality and cause of death among 1705 illicit drug users: a 37 year follow up. *Drug Alcohol Rev* 2010;**29**:21–27.

88. Cretzmeyer M, Sarrazin MV, Huber DL, Block RI, Hall JA. Treatment of methamphetamine abuse: research findings and clinical directions. *J Subst Abuse Treat* 2003;**24**:267–277.

89. Meredith CW, Jaffe C, Ang-Lee K, Saxon AJ. Implications of chronic methamphetamine use: a literature review. *Harv Rev Psychiatry* 2005;**13**:141–154.

90. Shearer J, Sherman J, Wodak A, van Beek I. Substitution therapy for amphetamine users. *Drug Alcohol Rev* 2002;**21**:179–185.

91. Jones CM, Compton WM, Mustaquim D. Patterns and characteristics of methamphetamine use among adults – United States, 2015–2018. Centre for Disease Control and Prevention. *Morb Mort Wkly Rep* 2020;**69**(12):317.

92. Won S, Hong RA, Shohet RV, Seto TB, Parikh NI. Methamphetamine-associated cardiomyopathy. *Clin Cardiol* 2013;**36**:737–742. https://doi.org/10.1002/clc.2219514

93. Darke S, Duflou J, Kaye S. Prevalence and nature of cardiovascular disease in methamphetamine-related death: a national study. *Drug Alcohol Depend* 2017;**179**:174–179. https://doi.org/10.1016/j.drugalcdep.2017.07.001

94. Voskoboinik A, Ihle JF, Bloom JE, Kaye DM. Amphetamine-induced cardiomyopathy: patterns and predictors of recovery. *Heart Lung Circ* 2015 (online). https://doi.org/10.1016/j.hlc.2015.06.198

95. Kiyatkin EA, Brown PL, Sharma HS. Brain edema and breakdown of the blood–brain barrier during methamphetamine intoxication: critical role of brain hyperthermia. *Eur J Neurosci* 2007;**26**:1242–1253.

96. Harris DS, Reus VI, Wolkowitz OM, Mendelson JE, Jones RT. Altering cortisol level does not change the pleasurable effects of methamphetamine in humans. *Neuropsychopharmacology* 2003;**28**:1677–1684.

97. Vearrier D, Greenberg MI, Miller SN, Okaneku JT, Haggerty DA. Methamphetamine: history, pathophysiology, adverse health effects, current trends, and hazards associated with the clandestine manufacture of methamphetamine. *Dis Mon* 2012;**58**(2):38–89. https://doi.org/10.1016/j.disamonth.2011.09.004

98. Richards JR, Bretz SW, Johnson EB, et al. Methamphetamine abuse and emergency department utilization. *West J Med* 1999;**170**(4):198–202.

99. Wijetunga M, Bhan R, Lindsay J, et al. Acute coronary syndrome and crystal methamphetamine use: a case series. *Hawaii Med J* 2004;**63**(1):8–13.

100. Turnipseed SD, Richards JR, Kirk JD, et al. Frequency of acute coronary syndrome in patients presenting to the emergency department with chest pain after methamphetamine use. *J Emerg Med* 2003;**24**(4):369–373.

101. Karch SB, Stephens BG, Ho CH. Methamphetamine-related deaths in San Francisco: demographic, pathologic, and toxicologic profiles. *J Forensic Sci* 1999;**44**(2):359–368.

102. Chen JP. Methamphetamine-associated acute myocardial infarction and cardiogenic shock with normal coronary arteries: refractory global coronary microvascular spasm. *J Invasive Cardiol* 2007;**19**(4):E89–92.

103. Kevil CG, Goeders NE, Woolard MD, et al. Methamphetamine use and cardiovascular disease: in search of answers. *Arterioscler Thromb Vasc Biol* 2019;**39**:1739–1746. https://doi.org/10.1161/ATVBAHA.119.312461

104. Farnsworth TL, Brugger CH, Malters P. Myocardial infarction after intranasal methamphetamine. *Am J Health Syst Pharm* 1997;**54**(5):586–587.

105. Hong R, Matsuyama E, Nur K. Cardiomyopathy associated with the smoking of crystal methamphetamine. *JAMA* 1991;**265**(9):1152–1154.

106. Karch SB. The unique histology of methamphetamine cardiomyopathy: a case report. *Forensic Sci Int* 2011;**212**(1–3):e1–4. https://doi.org/10.1016/j.forsciint.2011.04.028

107. Diercks DB, Fonarow GC, Kirk JD, et al. ADHERE Scientific Advisory Committee and Investigators. Illicit stimulant use in a United States heart failure population presenting to the emergency department (from the Acute Decompensated Heart Failure National Registry Emergency Module). *Am J Cardiol* 2008;**102**(9):1216–1219. https://doi.org/10.1016/j.amjcard.2008.06.045

108. Haning W, Goebert D. Electrocardiographic abnormalities in methamphetamine abusers. *Addiction* 2007;**102**(Suppl. 1):70–75.

109. Islam MN, Jesmine K, Kong Sn Molh A, et al. Histopathological studies of cardiac lesions after long term administration of methamphetamine in high dosage – Part II. *Leg Med* 2009;**11**(Suppl. 1):S147–150.

110. Swalwell CI, Davis GG. Methamphetamine as a risk factor for acute aortic dissection. *J Forensic Sci* 1999;**44**(1):23–26.

111. Kaye S, McKetin R, Duflou J, Darke S. Methamphetamine and cardiovascular pathology: a review of the evidence. *Addiction* 2007;**102**(8):1204–1211.

112. Zhu Z, Osman S, Stradling D, et al. Clinical characteristics and outcomes of methamphetamine-associated versus non-methamphetamine intracerebral hemorrhage. *Sci Rep* 2020;**10**:6375.

113. Albertson TE, Derlet RW, Van Hoozen BE. Methamphetamine and the expanding complications of amphetamines. *West J Med* 1999;**170**:214–219.

114. Darke S, Kaye S, McKetin R, Duflou J. Major physical and psychological harms of methamphetamine use. *Drug Alcohol Rev* 2008;**27**:253–262.

115. Perez Jr JA, Arsura EL, Strategos S. Methamphetamine-related stroke: four cases. *J Emerg Med* 1999;**17**:469–471.

116. Lappin JM, Darke S, Farrell M. Stroke and methamphetamine use in young adults: a review. *J Neurol Neurosurg Psychiatry* 2017;**88**(12):1079–1091.

117. Darke S, Lappin J, Kaye S, Duflou J. Clinical characteristics of fatal methamphetamine-related stroke: a national study. *J Forensic Sci* 2018;**63**(3):735–739. https://doi.org/10.1111/1556-4029.13620

118. Eliveha J, Vindhyal S, Vindhyal M. Cardiac and systemic thrombus caused by drug abuse. *Case Rep Cardiol* 2019; 2019. https://doi.org/10.1155/2019/5083624

119. European Monitoring Centre for Drugs and Drug Addiction (EMCDDA). The Levels of Use of Opioids, Amphetamines and Cocaine and Associated Levels of Harm: Summary of Scientific Evidence. Published March 2014.

120. Richards JR, Wang CG, Fontenette RW, Stuart RP, McMahon KF, Turnipseed SD. Rhabdomyolysis, methamphetamine, amphetamine and MDMA use: associated factors and risks. *J Dual Diagn* 2020;16(4):429–437.

121. Richards JR, Johnson EB, Stark RW, et al. Methamphetamine abuse and rhabdomyolysis in the ED: a 5-year study. *Am J Emerg Med* 1999;17(7):681–685.

122. Angrist B, Sathananthan G, Wilk S, Gershon S. Amphetamine psychosis: behavioral and biochemical aspects. *J Psychiatr Res* 1974;11:13–23.

123. Bell DS. The experimental reproduction of amphetamine psychosis. *Arch Gen Psychiatry* 1973;29(1):35–40.

124. Griffith JD. Experimental psychosis induced by the administration of d-amphetamine. In: E Costa, S Garattini, (eds.),*Amphetamine and Related Compounds*. New York, Raven Press, 1970.

125. Marshall BD, Werb D. Health outcomes associated with methamphetamine use among young people: a systematic review. *Addiction* 2010;105(6):991–1002.

126. Degenhardt L, Whiteford H, Hall WD. The Global Burden of Disease projects: what have we learned about illicit drug use and dependence and their contribution to the global burden of disease. *Drug Alcohol Rev* 2014;33(1):4–12.

127. McKetina R, Leunga J, Stockings E, et al.Mental health outcomes associated with the use of amphetamines: a systematic review and meta-analysis. *Clin Med* 2019; 16:81–97. https://doi.org/10.1016/j.eclinm.2019.09.014 2589-5370

128. Angrist B, Sathananthan G, Wilk S, Gershon S. Amphetamine psychosis: behavioral and biochemical aspects. *J Psychiatr Res* 1974;11:13–23.

129. Bell DS. The experimental reproduction of amphetamine psychosis. *Arch Gen Psychiatry* 1973;29(1):35–40.

130. Griffith JD. Experimental psychosis induced by the administration of d-amphetamine. In: E Costa, S Garattini, (eds.),*Amphetamine and Related Compounds*. New York, Raven Press, 1970.

131. McKetin R, Dawe S, Burns RA, et al. The profile of psychiatric symptoms exacerbated by methamphetamine use. *Drug Alcohol Depend* 2016;161:104–109.

132. See for example: Hoenigl M, Chaillon A, Moore DJ, Morris SR, Smith DM, Little SJ. Clear links between starting methamphetamine and increasing sexual risk behavior: a cohort study among men who have sex with men. *J Acquir Immune Defic Syndr* 2016;71(5):551–557. https://doi.org/10.1097/QAI.0000000000000888

133. Greenwood GL, White EW, Page-Shafer K, et al. Correlates of heavy substance use among young gay and bisexual men: the San Francisco Young Men's Health Study. *Drug Alcohol Depend* 2001;61:105–112.

134. Maxwell S, Shahmanesh M, Gafos M. Chemsex behaviours among men who have sex with men: a systematic review of the literature. *Int J Drug Policy* 2019;63: 74–89.

135. Maxwell S, Shahmanesh M, Gafos M. Chemsex behaviours among men who have sex with men: a systematic review of the literature. *Int J Drug Policy* 2019;63: 74–89.

136. Bourne A, Reid D, Hickson F, et al. Illicit drug use in sexual settings ('chemsex') and HIV/STI transmission risk behaviour among gay men in South London: findings from a qualitative study. *Sex Transm Infect* 2015;91(8):564–568.

137. Perelló R, Aused M, Saubí N, et al. Acute street drug poisoning in the patient with human immunodeficiency virus infection: the role of chemsex. *Emergencias: Revista de la Sociedad Espanola de Medicina de Emergencias* 2018;30 (6):405–407.

138. Graf N, Dichtl A, Deimel D, Sander D, Stöver H. Chemsex among men who have sex with men in Germany: motives, consequences and the response of the support system. *Sex Health* 2018;15:151–156. https://doi.org/10.1071/SH17142

139. Kenyon C, Wouters K, Platteau T, et al. Increases in condomless chemsex associated with HIV acquisition in MSM but not heterosexuals attending a HIV testing center in Antwerp, Belgium. *AIDS Res Ther* 2018;15:14. https://doi.org/10.1186/s12981-018-0201-3

140. Glynn RW, Byrne N, O'Dea S, Shanley A. Chemsex, risk behaviours and sexually transmitted infections among men who have sex with men in Dublin, Ireland. *Int J Drug Policy* 2017 (online). https://doi.org/10.1016/j.drugpo.2017.10.008

141. Anzillotti L, Calò A, Banchini et al. Mephedrone and chemsex: a case report. *Leg Med* 2020;42:101640.

142. Giorgetti R, Tagliabracci A, Schifano F, Zaami S, Marinelli E, Busardò FP. when 'chems' meet sex: a rising phenomenon called 'chemsex'. *Curr Neuropharmacol* 2017;15(5):762–770.

143. Bourne A, Reid D, Hickson F, et al. Illicit drug use in sexual settings ('chemsex') and HIV/STI transmission risk behaviour among gay men in South London: findings from a qualitative study. *Sex Transm Infect* 2015;91(8):564–568.

144. Perelló R, Aused M, Saubí N, et al. Acute street drug poisoning in the patient with human immunodeficiency virus infection: the role of chemsex. *Emergencias: Revista de la Sociedad Espanola de Medicina de Emergencias* 2018;30(6):405–407.

145. Kirby T, Thornber-Dunwell M. High-risk drug practices tighten grip on London gay scene. *Lancet* 2013;381 (9861):101–102.

146. Saxton P, Newcombe D, Ahmed A, Dickson N, Hughes A. Illicit drug use among New Zealand gay and bisexual men: prevalence and association with sexual health behaviours. *Drug Alcohol Rev* 2018;37:180–187. https://doi.org/10.1111/dar.12536

147. Semple SJ, Patterson TL, Grant I. Motivations associated with methamphetamine use among HIV men who have sex with men. *J Subst Abuse Treat* 2002;**22**(3):149–156.

148. Rhodes T, Quirk A. Drug users' sexual relationships and the social organization of risk: the sexual relationship as a site of risk management. *Soc Sci Med* 1998;**46**(2):157–169.

149. Colfax GN, Santos GM, Das M, et al. Mirtazapine to reduce methamphetamine use: a randomized controlled trial. *Arch Gen Psychiatry* 2011;**68**:1168–1175.

150. Mansergh G, Colfax GN, Marks G, Rader M, Guzman R, Buchbinder S. The Circuit Party Men's Health Survey: findings and implications for gay and bisexual men. *Am J Public Health* 2001;**91**:953–958.

151. Molitor F, Ruiz JD, Flynn N, Mikanda JN, Sun RK, Anderson R. Methamphetamine use and sexual and injection risk behaviors among out-of-treatment injection drug users. *Am J Drug Alcohol Abuse* 1999;**25**:475–493.

152. Shoptaw S, Reback CJ. Methamphetamine use and infectious disease-related behaviors in men who have sex with men: implications for interventions. *Addiction* 2007;**102**(Suppl. 1):130–135.

153. Drumright LN, Gorbach PM, Little SJ, Strathdee SA. Associations between substance use, erectile dysfunction medication and recent HIV infection among men who have sex with men. *AIDS Behav* 2009;**13**:328–336. https://doi.org/10.1007/s10461-007-9330-8

154. Plankey MW, Ostrow DG, Stall R, et al. The relationship between methamphetamine and popper use and risk of HIV seroconversion in the multicenter AIDS cohort study. *J Acquir Immune Defic Syndr* 2007;**45**(1):85–92. https://doi.org/10.1097/QAI.0b013e3180417c99

155. Shoptaw S, Reback CJ. Associations between methamphetamine use and HIV infection in men who have sex with men: a model for guiding public policy. *J Urban Health* 2006;**83**(6):1151–1157. https://doi.org/10.1007/s11524-006-9119-5

156. Rajasingham R, Mimiaga MJ, White JM, Pinkston MM, Baden RP, Mitty JA. A systematic review of behavioral and treatment outcome studies among HIV-infected men who have sex with men who abuse crystal methamphetamine. *AIDS Patient Care STDS* 2012;**26**(1):36–52. https://doi.org/10.1089/apc.2011.0153

157. Carey J, Mejia R, Bingham T, et al. Drug use, high-risk sex behaviors, and increased risk for recent HIV infection among men who have sex with men in Chicago and Los Angeles. *AIDS Behav* 2009;**13**:1084–1096.

158. Halkitis P, Mukherjee P, Palamar J. Longitudinal modelling of methamphetamine use and sexual risk behaviors in gay and bisexual men. *AIDS Behav* 2009;**13**:783–791.

159. Wong W, Chow JK, Kent CK, Klausner JD. Risk factors for early syphilis among gay and bisexual men seen in an STD clinic: San Francisco, 2002–2003. *Sex Transm Dis* 2005;**32** (7):458–463.

160. Reback CJ, Grella CE. HIV risk behaviors of gay and bisexual male methamphetamine users contacted through street outreach. *J Drug Issues* 1999;**29**:155–166.

161. Colfax GN, Mansergh G, Guzman R, et al. Drug use and sexual risk behavior among gay and bisexual men who attend circuit parties: a venue-based comparison. *J Acquir Immune Defic Syndr* 2001;**28**(4):373–379.

162. Colfax G, Vittinghoff E, Husnik MJ, et al. EXPLORE Study Team. Substance use and sexual risk: a participant- and episode-level analysis among a cohort of men who have sex with men. *Am J Epidemiol* 2004;**159**(10):1002–1012.

163. Frosch D, Shoptaw S, Huber A, Rawson RA, Ling W. Sexual HIV risk among gay and bisexual male methamphetamine abusers. *J Subst Abuse Treat* 1996;**13**(6):483–486.

164. Gorman EM, Morgan P, Lambert EY. Qualitative research considerations and other issues in the study of methamphetamine use among men who have sex with other men. *NIDA Res Monogr* 1995;**157**:156–181.

165. Halkitis PN, Parsons JT, Stirratt MJ. A double epidemic: crystal methamphetamine drug use in relation to HIV transmission among gay men. *J Homosexuality* 2001;**41**:17–35.

166. Paul JP, Stall R, Davis F. Sexual risk for HIV transmission among gay/bisexual men in substance abuse treatment. *AIDS Educ Prev* 1993;**5**:11–24.

167. Peck JA, Shoptaw S, Rotheram-Fuller E, Reback CJ, Bierman B. HIV-associated medical, behavioral, and psychiatric characteristics of treatment-seeking, methamphetamine-dependent men who have sex with men. *J Addict Dis* 2005;**24**:115–132.

168. Reback CJ, Larkins S, Shoptaw S. Changes in the meaning of sexual risk behaviors among gay and bisexual male methamphetamine abusers before and after drug treatment. *AIDS Behav* 2004;**8**:87–98.

169. Shoptaw S, Reback CJ, Frosch DL, Rawson RA. Stimulant abuse treatment as HIV prevention. *J Addict Dis* 1998;**17**:19–32.

170. Davis LE, Kalousek G, Rubenstein E. Hepatitis associated with illicit use of intravenous methamphetamine. *Public Health Rep* 1970;**85**:809–813.

171. Greenwell L, Brecht ML. Self-reported health status among treated methamphetamine users. *Am J Drug Alcohol Abuse* 2003;**29**:75–104.

172. Harkess J, Gildon B, Istre GR. Outbreaks of hepatitis A among illicit drug users, Oklahoma, 1984–98 [comment]. *Am J Public Health* 1989;**79**:463–466.

173. Hutin YJ, Sabin KM, Hutwagner LC, et al. Multiple modes of hepatitis A virus transmission among methamphetamine users. *Am J Epidemiol* 2000;**152**:186–192.

174. Koester S, Glanz J, Barón A. Drug sharing among heroin networks: implications for HIV and hepatitis B and C prevention. *AIDS Behav* 2005;**9**:27–39.

175. Meyer JM. Prevalence of hepatitis A, hepatitis B, and HIV among hepatitis C-seropositive state hospital patients: results from Oregon State Hospital. *J Clin Psychiatry* 2003;**64**:540–545.

176. Urbina A, Jones K. Crystal methamphetamine, its analogues, and HIV infection: medical and psychiatric aspects of a new epidemic. *Clin Infect Dis* 2004;**38**:890–894.

177. Vogt TM, Perz JF, Van Houten CKJ, et al. An outbreak of hepatitis B virus infection among methamphetamine injectors: the role of sharing injection drug equipment. *Addiction* 2006;**101**:726–730.

178. Rudy ET, Shoptaw S, Lazzar M, Bolan RK, Tilekar SD, Kerndt PR. Methamphetamine use and other club drug use differ in relation to HIV status and risk behavior among gay and bisexual men. *Sex Transm Dis* 2009;**36**:693–695.

179. Burcham JL, Tindall B, Marmor M, Cooper DA, Berry G, Penny R. Incidence and risk factors for human immunodeficiency virus seroconversion in a cohort of Sydney homosexual men. *Med J Aust* 1989;**150**(11):634–639.

180. Chesney MA, Barrett DC, Stall R. Histories of substance use and risk behavior: precursors to HIV seroconversion in homosexual men. *Am J Public Health* 1998;**88**(1):113–116.

181. Koblin BA, Husnik MJ, Colfax G, et al. Risk factors for HIV infection among men who have sex with men. *AIDS* 2006;**20** (5):731–739.

182. Menza TW, Hughes JP, Celum CL, Golden MR. Prediction of HIV acquisition among men who have sex with men. *Sex Transm Dis* 2009;**36**(9):547–555.

183. Bousman CA, Cherner M, Ake C, et al. Negative mood and sexual behavior among non-monogamous men who have sex with men in the context of methamphetamine and HIV. *J Affect Disord* 2009;**119**:84–91.

184. Mayer KH, O'Cleirigh C, Skeer M, et al. Which HIV-infected men who have sex with men in care are engaging in risky sex and acquiring sexually transmitted infections: findings from a Boston community health centre. *Sex Transm Infect* 2010;**86**:66–70.

185. Mansergh G, Shouse RL, Marks G, et al. Methamphetamine and sildenafil (Viagra) use are linked to unprotected receptive and insertive anal sex, respectively, in a sample of men who have sex with men. *Sex Transm Infect* 2006;**82**:131–134.

186. Halkitis P, Shrem M, Martin F. Sexual behavior patterns of methamphetamine-using gay and bisexual men. *Subst Use Misuse* 2005;**40**:703–719.

187. Marquez C, Mitchell SJ, Hare CB, John M, Klausner JD. Methamphetamine use, sexual activity, patient–provider communication, and medication adherence among HIV-infected patients in care, San Francisco 2004–2006. *AIDS Care* 2009;**21**:575–582.

188. Wohl A, Frye D, Johnson D. Demographic characteristics and sexual behaviors associated with methamphetamine use among MSM and non-MSM diagnosed with AIDS in Los Angeles County. *AIDS Behav* 2008;**12**:705–712.

189. Spindler HH, Scheer S, Chen SY, et al. Viagra, methamphetamine, and HIV risk: results from a probability sample of MSM, San Francisco. *Sex Transm Dis* 2007;**34**:586–591.

190. Semple S, Zians J, Grant I, Patterson T. Sexual compulsivity in a sample of HIV-positive methamphetamine-using gay and bisexual men. *AIDS Behav* 2006;**10**:587–598.

191. Hall W, Hando J. Route of administration and adverse effects of amphetamine use among young adults in Sydney, Australia. *Drug Alcohol Rev* 1994;**13**:277–284.

192. Klee H. HIV risks for women drug injectors: heroin and amphetamine users compared. *Addiction* 1993;**88**:1055–1062.

193. Bourne A, Reid D, Hickson F, Torres Rueda S, Steinberg P, Weatherburn P. A perfect storm? Modern technological and structural facilitators of drug use during sex among gay men in London. Poster presentation, 2014. Available at: https://sigmaresearch.org.uk/files/Adam_Bourne_IAS_Melbourne_2014e_poster.pdf [last accessed 25 April 2022].

194. Bourne A, Reid D, Torres Rueda S, Hickson F, Steinberg P, Weatherburn P. A perfect storm? Modern technological and structural facilitators of drug use during sex among gay men in London. XX International AIDS Conference, Melbourne, Australia, 20–25 July 2014 (poster). Available at: http://sigmaresearch.org.uk/presentations/item/talk2014e

195. Jennings J, Tilchin C, Schumacher C, et al. Sex, drugs and the Internet – the perfect storm for syphilis transmission among black gay and bisexual men (BMSM) 1. *Sex Transm Infect* 2019;**95**(Suppl. 1):A1–A376.

196. Hatfield LA, Horvath KJ, Jacoby SM, Simon Rosser BR. Comparison of substance use and risky sexual behaviour among a diverse sample of urban, HIV-positive men who have sex with men. *J Addict Dis* 2009;**28**:208–218.

197. Patterson T, Semple S, Zians J, Strathdee S. Methamphetamine-using HIV-positive men who have sex with men: correlates of polydrug use. *J Urban Health* 2005;**82**: i120–126.

198. Semple SJ, Strathdee SA, Zians J, Patterson TL. Sexual risk behavior associated with co-administration of methamphetamine and other drugs in a sample of HIV-positive men who have sex with men. *Am J Addict* 2009;**18**:65–72.

199. Semple SJ, Strathdee SA, Zians J, Patterson TL. Social and behavioral characteristics of HIV-positive MSM who trade sex for methamphetamine. *Am J Drug Alcohol Abuse* 2010;**36**:325–331.

200. Semple S, Zians J, Strathdee S, Patterson T. Sexual marathons and methamphetamine use among HIV-positive men who have sex with men. *Arch Sex Behav* 2009;**38**:583–590.

201. Semple S, Strathdee S, Zians J, Patterson T. Factors associated with sex in the context of methamphetamine use in different sexual venues among HIV-positive men who have sex with men. *BMC Public Health* 2010;**10**:178.

202. Semple SJ, Patterson TL, Grant I. Binge use of methamphetamine among HIV-positive men who have sex with men: pilot data and HIV prevention implications. *AIDS Educ Prev* 2003;**15**:133.

203. Halkitis PN, Mukherjee PP, Palamar JJ. Multi-level modelling to explain methamphetamine use among gay and bisexual men. *Addiction* 2007;**102**(Suppl. 1):76–83.

204. Waldo CR, McFarland W, Katz MH, MacKellar D, Valleroy LA. Very young gay and bisexual men are at risk for

HIV infection: the San Francisco Bay Area Young Men's Survey II. *J Acquir Immune Defic Syndr* 2000;**24**:168–174.

205. Woody GE, Donnell D, Seage GR, et al. Non-injection substance use correlates with risky sex among men having sex with men: data from HIVNET. *Drug Alcohol Depend* 1999;**53**:197–205.

206. Corsi KF, Booth RE. HIV sex risk behaviors among heterosexual methamphetamine users: literature review from 2000 to present. *Curr Drug Abuse Rev* 2008;**1**(3):292–296.

207. Molitor F, Truax SR, Ruiz JD, Sun RK. Association of methamphetamine use during sex with risky sexual behaviors and HIV infection among non-injection drug users. *West J Med* 1998;**168**(2):93–97.

208. Semple SJ, Patterson TL, Grant I. Determinants of condom use stage of change among heterosexually-identified methamphetamine users. *AIDS Behavior* 2004;**8**:391–400.

209. Semple SJ, Patterson TL, Grant I. The context of sexual risk behavior among heterosexual methamphetamine users. *Addict Behav* 2004;**29**:807–810.

210. Morb M. Methamphetamine use and HIV risk behaviors among heterosexual men – preliminary results from five northern California counties, December 2001– November 2003. *Morb Mort Wkly Rep* 2006;**55**(10):273–277.

211. Copeland AL, Sorensen JL. Differences between methamphetamine users and cocaine users in treatment. *Drug Alcohol Depend* 2001;**62**(1):91–95.

212. Maxwell JC, Rutkowski BA. The prevalence of methamphetamine and amphetamine abuse in North America: a review of the indicators, 1992–2007. *Drug Alcohol Rev* 2008;**27**:229–235.

213. Braine N, Des Jarlais DC, Goldblatt C, Zadoretzky C, Turner C. HIV risk behavior among amphetamine injectors at US syringe exchange programs. *AIDS Educ Prev* 2005;**17**:515–524.

214. Hall W, Darke S, Ross M, Wodak A. Patterns of drug use and risk-taking among injecting amphetamine and opioid drug users in Sydney, Australia. *Addiction* 1993;**88**:509–516.

215. Kaye S, Darke S. A comparison of the harms associated with the injection of heroin and amphetamines. *Drug Alcohol Depend* 2000;**58**:189–195.

216. McKetin R, Ross J, Kelly E, et al. Characteristics and harms associated with injecting versus smoking methamphetamine among methamphetamine treatment entrants. *Drug Alcohol Rev* 2008;**27**:277–285.

217. Fairbairn N, Wood E, Stoltz JA, Li K, Montaner JS, Kerr T. Crystal methamphetamine use associated with non-fatal overdose among a cohort of injection drug users in Vancouver. *Public Health* 2008;**122**:70–78.

218. Fairbairn N, Kerr T, Buxton JA, Li K, Montaner JS, Wood E. Increasing use and associated harms of crystal methamphetamine injection in a Canadian setting. *Drug Alcohol Depend* 2007;**88**:313–316.

219. Hayashi K, Wood E, Suwannawong P, Kaplan K, Qi J, Kerr T. Methamphetamine injection and syringe sharing among a community-recruited sample of injection drug users in Bangkok, Thailand. *Drug Alcohol Depend* 2011;**115**:145–149.

220. Lorvick J, Martinez A, Gee L, Kral AH. Sexual and injection risk among women who inject methamphetamine in San Francisco. *J Urban Health* 2006;**83**:497–505.

221. Semple SJ, Patterson TL, Grant I. A comparison of injection and non-injection methamphetamine using HIV-positive men who have sex with men. *Drug Alcohol Depend* 2004;**76**(2):203–212.

222. Hall W, Hando J, Darke S, Ross J. Psychological morbidity and route of administration among amphetamine users in Sydney, Australia. *Addiction* 1996;**91**:81–87.

223. Zweben JE, Cohen JB, Christian D, et al. Psychiatric symptoms in methamphetamine users. *Am J Addict* 2004;**13**:181–190.

224. Darke S, Kaye S, Duflou J, Lappin J. Completed suicide among methamphetamine users: a national study. *Suicide Life Threat Behav* 2019;**49**(1):328–337. https://doi.org/10.1111/sltb.12442

225. Glasner-Edwards S, Mooney LJ, Marinelli-Casey P, Hillhouse M, Ang A, Rawson R. Risk factors for suicide attempts in methamphetamine-dependent patients. *Am J Addict* 2008;**17**:24–27.

226. Marshall BD, Grafstein E, Buxton JA, et al. Frequent methamphetamine injection predicts emergency department utilization among street-involved youth. *Public Health* 2012;**126** (1):47–53. https://doi.org/10.1016/j.puhe.2011.09.011

227. Darke S, Hall W. Levels and correlates of polydrug use among heroin users and regular amphetamine users. *Drug Alcohol Depend* 1995;**39**(3):231–235.

228. Grant BF, Harford TC. Concurrent and simultaneous use of alcohol with cocaine: results of national survey. *Drug Alcohol Depend* 1990;**25**:97–104.

229. Druglnfo Clearinghouse. Methamphetamine. Prevention Research Quarterly: Current Evidence Evaluated. 2008;**24**(2). Available at: www.druginfo.adf.org.au

230. Cook CE, Jeffcoat AR, Sadler BM, et al. Pharmacokinetics of oral methamphetamine and effects of repeated daily dosing in humans. *Drug Metab Dispos* 1992;**20**:856–862.

231. Lai MW, Klein-Schwartz W, Rodgers GC, et al. 2005 Annual report of the American Association of Poison Control Centers' national poisoning and exposure database. *Clin Toxicol* 2006;**44**:803–932.

232. Chan P, Chen JH, Lee MH, Deng JF. Fatal and nonfatal methamphetamine intoxication in the intensive care unit. *J Toxicol Clin Toxicol* 1994;**32**:147–155.

233. Kerr T, Wood E, Grafstein E, et al. High rates of primary care and emergency department use among injection drug users in Vancouver. *J Public Health* 2005;**27**:62e6.

234. Hendrickson RG, Cloutier RL, Fu R. The association of controlling pseudoephedrine availability on methamphetamine-related emergency department visits. *Acad Emerg Med* 2010;**17**:1216–1222.

235. Hendrickson RG, Cloutier RL, McConnell KJ. Methamphetamine-related emergency department utilization and cost. *Acad Emerg Med* 2008;**15**:23–31.

236. Schep LJ, Slaughter RJ, Beasley MG. The clinical toxicology of methamphetamine. *Clin Toxicol* 2010;**48**:675–694.

237. Glasner-Edwards S, Mooney LJ, Marinelli-Casey P, et al. Clinical course and outcomes of methamphetamine-dependent adults with psychosis. *J Subst Abuse Treat* 2008;**35**:445–450.

238. Mahoney JJ, Kalechstein AD, De La Garza R, Newton TF. Presence and persistence of psychotic symptoms in cocaine-versus methamphetamine-dependent participants. *Am J Addict* 2008;**17**:83–98.

239. McKetin R, McLaren J, Lubman DI, Hides L. The prevalence of psychotic symptoms among methamphetamine users. *Addiction* 2008;**17**:24–27.

240. Iwanami A, Sugiyama A, Kuroki N, et al. Patients with methamphetamine psychosis admitted to a psychiatric hospital in Japan – a preliminary report. *Acta Psychiatr Scand* 1994;**89**:428–432.

241. Nakama H, Chang L, Cloak C, et al. Association between psychiatric symptoms and craving in methamphetamine users. *Am J Addict* 2008;**17**:441–446.

242. West PL, McKeown NJ, Hendrickson RG. Methamphetamine body stuffers: an observational case series. *Ann Emerg Med* 2010;**55**:190–197.

243. Glasner-Edwards S, Marinelli-Casey P, Hillhouse M, et al. Depression among methamphetamine users: association with outcomes from the Methamphetamine Treatment Project at 3-year follow-up. *J Nerv Ment Dis* 2009;**197**:225–231.

244. Sutcliffe CG, German D, Sirirohn B, et al. Patterns of methamphetamine use and symptoms of depression among young adults in northern Thailand. *Drug Alcohol Depend* 2009;**101**:146–151.

245. Pasic J, Russo JE, Ries RK, Roy-Byrne PP. Methamphetamine users in the psychiatric emergency services: a case-control study. *Am J Drug Alcohol Abuse* 2007;**33**:675–686.

246. Bunting PJ, Fulde GWO, Forster SL. Comparison of crystalline methamphetamine ('ice') users and other patients with toxicology-related problems presenting to a hospital emergency department. *Med J Austr* 2007;**187**:564–566.

247. Cloutier RL, Hendrickson RG, Fu RR, Blake B. Methamphetamine-related psychiatric visits to an urban academic emergency department: an observational study. *J Emerg Med* 2013;**45**(1):136–142. https://doi.org/10.1016/j.jemermed.2012.11.094

248. Isoardi KZ, Ayles SF, Harris K, Finch CJ, Page CB. Methamphetamine presentations to an emergency department: management and complications. *Emerg Med Australas* 2019;**31**:593–599.

249. Unadkat A, Subasinghe S, Harvey RJ, Castle DJ. Methamphetamine use in patients presenting to emergency departments and psychiatric inpatient facilities: what are the service implications? *Australas Psychiatry* 2019;**27**(1):14–17.

250. Isoardi KZ, Ayles SF, Harris K, Finch CJ, Page CB. Methamphetamine presentations to an emergency department: management and complications. *Emerg Med Australas* 2019;**31**:593–599.

251. McKetin R, Baker AL, Dawe S, Voce A, Lubman DI. Differences in the symptom profile of methamphetamine-related psychosis and primary psychotic disorders. *Psychiatry Res* 2017;**251**:349–354. https://doi.org/10.1016/j.psychres.2017.02.028

252. Shoptaw SJ, Kao U, Ling W. Treatment for amphetamine psychosis. *Cochrane Database Syst Rev* 2009;**1**:CD003026. https://doi.org/10.1002/14651858.CD003026.pub3

253. Wang G, Zhang Y, Zhang S, et al. Aripiprazole and risperidone for treatment of methamphetamine-associated psychosis in Chinese patients. *J Subst Abuse Treat* 2016;**62**:84–88. https://doi.org/10.1016/j.jsat.2015.11.009

254. Chiang M, Lombardi D, Du J, et al. Methamphetamine-associated psychosis: clinical presentation, biological basis, and treatment options. *Hum Psychopharmacol Clin Exp* 2019;**2019**:e2710. https://doi.org/10.1002/hup.2710

255. McKetina R, Leunga J, Stockings E, et al. Mental health outcomes associated with the use of amphetamines: a systematic review and meta-analysis. *Clin Med* 2019; **16**: 81–97. https://doi.org/10.1016/j.eclinm.2019.09.014 2589-5370

256. Jones CM, Compton WM, Mustaquim D. Patterns and characteristics of methamphetamine use among adults – United States, 2015–2018. Centre for Disease Control and Prevention. *Morb Mort Wkly Rep* 2020;**69**(12):317.

257. Bruehl AM, Lende DH, Schwartz M, Sterk CE, Elifson K. Craving and control: methamphetamine users' narratives. *J Psychoactive Drugs* 2006;Suppl. **3**:385–392.

258. Newton TF, Roache JD, De La Garza R, et al. Bupropion reduces methamphetamine-induced subjective effects and cue-induced craving. *Neuropsychopharmacology* 2006;**31**(7):1537–1544.

259. Tolliver BK, McRae-Clark AL, Saladin M, et al. Determinants of cue-elicited craving and physiologic reactivity in methamphetamine-dependent subjects in the laboratory. *Am J Drug Alcohol Abuse* 2010;**36**:106–113.

260. Hartz DT, Frederick-Osborne SL, Galloway GP. Craving predicts use during treatment for methamphetamine dependence: a prospective, repeated measures, within-subject analysis. *Drug Alcohol Depend* 2001;**63**(3):269–276.

261. Sadek JR, Vigil O, Grant I, Heaton RK. The impact of neuropsychological functioning and depressed mood on functional complaints in HIV-1 infection and methamphetamine dependence. *J Clin Exp Neuropsychol* 2007;**29**(3):266–276.

262. Rendell PG, Mazur M, Henry JD. Prospective memory impairment in former users of methamphetamine. *Psychopharmacology* 2009;**203**(3):609–616.

263. Cheng M, Liu Q, Wang Y, et al. MMP-9-BDNF pathway is implicated in cognitive impairment of male individuals with methamphetamine addiction during early withdrawal. *Behav Brain Res* 2019;**366**:29–35. doi.org/10.1016/j.bbr.2019.03.020

264. Kalechstein AD, Newton TF, Green M. Methamphetamine dependence is associated with neurocognitive impairment in the initial phases of abstinence. *J Neuropsychiatry Clin Neurosci* 2003;**15**:215–220.

265. Simon SL, Dacey J, Glynn S, Rawson R, Ling W. The effect of relapse on cognition in abstinent methamphetamine abusers. *J Subst Abuse Treat* 2004;**27**:59–66.

266. Simon SL, Domier CP, Sim T, Richardson K, Rawson RA, Ling W. Cognitive performance of current methamphetamine and cocaine abusers. *J Addict Dis* 2002;**21**:61–74.

267. Kamei H, Nagai T, Nakano H, et al. Repeated methamphetamine treatment impairs recognition memory through a failure of novelty-induced ERK1/2 activation in the prefrontal cortex of mice. *Biol Psychiatry* 2006;**59**:75–84.

268. Kitanaka J, Kitanaka N, Takemura M. Neurochemical consequences of dysphoric state during amphetamine withdrawal in animal models: a review. *Neurochem Res* 2008;**33**:204–219.

269. Marshall JF, Belcher AM, Feinstein EM, O'Dell SJ. Methamphetamine-induced neural and cognitive changes in rodents. *Addiction* 2007;**102**:61–69.

270. Nordahl TE, Salo R, Leamon M. Neuropsychological effects of chronic methamphetamine use on neurotransmitters and cognition. *J Neuropsychiatry Clin Neurosci* 2003;**15**:317–325.

271. European Monitoring Centre for Drugs and Drug Addiction (EMCDDA). Exploring Methamphetamine Trends in Europe (EMCDDA Paper). Lisbon, Publications Office of the European Union, 2014.

272. Henry BL, Minassian A, Perry W. Effect of methamphetamine dependence on everyday functional ability. *Addict Behav* 2010;**35**(6):593–598. https://doi.org/10.1016/j.addbeh.2010.01.013

273. Fitzpatrick RE, Rubenis AJ, Verdejo-Garcia A. Cognitive deficits in methamphetamine addiction: independent contributions of dependence and intelligence. *Drug Alcohol Depend* 2020;**209**:107891.

274. Shoptaw SJ, Kao U, Heinzerling K, Ling W. Treatment for amphetamine withdrawal (review). *Cochrane Database Syst Rev* 2009;(2):CD003021. https://doi.org/10.1002/14651858.CD003021.pub2

275. McGregor C, Srisurapanont M, Jittiwutikarn J, Laobhripatr S, Wongtan T, White JM. The nature, time course and severity of methamphetamine withdrawal. *Addiction* 2005;**100**(9):1320–1329.

276. Homer BD, Solomon TM, Moeller RW, Mascia A, DeRaleau L, Halkitis PN. Methamphetamine abuse and impairment of social functioning: a review of the underlying neurophysiological causes and behavioral implications. *Psychol Bull* 2008;**134**:301–310.

277. Sekine Y, Ouchi Y, Takei N, et al. Brain serotonin transporter density and aggression in abstinent methamphetamine abusers. *Arch Gen Psychiatry* 2006;**63**:90–100.

278. Srisurapanont M, Jarusuraisin N, Jittiwutikan J. Amphetamine withdrawal: I. Reliability, validity and factor structure of a measure. *Aust NZ J Psychiatry* 1999;**33**:89–93.

279. Dyer KR, Cruickshank CC. Depression and other psychological health problems among methamphetamine-dependent patients in treatment: implications for assessment and treatment outcomes. *Aust Psychologist* 2003;**40**:96–108.

280. Scott JC, Woods SP, Matt GE, et al. Neurocognitive effects of methamphetamine: a critical review and meta-analysis. *Neuropsychol Rev* 2007;**17**(3):275–297.

281. Werb D, Kerr T, Zhang R, Montaner JS, Wood E. Methamphetamine use and malnutrition among street-involved youth. *Harm Reduct J* 2010;**7**:5.

282. Bhave PD, Goldschlager N. An unusual pattern of ST-segment elevation. *Arch Intern Med* 2011;**171**(13):1146 (discussion 1147–1148).

283. Bindoli A, Rigobello MP, Deeble DJ. Biochemical and toxicological properties of the oxidation products of catecholamines. *Free Radic Biol Med* 1992;**13**(4):391–405.

284. Ito H, Yeo KK, Wijetunga M, Seto TB, Tay K, Schatz IJ. A comparison of echocardiographic findings in young adults with cardiomyopathy: with and without a history of methamphetamine abuse. *Clin Cardiol* 2009;**32**(6):E18–22.

285. Jacobs LJ. Reversible dilated cardiomyopathy induced by methamphetamine. *Clin Cardiol* 1989;**12**(12):725–727.

286. Yeo K-K, Wijetunga M, Ito H, et al. The association of methamphetamine use and cardiomyopathy in young patients. *Am J Med* 2007;**120**(2):165–171.

287. Nishimura M, Ma J, Maisel AS, et al. characteristics and outcomes of methamphetamine abuse among veterans with heart failure. *Am J Cardiol* 2019;**124**(6);907–911. doi.org/10.1016/j.amjcard.2019.05.068

288. Voskoboinik A, Ihle JF, Bloom JE, Kaye DM. Methamphetamine-associated cardiomyopathy: patterns and predictors of recovery. *Intern Med J* 2016;**46**(6):723–727. https://doi.org/10.1111/imj.13050

289. Callaghan RC, Cunningham JK, Sykes J, Kish SJ. Increased risk of Parkinson's disease in individuals hospitalized with conditions related to the use of methamphetamine or other amphetamine-type drugs. *Drug Alcohol Depend* 2012;**120**(1–3):35–40. https://doi.org/10.1016/j.drugalcdep.2011.06.013

290. Chin KM, Channick RN, Rubin LJ. Is methamphetamine use associated with idiopathic pulmonary arterial hypertension? *Chest* 2006;**130**(6):1657–1663.

291. Kamijo Y, Soma K, Nishida M, et al. Acute liver failure following intravenous methamphetamine. *Vet Hum Toxicol* 2002;**44**(4):216–217.

292. Brannan TA, Soundararajan S, Houghton BL. Methamphetamine-associated shock with intestinal infarction. *Med Gen Med* 2004;**6**(4):6.

293. Garcia E, Waksman J, Benowitz N. Methamphetamine-induced pseudovasculitis. *Clin Toxicol* 2019;**57**(10):896. doi.org/10.1080/15563650.2019.1636569

294. Johnson TD, Berenson MM. Methamphetamine-induced ischemic colitis. *J Clin Gastroenterol* 1991;**13**(6):687–9.

295. Gonzales R, Marinelli-Casey P, Hillhouse M, et al. Hepatitis A and B infection among methamphetamine-dependent users. *J Subst Abus Treat* 2008;**35**(3):351–352.

296. Scheinmann R, Hagan H, Lelutiu-Weinberger C, et al. Non-injection drug use and hepatitis C virus: a systematic review. *Drug Alcohol Depend* 2007;**89**(1):1–12.

297. Howe CJ, Fuller CM, Ompad DC, et al. Association of sex, hygiene and drug equipment sharing with hepatitis C virus infection among non-injecting drug users in New York City. *Drug Alcohol Depend* 2005;**79**(3):389–395.

298. Banooni P, Rickman LS, Ward DM. Pott puffy tumor associated with intranasal methamphetamine. *JAMA* 2000;**283**(10):1293.

299. Wijaya J, Salu P, Leblanc A, et al. Acute unilateral visual loss due to a single intranasal methamphetamine abuse. *Bull Soc Belge Ophthalmol* 1999;**271**:19–25.

300. Shaw HE Jr, Lawson JG, Stulting RD. Amaurosis fugax and retinal vasculitis associated with methamphetamine inhalation. *J Clin Neuro Ophthalmol* 1985;**5**(3):169–176.

301. Baker A, Lee NK, Claire M, et al. Brief cognitive behavioural interventions for regular amphetamine users: a step in the right direction. *Addiction* 2005;**100**(3):367–378.

302. Glasner-Edwards S, Mooney LJ, Marinelli-Casey P, Hillhouse M, Ang A, Rawson RA. Psychopathology in methamphetamine-dependent adults 3 years after treatment. *Drug Alcohol Rev* 2010;**29**:12–20.

303. McKetina R, Leunga J, Stockings E, et al. Mental health outcomes associated with the use of amphetamines: a systematic review and meta-analysis. *Clin Med* 2019;**16**:81–97. https://doi.org/10.1016/j.eclinm.2019.09.014 2589-5370

304. Stinson FS, Grant BF, Dawson DA, Ruan WJ, Huang B, Saha T. Comorbidity between DSM-IV alcohol and specific drug use disorders in the United States: results from the National Epidemiologic Survey on Alcohol and Related Conditions. *Drug Alcohol Depend* 2005;**80**:105–116.

305. Conway KP, Compton W, Stinson FS, Grant BF. Lifetime comorbidity of DSM-IV mood and anxiety disorders and specific drug use disorders: results from the National Epidemiologic Survey on Alcohol and Related Conditions. *J Clin Psychiatry* 2006;**67**:247–257.

306. Sommers I, Baskin D, Baskin-Sommers A. Methamphetamine use among young adults: health and social consequences. *Addict Behav* 2006;**31**:1469–1476.

307. Semple SJ, Zians J, Strathdee SA, Patterson TL. Psychosocial and behavioural correlates of depressed mood among female methamphetamine users. *J Psychoactive Drugs* 2007;Suppl. 4:353–366.

308. Regier DA, Farmer ME, Rae DS, et al. Comorbidity of mental disorders with alcohol and other drug abuse. Results from the Epidemiologic Catchment Area (ECA) Study. *JAMA* 1990;**264**:2511–2518.

309. McKetin R, Lubman DI, Lee NM, Ross JE, Slade TN. Major depression among methamphetamine users entering drug treatment programs. *Med J Aust* 2011;**195**(Suppl. 3):S51–SS5.

310. Rawson RA, Ling W. Clinical management: methamphetamine. In: M Galanter, HD Kleber, eds., *Textbook of Substance Abuse Treatment*, 4th ed., pp. 169–179. Washington, DC, American Psychiatric Publishing, 2008.

311. McKetina R, Leunga J, Stockings E, et al. Mental health outcomes associated with the use of amphetamines: a systematic review and meta-analysis. *Clin Med* 2019; **16**:81–97. https://doi.org/10.1016/j.eclinm.2019.09.0142589-5370

312. Sommers I, Baskin D. Methamphetamine use and violence. *J Drug Issues* 2006;**36**:77–96.

313. Bramness JG, Gundersen OH, Guterstam J, et al. Amphetamine-induced psychosis: a separate diagnostic entity or primary psychosis triggered in the vulnerable? *BMC Psychiatry* 2012;**12**:221.

314. McKetin R. Methamphetamine psychosis: insights from the past. *Addiction* 2018;**113**:1522–1527.

315. McKetin R, Dawe S, Burns RA, et al. The profile of psychiatric symptoms exacerbated by methamphetamine use. *Drug Alcohol Depend* 2016;**161**:104–109.

316. Chen CK, Lin SK, Sham PC, et al. Pre-morbid characteristics and co-morbidity of methamphetamine users with and without psychosis. *Psychol Med* 2003;**33**(8):1407–1414. https://doi.org/10.1017/S0033291703008353

317. Bramness JG, Gundersen OH, Guterstam J, et al. Amphetamine-induced psychosis: a separate diagnostic entity or primary psychosis triggered in the vulnerable? *BMC Psychiatry* 2012;**12**:221.

318. Glasner-Edwards S, Mooney LJ, Marinelli-Casey P, Hillhouse M, Ang A, Rawson R. Methamphetamine Treatment Project Corporate, A. Clinical course and outcomes of methamphetamine-dependent adults with psychosis. *J Subst Abuse Treat* 2008;**35**(4):445–450. https://doi.org/10.1016/j.jsat.2007.12.004

319. Brown ES, Gabrielson B. A randomized, double-blind, placebo-controlled trial of citicoline for bipolar and unipolar depression and methamphetamine. *J Affect Disord* 2012;**143**(1–3):257–260. https://doi.org/10.1016/j.jad.2012.05.006

320. Roberts AR, Yeager K, Siegel A. Obsessive-compulsive disorder, comorbid depression, substance abuse, and suicide attempts: clinical presentations, assessments, and treatment. *Brief Treat Crisis Interv* 2003;**3**:145–167.

321. Shoptaw S, Peck J, Reback CJ, Rotheram-Fuller E. Psychiatric and substance dependence comorbidities, sexually transmitted diseases, and risk behaviors among methamphetamine-dependent gay and bisexual men seeking outpatient drug abuse treatment. *J Psychoactive Drugs* 2003;**35**:161–168.

322. Yen CF, Shieh BL. Suicidal ideation and correlates in Taiwanese adolescent methamphetamine users. *J Nerv Ment Dis* 2005;**193**:444–449.

323. Bramness JG, Gundersen OH, Guterstam J, et al. Amphetamine-induced psychosis: a separate diagnostic entity or primary psychosis triggered in the vulnerable? *BMC Psychiatry* 2012;**12**:221.

324. Glasner-Edwards S, Mooney LJ, Marinelli-Casey P, Hillhouse M, Ang A, Rawson R. Methamphetamine Treatment Project Corporate, A. Clinical course and outcomes of methamphetamine-dependent adults with psychosis. *J Subst Abuse Treat* 2008;**35**(4):445–450. https://doi.org/10.1016/j.jsat.2007.12.004

325. McKetin R, Dawe S, Burns RA, et al. The profile of psychiatric symptoms exacerbated by methamphetamine use. *Drug Alcohol Depend* 2016;**161**:104–109.

326. Christian DR, Huber A, Brecht ML, et al. Methamphetamine users entering treatment: characteristics of the methamphetamine treatment project sample. *Subst Use Misuse* 2007;**42**(14):2207–2222. https://doi.org/10.1080/10826080701209341

327. Fujii D. Risk factors for treatment-resistive methamphetamine psychosis. *J Neuropsychiatry Clin Neurosci* 2002;**14**(2):239–240.

328. Arunogiri S, Foulds JA, McKetin R, Lubman DI. A systematic review of risk factors for methamphetamine-associated psychosis. *Aust N Z J Psychiatry* 2018;**52**:514–529. https://doi.org/10.1177/0004867417748750

329. Lecomte T, Dumais A, Dugre JR, Potvin S. The prevalence of substance-induced psychotic disorder in methamphetamine misusers: a meta-analysis. *Psychiatry Res* 2018;**268**:189–192. https://doi.org/ 10.1016/j.psychres.2018.05.033

330. Ujike H, Sato M. Clinical features of sensitization to methamphetamine observed in patients with methamphetamine dependence and psychosis. *Ann N Y Acad Sci* 2004;**1025**:279–287. https://doi.org/10.1196/annals.1316.035

331. Srisurapanont M, Ali R, Marsden J, Sunga A, Wada K, Monteiro M. Psychotic symptoms in methamphetamine psychotic in-patients. *Int J Neuropsychopharmacol* 2003;**6**(4):347–352.

332. Arunogiri S, Foulds JA, McKetin R, Lubman DI. A systematic review of risk factors for methamphetamine-associated psychosis. *Aust N Z J Psychiatry* 2018;**52**(6:514–529. https://doi.org/10.1177/0004867417748750

333. Lecomte T, Dumais A, Dugré JR, Potvin S. The prevalence of substance-induced psychotic disorder in methamphetamine misusers: a meta-analysis. *Psychiatry Res* 2018;**268**:189–192,

334. Akiyama K. Longitudinal clinical course following pharmacological treatment of methamphetamine psychosis which persists after long-term abstinence. *Ann N Y Acad Sci* 2006;**1074**:125–134.

335. Chen CK, Lin SK, Sham PC, et al. Pre-morbid characteristics and co-morbidity of methamphetamine users with and without psychosis. *Psychol Med* 2003;**33**:1407–1414.

336. Dore G, Sweeting M. Drug-induced psychosis associated with crystalline methamphetamine. *Australas Psychiatry* 2006;**14**:86–89.

337. Harris D, Batki SL. Stimulant psychosis: symptom profile and acute clinical course. *Am J Addict* 2000;**9**:28–37.

338. Srisurapanont M, Ali R, Marsden J, Sunga A, Wada K, Monteiro M. Psychotic symptoms in methamphetamine psychotic in-patients. *Int J Neuropsychopharmcol* 2003;**6**:347–352.

339. Arunogiri S, McKetin R, Verdejo-Garcia A, Lubman DI. The methamphetamine-associated psychosis spectrum: a clinically focused review. *Int J Ment Health Addict* 2018 (online). https://doi.org/10.1007/s11469-018-9934-4.

340. McKetin R. Methamphetamine psychosis: insights from the past. *Addiction* 2018;**113**:1522–1527.

341. Akiyama K. Longitudinal clinical course following pharmacological treatment of methamphetamine psychosis which persists after long-term abstinence. *Ann N Y Acad Sci* 2006;**1074**:125–134.

342. Grelotti DJ, Kanayama G, Pope HG Jr. Remission of persistent methamphetamine-induced psychosis after electroconvulsive therapy: presentation of a case and review of the literature. *Am J Psychiatry* 2010;**167**(1):17–23. https://doi.org/10.1176/appi.ajp.2009.08111695

343. Harris D, Batki SL. Stimulant psychosis: symptom profile and acute clinical course. *Am J Addict* 2000;**9**:28–37.

344. Sato M. Acute exacerbation of methamphetamine psychosis and lasting dopaminergic supersensitivity: a clinical survey. *Psychopharmacol Bull* 1986;**22**:751–756.

345. Sato M. A lasting vulnerability to psychosis in patients with previous methamphetamine psychosis. *Ann N Y Acad Sci* 1992;**654**:160–170.

346. Sato M, Chen CC, Akiyama K, Otsuki S. Acute exacerbation of paranoid psychotic state after long-term abstinence in patients with previous methamphetamine psychosis. *Biol Psychiatry* 1983;**18**:429–440.

347. Yui K, Goto K, Ikemoto S, Nishijima K, Yoshino T, Ishiguro T. Susceptibility to subsequent episodes of spontaneous recurrence of methamphetamine psychosis. *Drug Alcohol Depend* 2001;**64**:133–142.

348. Takezaki H, Inotani T, Ikeda T, Yasuoka T. A case of acute recurrent methamphetamine psychosis characterized by fancy delusions of grandeur. *Seishin Shinkeigaku Zasshi* 1984;**86**:621–630 [in Japanese].

349. Teraoka A. A study on methamphetamine psychosis in a psychiatric clinic: comparison of acute and chronic-type cases. *Seishin Shinkeigaku Zasshi* 1998;**100**:425–468 [in Japanese].

350. Bortolato M, Frau R, Piras AP, et al. Methamphetamine induces long-term alterations in reactivity to environmental stimuli: correlation with dopaminergic and serotonergic toxicity. *Neurotox Res* 2009;**15**:232–245.

351. Wood DM, Button J, Ashraf T, et al. What evidence is there that the UK should tackle the potential emerging threat of methamphetamine toxicity rather than established recreational drugs such as MDMA ('ecstasy')? *QJM* 2008;**101**(3):207–213. https://doi.org/10.1093/qjmed/hcm133

352. Hall MG, Hauson AO, Wollman SC, et al. Neuropsychological comparisons of cocaine versus methamphetamine users: a research synthesis and meta-analysis. *Am J Drug Alcohol Abuse* 2018;**44**(3):277–293. https://doi.org/10.1080/00952990.2017.1355919

353. Jernigan TL, Gamst AC, Archibald SL, et al. Effects of methamphetamine dependence and HIV infection on cerebral morphology. *Am J Psychiatry* 2005;**162**:1461–1472.

354. Reback C, Larkins S, Shoptaw S. Methamphetamine abuse as a barrier to HIV medication adherence among gay and bisexual men. *AIDS Care* 2003;**15**:775–785.

355. Ellis RJ, Childers ME, Cherner M, Lazzaretto D, Letendre S, Grant I. HIV Neurobehavioral Research Center Group. Increased human immunodeficiency virus loads in active methamphetamine users are explained by reduced effectiveness of antiretroviral therapy. *J Infect Dis* 2003;**188**(12):1820–1826.

356. Cherner M, Letendre S, Heaton RK, et al. Hepatitis C augments cognitive deficits associated with HIV infection and methamphetamine. *Neurology* 2005;**64**(8):1343–1347.

357. Quinn B, Stoové M, Dietze P. One-year changes in methamphetamine use, dependence and remission in a community-recruited cohort. *J Subst Use* 2015 (online). https://doi.org/10.3109/14659891.2015.10189729

358. Borders TF, Booth BM, Han X, et al. Longitudinal changes in methamphetamine and cocaine use in untreated rural stimulant users: racial differences and the impact of methamphetamine legislation. *Addiction* 2008;**103**:800–808.

359. Lanyon C, Nambiar D, Higgs P, Dietze P, Quin B. Five-year changes in methamphetamine use, dependence, and remission in a community-recruited cohort. *J Addict Med* 2019;**13**(2):159–165. https://doi.org/10.1097/ADM.0000000000000469

360. Mimiaga MJ, Pantalone DW, Biello KB. et al. An initial randomized controlled trial of behavioral activation for treatment of concurrent crystal methamphetamine dependence and sexual risk for HIV acquisition among men who have sex with men. *AIDS Care* 2019;**31**(9):1083–1095. doi.org/10.1080/09540121.2019.1595518

361. Ciketic S, Hayatbakhsh R, McKetin R, Doran CM, Najman JM. Cost-effectiveness of counselling as a treatment option for methamphetamine dependence. *J Subst Use* 2015;**20**(4):239–246.

362. Vocci FJ, Montoya ID. Psychological treatments for stimulant misuse, comparing and contrasting those for amphetamine dependence and those for cocaine dependence. *Curr Opin Psychiatry* 2009;**22**:263–268.

363. Shoptaw S, Reback CJ, Peck JA, et al. Behavioral treatment approaches for methamphetamine dependence and HIV-related sexual risk behaviors among urban gay and bisexual men. *Drug Alcohol Depend* 2005;**78**(2):125–134.

364. Shoptaw S, Klausner JD, Reback CJ, et al. A public health response to the methamphetamine epidemic: the implementation of contingency management to treat methamphetamine dependence. *BMC Public Health* 2006;**6**:214.

365. Rawson RA, Marinelli-Casey P, Anglin MD, et al. A multisite comparison of psychosocial approaches for the treatment of methamphetamine dependence. *Addiction* 2004;**99**:708–717.

366. Reback CJ, Peck JA, Dierst-Davies R, Nuno M, Kamien JB, Amass L. Contingency management among homeless, out-of-treatment men who have sex with men. *J Subst Abuse Treat* 2010;**39**:255–263.

367. Roll JM, Petry NM, Stitzer ML, et al. Contingency management for the treatment of methamphetamine use disorders. *Am J Psychiatry* 2006;**163**:1993–1999.

368. Rawson RA, McCann MJ, Flammino F, et al. A comparison of contingency management and cognitive-behavioral approaches for stimulant-dependent individuals. *Addiction* 2006;**101**:267–274. https://doi.org/10.1111/j.1360-0443.2006.01312.x

369. Knapp WP, Soares B, Farrell M, Silva de Lima M. Psychosocial interventions for cocaine and psychostimulant amphetamines related disorders (review). *Cochrane Database Syst Rev* (online) 2008;**2008**:3. https://doi.org/10.1002/14651858.CD003023.

370. Higgins ST, Budney AJ, Bickel WK, Foerg FE, Donman R, Badger GJ. Incentives improve outcome in outpatient behavioural treatment of cocaine dependence. *Arch Gen Psychiatry* 1994;**51**:568–576.

371. Roll JM, Huber A, Sodano R, et al. A comparison of five reinforcement schedules for use in contingency management-based treatment of methamphetamine users. *Psychological Record* 2006;**56**(winter):1.

372. Ling Murtaugh K, Krishnamurti T, Davis AL, Reback CJ, Shoptaw S. Spend today, clean tomorrow: predicting methamphetamine abstinence in a randomized controlled trial. *Health Psychol* 2013;**32**(9):958–966. https://doi.org/10.1037/a0032922

373. Stuart A, Baker AL, Bowman J, et al. Protocol for a systematic review of psychological treatment for methamphetamine use: an analysis of methamphetamine use and mental health symptom outcomes. *BMJ Open* 2017;**7**(9):e015383. https://doi.org/10.1136/bmjopen-2016-015383

374. Menza TW, Jameson DR, Hughes JP, Colfax GN, Shoptaw S, Golden MR. Contingency management to reduce methamphetamine use and sexual risk among men who have sex with men: a randomized controlled trial. *BMC Public Health* 2010;**10**:774. https://doi.org/10.1186/1471-2458-10-774

375. McKetina R, Leunga J, Stockings E, et al. Mental health outcomes associated with the use of amphetamines: a systematic review and meta-analysis. *Clin Med* 2019;**16**:81–97. https://doi.org/10.1016/j.eclinm.2019.09.014 2589-5370

376. Graves SM, Rafeyan R, Watts J, Napier TC. Mirtazapine, and mirtazapine-like compounds as possible pharmacotherapy for substance abuse disorders: evidence from the bench and the bedside. *Pharmacol Ther* 2012;**136**(3):343–353. https://doi.org/10.1016/j.pharmthera.2012.08.013

377. Lee NK, Rawson RA. A systematic review of cognitive and behavioural therapies for methamphetamine dependence. *Drug Alcohol Rev* 2008;**27**:309–317.

378. Lea T, Kolstee J, Lambert S, Ness R, Hannan S, Holt M. Methamphetamine treatment outcomes among gay men attending a LGBTI-specific treatment service in Sydney, Australia. *PLOS ONE* 2017 (online). https://doi.org/10.1371/journal.pone.0172560

379. Marshall BD, Wood E, Shoveller JA, et al. Individual, social, and environmental factors associated with initiating methamphetamine injection: implications for drug use and HIV prevention strategies. *Prev Sci* 2011;**12**:173–180. https://doi.org/10.1007/s11121-010-0197-y

380. Degenhardt L, Roxburgh A, Black E, et al. The epidemiology of methamphetamine use and harm in Australia. *Drug Alcohol Rev* 2008;**27**:243–252. https://doi.org/10.1080/09595230801950572

381. Damon W, McNeil R, Milloy M-J, Nosova E, Kerr T, Hayashi K. Residential eviction predicts initiation of or relapse into crystal methamphetamine use among people who inject drugs: a prospective cohort study. *J Public Health* 2019;**41**(1):36–45. https://doi.org/10.1093/pubmed/fdx187

382. Morris L, Stander J, Ebrahim W, et al. Effect of exercise versus cognitive behavioural therapy or no intervention on anxiety, depression, fitness and quality of life in adults with previous methamphetamine dependency: a systematic review. *Addict Sci Clin Pract* 2018;**13**:4.

383. Ahmadi J. Comparison of electroconvulsive therapy, buprenorphine and methadone in the management of methamphetamine dependency and withdrawal craving. *J Addict Depend* 2016;**2**:1–3. https://doi.org/10.15436/2471-061X-16-031

384. Ahmadi J, Ekramzadeh S, Pridmore S. Remission of methamphetamine-induced withdrawal delirium and craving after electroconvulsive therapy. *Iran J Psychiatr Behav Sci* 2015;**9**(4):e1793.https://doi.org/10.17795/ijpbs-1793

385. Grelotti DJ, Kanayama G, Pope HG. Jr. Remission of persistent methamphetamine-induced psychosis after electroconvulsive therapy: presentation of a case and review of the literature. *Am J Psychiatry* 2010;**167**(1):17–23. https://doi.org/10.1176/appi.ajp.2009.08111695

386. Zeng L, Tao Y, Hou W, Zong L, Yu L. Electro-acupuncture improves psychiatric symptoms, anxiety and depression in methamphetamine addicts during abstinence: a randomized controlled trial. *Medicine* 2018;**97**(34):e11905. https://doi.org/10.1097/MD.0000000000011905

387. Liang Y, Zhang X, Xu B, Zong L. Clinical observation of electroacupuncture for withdrawal symptoms in methamphetamine addicts. *Int J Clin Acupunct* 2015;**24**(4):236–241.

388. Zemestani M, Ottaviani C. Effectiveness of mindfulness-based relapse prevention for co-occurring substance use and depression disorders. *Mindfulness*2016;**7**(6):1347–1355. https://doi.org/10.1007/s12671-016-0576-y

389. Glasner S, Mooney LJ, Ang A, et al. Mindfulness-based relapse prevention for stimulant-dependent adults: a pilot randomized clinical trial. *Mindfulness* 2017;**8**(1):126–135.

390. National Institute of Drug Abuse (NIDA). What treatments are effective for people who abuse methamphetamine? Available at: www.drugabuse.gov/publications/research-reports/methamphetamine/what-treatments-are-effective-methamphetamine-abusers [last accessed 15 March 2022].

391. Collins KC, Schlosburg JE, Bremer PT, Janda KD. Methamphetamine vaccines: improvement through hapten design. *J Med Chem* 2016;**59**:3878–3885.

392. Elkashef A, Kahn R, Yu E, et al. Topiramate for the treatment of methamphetamine addiction: a multi-center placebo-controlled trial. *Addiction* 2012;**107**(7):1297–1306. https://doi.org/10.1111/j.1360-0443.2011.03771.x

393. McElhiney MC, Rabkin JG, Rabkin R, Nunes EV. Provigil (modafinil) plus cognitive behavioral therapy for methamphetamine use in HIV+ gay men: a pilot study. *Am J Drug Alcohol Abuse* 2009;**35**(1):34–7. https://doi.org/10.1080/00952990802342907

394. Piasecki M, Steinagel G, Thienhaus O, Kohlenberg B. An exploratory study: the use of paroxetine for methamphetamine craving. *J Psychoactive Drugs* 2002;**34**:301–304.

395. Elkashef AM, Rawson RA, Anderson AL, et al. Bupropion for the treatment of methamphetamine dependence. *Neuropsychopharmacology* 2008;**33**(5):1162–1170.

396. Shoptaw S, Huber A, Peck J, et al. Randomized, placebo-controlled trial of sertraline and contingency management for the treatment of methamphetamine dependence. *Drug Alcohol Depend* 2006;**85**:12–18.

397. Shoptaw S, Heinzerling KG, Rotheram-Fuller E, et al. Randomized, placebo-controlled trial of bupropion for the treatment of methamphetamine dependence. *Drug Alcohol Depend* 2008;**96**:222–232.

398. McCann DJ, Li SH. A novel, nonbinary evaluation of success and failure reveals bupropion efficacy versus methamphetamine dependence: reanalysis of a multisite trial. *CNS Neurosci Ther* 2012;**18**(5):414–418. https://doi.org/10.1111/j.1755-5949.2011.00263.x

399. Brensilver M, Heinzerling KG, Swanson A-N, Shoptaw SJ. A retrospective analysis of two randomized trials of bupropion for methamphetamine dependence: suggested guidelines for treatment discontinuation/augmentation. *Drug Alcohol Depend* 2012;**125**:169–172.

400. Kenford SL, Fiore MC, Jorenby DE, Smith SS, Wetter D, Baker TB. Predicting smoking cessation. *JAMA* 1994;**271**:589.

401. Plebani JG, Kampman KM, Lynch KG. Early abstinence in cocaine pharmacotherapy trials predicts successful treatment outcomes. *J Subst Abuse Treat* 2009;**37**:313–317.

402. Urschel HC III, Hanselka LL, Baron M. A controlled trial of flumazenil and gabapentin for initial treatment of methylamphetamine dependence. *J Psychopharmacol* 2011;**25**:254–262.

403. Grant JE, Odlaug BL, Kim SW. A double-blind, placebo-controlled study of N-acetylcysteine plus naltrexone for methamphetamine dependence. *Eur Neuropsychopharmacol* 2010;**20**:823–828.

404. McGregor C, Srisurapanont M, Mitchell A, Wickes W, White JM. Symptoms and sleep patterns during inpatient treatment of methamphetamine withdrawal: a comparison of mirtazapine and modafinil with treatment as usual. *J Subst Abuse Treat* 2008;**35**:334–342.

405. Cruickshank CC, Montebello ME, Dyer KR, et al. A placebo-controlled trial of mirtazapine for the management of methamphetamine withdrawal. *Drug Alcohol Rev* 2008;**27** (3):326–333.

406. Laqueille X, Dervaux A, El Omari F, Kanit M, Bayle FJ. Methylphenidate effective in treating amphetamine abusers with no other psychiatric disorder. *Eur Psychiatry* 2005;**20**:456–457.

407. De La Garza R II, Newton TF, Haile CN, et al. Rivastigmine reduces 'likely to use methamphetamine' in methamphetamine-dependent volunteers. *Prog Neuropsychopharmacol Biol Psychiatry* 2012;**37**:141–146.

408. Siefried KJ, Acheson LS, Lintzeris N, et al. Pharmacological treatment of methamphetamine/amphetamine dependence: a systematic review. *CNS Drugs* 2020;**34**:337–365. https://doi.org/10.1007/s40263-020-00711-x

409. Siefried KJ, Acheson LS, Lintzeris N, et al. Pharmacological treatment of methamphetamine/amphetamine dependence: a systematic review. *CNS Drugs* 2020;**34**:337–365. https://doi.org/10.1007/s40263-020-00711-x

410. Morley KC, Cornish JL, Faingold A, Wood K, Haber PS. Pharmacotherapeutic agents in the treatment of methamphetamine dependence. *Exp Opin Investig Drugs* 2017;**26**(5):563–578. https://doi.org/10.1080/13543784.2017.1313229

411. Chan B, Kansagara D, Kondo K, et al. Amphetamine use disorder: a systematic review and meta-analysis. *J Gen Intern Med* 2019;**34**(2):2122–2136. doi.org/10.1007/11606.1525-1497

412. Chan B, Kansagara D, Kondo K, et al. Amphetamine use disorder: a systematic review and meta-analysis. *J Gen Intern Med* 2019;**34**(2):2122–2136.

413. Chan B, Freeman M, Kondo K, et al. Pharmacotherapy for methamphetamine/amphetamine use disorder: a systematic review and meta-analysis. *Addiction* 2019 (online). https://doi.org/10.1111/add.14755

414. Ahmadi J, Sahraian A, Biuseh M. A randomized clinical trial on the effects of bupropion and buprenorphine on the reduction of methamphetamine craving. *Trials* 2019;**20**:468. https://doi.org/10.1186/s13063-019-3554-6

415. Pérez-Mañá C, Castells X, Torrens M, Capellà D, Farre M. Efficacy of psychostimulant drugs for amphetamine abuse or dependence (review). *Cochrane Database Syst Rev* 2013;**9**: CD009695. https://doi.org/10.1002/14651858.CD009695.pub2

416. Siefried KJ, Acheson LS, Lintzeris N, et al. Pharmacological treatment of methamphetamine/amphetamine dependence:

417. Chan B, Freeman M, Kondo K, et al. Pharmacotherapy for methamphetamine/amphetamine use disorder: a systematic review and meta-analysis. *Addiction* 2019 (online). https://doi.org/10.1111/add.14755

418. Coffin PO, Santos GM, Hern J, et al. Extended-release naltrexone for methamphetamine dependence among men who have sex with men: a randomized placebo-controlled trial. *Addiction* 2018;**113**:268–278.

419. Trivedi MH, Walker R, Ling W, et al. Bupropion and naltrexone in methamphetamine use disorder. *N Engl J Med* 2021;**384**:2.

420. Lim AC, Grodin EN, Green R, et al. Executive function moderates naltrexone effects on methamphetamine-induced craving and subjective responses. *Am J Drug Alcohol Abuse* 2020 (online). https://doi.org/10.1080/00952990.2020.1741002

421. Batki SL, Moon J, Bradley M, et al. Fluoxetine in methamphetamine dependence. A controlled trial: a preliminary analysis. CPDD 61st Annual Scientific Meeting. Acapulco, June 1999.

422. Batki SL, Moon J, Delucchi K, et al. Methamphetamine quantitative urine concentrations during a controlled trial of fluoxetine treatment. Preliminary analysis. *Ann N Y Acad Sci* 2000;**909**:260–263.

423. Kongsakon R, Papadopoulos KI, Saguansiritham R. Mirtazapine in amphetamine detoxification: a placebo-controlled pilot study. *Int Clin Psychopharmacol* 2005;**20**:253–256.

424. Ling W, Shoptaw S, Hillhouse M, et al. Double-blind placebo-controlled evaluation of the PROMETA™ protocol for methamphetamine dependence. *Addiction* 2012;**107** (2):361–369. https://doi.org10.1111/j.1360-0443.2011.03619.x

425. Bhatt M, Zielinski L, Baker-Beal L, et al. Efficacy and safety of psychostimulants for amphetamine and methamphetamine use disorders: a systematic review and meta-analysis. *Syst Rev* 2016;**5**:189. https://doi.org/10.1186/s13643-016-0370-x

426. Chan B, Kansagara D, Kondo K, et al. Amphetamine use disorder: a systematic review and meta-analysis. *J Gen Int Med* 2019;**34**(2):2122–2136. doi.org/10.1007/11606.1525-1497

427. Brecht ML, Greenwell L, Anglin MD. Methamphetamine treatment: trends and predictors of retention and completion in a large state treatment system (1992–2002). *J Subst Abuse Treat* 2005;**29**(4):295–306.

428. Otero C, Boles S, Young N, Dennis K. *Methamphetamine Addiction, Treatment, and Outcomes: Implications for Child Welfare Workers.* Washington, DC, Substance Abuse and Mental Health Services Administration (SAMSHA), Center for Substance Abuse Treatment, 2006.

429. Rawson R, Huber A, Brethen P, et al. Methamphetamine and cocaine users: differences in characteristics and treatment retention. *J Psychoactive Drugs* 2000;**32**:233–238.

430. Embry D, Hankins M, Biglan A, Boles S. Behavioral and social correlates of methamphetamine use in a population-based sample of early and later adolescents. *Addict Behav* 2009;**34**:343–351.

431. Šefránek M, Miovský M. Treatment outcome evaluation in therapeutic communities in the Czech Republic: alcohol consumption and other results one year after discharge. *Alcohol Treat Q* 2018;**36**(1):54–71.

432. Kamp F, Proebst L, Hager L, et al. Effectiveness of methamphetamine abuse treatment: predictors of treatment completion and comparison of two residential treatment programs. *Drug Alcohol Depend* 2019;**201**:8–15

433. Jaffe A, Shoptaw S, Stein J, Reback CJ, Rotheram-Fuller E. Depression ratings, reported sexual risk behaviors, and methamphetamine use: latent growth curve models of positive change among gay and bisexual men in an outpatient treatment program. *Exp Clin Psychopharmacol* 2007;**15**(3):301–307.

434. Rawson RA, Gonzales R, Pearce V, Ang A, Marinelli-Casey P, Brummer J. Methamphetamine Treatment Project Corporate Authors. Methamphetamine dependence and human immunodeficiency virus risk behaviour. *J Subst Abuse Treat* 2008;**35**(3):279–284. https://doi.org/10.1016/j.jsat.2007.11.003

435. Brecht ML, Greenwell L, von Mayrhauser C, Anglin MD. Two-year outcomes of treatment for methamphetamine use. *J Psychoactive Drugs* 2006;Suppl. 3:415–426.

436. Hillhouse MP, Marinelli-Casey P, Gonzales R, Ang A, Rawson RA. Predicting in-treatment performance and post-treatment outcomes inmethamphetamine users. *Addiction* 2007;**102**(Suppl. 1):84–95.

437. Brecht ML, von Mayrhauser C, Anglin MD. Predictors of relapse after treatment for methamphetamine use. *J Psychoactive Drugs* 2000;**32**:211–220.

438. Maglione M, Chao B, Anglin MD. Correlates of outpatient drug treatment drop-out among methamphetamine users. *J Psychoactive Drugs* 2000;**32**:221–228.

439. Maglione M, Chao B, Anglin D. Residential treatment of methamphetamine users: correlates of drop-out from the California alcohol and drug data system (CADDS). *Addict Res* 2000;**8**:65–79.

440. Quinn B, Stoové M, Dietze P. One-year changes in methamphetamine use, dependence and remission in a community-recruited cohort. *J Subst Use* 2015 (online). https://doi.org/10.3109/14659891.2015.1018972

441. Quinn B, Stoové M, Dietze P. One-year changes in methamphetamine use, dependence and remission in a community-recruited cohort. *J Subst Use* 2015 (online). https://doi.org/10.3109/14659891.2015.1018972

442. Quinn B, Stoové M, Dietze P. One-year changes in methamphetamine use, dependence and remission in a community-recruited cohort. *J Subst Use* 2015 (online). https://doi.org/10.3109/14659891.2015.1018972

443. Quinn B, Stoové M, Dietze P. One-year changes in methamphetamine use, dependence and remission in

a community-recruited cohort. *J Subst Use* 2015 (online). https://doi.org/10.3109/14659891.2015.1018972

444. Gonzales R, Ang A, Marinelli-Casey P, Glik DC, Iguchi MY, Rawson RA. Methamphetamine Treatment Project Corporate Authors. Health-related quality of life trajectories of methamphetamine-dependent individuals as a function of treatment completion and continued care over a 1-year period. *J Subst Abuse Treat* 2009;**37**(4):353–361. https://doi.org/10.1016/j.jsat.2009.04.001

445. Dean AC, London ED, Sugar CA, et al. Predicting adherence to treatment for methamphetamine dependence from neuropsychological and drug use variables. *Drug Alcohol Depend* 2009;**105**(1–2):48–55. https://doi.org/10.1016/j.drugalcdep.2009.06.008

446. Peterson JD, Wolf ME, White FJ. Repeated amphetamine administration decreases D1 dopamine receptor-mediated inhibition of voltage-gated sodium currents in the prefrontal cortex. *J Neurosci* 2006;**26**:3164–3168.

447. Lee N, Pennay A, Kenny P, Harney A, Johns L. Methamphetamine withdrawal: natural history and options for intervention. Australasian Society for Psychiatric Research Annual Meeting. Sydney, Brainwaves, 2006.

448. Gonzalez Castro F, Barrington EH, Walton MA, Rawson RA. Cocaine and methamphetamine: differential addiction rates. *Psychol Addict Behav* 2000;**14**(4):390–396.

449. Simon S, Richardson K, Dacey J, et al. A comparison of patterns of methamphetamine and cocaine use. *J Addict Dis* 2002;**21**(1):35–44.

450. Kenny P, Harney A, Lee NK, Pennay A. Teatment utilization and barriers to treatment: results of a survey of dependent methamphetamine users. *Subst Abuse Treat Prevent Policy* 2011;**6**:3.

451. McKetin R, McLaren J, Kelly E, Hall W, Hickman M. Estimating the Number of Regular and Dependent Methamphetamine Users in Australia (Technical Report No. 230). Sydney, NDARC, UNSW, 2005.

452. Australian Institute of Health and Welfare. Alcohol and Other Drug Treatment Services in Australia 2007–2009: Report on the National Minimum Data Set (Drug treatment series no. 9. Cat. no. HSE 73). Canberra, AIHW, 2009.

453. Pennay A, Lee N. Barriers to methamphetamine withdrawal treatment in Australia: findings from a survey of AOD service providers. *Drug Alcohol Rev* 2009;**28**(1):636–640.

454. Saltman DC, Newman CE, Mao L, Kippax SC, Kidd MR. Experiences in managing problematic crystal methamphetamine use and associated depression in gay men and HIV positive men: in-depth interviews with general practitioners in Sydney, Australia. *BMC Fam Pract* 2008;**9**(45):1–7.

455. Quinn B, Stoové M, Dietze P. Factors associated with professional support access among a prospective cohort of methamphetamine users. *J Subst Abuse Treat* 2013;**45**:235–241.

456. Darke S, Ross J, Teesson M, Lynskey M. Health service utilization and benzodiazepine use among heroin users:

findings from the Australian Treatment Outcome Study (ATOS). *Addiction* 2003;**98**(8):1129–1135.

457. Pennay A, Ferris J, Reed M, Devaney M, Lee N. Evaluation of 'Access Point' Specialist Methamphetamine Clinic. Fitzroy, Melbourne, Turning Point Alcohol and Drug Centre, 2010.

458. Kelly E, McKetin R, McLaren J. Health Service Utilisation Among Regular Methamphetamine Users (Vol. Technical Report No. 233). Sydney, National Drug and Alcohol Research Centre, 2005.

459. McKetin R, Kelly E. Socio-demographic factors associated with methamphetamine treatment contact among dependent methamphetamine users in Sydney, Australia. *Drug Alcohol Rev* 2007;**26**:161–168.

460. Lea T, Mao L, Hopwood M, et al. Methamphetamine use among gay and bisexual men in Australia: trends in recent and regular use from the Gay Community Periodic Surveys. *Int J Drug Policy* 2016;**29**:66–72.

461. Hando J, Topp L, Hall W. Amphetamine-related harms and treatment preferences of regular amphetamine users in Sydney, Australia. *Drug Alcohol Depend* 1997;**46**:105–113.

462. Degenhardt L, Sara G, Mcketin R, et al. Crystalline methamphetamine use and methamphetamine-related harms in Australia. *Drug Alcohol Rev* 2016 (online). https://doi.org/10.1111/dar.12426

463. Degenhardt L, Sara G, Mcketin R, et al. Crystalline methamphetamine use and methamphetamine-related harms in Australia. *Drug Alcohol Rev* 2016 (online). https://doi.org/10.1111/dar.12426

464. Lemos NP. Methamphetamine and driving. *Social Sci Justice* 2009;**49**:247–249.

465. Degenhardt L, Sara G, Mcketin R, et al. Crystalline methamphetamine use and methamphetamine-related harms in Australia. *Drug Alcohol Rev* 2016 (online). https://doi.org/10.1111/dar.12426

Synthetic Cathinones

The natural analogue to synthetic cathinones is the active compound in the leaves of the khat plant (*Catha edulis*), which have been chewed for centuries in parts of Africa and the Arabian Peninsula for their stimulant properties.[1] Synthetic cathinones are also prescribed medications, such as bupropion, Wellbutrin®.

Synthetic cathinones form a significant proportion of novel psychoactive substances (NPS) with stimulant effects that have appeared in the last decade or so.[2,3] By 2019, the EMCDDA was monitored 138 synthetic cathinones, including eight reported for the first time in 2018.[4] Police seizures of new psychoactive substances continue to be typically dominated by synthetic cathinones (and synthetic cannabinoids).[5] There is concern over the use of synthetic cathinones by opioid and stimulant injectors, as this has been linked to health and social problems in some European countries.[6]

Synthetic cathinones appeared on the recreational drug scene more than a decade ago. The first synthetic cathinones to appear included 4-methylmethcathinone (mephedrone), 3,4-methylenedioxy-N-methylcathinone (methylone), and 4-methylenedioxypyrovalerone (MDPV).[7]

Mephedrone and its derivatives, as well as MDPV, are some of the NPS that have been reported every year since 2009[8] and have been detected in many parts of the world. However, in more recent years, MDPV and mephedrone are no longer as prevalent as they have been in previous years and new generations of synthetic cathinones have emerged on drug markets.[9,10]

Newer generations of synthetic cathinones are often more potent and associated with greater levels of harms. An animal study has suggested for example that the second generation cathinones pentylone and pentedrone have abuse liability greater than that of methylone.[11] There may also have been a shift in the use of synthetic cathinones from 'clubbers' to marginalised populations.

The second generation of synthetic cathinones, such as naphyrone and 4- methyl-N-ethcathinone

(4-MEC), emerged as replacements for mephedrone, methylone (3,4-methylenedioxy-N-methylcathinone) and MDPV (3,4 Methylenedioxypyrovalerone) when these came under legal controlled in 2010.[12] Similarly, 'second generation' pyrovalerone-cathinones compounds such as α-PVP, (α-pyrrolidinovalerophenone; α-pyrrolidinopentiophenone) were developed, sharing a very similar chemical structure with MDPV. New pyrovalerone drugs were also identified and include the following substances: 4F-α-PVP, α-PHP, PV8, 4Me-PPP, α-PBP, 4F-PV8, α-PPP, MDPHP, α-PVT, 4Cl-α-PVP, 4F-α-PHP MDPHP, and 4F-α-PVP.[13]

A so-called third-generation of synthetic cathinones also began to emerge including: 3,4-DMMC (3,4-dimethylmethcathinone), then pentedrone (α-methylaminovalerophenone)[14] [2-(methylamino)-1-phenylpentan-1-one], 4-methylethcathinone (4-MEC), butylone, ethcathinone, ethylone, 3- and 4-fluoromethcathinone, methedrone, methylone, pyrovalerone, 3-MeOMC; 3-MMC; 4-BMC; 4-MEC; 4-MeO-a-PVP; 4-MeO-PBP; 4-MeO-PV9; 4-MPD; 4F-PV8; 4FPV9; 4F-PVP; a-PBT; a-PHP; a-PVT; dibutylone; DL-4662; ethylone; MDPPP; MOPPP; NEB; pentedrone; PV-8, 4-CMC and alpha-PVP, 4-CEC α-pyrrolidinohexanophenone (α-PHP)

Other new synthetic cathinones identified include iso-4-BMC, β-TH-naphyrone, mexedrone, and 4-MDMC: (1) 1-(4-bromophenyl)-1-(methylamino) propan-2-one (iso-4-BMC or iso-brephedrone), (2) 2-(pyrrolidin-1- yl)-1-(5,6,7,8-tetrahydronaphthalen-2-yl)pentan-1-one (β-TH-naphyrone), (3) 3-methoxy-2-(methylamino)-1-(4-methylphenyl) propan-1-one (mexedrone), and (4) 2-(dimethylamino)-1-(4-methylphenyl)propan-1-one (4-MDMC),[15] 4-Chloromethcathinone (4-CMC, also known as clephedrone).

11.1 Street Names

Street names will of course vary by country, time and type of synthetic cathinones used. For example, 3-MMC, is referred to as 'ice cream' in Slovenia,[16]

while in the UK mephedrone is referred to as Bubble(s), Miaow, Meow Meow and Mcat.[17] In Hungary mephedrone is referred to as 'mefedron', 'kati'), MDPV ('MP', 'MP3', 'MP4'), 4-MEC ('formek'), and pentedrone ('penta', 'pentakristály', 'kristály').[18]

The term 'bath salts' is mainly used in the US to refer to synthetic cathinones (often MDPV) and will appear in the American literature.

11.2 Legal Status

Although the plant itself is not under international control, the principal psychoactive substances that the plant contains, cathine and cathinone, are controlled. Cathinone was included in Schedule I of the UN Convention on Psychotropic Substances in 1988, and cathine was then included in Schedule III of this Convention.

Some synthetic cathinones are now under international control including 3,4- methylenedioxypyrovalerone (MDPV), mephedrone and methylone and α-pyrrolidinovalerophenone (α-PVP); ethylone, pentedrone and 4-methylethcathinone (4-MEC) under Schedule II of the 1971 Convention on Psychotropic Substances (UNODC, 2017a).

In the US, MDPV, mephedrone and methylone come within the realm of Schedule I of the Controlled Substances Act 1970. In the EU, mephedrone was submitted to control by the European Council's decision of 2 December 2010 (2010/759/ EU). At national levels, other cathinone derivatives are caught by drug control or equivalent legislation, for example:

- mephedrone (Belgium, Crotia, Denmark, Estonia, France, Germany, Ireland, Italy, Lithuania, Norway, Romania and Sweden);
- methylone (Denmark, Ireland, Romania and Sweden);
- butylone (Denmark, Ireland, Norway, Romania and Sweden);
- MDPV (Denmark, Ireland, Finland and Sweden);
- flephedrone (Denmark, Ireland and Romania).
- Medicines' legislation is used in Finland and the Netherlands to control mephedrone. In the UK context, several generations/classes of synthetic cathinones and derivatives have been dealt with by means of generic definitions under the 1971 Act as Class B drugs and under Schedule 1 of the Misuse

of Drugs Regulations (2003, as amended) and the Psychoactive Substances Act 2016.[19]

11.3 Quality of the Research Evidence

Our knowledge of synthetic cathinones continues to be limited, although a number of pre-clinical, animal and laboratory studies have been conducted in recent years. Much of the literature on the harm associated with the use of synthetic cathinones and the management of those harms focuses on mephedrone and MDPV (often referred to in the American literature as 'bath salts'), reflecting their higher prevalence of use relative to other synthetic cathinones. We know less about the clinical effects of other synthetic cathinones, especially newer ones.

In addition to the lack of robust research evidence, not all studies of the clinical harms have analytical confirmation of cathinone use, reducing the ability to draw robust conclusions and make recommendations. US studies generally refer to the whole group of so-called 'bath salts'. Although it is not always clear what these are, they tend to include findings relating to methylenedioxypyrovalerone (MDPV) in particular, as well as mephedrone and other synthetic cathinones.

11.4 Brief Summary of Pharmacology

It has been argued that because cathinones present structural differences in their backbone and in the substitute groups, this makes them a unique family of drugs.[20]

Synthetic cathinones are beta-keto phenethylamines. Typically, they have an amphetamine-type analogue, which means that they are structurally related to amphetamine, methamphetamine and MDMA. Some synthetic cathinones are analogues of pyrovalerone (3,4-methylenedioxypyrovalerone or MDPV and naphyrone)[21] and have a slightly different mode of action.

Synthetic cathinones are amphetamine-like stimulants. Like amphetamines, cathinones act as central nervous system stimulants, although they are generally less potent than amphetamine.[22,23]

Synthetic cathinones are generally less able than amphetamines to cross the blood–brain barrier because the beta-keto group causes an increase in polarity.[24]

There are considerable variations between the different synthetic cathinones in their chemistry, modes of action, potency, and toxicity.[25] The most commonly used are the first-generation cathinones such as mephedrone, methylone and MDPV, which have been described as drugs with euphoric effects, because they act through the monoamine transporters (nor-adrenaline, dopamine or serotonin transporters). However, they do so in two ways: either as monoamine uptake inhibitors, or as transporter substrates that increase the release of these neurotransmitters.[26,27]

For example, mephedrone acts primarily (but not exclusively) as a releasing agent of dopamine, whereas MDPV is an uptake inhibitor at the same transporter. In other words, mephedrone and MDPV behave in an opposite manner at the level of dopamine transporter (DAT and NET). Like amphetamine and metham-phetamine, mephedrone is a DAT releasing agent whereas, like cocaine, MDPV is an uptake inhibitor at DAT.[28] Methylone shows a pharmacological profile that more closely resembles 3,4- methylenedioxy-methamphetamine (MDMA).[29]

A classification based on the pharmacological action of cathinones (i.e., Dopamine Transporter; DAT/Serotonin Transporter SERT inhibition ratio) and comparability to traditional drugs of abuse, in particular has been proposed.[30,31] Also see:[32]

1. Cocaine-MDMA-mixed cathinones, for example, mephedrone, 4-MEC, methylone, etylone, butylone and naphyrone. These substances are associated with an entactogenic, MDMA-like effect when ingested orally, and have a psychostimulant cocaine-like effect when taken intranasally.

2. Methamphetamine-like cathinones, for example, cathinone, methcathinone, flephedrone, ethcathinone, and 3-FMC.

3. MDMA-like cathinones, for example, methedrone and 4- trifluoromethylmethcathinone. These have effects broadly similar to MDMA and include NPS such as paramethoxymethamphetamine (PMMA), paramethoxyamphetamine, 4-ethylthioamphetamine.

4. Pyrovalerone-cathinones: for example, pyrovalerone, MDPV (see Box 11.1), and α-PVP. These molecules are non-substrate transporter inhibitors. All pyrovalerone-cathinones present with similar pharmacological profiles. They all exhibit inhibitory potencies at DAT and NET equal or greater than cocaine or methamphetamine, do not induce monoamine release, and readily cross the blood–brain barrier (BBB) owing to their high lipophilicity. Due to

these characteristics, these molecules may present with a high abuse potential.

Box 11.1 looks at mephedrone and MDVP in more detail.

Box 11.1 Mephedrone and MDVP

Mephedrone

Mephedrone is an example of the fact a 'novel' or 'new' substance is not always a new invention. Whereas mephedrone appeared as a recreational drug in 2007 in mainland Europe, it was synthetised in 1929.

Mephedrone is produced by replacement of the 4-position aromatic hydrogen of cathinone with a methyl group, and carries a similar molecular structure to many common street drugs, including amphetamine and MDMA.[33,34]

The ability of mephedrone to cause subjective effects resembling those of MDMA is likely to have contributed to its relatively widespread use. However, its ability to cause dopamine release may be problematic, inasmuch as in comparison with MDMA, mephedrone may have a greater liability to misuse, resembling that of dopamine releasing agents, such as methamphetamine.[35]

MDPV

Information obtained from studies carried out *in vitro* and *in vivo* in animal models suggests that the psychopharmacological and behavioural profile observed for MDPV is similar to cocaine. However, it appears that MDPV is more potent and longer lasting and it has been described as having powerful cocaine-like actions.[36]

It has also been suggested that in comparison to other synthetic cathinones, MDPV displays a novel pharmacological profile in as much as it is a potent uptake blocker at dopamine and norepinephrine transporters.[37] It has been suggested that the potency of MDPV at the DAT and NET and high blood–brain barrier permeability could result in high sympathomimetic toxicity.

Animal studies suggest that despite some of the structural similarities and similarities in behavioural effect with classical psychostimulants, MDPV shows greater potency, selectivity and functional upregulation of DAT[38] and induces greater locomotor activation, tachycardia and hypertension than cocaine in rats.[39]

Box 11.1 (cont.)

A study of *in vivo* locomotor activity testing and assessment of cardiovascular parameters (heart rate and blood pressure) found that MPDV is at least tenfold more potent than cocaine in inducing locomotor activation, tachycardia and hypertension. The authors concluded that the 'potent blockade of dopamine uptake caused by MDPV predicts that the drug has a high risk for abuse, whereas the potent blockade of norepinephrine uptake portends dangerous cardiovascular stimulation.[40]

Simmler et al. (2013) also argued that the potency of MDPV at the dopamine and noradrenaline transporters and high blood–brain barrier permeability could not only result in high sympathomimetic toxicity, but that there is also a risk of addiction in humans.[41]

Mephedrone and MDPV Combinations

Some synthetic cathinone products available appear to contain both mephedrone and MDPV. Some have argued that this combination of both is likely to be similar to ingestion of methamphetamine followed by ingestion of cocaine[42] – but in a more potent fashion.[43]

11.5 Clinical Uses of Synthetic Cathinones

Bupropion, a cathinone derivative, carries a medical indication in the US and Europe. It is used for the treatment of depression and as a smoking cessation aid.[44]

Some synthetic cathinones were originally developed as drug candidates, but later appeared on the NPS market.[45,46] Others, such as pyrovalerone for example, were developed in the late 1960s and are structurally related to MDPV. Pyrovalerone was used in the clinical treatment of chronic fatigue and lethargy but was later withdrawn and banned as a narcotic substance, as a result of misuse.[47,48,49,50,51]

11.6 Prevalence and Patterns of Use

Synthetic cathinones appeared as recreational drugs in Europe in 2004. By 2019, seizures of new psychoactive substances in Europe were typically dominated by synthetic cathinones (as well as synthetic cannabinoids) although more diversity can be seen in recent years, with other groups of substances becoming more prominent, including opioid and benzodiazepine NPS.[52]

Widely used synthetic cathinones in the European Union are mephedrone, 3-MMC, 4-methylethcathinone, pentedrone and pyrovalerone derivatives, such as MDPV and alpha-PVP.[53,54]

As mentioned above, synthetic cathinones have appeared on the recreational drug scene for over a decade. There was initially a rapid increase in the use of mephedrone in 2009 in some countries[55,56] and there are suggestions that in the UK and Holland, this was associated with the poor quality of cocaine and ecstasy/MDMA at the time. Its popularity was also enhanced by its relative low cost, availability and its desired effects.[44,55,57]

There is a mixed picture of its availability and prevalence of use after mephedrone was controlled.[58] Studies have suggested that there was a marked general decline in the use of 'bath salts' among young people in the US after the sale of such stimulants was outlawed in 2011. In the UK, the use of mephedrone declined sharply in the years after it was placed under national control in 2010,[59] and continues to do so.[60] Some studies have suggested the control of the drug in 2010 did not stop the spread of its use,[61,62] while others have suggested it did.[63]

Evidence from elsewhere shows that legal control may lead users to seek new drugs. For example, in Slovenia, after the ban on mephedrone, users continued to seek the same effects in other NPS and were reported to have shifted to 3-MMC, methylone, 4-methylethcathinone and pentedrone, which were believed to have similar effects as mephedrone.[64]

In some countries, the use of synthetic cathinones has been particularly associated with public health crisis. A study found for example that synthetic cathinones were found in a majority of syringes from Budapest. Synthetic cathinones in this country first appeared on the local drug market after the heroin shortage in 2011, and cathinones have since presented a substantial challenge for harm reduction services. The shift towards cathinones was linked to increased frequency of injecting, reuse and sharing of syringes, and higher HCV prevalence among stimulant users. The main cathinones injected were pentedrone and MDPV.[65]

In the Czech Republic, the increase in the use of synthetic cathinones was identified by a study as another drug used by marginalised people. Synthetic cathinone use was associated with poly-drug use and homelessness. In addition, as synthetic cathinones have an inferior status among IDUs, their users face a risk of stigmatisation and further marginalisation.[66]

11.6.1 Population Sub-groups More Likely to Use Synthetic Cathinones

Different people will use synthetic cathinones for different reasons and there are geographic differences between the various European countries of the groups of people most likely to use synthetic cathinones.

Nonetheless, the following groups have been associated with higher levels of risk of using synthetic cathinones, with a shift in recent years to use by marginalised groups.

11.6.1.1 'Clubbers' and People who Frequent Night-time Venues

As with other club drugs, there is evidence that use of mephedrone is associated with lifestyle.

For example, UK population-level data showed that the use of mephedrone in the previous year was around 20 times higher among those who had visited a nightclub four or more times in the past month (5.8%) than among those who had not visited a nightclub in the past month (0.3%).[67]

11.6.1.2 Synthetic Cathinone Use by Problem Drug Users

There is evidence that synthetic stimulants, especially cathinones, are replacing opioids in some countries reporting heroin shortages. The motive for the transition from injecting heroin to cathinones is unclear, but may be linked to easy availability and perceived high quality of the new drugs.[68] There have been reports of mephedrone injecting from Romania, Slovenia and Ireland,[69] as well as the Channel Islands. The practice of injecting synthetic cathinones is also reported by other countries in Europe, namely Austria, Finland, Germany, Latvia, Slovenia, Sweden and the UK.[70]

In Hungary, probably owing to the limited availability, low purity and high prices of 'traditional' drugs such as heroin, amphetamines and cocaine, there has been a shift among street drug users from the use of heroin to mephedrone injection, potentially increasing the risk of severe psychiatric symptoms.[71] Dependence and high rates of cathinone injecting have been reported.[72] It has been shown that among people who inject drugs, the proportion of those who injected amphetamine or heroin decreased from 95%

in 2009 to 13% in 2015, while cathinones, such as MDPV, mephedrone, pentedrone and methylone, became the main substances injected in that country.[73]

This was reflected in patients of drug treatment services. In Hungary, where there was a significant decrease in heroin injecting, this was followed by a rise in the proportion of patients of drug treatment services who injected 'amphetamine', 'other stimulant' and 'other (unclassifiable) drugs'. The proportion of 'other stimulant' and 'other drug' injector clients increased in total from 1% (2008 and 2009) to 21% by 2012. Although the authors were not able to determine the exact proportion of synthetic cathinone injectors, it was assumed that the vast majority of clients reported as 'other stimulant' and 'other (unclassifiable) drug' injectors were cathinone users.[74]

Cathinones continue to be widely available on the drug markets of many East European countries and Russia.[75]

Problem drug users sometimes inject synthetic cathinones as part of poly-drug use. In Finland for example, the use of synthetic cathinones such as alpha-PVP and MDPV, along with a primary substance, such as amphetamines, has been reported.[76] Similarly, a study carried out in Ireland through the analysis of urine collected from attendees of a methadone maintenance clinic, found that 14% were positive for mephedrone and 3% for methylone.[77]

Synthetic cathinones can be associated with compulsive patterns of injecting. One qualitative Irish study of 11 attendees of low-threshold harm-reduction services reported that compulsive re-injecting with excessive binge use over long periods was common, despite the fact that respondents were aware of the risks of injecting and of safer injecting practices. In this small cohort, 7 of the 11 were homeless, and injecting in public spaces and groin injecting were common. Mephedrone was not the first drug injected and its use appears to be an extension to other drugs also injected.[78]

11.6.1.3 Men Who Have Sex with Men and Pro-sexual Effects of Some Cathinones

The use of mephedrone has been associated with men who have sex with men (MSM) in some countries such as the UK, although in recent years this appears to be less prevalent.

Bourne et al. have shown that in the UK the use of mephedrone, as well as methamphetamine, GHB/GBL and ketamine, was associated with attendance of gay cafes, bars, pubs and clubs. Gay and bisexual men who used any or all of these substances were more frequent attenders of these venues than gay and bisexual men who used none of them.[79] Mephedrone was one of the drugs associated with 'chemsex', or the use of drugs in a sexual context. The practice of injecting mephedrone has also been noted.[80]

Factors associated with the use of cathinones in a sexual context include its dis-inhibitory effects as well as its pro-sexual effects (see also Section 10.7.3). There are some user reports of heightened sensuality, disinhibition, prolonged performance in males and ability to reach climax for females; users have also reported engaging in sexual behaviours when under the influence of mephedrone that they would not have engaged in while sober.[81,82,83,84,85,86]

11.6.1.4 Polydrug Use: Use of Synthetic Cathinones as Part of a Wider Repertoire of Drugs

Among most synthetic cathinone users, the drug is often taken as part of a wider repertoire of substances. Mixing cathinones with other drugs is common,[87] including with alcohol,[88] cannabis,[89,90] cocaine, ecstasy and ketamine,[91] as well as methamphetamine and GHB/GBL.

Many users will co-ingest cathinones with other substances. For example, a US study showed that a high percentage of 'bath salts' or synthetic cathinone users (94%) also tested positive for other common drugs such as cannabis, opiates, benzodiazepines, cocaine, or amphetamines,[92] a finding also made by numerous other studies.[93,94,95,96]

There is also evidence that mephedrone was used in combination with methamphetamine and HGB by MSM in particular.

There is evidence that some users co-ingest more than one substance not only to enhance the desired effects but also to attempt to reduce the harmful effects. Popular combinations reported are mephedrone or MDPV in combination with the following drugs:[78,84,86,97,98,99,100,101,102]

- alcohol, propranolol or another beta-blocker to offset tachycardia;
- cannabis, diazepam or alprazolam for anxiety and overstimulation;
- famotidine, omeprazole or domperidone for stomach pain;
- other psychostimulants such as cocaine, amphetamine, modafinil,

trifluoromethylphenylpiperazine, benzylpiperazine, butylone, methylone or pentylone to enhance stimulant and entactogenic effects;
- opiates, such as morphine or tramadol, to create 'speedball'-like effects;
- GHB/GBL to enhance sexual stimulation;
- ketamine or zopiclone to enhance visual hallucinations.

11.7 Routes of Ingestion, Dosing and Frequency of Dosing

Synthetic cathinones are typically misused as a fine white, off-white or yellowish powder, but some can be brown in colour. Cathinones are usually used intranasally or wrapped in paper and swallowed. They can also be found as capsules and pills and can be smoked. Synthetic cathinones can also be injected.

Although broadly similar, there are some differences between them, including their half-life and duration of effects. Nonetheless, there are similar patterns of risk associated with patterns of synthetic cathinone use. The short half-life and duration of effects of some synthetic cathinones have been reported, which means that users may redose and even binge.

In-depth interviews with people who have used 3-MMC in Slovenia showed binge use spanning several days being a prominent feature of drug use.[103] The compulsive and repeated injecting of synthetic cathinones is discussed in Section 11.6.2.

Boxes 11.2 and 11.3 look in more detail at mephedrone and MDPV.

11.8 Desired and Unwanted Effects for Recreational Use

Some users reported that a cathinone-induced stimulant effect is comparable to methylphenidate at low doses or to a combined effect of both amphetamine and cocaine at high doses.[130] Others consider cathinones to be pharmacologically similar to and as potent as amphetamine, cocaine, and MDMA.[131]

Overall, acute administration of low doses of synthetic cathinones produces euphoria and increases alertness. Users reported being motivated to consume synthetic cathinones for their euphoric properties, out of curiosity, and because these drugs are inexpensive and easy to obtain.[132] In a study where 104 respondents were asked about the reasons for taking synthetic cathinones, the given reasons for use included

Box 11.2 Mephedrone

Mephedrone is typically sold as a white or off-white crystalline powder, with a light-yellow hue.[104] Some users have reported its distinctive unpleasant smell[93] and some that their body sweat developed a 'chemical smell' as a result of its use.

Mephedrone powder is often sold in small plastic bags (typically 1 g doses), but there are reports of its sale as tablets pressed from the powder, or as capsules containing the powder. Mephedrone is water soluble. It is typically either snorted or swallowed (usually wrapped in a cigarette paper) or added to a drink. It is also used by rubbing on the gum, rectally, by smoking, or by injection (intramuscular and intravenous).[55,85,105] Users have also reported multiple concomitant routes of use.[1,21,22,23,24,33,34,35,44,55,56,57,58,61,62,63,68,69,77,78,84,85,86,89,90,91,92,93,94,96,97,106-120]

A cross-sectional anonymous online survey of mephedrone users associated with the dance music scene suggested that the most common route of use was intra-nasally (65.9%), with women significantly more likely than men to use the drug through snorting (76.2% and 67.2% respectively).[113]

Snorting is sometimes carried out through the 'keying' method, whereby a user will dip a key in the powder and snort the powder off the key (it is estimated that five to eight keys would represent a 1 g dose).[44] There are suggestions that the insufflation of mephedrone is associated with significant nasal irritation, which has led some users to switch to oral ingestion.[121]

Intranasal use may be associated with greater liability to misuse than oral use.[113,122] A survey carried out among 947 UK mephedrone users, reported that the amount of drug used in a typical session was significantly larger for those snorting (mean 0.97 g, SD 0.91) than for those using it orally (mean 0.74 g, SD 0.64). Those who snorted the drug reported significantly more days of use per month (mean 4.85, SD 5.11) than those who used it orally (mean 3.21 days, SD 3.01). Those who snorted the drug were significantly more likely to use it more frequently than those who did not, with 59.2% having used it at least monthly over the last 12 months.[113]

The onset of the desired effects of mephedrone is linked to the route of administration, being within a few minutes through nasal insufflation or intravenous injection and 15–45 minutes following oral ingestion. The onset of the effects following oral use can be delayed in the presence of food.[123] Rectal administration has been described by users as having a faster onset and the effects require lower doses.[93]

The duration of the effects is also linked to mode of use. The effects last up to 2–3 hours following nasal or oral use, albeit with a shorter duration where ingested through nasal insufflation, but only 15–30 minutes following intravenous use. Some users combine routes of use in a single session, for instance first snorting and then using orally in order to achieve both a fast effect and a longer-lasting effect.[117]

Typically, users ingest mephedrone in staggered doses, between 0.5 g and 1 g per session. Although a UK survey of clubbers found that approximately a quarter of mephedrone users took more than 1 g in a typical session,[113] other studies reported oral doses of 1–2 g[124] or even higher.[44] The same survey respondents reported that the average duration of a single session was 10.4 hours and that there was a correlation between total amount used and the duration of a session.[113]

The relatively short duration of the effects of mephedrone is associated with repeated dosing during a single session.[117] Regardless of the route of ingestion, the majority of mephedrone users will repeatedly re-dose within a single session to maintain the desired effect, leading to 'bingeing'.[125] Cathinones are associated with compulsive use and frequent, repeated injecting.

An animal study has reported vigorous mephedrone self-administration behaviour in rats, eliciting response levels that appear to match, or even exceed, those seen with other drugs of misuse.[126]

Box 11.3 MDPV

The hydrochloride salt form of MDPV is white but has also been described as a white-tan coloured powder.

MDPV is typically found in powder form, but there are reports of tablet, capsule and liquid form. It is used nasally, orally, and by intravenous injection; other reported routes of use include rectal insertion, smoking and subcutaneous injection.[127] There are also reports of MDPV detected in paper blotters (like LSD) and therefore buccal or sublingual administration may also occur. Similarly, the presence of MDPV in vegetable material suggested that this product would most probably be smoked.[128]

The onset of desired effects of MDPV is typically seen within 5–30 minutes, with desired effects lasting 2–7 hours for the common routes of administration (oral and nasal).[129]

curiosity (79%), liking the effect (52%), mind/brain exploration (52%), avoiding a positive test for another drug (26%), staying awake (22%), and improved sexual experience (21%). The most commonly reported acute subjective effects were stimulation and increased energy. Fewer than one quarter reported hallucinations, paranoia, or having an urge to act violently.[133]

In this study, respondents reviewed a list of 53 potential acute subjective effects and indicated (Yes/No) which effects, if any, they had personally experienced while 'high' on synthetic cathinones The most prevalent effects included a mixture of desirable and undesirable effects: increased energy (94%), fast heart beat (91%), rapid thoughts (91%), difficulty sleeping (89%), rush of euphoria (88%), decreased hunger (88%), feeling more open-minded (87%), increased sweating (86%), feeling happy (85%), dry mouth or thirsty (85%), increased sex drive (79%), grinding teeth (79%), feeling loving toward others (78%), feeling closer to others (75%), feeling that time seemed faster (66%), having hot flushes (62%), and body tension (60%).[134]

Box 11.4 looks in more detail at mephedrone and MDPV.

Box 11.4 Mephedrone

The reported desired effects of mephedrone include its stimulant and sympathomimetic effects, similar to those of MDMA (ecstasy) and cocaine.[55,93,113,118,135,136]

Reasons for its appeal include the fact that it is relatively non-potent and short-acting. Mephedrone is used for both its mood-enhancing properties and its role as a psychomotor stimulant in social situations.[113] Users report stimulant-related subjective effects such as euphoria, increased concentration, the urge to move, talkativeness, reduced appetite and wakefulness.

Desired effects also include stimulation, mood elevation, reduced hostility, improved mental function and increased energy.[55,61,86,113] At higher doses, perceptual distortions or hallucinations and the empathogenic properties of mephedrone have been reported.[55,61,113]

Synthetic cathinones can increase sexual desire and sexual risk-taking behaviour. There is evidence that some users ingest stimulants to increase sexual thoughts, intensify sexual desire, enhance sensuality, improve sexual functioning and prolong sexual performance.[137]

Users have reported heightened sensuality, disinhibition, prolonged performance for males, the ability to reach climax for females and sexual

Box 11.4 (cont.)

behaviours which they would not engage in while sober.[138,139,140,141,142,143]

A dose–response relationship between mephedrone and heightened sex drive has been reported.[113,132] However, the effects of mephedrone also depend on combinations and types of drugs used, length of time used, sexual roles, normative risk, settings and the individual's experiences and expectation.[134,144]

Despite the desired effects of mephedrone, there is also evidence that many users prefer other drugs with broadly similar effects to cathinones. For example, compared to cocaine and MDMA, mephedrone had some less favourable effects. Winstock[145] reports that users ceased their 'love affair' with mephedrone, in part, due to its higher scores for extreme agitation, headaches, tremors, nausea and feeling depressed after use, and to a lesser extent paranoia and chest pain. In terms of positive effects of using drugs, mephedrone came second out of ten drugs for increased pleasure from social interactions, but had more negative effects, which included not being able to function normally in the days after use and negative effects on mental health. Negative effects included its impact on ability to work/study/progress; negative effects on physical health; and unpleasant physical and psychological effects when intoxicated.[146]

A survey of 900 clubbers using mephedrone suggested that the frequency of specific unwanted effects (predetermined by the study) is as follows: excessive sweating (67.2%), headaches (50.7%), palpitations (43.4%), nausea (37%) and cold, blue fingers and toes (15.3%).[113] Similarly, in a Scottish student survey, more than half (56%) of those who had used mephedrone reported having at least one unwanted effect, at the following frequency: bruxism (teeth grinding) (28.3%), paranoia (24.9%), sore nasal passages (24.4%), hot flushes (23.4%), sore mouth/throat (22.9%), nose bleeds (22.4%), suppressed appetite (21.5%), blurred vision (21.0%), palpitations (20.5%), insomnia (19.5%), hallucinations (18.0%), nausea/vomiting (17.1%) and blue/cold extremities (14.6%).[147] Other unwanted effects include difficulties with urination, poor concentration and aggression.

Surveys suggest that approximately 20–56% of users of mephedrone have experienced adverse effects[84,141] and these are similar to those reported for amphetamine, methamphetamine and MDMA.[148] There is evidence that the most severe

Box 11.4 (cont.)

unwanted effects may be associated with high doses and/or prolonged use.[117]

However, there are important individual variations and similar doses may have significantly different effects and consequences in different individuals.[149] It has been suggested that it is impossible to determine what a 'safe' dose is, as negative effects may present with any dosage consumed.[150]

The most common unwanted effects of mephedrone and MDPV reported by users are summarised in Boxes 11.5 and 11.6 [57,77,93,113,117,130,141]

For acute harms see Section 11.9.

Box 11.5 Some Common Unwanted Effects of Mephedrone, as Reported by Users

Jaw clenching

Reduced appetite

Nasal irritation and nose bleeds

Nausea and vomiting

Discolouration of extremities and joints

Insomnia and/or nightmares

'Head rush'

Inability to concentrate and/or to focus visually

Memory problems

Altered conscious levels

Anxiety

Agitation

Hallucinations and delusions

Headaches, tremors and convulsions

Raised body temperature

Chest pains

Elevated heart rate

11.9 Acute Harms

11.9.1 Acute Toxicity

As mentioned above in the discussion of unwanted effects of synthetic cathinones, acute toxic effects of synthetic cathinones are common, with psychiatric and physical effects often manifesting together. (also see box 11.6 and 11.7)

Box 11.6 MDVP

Acute intoxication associated with MDPV produces typical stimulant-like effects, including increased energy, euphoria, and elevated feelings of empathy, and sociability.

Like other amphetamine-type substances, MDPV use is also associated with a 'crash' that follows use. This typically involves negative affective states, such as depression, suicidal thoughts, anxiety, panic attacks, excited delirium, bouts of violent aggression towards self and others, and combativeness that resemble a severe psychotic episode.[151]

For acute harms see Box 11.7 and Section 11.9.

α-pyrrolidinohexanophenone (α-PHP)

The long-lasting psychotic symptoms induced by synthetic cathinones appear to be correlated with their toxicokinetic characteristics, such as their long half-lives.[152] It has been suggested that a-PVP has been associated with strong stimulation, euphoria, and empathy at first, followed by restlessness and anxiety after about 20 minutes. Pleasant and unpleasant results alternate throughout the whole duration of a-PVP action. In the last stage of action, users develop paranoia, anxiety, and aggression.[153,154,155,156,157,158,159,160,161,162]

Box 11.7 Features of Acute Mephedrone Toxicity

Cardiovascular
Hypertension, tachycardia, chest pain, diaphoresis, hot flushes, shortness of breath, palpitations, cardiac arrest, peripheral vasoconstriction

Cognitive
Confusion, improved concentration, alertness, amnesia, cravings, empathy/feelings of closeness, dysphoria

Dermatological
Unusual sweat odour, rash

ENT
Sore nasal passages, mouth/throat pain, epistaxis

Gastrointestinal
Nausea/vomiting, anorexia, dry mouth, abdominal pain, sore mouth/throat

Metabolic
Elevated creatinine, metabolic acidosis

Box 11.7 (cont.)

Neurological/Psychiatric/Psychological

Anxiety, panic, depression, irritability, lack of motivation, anhedonia, sexual arousal, sociability, euphoria, insomnia, bruxism, headache, dizziness/light-headedness, tinnitus, seizures, nystagmus, mydriasis, blurred vision, numbness, blue/cold extremities, fever, paraesthesias, visual and auditory hallucinations, paranoid delusions, intensification of sensory experiences, reduced consciousness, agitation, aggression, short-term psychosis, short-term mania

Musculoskeletal

Increase in muscle tone, trismus

Respiratory

Dyspnoea

Serotonin Syndrome

Synthetic cathinone exposure has also resulted in many cases of seizures in the paediatric population.[229]

Box 11.8 MDPV Acute Harms

There is some evidence from animal studies on the acute adverse effects and the potential for toxicity associated with MDPV (both dose- and time-dependent), can cause cardiovascular stimulation and hyperpyrexia (particularly at increased ambient temperature). It has been suggested that the stimulant effects of MDPV appear to be intermediate between the stimulant effects of cocaine and methamphetamine.[230] MDPV acts as a dopamine reuptake inhibitor; it is more potent than cocaine.[231]

Data from a small number of cases in Europe, along with information from user self-reports, suggest that individuals typically present to emergency services with stimulant features including agitation/aggression, psychosis, delirium, tachycardia, hypertension and convulsions; there are also reports of more severe toxicity including hyperpyrexia, rhabdomyolysis, acute kidney injury and stroke.[232]

A study looking at the medical records and clinical data of 193 MDPV-positive cases found that the main clinical manifestations reported in patients testing positive for MDPV included agitation, tachycardia (100/min), and hypertension (systolic blood pressure 140 mmHg), which were observed in 130 (69%), 106 (56%), and 65 (34%) cases, respectively. Other symptoms included hallucinations (16%), delirium (15%), hyperthermia (10%), and rhabdomyolysis (8%).[233]

Box 11.8 (cont.)

The health burden caused by MDPV includes serious intoxications requiring intensive care treatment and fatalities.[234,235,236,237,238] In addition, it has been argued adverse effects do not only concern acute toxicity but also chronic toxicity.[239] There are also acute and longer-term problems associated with the injecting of MDPV[240] and other cathinones, as will be discussed in the next section.

α-pyrrolidinohexanophenone (α-PHP)

Symptoms of intoxication with α-PVP include hypertension, tachycardia, agitation, psychosis, visual and/or auditory hallucinations, and potentially death as a result of heart failure.[241,242,243,244,245,246,247,248,249,250]

Synthetic cathinones produce sympathomimetic clinical effects consistent with stimulant intoxication.[163–179] Cardiovascular effects (tachycardia, hypertension) and hallucinations are the most common medical complications of synthetic cathinone use.[180]

Case reports and case series relating to hospital presentations with acute mephedrone toxicity[85,97,114,181,182] describe sympathomimetic clinical features[114] and clinical effects consistent with stimulant intoxication.[183] Triangulation of data from a number of sources presents a picture of mephedrone acute toxicity (Box 11.6) that is consistent with that seen with the use of other sympathomimetic recreational drugs, such as amphetamine, cocaine and MDMA.[184]

People with synthetic cathinone poisoning will present to hospital with psychiatric, neurological, gastrointestinal, cardiovascular and muscular symptoms,[185] with cardiac, psychiatric and neurological symptoms the most common reported effects that require medical care.[175,186,187]

Synthetic cathinones can be associated with serotonin syndrome, especially if other serotonergic illicit drugs or medications are also used.[188,189] The use of synthetic cathinones has been associated with hyperthermia, similar to that linked to MDMA use.[190,191,192] (See Chapter 8 and Section 9.14 on serotonin syndrome.)

A range of adverse effects are associated with synthetic cathinones toxicity. Case reports have described for example mephedrone-induced euvolaemic hypoosmotic hyponatraemia with encephalopathy and raised intracranial pressure;[176] posterior reversible encephalopathy syndrome (PRES);[193] spontaneous subcutaneous emphysema associated with mephedrone use, which did not require airway support;[194] and a case report of methaemoglobinaemia, a serious complication caused by a number of oxidising drugs.[195] A case of prolonged hypoglycaemia associated with the use of synthetic cathinones has also been reported.[196]

A case report highlighted the potential danger of mephedrone to people with diabetes. A patient with type 1 diabetes developed ketoacidosis following self-reported mephedrone use. Cathinone compounds may directly increase the risk of diabetic ketoacidosis by stimulating the central nervous system. They may also indirectly impair an individual's ability to manage diabetes through changes in cognitive function and behaviour.[197]

As with other 'traditional' psychostimulants, synthetic cathinones appear to be linked to neurocognitive dysfunction and cytotoxicity (toxicity to cells), which are dependent on drug type, dose, frequency, and time after use.[198] Synthetic cathinones may be associated with enhanced neurotoxicity in comparison to traditional stimulants.[199–215] There is emerging evidence that when intoxicated, mephedrone use can impair working memory acutely[119] and a case report of catatonia.[216]

A wide spectrum of psychiatric effects of synthetic cathinones has been described. As with other stimulants, these affect in particular, but not exclusively, people with mental health co-morbidities. The most commonly reported are agitation, insomnia, impaired concentration, transient paranoid and perceptual disturbances, anxiety, temporary mood disturbances, and also delirium.[217,218,219] Repeated use of synthetic cathinones is associated with paranoia and hallucinations.[220]

Psychosis and suicidality have also been reported,[221,222,223] with studies on 'bath salts' describing psychotic symptoms and 'bath-salt'-induced psychosis,[224,225,226,227] similar to other cathinones, such as pentedrone.[228]

It is not possible to quantify accurately how common these presentations are. A US case series of 35 patients presenting at an emergency department with toxicity relating to synthetic cathinones reported that:

- 91% had neurological symptoms;
- 77% had cardiovascular symptoms;
- 49% had psychological symptoms.[177]

In the UK, a report of a case series of 72 patients with self-reported acute mephedrone toxicity indicated that the most common symptoms on presentation to hospital, or before, were: agitation (38.9%); tachycardia (36.1%); palpitations (25.0%); vomiting (13.9%); clinically significant hypertension (13.9%); chest pain (12.5%); severe tachycardia (8.3%); headaches (7.2%); self-limiting pre-hospital seizures (6.9%).[96]

11.9.2 Harms from High-risk Injecting and Sexual Behaviour

Synthetic cathinones can be associated with frequent and compulsive injecting, increasing the risk of blood-borne infections as well as systemic and bacterial infections.

Injecting synthetic cathinones has been a challenge for some countries, notably Hungary and Romania, where it seems to be widespread among injecting drug users.[251,252,253,254]

The injection of synthetic cathinones has been linked with increased transmission of HIV and hepatitis C in many countries in Europe, including Hungary, Ireland and the UK; in Greece and Romania, the injection of these substances was identified in 2012 as a possible factor linked to outbreaks of HIV infection.[255]

The limited research describing this practice strongly suggests its potential for unpleasant side-effects. Intravenous users of mephedrone report paracitosis (leading to scratching and gouging of the skin of the face, neck and arms in particular), paranoia, suicidal ideation and severe insomnia, especially after prolonged use.[117]

In a small qualitative Irish study, participants reported unwanted effects which included intense paranoia, violent behaviour and aggression, and the emergence of Parkinson-type symptoms, in the form of spasm, 'wobbling' and permanent numbness in the extremities. Injectors also report intense burning sensations at injection sites, limb abscesses, and vein clotting, damage and recession. These result from drug toxicity, crystallisation of the drug when diluted and syringe flushing practices. They also report multi-drug and serial drug injecting. Heroin is used in an attempt to manage the intense 'rush' and avoid an unpleasant come-down from mephedrone.[78]

As with other club drugs, mephedrone use has been linked to high-risk sexual behaviours among heterosexual men and men who have sex with men.[86,137] There is some anecdotal evidence of mephedrone injecting among MSM in London (referred to as 'slamming'), sometimes in combination with methamphetamine and injecting behaviours that put users at high risk of HIV and hepatitis.[110]

11.9.3 Acute Withdrawal

For withdrawal see Section 11.12.2.

11.9.4 Poly-drug Use and Drug Interaction

The co-ingestion of other substances alongside synthetic cathinones appears to increase harm.

For example, the reports of many mephedrone-associated deaths in the UK indicate poly-drug use.[256] Alcohol in particular may potentiate the effects of mephedrone.[257,258]

A two-patient case study found that large quantities of alcohol ingested with mephedrone may lead to serious cardiac arrhythmias.[259] The co-ingestion of two stimulants is likely to increase mephedrone toxicity, as well as its potential harm,[90] including the risk of serotonin syndrome or toxicity (see Chapter 8 and Section 9.14).

An animal study found that mephedrone enhances the neurotoxicity of methamphetamine, amphetamine and MDMA, substances that are commonly used alongside mephedrone.[260] There is also one reported death resulting from a combination of GHB and mephedrone, albeit with no analytical confirmation of the substances used.[261]

As CYP2D6 and CYP3A4 may be involved in mephedrone metabolism, inhibitors of these metabolic enzymes could increase the systemic exposure to mephedrone and lead to increased toxicity. In terms of HIV treatment medications, among the antiretroviral drugs, these would be ritonavir (a CYP3A4 inhibitor at low boosting doses) and cobicistat (a CYP3A4 and CYP2D6 inhibitor). The role of ritonavir's inducing effect on glucuronidation and its impact on mephedrone exposure remains unclear.

Care should also be given to the prescribing of medications with serotonergic effects.

11.9.5 Mortality

Deaths associated with a range of synthetic cathinones have been reported. The medical literature presents numerous fatal case reports associated with the range of synthetic cathinones.[262,263]

There are numerous reports of deaths where synthetic cathinones were implicated. This includes, but is not limited to, deaths where mephedrone was implicated,[250] as well as MDPV,[264] alpha-PVP,[265] N-ethylpentylone,[266] α-propyloaminopentiophenone,[267] n-Ethyl pentylone (NEP),[268] α-pyrrolidinoheptiophenone (PV8)[269] and pentedrone and a-pyrrolidinovalerophenone.[270]

It has been shown by one study on deaths where mephedrone was implicated that most deaths occurred when more than one substance was ingested, and especially when alcohol was one of these.[250] Nonetheless, in a small number of cases, death was directly related to mephedrone on its own, which confirms the concerns regarding the acute toxicity potential of the drug itself.[250] In the same study, Schifanno et al. found that factors associated with mephedrone-associated death were young age (mean age 29 years), male and previous history of substance misuse.[250]

11.10 Management of Acute Harms

11.10.1 Identification and Assessment of Mephedrone Toxicity

Toxicological screening is not usually carried out for patients presenting to emergency departments with harms associated with synthetic cathinones because the results are typically not available in time to inform the patient's management. It is recommended that diagnosis is made on clinical assessment, with other causes of presentation excluded and recognition of the associated clinical toxidrome.

It is not possible to determine accurately the numbers of presentations to hospital associated with mephedrone toxicity or indeed admissions resulting from the use of any recreational drug, not least because presentations with acute toxicity are assigned a wide variety of primary codes, which are likely to relate to symptoms rather than cause.[271] In addition, synthetic cathinones are also often used as part of a wider repertoire of drug use and thus effects may be due to other substances.[117]

Two case series of presentations to an emergency department (ED) for acute mephedrone toxicity provide some insight. In a study of 89 cases in the ED of Aberdeen Royal Infirmary, self-reports suggested that 33% had ingested mephedrone only, 30% mephedrone and alcohol, and 35% co-ingestion of other substances.[272]

11.10.2 Management of Acute Toxicity

There are no large robust studies that have looked at the management of acute synthetic cathinone intoxication, but there is consistency from case series and reports that treatment should consist of symptom-directed supportive care. It has been argued that, given the similarities with cocaine and amphetamine, management strategies similar to those recommended for intoxication with those drugs might be useful.[180]

Symptom-directed supportive care for acute stimulant intoxication may include the management of agitation, convulsions, metabolic acidosis, hypertension, hypothermia and rhabdomyolysis. The management of serotonin syndrome may also be indicated.

It also suggests that agitated adults be sedated with an initial dose of oral or intravenous diazepam (0.1–0.3 mg/kg body weight). Larger doses may be required.

For agitation and psychiatric symptoms associated with mephedrone, the use of benzodiazepine is commonly reported. Case reports described the use of antidepressants, hypnotic-sedatives including midazolam, lorazepam, diazepam, and etomidate given for agitation.[273] One report described lorazepam as effective for agitation and various sympathomimetic features of mephedrone use.[114]

Case studies have reported the use of propofol, haloperidol, as well as quetiapine and other antipsychotics for paranoid ideation, agitation and anxiety.[90,274] Antipsychotics should be used cautiously with synthetic cathinone intoxication, as they increase seizure activity[275] and decrease heat dissipation.

11.10.3 Treatment Outcome

A study looking into pharmacological treatment in acute hospital settings of 201 analytically confirmed MDPV-positive patients reported that medication used primarily included benzodiazepines, haloperidol and propofol (n = 16; 8%). Only seven (4%) patients required intubation. The number of days in hospital care was 1 day for 76 (40%) patients, 2 days for 79 (42%) patients, and 3 days for 21 (11%) patients.[276]

People who present to hospitals generally make a good recovery. The majority (84.7%) of the 72 patients presenting to hospital with acute toxicity described in one case series[96] were discharged either directly from the ED or from a short-stay observation ward; the other 15.3% were admitted to hospital, with 11.1% admitted for observation/management on a general internal medicine ward, and 4.2% required admission to intensive care. Overall, 13.9% required benzodiazepines (oral or intravenous) for ongoing agitation at, or after, presentation to the hospital. All but one patient were discharged with no long-term sequelae at the time of discharge. The length of stay following presentation ranged from 0.3 to 30 hours (a mean of 6.7 hours, SD 7.3 hours).[96]

11.10.4 Management of Acute Withdrawal

See section 11.12.2.

11.11 Harms Associated with Chronic Use

11.11.1 Dependence

There is some evidence that mephedrone has a dependence potential. It has been argued that the ability of mephedrone to cause striatal dopamine release may be problematic inasmuch as, in comparison with MDMA, mephedrone may have an enhanced liability to misuse, more resembling that of dopamine-releasing agents such as methamphetamine.[35] One animal study suggests that the dopaminergic effects of mephedrone may contribute to its addictive potential.[277]

It has been suggested that, because of the similarity of synthetic cathinones to amphetamine, they carry a similar risk of dependence, with chronic use leading to dependence and a cycle of bingeing and periods of recovery associated with depression.[44] Cases of dependence have been reported.[86,278] In a Scottish school survey, 17.6% of those who had used mephedrone reported 'addiction/dependency' symptoms relating to their use of mephedrone.[141] Similarly, a survey of 797 clubbers who had used mephedrone reported that it was 'as or more addictive' than cocaine.[113] In another survey, 50% of 1,500 mephedrone users considered it to be addictive.[84]

MDPV is also associated with a risk of harmful and dependent use,[279] with associated health care utilisation and social costs.[280] It has also been shown that the regular use of α-PVP may lead to dependence, tolerance and withdrawal syndrome.[281,282,283,284,285,286,287,288,289,290]

Synthetic cathinone dependence is a disorder of regulation of synthetic cathinone use arising from repeated or continuous use of synthetic cathinones. The characteristic feature is a strong internal drive to use synthetic cathinones, which is manifested by impaired ability to control use, increasing priority given to use over other activities and persistence of use despite harm or negative consequences.

These experiences are often accompanied by a subjective sensation of urge or craving to use synthetic cathinones. Physiological features of dependence may also be present, including tolerance to the effects of synthetic cathinones, withdrawal symptoms following cessation or reduction in use of synthetic cathinones, or repeated use of synthetic cathinones or pharmacologically similar substances to prevent or alleviate withdrawal symptoms. The features of dependence are usually evident over a period of at least 12 months but the diagnosis may be made if synthetic cathinone use is continuous (daily or almost daily) for at least 1 month.

α-PVP appears to give rise to extreme craving and risk of binge consumption and it seems that it has abuse liability and possibly a dependency potential in humans.[291]

Diagnostic criteria for dependence on synthetic cathinones have been described by IDC-11 (see Box 11.9).

There is increasing evidence that mephedrone causes a strong and repeated compulsion to use,[57,141] that tolerance to mephedrone develops quickly and that users tend to consume higher doses more frequently. Subjective reports of craving suggest that mephedrone may have a greater potential for repetitive and compulsive use than MDMA,[57,84,141] although these observations are made on the basis of self-reports. Emerging evidence on the subjective effects of mephedrone suggests that its ingestion is associated with 'wanting more',[57,86,119] and this was shown to be elevated significantly when users were sober but anticipated use in the near future.[119]

The development of substance use disorder symptoms associated with synthetic cathinones, such as tolerance, have been described,[293] as well as withdrawal after repeated use. The withdrawal symptoms reported include depression, concentration difficulties, feelings of fear and anxiety, irritability, tiredness, insomnia, and, in some cases, cravings followed in response to compulsive drug use.[294,295]

11.11.2 Withdrawal

Reports have been published of craving for mephedrone and of withdrawal.[55,93,141] There are users' reports that the development of cravings for mephedrone may be linked to increased frequency of use.[113] A survey of users also suggested that those who ingested the drug through nasal insufflation were more likely than those who used it orally to rate it as more addictive than cocaine,[113] possibly reflecting the more rapid onset and shorter duration of desired effects of mephedrone when it is used nasally. Craving for mephedrone has been described as stronger than for ecstasy.[57]

Studies have shown that unpleasant physical and mental symptoms may be experienced when going through withdrawal from synthetic cathinones. They have not described a physical withdrawal syndrome following the abrupt stopping of chronic use of synthetic cathinones, but psychological dependency is possible. Reported symptoms include anxiety and depression, craving, anhedonia, anergia and insomnia associated with mephedrone, methcathinone and MDPV for example.[296]

A study of 100 users suggested that the most frequent effects related to withdrawal after a session of mephedrone use were tiredness, insomnia, nasal congestion and impaired concentration. Other withdrawal symptoms include depression, anxiety, increased appetite, irritability, unusual sweat odours and urge or craving to use.[86]

There may be some differences between the various synthetic cathinones, but more research is needed. For example, Van Hout (2014) noted that 4-MEC users did not report withdrawal symptoms akin to those of mephedrone.[297] Mephedrone was described by a frequent and heavy user in a case report as providing a more intense initial euphoria and a more severe withdrawal syndrome than MDPV.[298] In this case report, the user, who also reported a history of opiate and methamphetamine use, reported mephedrone withdrawal as the most unpleasant drug withdrawal he had experienced. He reported that discontinuation of mephedrone resulted in agitation and dysphoria within a few hours, which was more severe than that of cocaine or methamphetamine, and which was accompanied by an increase in muscle tone, the alleviation of which required constant movement.[293] He reported that only methamphetamine gave some degree of relief to the withdrawal.[293]

11.11.3 Other Harms

11.11.3.1 Risk of Systemic and Viral Infections

Like other club drugs, the impact of mephedrone on sexual behaviour can affect the transmission of blood-borne viruses and sexually transmitted infections.[137] Moreover, mephedrone is associated with compulsive and frequent injecting, making its users at particular risk of the acquisition and transmission of blood-borne viruses. To this are added the risks specifically linked to the injection of mephedrone, which can include limb abscesses and vein clotting, damage and recession. This places injectors at risk of septicaemia, endocarditis, deep-vein thrombosis and other complications.

11.12 Management of Harms Related to Chronic Use and Dependence

11.12.1 Clinical Management of Chronic Use and Dependence

See Chapter 8 on the identification and assessment of dependence on ATS in general (Section 8.10.1), which apply to mephedrone, as does the guidance on psychosocial and pharmacological support and intervention (Chapter 2 and Section 8.10.3).

11.12.2 Management of Withdrawal

Psychosocial interventions constitute the main interventions for dependence on synthetic cathinones, as with other stimulants as discussed in Chapter 2. Ongoing psychological support may be required, including for the prevention of relapse.[117]

There are no recognised pharmacological regimens for the management of synthetic cathinone withdrawal, as with other stimulants (also see Chapter 8, Section 8.14.3.2). Some have suggested bupropion,[299,300] but more research is needed.

Nonetheless, patients may require medical treatment for their symptoms on discontinuation. Reports suggest supportive treatment with low to moderate doses of benzodiazepines for agitation and paranoia. A treatment regimen of olanzapine[272] was described

in a case report of dependence on mephedrone (diagnosis based on ICD-10 criteria) and where dependence had led to psychotic symptoms. Another case report described a patient prescribed antidepressants for residual symptoms of depressed mood, anhedonia and hopelessness present in all his periods of abstinence.[293] A further case report described a pharmacological intervention for MPDV withdrawal involving risperidone, which was effective for symptoms of disorganisation, delusions and hallucinations.[301]

11.12.3 Aftercare and Support

As is the case with many people who use drugs in general, some people who use synthetic cathinones will sometimes use harm reduction strategies to minimise risk. For example, 3-MMC users in Slovenia report obtaining information beforehand, using their own injecting equipment and paraphernalia and using only small quantities of unknown substances.[302]

11.12.4 Public Health and Harm Reduction

Winstock et al. recommend as harm reduction[116]:

- Avoiding using regularly to prevent developing tolerance;
- Not using with stimulants or large amounts of alcohol and/or other depressants;
- Not injecting;
- Avoiding dehydration;
- Avoiding overheating.

See also Chapter 8.

11.12.5 Public Safety: Driving

Mephedrone can affect driving inasmuch as it can produce poor concentration, hallucinations and psychosis.[303]

References

1. Warfa N, Klein A, Bhui K, Leavey G, Craig T, Alfred Stansfeld S. Khat use and mental illness: a critical review. *Soc Sci Med* 2007;**65**(2):309–318.

2. World Drug Report 2019 (United Nations publication, Sales No. E.19.XI.9)

3. World Drug Report 2020 (United Nations publication, Sales No. E.20.XI.6).

4. European Monitoring Centre for Drugs and Drug Addiction and Europol. EU Drug Markets Report 2019. Luxembourg, Publications Office of the European Union, 2019.

5. European Monitoring Centre for Drugs and Drug Addiction. European Drug Report 2020: Trends and Developments. Luxembourg, Publications Office of the European Union, 2020.

6. European Monitoring Centre for Drugs and Drug Addiction and Europol. EU Drug Markets Report 2019. Luxembourg, Publications Office of the European Union, 2019.

7. Lopez-Rodriguez AB, Viveros M-P. Bath salts and polyconsumption: in search of drug-drug interactions. *Psychopharmacology* 2019;**236**:1001–1014. https://doi.org/10.1007/s00213-019-05213-3

8. Corkery JM, Guirguis A, Papanti DG, Orsolini L, Schifano F. Synthetic cathinones: prevalence and motivations for use. In: J Zawilska (ed.), *Synthetic Cathinones. Current Topics in Neurotoxicity*, volume 12. Cham, Springer.

9. Baumann MH, Volkow ND. Abuse of new psychoactive substances (NPS): threats and solutions. *Neuropsychopharmacology* 2016;**41**(3):663–665. https://doi.org/10.1038/npp.2015.260

10. Baumann MH, Ayestas MA Jr, Partilla JS, et al. The designer methcathinone analogs, mephedrone and methylone, are substrates for monoamine transporters in brain tissue. *Neuropsychopharmacology* 2012;**37**:1192–1203. https://doi.org/10.1038/npp.2011.304

11. Javadi-Paydar M, Nguyen JD, Vandewater SA, Dickerson TJ, Taffe MA. Locomotor and reinforcing effects of pentedrone, pentylone and methylone in rats.*Neuropharmacology* 2018;**134**(Pt A):57–64. https://doi.org/10.1016/j.neuropharm.2017.09.002

12. Valente MJ, Guedes de Pinho P, de Lourdes Bastos M, Carvalho F, Carvalho M. Khat and synthetic cathinones: a review. *Arch Toxicol* 2014;**88**(1):15–45. https://doi.org/10.1007/s00204-013-1163-9

13. Beck O, Helander A, Signell P, Backberg M. Intoxications in the STRIDA project involving a panorama of psychostimulant pyrovalerone derivatives, MDPV. *Clin Toxicol* 2018;**56**(4):256–263.https://doi.org/10.1080/15563650.2017.1370097

14. Valente MJ, Guedes de Pinho P, de Lourdes Bastos M, Carvalho F, Carvalho M. Khat and synthetic cathinones: a review. *Arch Toxicol* 2014;**88**(1):15–45. https://doi.org/10.1007/s00204-013-1163-9

15. Qian Z, Jia W, Li T, Liu C, Hua Z. Drug identification and analytical characterization of four synthetic cathinone derivatives iso-4-BMC, β-TH-naphyrone, mexedrone, and 4-MDMC test. *Analysis* 2017;**9**:274–281.

16. Sande M. Characteristics of the use of 3-MMC and other new psychoactive drugs in Slovenia, and the perceived problems experienced by users. *Int J Drug Policy* 2016;**27**:65–73.

17. Mecham F, Measham F, Moore K, Østergaard J. Mephedrone, 'Bubble' and unidentified white powders: the contested identities of synthetic 'legal highs'. *Drugs Alcohol Today* 2011;**11**(3):137–146.

18. Péterfi A, Tarján A, Csaba Horváth G, Csesztregi T, Nyírádya A. Changes in patterns of injecting drug use in Hungary: a shift to synthetic cathinones. *Drug Test Analysis* 2014 (online. https://doi.org/10.1002/dta.1625

19. Corkery JM, Guirguis A, Papanti DG, Orsolini L, Schifano F. Synthetic cathinones: prevalence and motivations for use. In: J Zawilska (ed.), *Synthetic Cathinones. Current Topics in Neurotoxicity*, volume 12. Cham, Springer.

20. Baumann MH, Partilla JS, Lehner KR, et al. Powerful cocaine-like actions of 3,4-methylenedioxypyrovalerone (MDPV), a principal constituent of psychoactive 'bath salts' products. *Neuropsychopharmacology* 2013;**38**:552–562. https://doi.org/10.1038/npp.2012.204

21. United Nations Office on Drugs and Crime (UNODC), Laboratory and Scientific Section. Details for Synthetic Cathinones. Available at: www.unodc.org/LSS/SubstanceGroup/Details/67b1ba69-1253-4ae9-bd93-fed1ae8e6802 [last accessed 16 March 2022].

22. Fleckenstein AE, Volz TJ, Riddle EL, Gibb JW, Hanson GR. New insights into the mechanism of action of amphetamines. *Annu Rev Pharmacol Toxicol* 2007;**47**:681–698.

23. Cozzi NV, Sievert MK, Shulgin AT, Jacob P 3rd, Ruoho AE. Inhibition of plasma membrane monoamine transporters by beta-ketoamphetamines. *Eur J Pharmacol* 1999;**381**(1):63–69.

24. Coppola M, Mondola R. Synthetic cathinones: chemistry, pharmacology and toxicology of a new class of designer drugs of abuse marketed as 'bath salts' or 'plant food'. *Toxicol Lett* 2012;**211**(2):144–149. https://doi.org/10.1016/j.toxlet.2012.03.009

25. Baumann MH, Partilla JS, Lehner KR. Psychoactive 'bath salts': Not so soothing. *Eur J Pharmacol* 2013;**698**:1–5. https://doi.org/10.1016/j. ejphar.2012.11.020

26. Luethi D, Liechti ME. Monoamine transporter and receptor interaction profiles in vitro predict reported human doses of novel psychoactive stimulants and psychedelics. *Int J Neuropsychopharmacol* 2018;**21**:926–931.

27. Lopez-Rodriguez AB, Viveros MP. Bath salts and polyconsumption: in search of drug-drug interactions. *Psychopharmacology*2019;**236**:1001–1014. https://doi.org/10.1007/s00213-019-05213-3

28. Glennon RA, Dukat M. Synthetic cathinones: a brief overview of overviews with applications to the forensic sciences. *Ann Forensic Res Anal* 2017;**4**(2):1040.

29. Lopez-Rodriguez AB, Viveros M-P. Bath salts and polyconsumption: in search of drug-drug interactions. *Psychopharmacology* 2019;**236**:1001–1014. https://doi.org/10.1007/s00213-019-05213-3

30. Guirguis A, Corkery JM, Stair JL, Kirton SB, Zloh M, Schifano F. Intended and unintended use of cathinone mixtures. *Hum Psychopharmacol Clin Exp* 2017;**32**:e2598. https://doi.org/10.1002/hup.2598

31. Simmler TA, Buser M, Donzelli Y, et al. Pharmacological characterization of designer cathinones in vitro. *Br J Pharmacol* 2013;**168**:458–470.

32. Schifano F, Papanti GD, Orsolini L, Corkery JM. Novel psychoactive substances: the pharmacology of stimulants and hallucinogens. *Exp Rev Clin Pharmacol* 2016;**9**(7):943–954.

33. Carroll FI, Lewin AH, Mascarella SW, Seltzman HH, Reddy PA. Designer drugs: a medicinal chemistry perspective. *Ann NY Acad Sci* 2012;**1248**:18–38.

34. Iversen L, White M, Treble R. Designer psychostimulants: pharmacology and differences. *Neuropharmacology* 2014;**87**:59–65. https://doi.org/10.1016/j.neuropharm.2014.01.015

35. Hadlock GC, Webb KM, McFadden LM, et al. 4-Methylmethcathinone (mephedrone): neuropharmacological effects of a designer stimulant of abuse. *J Pharmacol Exp Ther* 2011;**339**(2):530–536. https://doi.org/10.1124/jpet.111.184119

36. Baumann MH, Partilla JS, Lehner KR, et al. Powerful cocaine-like actions of 3,4-Methylenedioxypyrovalerone (MDPV), a principal constituent of psychoactive 'bath salts' products. *Neuropsychopharmacology* 2013;38(4):552–562.

37. Baumann MH, Partilla JS, Lehner KR, et al. Powerful cocaine-like actions of 3,4-methylenedioxypyrovalerone (MDPV), a principal constituent of psychoactive 'bath salts' products. *Neuropsychopharmacology* 2013;**38**(4):552–562.

38. López-Arnau R, Buenrostro-Jáuregui M, Camarasa J, et al. Effect of the combination of mephedrone plus ethanol on serotonin and dopamine release in the nucleus accumbens and medial prefrontal cortex of awake rats. *Naunyn Schmiedebergs Arch Pharmacol* 2018;**391**:247–254. https://doi.org/10.1007/s00210-018-1464-x

39. Baumann MH, Partilla JS, Lehner KR, et al. Powerful cocaine-like actions of 3,4-methylenedioxypyrovalerone (MDPV), a principal constituent of psychoactive 'bath salts' products. *Neuropsychopharmacology* 2013;**38**:552–562. https://doi.org/10.1038/npp.2012.204

40. Baumann MH, Partilla JS, Lehner KR, et al. Powerful cocaine-like actions of 3,4-methylenedioxypyrovalerone (MDPV), a principal constituent of psychoactive 'bath salts' products. *Neuropsychopharmacology* 2013;**38**:552–562. https://doi.org/10.1038/npp.2012.204

41. Simmler LD, Buser TA, Donzelli M, et al. Pharmacological characterization of designer cathinones in vitro. *Br J Pharmacol* 2013;**168**:458–470.

42. Cameron K, Kolanos R, Verkariya R, De Felice L, Glennon RA. Mephedrone and Methylenedioxypyrovalerone (MDPV), major constituents of bath salts, produce opposite effects at the human dopamine transporter. *Psychopharmacology* 2013;**227**(3):493–499. https://doi.org/10.1007/s00213-013-2967-2

43. Glennon RA, Dukat M. Synthetic cathinones: a brief overview of overviews with applications to the forensic sciences. *Ann Forensic Res Anal* 2017;**4**(2):1040.

44. Advisory Council on the Misuse of Drugs (ACMD). Consideration of the Cathinones. London, Home Office, 2010.

45. Beck O, Bäckberg M, Signell P, Helander A. Intoxications in the STRIDA project involving a panorama of psychostimulant pyrovalerone derivatives: MDPV copycats. *Clin Toxicol*

46. Meltzer PC, Butler D, Deschamps JR, et al. 1-(4-Methylphenyl)-2- pyrrolidin-1-yl-pentan-1-one (Pyrovalerone) analogues: a promising class of monoamine uptake inhibitors. *J Med Chem* 2006;**49**:1420–1432.

47. Beck O, Bäckberg M, Signell P, Helander A. Intoxications in the STRIDA project involving a panorama of psychostimulant pyrovalerone derivatives: MDPV copycats. *Clin Toxicol* 2018;**56**(4):256–263. https://doi.org/10.1080/15563650.2017.1370097

48. Meltzer PC, Butler D, Deschamps JR, et al. 1-(4-Methylphenyl)-2- pyrrolidin-1-yl-pentan-1-one (Pyrovalerone) analogues: a promising class of monoamine uptake inhibitors. *J Med Chem* 2006;**49**:1420–1432.

49. Gardos G, Cole JO. Evaluation of pyrovalerone in chronically fatigued volunteers. *Curr Ther Res Clin Exp* 1971;**13**:631–635.

50. Fung M, Thornton A, Mybeck K, et al. Evaluation of the characteristics of safety withdrawal of prescription drugs from worldwide pharmaceutical markets – 1960 to 1999. *Drug Inf J* 2001;**35**:293–317.

51. World Health Organization. Convention on psychotropic substances, 1971. Available at: www.who.int/data/gho/indicator-metadata-registry/imr-details/3384 [last accessed 26 April 2022].

52. European Monitoring Centre for Drugs and Drug Addiction and Europol. EU Drug Markets Report 2019. Luxembourg, Publications Office of the European Union, 2019.

53. World Drug Report 2019 (United Nations publication, Sales No. E.19.XI.9).

54. European Monitoring Centre for Drugs and Drug Addiction. European Drug Report 2020: Trends and Developments. Luxembourg, Publications Office of the European Union, 2020.

55. Measham F, Moore K, Newcombe R, Welch Z. Tweaking, bombing, dabbing and stockpiling: the emergence of mephedrone and the perversity of prohibition. *Drugs Alcohol Today* 2010;**10**(1):14–21.

56. Measham F, Wood DM, Dargan PI, Moore K. The rise in legal highs: prevalence and patterns in the use of illegal drugs and first- and second-generation 'legal highs' in South London gay dance clubs. *J Subst Use* 2011;**16**(4):263–272.

57. Brunt TM, Poortman A, Niesink RJ, van den Brink W. Instability of the ecstasy market and a new kid on the block: mephedrone. *J Psychopharmacol* 2011;**25**(11):1543–1547. https://doi.org/10.1177/0269881110378370

58. Measham F, Moore K, Østergaard J. Mephedrone, 'Bubble' and unidentified white powders: the contested identities of synthetic 'legal highs'. *Drugs Alcohol Today* 2011;**11**(3):137–146.

59. World Drug Report 2019 (United Nations publication, Sales No. E.19.XI.9).

60. Home Office. Drugs Misuse: Findings from the 2018/19 Crime Survey for England and Wales Statistical Bulletin. Published 19 September 2019.

61. Winstock A, Mitcheson L, Marsden J. Mephedrone: still available and twice the price. *Lancet* 2010;**376**:1537.

62. Dybdal-Hargreaves NF, Holder ND, Ottoson PE, Sweeney MD, Williams T. Mephedrone: public health risk, mechanisms of action, and behavioural effects. *Eur J Pharmacol* 2013;**714**(1–3):32–40. https://doi.org/10.1016/j.ejphar.2013.05.024

63. Wood DM, Greene SL, Dargan PI. Emergency department presentations in determining the effectiveness of drug control in the United Kingdom: mephedrone (4-methylmethcathinone) control appears to be effective using this model. *Emerg Med J* 2013;**30**:70–71.

64. Sande M. Characteristics of the use of 3-MMC and other new psychoactive drugs in Slovenia. *Int J Drug Policy* 2016;27:65–73.

65. Tarján A, Dudás M, Gyarmathy VA, Rusvai E, Tresó B, Csohán Á. Emerging risks due to new injecting patterns in Hungary during austerity times. *Subst Use Misuse* 2015;**50**(7):848–858.

66. Belackova V, Vacek J, Janikova B, et al. 'Just another drug' for marginalized users: the risks of using synthetic cathinones among NSP clients in the Czech Republic. *J Subst Use* 2017;**22**(6):567–573. doi.org/10.1080/14659891.2016.1271034

67. Home Office. Drug Misuse: Findings from the 2013/14 Crime Survey for England and Wales. London, Home Office. Published July 2014.

68. European Monitoring Centre for Drugs and Drug Addiction (EMCDDA). European Drugs Report 2014. Trends and Developments. Luxembourg, Publications Office of the European Union, 2014.

69. Colfax G, Santos GM, Chu P, et al. Amphetamine-group substances and HIV. *Lancet* 2010;**376**:458–474.

70. World Drug Report 2019 (United Nations publication, Sales No. E.19.XI.9).

71. Péterfi A, Tarján A, Horváth GC, Csesztregi T, Nyírády A. Changes in patterns of injecting drug use in Hungary: a shift to synthetic cathinones. *Drug Test Anal* 2014;**6**(7–8):825–831. https://doi.org/10.1002/dta.1625

72. Kapitány-Fövény M, Rácz J. Synthetic cannabinoid and synthetic cathinone use in Hungary: a literature review. *Dev Health Sci* 2018;**1**(3):63–69. https://doi.org/10.1556/2066.2.2018.18

73. Kapitány-Fövény M, Rácz J. Synthetic cannabinoid and synthetic cathinone use in Hungary: a literature review. *Dev Health Sci* 2018;**1**(3):63–69. https://doi.org/10.1556/2066.2.2018.18

74. Péterfi A, Tarján A, Csaba Horváth G, Csesztregi T, Nyírády A. Changes in patterns of injecting drug use in Hungary: a shift to synthetic cathinones. *Drug Test Anal* 2014 (online). https://doi.org/10.1002/dta.1625

75. World Drug Report 2020 (United Nations publication, Sales No. E.20.XI.6).

76. European Monitoring Centre for Drugs and Drug Addiction (EMCDDA). European Drug Report 2018: Trends and Developments. Luxembourg, Publications Office of the European Union, 2018.

77. McNamara S, Stokes S, Coleman N. Head shop compound abuse amongst attendees of the Drug Treatment Centre Board. *Int Med J* 2010;**103**(5):134–137.

78. Van Hout MC, Bingham T. 'A costly turn on': patterns of use and perceived consequences of mephedrone-based head shop products amongst Irish injectors. *Int J Drug Policy* **23**;2012:188–197.

79. Bourne A, Reid D, Hickson F, Torres Rueda S, Weatherburn P. The chemsex study: drug use in sexual settings among gay and bisexual men in Lambeth, Southwark and Lewisham. London, Sigma Research, London School of Hygiene & Tropical Medicine. Available at: www.sigmaresearch.org.uk/chemsex [last accessed 17 March 2022].

80. Public Health England. Substance Misuse Services for Men Who Have Sex with Men Involved in Chemsex. London, Public Health England, 2015.

81. Semple SJ, Patterson TL, Grant I. A comparison of injection and non-injection methamphetamine using HIV positive men who have sex with men. *Drug Alcohol Depend* 2004;**76**:203–212.

82. Van Hout MC, Brennan R. 'Bump and grind': an exploratory study of mephedrone users' perceptions of sexuality and sexual risk. *Drugs Alcohol Today* 2012;**11**(2):93–103.

83. Frohmader KS, Pitchers KL, Balfour M, Coolen LM. Mixing pleasures: review of the effects of drugs on sex behavior in humans and animal models. *Hormones Behav* 2010;**58**:149–162.

84. Pfaus JG. Pathways of sexual desire. *J Sex Med* 2009;**6**:1506–1533.

85. Raj A, Saitz R, Cheng DM, Winter M, Samet JH. Associations between alcohol, heroin, and cocaine use and high-risk sexual behaviors among detoxification patients. *Am J Drug Alcohol Abuse* 2007;**33**:169–178.

86. Mitcheson L, McCambridge J, Byrne A, Hunt N, Winstock A. Sexual health risk among dance drug users: cross-sectional comparisons with nationally representative data. *J Drug Policy* 2008;**19**:304–310.

87. Sande M, Paš M, Nahtigal K, Šabić S. Patterns of NPS use and risk reduction in Slovenia. *Subst Use Misuse* 2018;**53**(9):1424–1432. doi.org/10.1080/10826084.2017.1411366

88. Ciudad-Roberts A, Duart-Castells L, Camarasa J, Pubill D, Escubedo E. The combination of ethanol with mephedrone increases the signs of neurotoxicity and impairs neurogenesis and learning in adolescent CD-1 mice. *Toxicol Appl Pharmacol* 2016;**293**:10–20. https://doi.org/10.1016/j.taap.2015.12.019.

89. Carhart-Harris RL, King LA, Nutt DJ. A web-based survey on mephedrone. *Drug Alcohol Depend* 2011;**118**:19–22.

90. Wood DM, Greene SL, Dargan PI. Clinical pattern of toxicity associated with the novel synthetic cathinone mephedrone. *Emergency Med J* 2010;**28**:280–282. https://doi.org/0:10.1136/emj.2010.092288

91. Winstock A, Mitcheson L, Ramsey J, Davies S, Puchnarewicz M, Marsden J. Mephedrone: use, subjective effects and health risks. *Addiction* 2011;**106**(11):1991–1996.

92. Centre for Disease Control and Prevention. Emergency department visits after use of a drug sold as 'bath salts'. *Morb Mort Wkly Rep* 2011;60(19):624–627.

93. Spiller HA, Ryan ML, Weston RG, Jansen J. Clinical experience with and analytical confirmation of 'bath salts' and 'legal highs' (synthetic cathinones) in the United States. *Clin Toxicol* 2011;**49**:499–505. https://doi.org/10.3109/15563650.2011.590812

94. Winstock A, Mitcheson L, Ramsey J, et al. Mephedrone: use, subjective effects and health risks. *Addiction* 2011;**106**:1991–1996. https://doi.org/10.1111/j.1360-0443.2011.03502.x

95. Assi S, Gulyamova N, Ibrahim K, et al. Profile, effects, and toxicity of novel psychoactive substances: a systematic review of quantitative studies. *Hum Psychopharmacol Clin Exp* 2017;**32**:e2607. https://doi.org/10.1002/hup.2607

96. Assi S, Gulyamova N, Kneller P, Osselton D. The effects and toxicity of cathinones from the users' perspectives: a qualitative study. *Hum Psychopharmacol Clin Exp* 2017;**32**:e2610. https://doi.org/10.1002/hup.2610

97. Zuba D, Byrska B. Prevalence and co-existence of active components of 'legal highs'. *Drug Test Anal* 2013;**5**(6):420–429. https://doi.org/10.1002/dta.1365

98. Schifano F, Albanese A, Fergus S, et al. Psychonaut Web Mapping; ReDNet Research Groups. *Mephedrone (4-methylmethcathinone; 'meow meow'): chemical, pharmacological and clinical issues. Psychopharmacology* 2011;**214**(3):593–602. https://doi.org/10.1007/s00213-010-2070-x

99. Marinetti LJ, Antonides HM. Analysis of synthetic cathinones commonly found in bath salts in human performance and post-mortem toxicology: method development, drug distribution and interpretation of results. *J Anal Toxicol* 2013;**37**(3):135–146. https://doi.org/10.1093/jat/bks136

100. McElrath K, O'Neill C. Experiences with mephedrone pre- and post-legislative control: perceptions of safety and sources of supply. *Int J Drug Policy* 2011;**22**:120–127.

101. Deluca P, Schifano F, Davey Z, Corazza O, Di Furia L. The Psychonaut Web Mapping Research Group. Mephedrone Report. London, Institute of Psychiatry, King's College London, 2009. Available at: www.psychonautproject.eu [last accessed 17 March 2022].

102. Karila L, Reynaud M. GHB and synthetic cathinones: clinical effects and potential consequences. *Drug Test Anal* 2011;**3**:552–559.

103. Sande M, Paš M, Nahtigal K, Šabić S. Patterns of NPS use and risk reduction in Slovenia. *Subst Use Misuse* 2018;**53**(9):1424–1432. doi.org/10.1080/10826084.2017.1411366

104. Dargan PI, Wood DM. Annex 1 to the risk assessment report Technical Report on Mephedrone. EMCDDA contract CT.10.EPI.057. Guy's and St Thomas' NHS Foundation Trust, London, 2010. Available at: www.emcdda.europa.eu [last accessed 17 March 2022].

105. Wood DM, Davies S, Greene SL, et al. Case series of individuals with analytically confirmed acute mephedrone toxicity. *Clin Toxicol* 2010;**48**:924–927.

106. Martínez-Clemente J, López-Arnau R, Carbó M, Pubill D, Camarasa J, Escubedo E. Mephedrone pharmacokinetics after intravenous and oral administration in rats: relation to pharmacodynamics. *Psychopharmacology* 2013;**229**(2):295–306.

107. Yanagihara Y, Kariya S, Ohtani M, et al. Involvement of CYP2B6 in n-demethylation of ketamine in human liver microsomes. *Drug Metab Dispos* 2001;**29**:887–890.

108. Hijazi Y, Boulieu R. Contribution of CYP3A4, CYP2B6, and CYP2C9 isoforms to N-demethylation of ketamine in human liver microsomes. *Drug Metab Dispos* 2002,**30**:853–858.

109. Office for National Statistics. Drug Misuse Declared: Findings from the 2011/12 Crime Survey for England and Wales (2nd ed.). London, Home Office, July 2012.

110. Archer JRH, Dargan PI, Hudson S, Wood DM. Analysis of anonymous pooled urine from portable urinals in central London confirms the significant use of novel psychoactive substances. *Q J Med* 2013;**106**:147–152.

111. National Poisons Information Service (NIPS). Annual Report 2010/11. Health Protection Agency, 2011.

112. National Poisons Information Service (NIPS). Annual Report 2011/12. Health Protection Agency, 2012.

113. Wood DM, Measham F, Dargan PI. 'Our favourite drug': prevalence of use and preference for mephedrone in the London night-time economy 1 year after control. *J Subst Use* 2012;**17**(2):91–97.

114. Welsh Government. Working Together to Reduce Harm. Substance Misuse Annual Report 2013.

115. Moore K, Dargan PI, Wood DM, Measham F. Do novel psychoactive substances displace established club drugs, supplement them or act as drugs of initiation? The relationship between mephedrone, ecstasy and cocaine. *Eur Addict Res* 2013;**19**(5):276–282.

116. DrugScope. DrugScope street drug trends survey highlights growing problems with mephedrone. Published 22 November 2012.

117. Kirby T, Thornber-Dunwell M. High-risk drug practices tighten grip on London gay scene. *Lancet* 2013;**381**(9861):101–102. https://doi.org/10.1016/S0140-6736(13)60032-X

118. James D, Adams RD, Spears R, et al. National Poisons Information Service. Clinical characteristics of mephedrone toxicity reported to the UK National Poisons Information Service. *Emerg Med J* 2011;**28**(8):686–689. https://doi.org/10.1136/emj.2010.096636

119. Winstock AR, Mitcheson LR, Deluca P, et al. Mephedrone, new kid for the chop? *Addiction* 2011;**106**(1):154–161.

120. Wood DM, Davies S, Puchnarewicz M, et al. Recreational use of mephedrone (4-methylmethcathinone, 4-MMC) with associated sympathomimetic toxicity. *J Med Toxicol* 2010;**6**(3):327–330.

121. Newcombe R. Mephedrone: Use of Mephedrone (M-Cat, Meow) in Middlesbrough. Lifeline, Manchester, 2009.

122. Winstock AR, Marsden J, Mitcheson L. What should be done about mephedrone? *Br Med J* 2010;**340**:c1605.

123. Dargan PI, Sedefov R, Gallegos A, Wood DM. The pharmacology and toxicology of the synthetic cathinonemephedrone (4-methylmethcathinone). *Drug Test Anal* 2011;**3**(7–8):454–463. https://doi.org/10.1002/dta.312

124. Rosenbaum CD, Carreiro SP, Babu KM. Here today, gone tomorrow . . . and back again? A review of herbal marijuana alternatives (K2, Spice), synthetic cathinones (bath salts), kratom, Salvia divinorum, methoxetamine, and piperazines. *J Med Toxicol* 2012;**8**(1):15–32. https://doi.org/10.1007/s13181-011-0202-2

125. Freeman TP, Morgan CJ, Vaughn-Jones J, Hussain N, Karimi K, Curran HV. Cognitive and subjective effects of mephedrone and factors influencing use of a 'new legal high'. *Addiction* 2012;**107**(4):792–800. https://doi.org/10.1111/j.1360-0443.2011.03719.x

126. Motbey CP, Clemens KJ, Apetz N, et al. High levels of intravenous mephedrone (4-methylmethcathinone) self-administration in rats: neural consequences and comparison with methamphetamine. *J Psychopharmacol* 2013;**27**(9):823–836. https://doi.org/10.1177/0269881113490325

127. Annex 2. Technical Report on 1-(1,3-benzodioxol-5-yl)-2-(pyrrolidin-1-yl)pentan-1-one (3,4-methylenedioxypyrovalerone, MDPV). Prepared by Ms Alison M Dines, Dr David M Wood and Dr Paul I Dargan.

128. European Monitoring Centre for Drugs and Drug Addiction and Europol. Joint Report on a New Psychoactive Substance: MDPV (3,4-methylenedioxypyrovalerone). Available at: www.emcdda.europa.eu/system/files/publications/819/TDAS14001ENN_466653.pdf[last accessed 17 March 2022].

129. Annex 2. Technical Report on 1-(1,3-benzodioxol-5-yl)-2-(pyrrolidin-1-yl)pentan-1-one (3,4-methylenedioxypyrovalerone, MDPV). Prepared by Ms Alison M Dines, Dr David M Wood and Dr Paul I Dargan.

130. Coppola M, Mondola R. Synthetic cathinones: chemistry, pharmacology and toxicology of a new class of designer drugs of abuse marketed as 'bath salts' or 'plant food'. *Toxicol Lett* 2012;**211**(2):144–149. https://doi.org/10.1016/j.toxlet.2012.03.009

131. European Monitoring Centre for Drugs and Drug Addiction (EMCDDA). The state of the drugs problem in Europe – Annual report 2012. Luxembourg: Publications Office of the European Union, 2012. https://doi.org/10.2810/64775. Available at: www.emcdda.europa.eu/attachements.cfm/at

t_190854_EN_TDAC12001ENC_.pdf [last accessed 17 March 2022].

132. Ashrafioun L, Bonadio FA, Baik KD, et al. Patterns of use, acute subjective experiences, and motivations for using synthetic cathinones ('bath salts') in recreational users. *J Psychoactive Drugs* 2016;**48**(5):336–343. https://doi.org/10.1080/02791072.2016.1229875

133. Ashrafioun L, Bonadio FA, Baik KD, et al. Patterns of use, acute subjective experiences, and motivations for using synthetic cathinones ('bath salts') in recreational users. *J Psychoactive Drugs* 2016;**48**(5):336–343. https://doi.org/10.1080/02791072.2016.1229875

134. Ashrafioun L, Bonadio FA, Baik KD, et al. Patterns of use, acute subjective experiences, and motivations for using synthetic cathinones ('bath salts') in recreational users. *J Psychoactive Drugs* 2016;**48**(5):336–343. https://doi.org/10.1080/02791072.2016.1229875

135. Wood DM, Dargan PI. Mephedrone (4-methylmethcathinone): what is new in our understanding of its use and toxicity. *Prog Neuropsychopharmacol Biol Psychiatry* 2012;**39**(2):227–233. https://doi.org/10.1016/j.pnpbp.2012.04.020

136. Dick D, Torrance C. Drugs survey. *MixMag* 2010;**225**:44.

137. Weinstein AM, Rosca P, Fattore L. London ED. Synthetic cathinone and cannabinoid designer drugs pose a major risk for public health. *Front Psychiatry* 2017;**8**:156.

138. Van Hout MC, Brennan R. 'Bump and grind': an exploratory study of mephedrone users' perceptions of sexuality and sexual risk. *Drugs Alcohol Today* 2012;**11**(2):93–103.

139. Semple SJ, Patterson TL, Grant I. Motivations associated with methamphetamine use among HIV men who have sex with men. *J Subst Abuse Treat* 2002;**22**:149–156.

140. Frohmader KS, Pitchers KL, Balfour M, Coolen LM. Mixing pleasures: review of the effects of drugs on sex behavior in humans and animal models. *Horm Behav* 2010;**58**:149–162.

141. Pfaus JG. Pathways of sexual desire. *J Sex Med* 2009;**6**:1506–1533.

142. Raj A, Saitz R, Cheng DM, Winter M, Samet JH. Associations between alcohol, heroin, and cocaine use and high-risk sexual behaviors among detoxification patients. *Am J Drug Alcohol Abuse* 2007;**33**:169–178.

143. Mitcheson L, McCambridge J, Byrne A, Hunt N, Winstock A. Sexual health risk among dance drug users: cross-sectional comparisons with nationally representative data. *J Drug Policy* 2008;**19**:304–310.

144. Rhodes T, Quirk A. Drug users' sexual relationships and the social organization of risk: the sexual relationship as a site of risk management. *Soc Sci Med* 1998;**46**(2):157–169.

145. Winstock A. The Mixmag Drugs Survey. Mixmag, April 2012. Available at: https://issuu.com/mixmagfashion/docs/drugs_survey_2012_2 [last accessed 17 March 2022].

146. Winstock A. The Mixmag Drugs Survey. Mixmag, April 2012. Available at: https://issuu.com/mixmagfashion/docs/drugs_survey_2012_2 [last accessed 17 March 2022].

147. Dargan PI, Albert S, Wood DM. Mephedrone use and associated adverse effects in school and college/university students before the UK legislation change. *QJM* 2010;**103**(11):875–879.

148. Schifano F, Corkery J, Naidoo V, Oyefeso A, Ghodse AH. Comparison between amphetamine/methylamphetamine and ecstasy (MDMA, MDEA, MDA, 4-MTA) mortality data in the UK (1997–2007). *Neuropsychobiology* 2010;**61**:122–130.

149. Dickson AJ, Vorce SP, Levine B, Past MR. Multiple-drug toxicity caused by the coadministration of 4-methylmethcathinone (mephedrone) and heroin. *J Analytic Toxicol* 2010;**34**:162–168.

150. Corkery JM, Schifano F, Ghodse AH. Mephedrone-related fatalities in the United Kingdom: contextual, clinical and practical issues. InTech-Open Access Publisher, 14 March 2012.

151. Colon-Perez LM, Tran K, Thompson K, et al. The psychoactive designer drug and bath salt constituent MDPV causes widespread disruption of brain functional connectivity. *Neuropsychopharmacology* 2016;41:2352–2365.

152. Fujita Y, Mita T, Usui K, et al. Toxicokinetics of the synthetic cathinone α-Pyrrolidinohexanophenone. *J Anal Toxicol* 2018;**42**:e1–e5. https://doi.org/10.1093/jat/bkx080

153. Antonowicz JL, Metzger AK, Ramanujam SL. Paranoid psychosis induced by consumption of methylenedioxypyrovalerone: two cases. *Gen Hosp Psych* 2011;**33**(640):e5.

154. Boulanger-Gobeil C, St-Onge M, Laliberte M, Auger PL. Seizures and hyponatremia related to ethcathinone and methylone poisoning. *J Med Toxicol* 2012;**8**(1):59–61.

155. European Monitoring Centre for Drugs and Drug Addiction. Drug profiles. Synthetic cathinones, 2012. Availableat:www.emcdda.europa.eu/publications/drug-profiles/synthetic-cathinones[last accessed 17 March 2022].

156. Derungs A, Schietzel S, Meyer MR, Maurer HH, Kr€ahenb€uhl S, Liechti ME. Sympathomimetic toxicity in a case of analytically confirmed recreational use of naphyrone (naphthylpyrovalerone). *Clin Toxicol* 2011;**49**(7):691–693.

157. Winder GS, Stern N, Hosanagar A. Are 'bath salts' the next generation of stimulant abuse? *J Subst Abuse Treat* 2013;**44**(1):42–45.

158. Spiller HA, Ryan ML, Weston RG, Jansen J. Clinical experience with and analytical confirmation of 'bath salts' and 'legal highs' (synthetic cathinones) in the United States. *Clin Toxicol* 2011;**49**(6):499–505.

159. Centers for Disease Control and Prevention (CDC). Emergency department visits after use of a drug sold as bath salts – Michigan, November 13, 2010 to March 31, 2011. *MMWR Morb Mortal Wkly Rep* 2011;**60**(19):624–627.

Available at: www.cdc.gov/mmwr/preview/mmwrhtml/mm6019a6.htm [last accessed 17 March 2022].

160. Zawilska JB, Słomiak K, Wasiak M, et al. Beta-cathinone derivatives – a new generation of dangerous psychostimulant 'designer drugs'. *Przegl Lek* 2013;**70**(6):386–391.

161. Kelly JP. Cathinone derivatives: a review of their chemistry, pharmacology and toxicology. *Drug Test Anal* 2011;**3**(7–8):43953.

162. Thornton SL, Gerona RR, Tomaszewski CA. Psychosis from a bath salt product containing flephedrone and MDPV with serum, urine, and product quantification. *J Med Toxicol* 2012;**8**(3):310–313.

163. Wood DM, Davies S, Greene SL, et al. Case series of individuals with analytically confirmed acute mephedrone toxicity. *Clin Toxicol* 2010;**48**:924–927.

164. Wood DM, Davies S, Puchnarewicz M, et al. Recreational use of mephedrone (4-methylmethcathinone, 4-MMC) with associated sympathomimetic toxicity. *J Med Toxicol* 2010;**6**(3):327–330.

165. Wood DM, Greene SL, Dargan PI. Clinical pattern of toxicity associated with the novel synthetic cathinone mephedrone. *Emergency Med J* 2010;**28**:280–282. https://doi.org/0:10.1136/emj.2010.092288

166. Nicholson PJ, Quinn MJ, Dodd JD. Headshop heartache: acute mephedrone meow myocarditis. *Heart* 2010;96:2051.

167. Sammler EM, Foley PL, Lauder GD, Wilson SJ, Goudie AR, O'Riordan JI. A harmless high? *Lancet* 2010;**376**:742.

168. Benzie F, Hekman K, Cameron L, et al. Emergency department visits after use of a drug sold as 'bath salts' – Michigan, November 13, 2010 to March 31, 2011. *Morb Mort Wkly Rep* 2011;**60**(19):624–627.

169. Hadlock GC, Webb KM, McFadden LM, et al. 4-Methylmethcathinone (mephedrone): neuropharmacological effects of a designer stimulant of abuse. *J Pharmacol Exp Ther* 2011;**339**(2):530–536. https://doi.org/10.1124/jpet.111.184119

170. Winstock AR, Mitcheson LR, Deluca P, et al. Mephedrone, new kid for the chop? *Addiction* 2011;**106**(1):154–161.

171. Dargan PI, Sedefov R, Gallegos A, Wood DM. The pharmacology and toxicology of the synthetic cathinonemephedrone (4-methylmethcathinone). *Drug Test Anal* 2011;**3**(7–8):454–463. https://doi.org/10.1002/dta.312

172. Wood DM, Dargan PI. Understanding how data triangulation identifies acute toxicity of novel psychoactive drugs. *J Med Toxicol* 2012;**8**:300–303. https://doi.org/10.1007/s13181-012-0241-3

173. Dybdal-Hargreaves N, Holder N, Ottoson P, Sweeney M, Williams T. Mephedrone: public health risk, mechanisms of action and behaviorial effects. *Eur J Pharmacol* 2013;**714**:32–40.

174. Zawilska J, Wojcieszak J. Designer cathinone—an emerging class of novel recreational drugs. *Forensic Sci Int* 2013;**231**:42–53.

175. Fleckenstein AE, Volz TJ, Riddle EL, Gibb JW, Hanson GR. New insights into the mechanism of action of amphetamines. *Annu Rev Pharmacol Toxicol* 2007;**47**:681–698.

176. Coppola M, Mondola R. Synthetic cathinones: chemistry, pharmacology and toxicology of a new class of designer drugs of abuse marketed as 'bath salts' or 'plant food'. *Toxicol Lett* 2012;**211**(2):144–149. https://doi.org/10.1016/j.toxlet.2012.03.009. 8

177. Carroll FI, Lewin AH, Mascarella SW, Seltzman HH, Reddy PA. Designer drugs: a medicinal chemistry perspective. *Ann NY Acad Sci* 2012;**1248**:18–38.

178. Iversen L, White M, Treble R. Designer psychostimulants: pharmacology and differences. *Neuropharmacology* 2014;**87**:59–65. https://doi.org/10.1016/j.neuropharm.2014.01.015

179. Luethi D, Kolaczynska KE, Docci L, Krahenbuhl S, Hoener MC, Liechti ME. Pharmacological profile of mephedrone analogs and related new psychoactive substances. *Neuropharmacology* 2017;**26**:4–12.

180. Weinstein AM, Rosca P, Fattore L, London ED. Synthetic cathinone and cannabinoid designer drugs pose a major risk for public health. *Front Psychiatry* 2017;**8**:156.

181. Nicholson PJ, Quinn MJ, Dodd JD. Headshop heartache: acute mephedrone meow myocarditis. *Heart* 2010;**96**:2051.

182. Sammler EM, Foley PL, Lauder GD, Wilson SJ, Goudie AR, O'Riordan JI. A harmless high? *Lancet* 2010;**376**:742.

183. Benzie F, Hekman K, Cameron L, et al. Emergency department visits after use of a drug sold as 'bath salts' – Michigan, November 13, 2010–March 31, 2011.*Morb Mort Wkly Rep* 2011;**60**(19):624–627.

184. Wood DM, Dargan PI. Understanding how data triangulation identifies acute toxicity of novel psychoactive drugs. *J Med Toxicol* 2012;**8**:300–303. https://doi.org/10.1007/s13181-012-0241-3

185. Fujita Y, Mita T, Usui K, et al. Toxicokinetics of the synthetic cathinone α-pyrrolidinohexanophenone. *J Anal Toxicol* 2018;**42**:e1–e5. https://doi.org/10.1093/jat/bkx080

186. Prosser JM, Nelson LS. The toxicology of bath salts: a review of synthetic cathinones. *J Med Toxicol* 2012;**8**:33–42.

187. Chhabra JS, Nandalan S, Saad R. Mephedrone poisoning – a case of severe refractory left ventricular failure. Poster Presentation 33. In: The State of the Art Meeting, London, 13–14 December 2010, pp. 74–75.

188. Garrett G, Sweeney M. The serotonin syndrome as a result of mephedrone toxicity. *BMJ Case Rep* 2010;2010: bcr0420092925. https://doi.org/10.1136/bcr.04.2010.2925

189. Mugele J, Nañagas KA, Tormoehlen LM. Serotonin syndrome associated with MDPV use: a case report. *Ann Emerg Med* 2012;**60**(1):100–102. https://doi.org/10.1016/j.annemergmed.2011.11.033

190. German CL, Fleckenstein AE, Hanson GR. Bath salts and synthetic cathinones: an emerging designer drug phenomenon. *Life Sci* 2014;**97**:2–8.

191. Angoa-Perez M, Kane MJ, Francescutti DM, et al. Mephedrone, an abused psychoactive component of 'bath salts' and methamphetamine congener, does not cause neurotoxicity to dopamine nerve endings of the striatum. *J Neurochem* 2012;**120**(6):1097–1107.

192. Fass JA, Fass AD, Garcia AS. Synthetic cathinones (bath salts): legal status and patterns of abuse. *Ann Pharmacother* 2012;**46**(3):436–441.

193. Omer TA, Doherty C. Posterior reversible encephalopathy syndrome (PRES) complicating the 'legal high' mephedrone. *BMJ Case Rep* 2011;2011:bcr0220113904. https://doi.org/10.1136/bcr.02.2011.3904

194. Maan ZN, D'Souza AR. Spontaneous subcutaneous emphysema associated with mephedrone usage. *Ann R Coll Surg Engl* 2012;**94**(1):e38–40. https://doi.org/10.1308/003588412X13171221499108

195. Ahmed N, Hoy BP, McInerney J. Methaemoglobinaemia due to mephedrone ('snow'). *BMJ Case Rep* 2010;2010: bcr0420102879. https://doi.org/10.1136/bcr.04.2010.2879

196. Ramirez Berlioz A, Gardner M. MON-146 prolonged hypoglycemia in the setting of synthetic cathinone abuse. *J Endocr Soc* 2019;3(Suppl. 1):146. https://doi.org/10.1210/js.2019-MON-146

197. Wong ML, Holt RI. The potential dangers of mephedrone in people with diabetes: a case report. *Drug Test Anal* 2011;**3**(7–8):464–465. https://doi.org/10.1002/dta.316

198. Leyrer-Jackson JM, Nagy EK, Olive MF. Cognitive deficits and neurotoxicity induced by synthetic cathinones: is there a role for neuroinflammation? *Psychopharmacology* 2019;**236**(3):1079–1095. 10.1007/s00213-018-5067-5doi.org/

199. Wood DM, Davies S, Greene SL, et al. Case series of individuals with analytically confirmed acute mephedrone toxicity. *Clin Toxicol* 2010;**48**:924–927.

200. Wood DM, Davies S, Puchnarewicz M, et al. Recreational use of mephedrone (4-methylmethcathinone, 4-MMC) with associated sympathomimetic toxicity. *J Med Toxicol* 2010;**6**(3):327–330.

201. Wood DM, Greene SL, Dargan PI. Clinical pattern of toxicity associated with the novel synthetic cathinone mephedrone. *Emergency Med J* 2010;**28**:280–282. https://doi.org/0:10.1136/emj.2010.092288

202. Nicholson PJ, Quinn MJ, Dodd JD. Headshop heartache: acute mephedrone meow myocarditis. *Heart* 2010;96:2051.

203. Sammler EM, Foley PL, Lauder GD, Wilson SJ, Goudie AR, O'Riordan JI. A harmless high? *Lancet* 2010;**376**:742.

204. Benzie F, Hekman K, Cameron L, et al. Emergency department visits after use of a drug sold as 'bath salts' – Michigan, November 13, 2010–March 31, 2011. *Morb Mort Wkly Rep* 2011;**60**(19):624–627.

205. Hadlock GC, Webb KM, McFadden LM, et al. 4-Methylmethcathinone (mephedrone): neuropharmacological effects of a designer stimulant of abuse. *J Pharmacol Exp Ther* 2011;**339**(2):530–536. https://doi.org10.1124/jpet.111.184119

206. Winstock A, Mitcheson L, Ramsey J, Davies S, Puchnarewicz M, Marsden J. Mephedrone: use, subjective effects and health risks. *Addiction* 2011;**106**:1991–1996.

207. Papaseit E, Olesti E, de la Torre R, Torrens M, Farre M. Mephedrone concentrations in cases of clinical intoxication. *Curr Pharm Des* 2017;4:5511–5522.

208. Wood DM, Davies S, Puchnarewicz M, et al. Recreational use of mephedrone (4-methylmethcathinone, 4-MMC) with associated sympathomimetic toxicity. *J Med Toxicol* 2010;**6** (3):327–330.

209. Winestock AR, Mitcheson LR, Deluca P, et al. Mephedrone, new kid for the chop? *Addiction* 2011;**106**(1):154–161.

210. Dargan PI, Sedefov R, Gallegos A, Wood DM. The pharmacology and toxicology of the synthetic cathinone mephedrone (4-methylmethcathinone). *Drug Test Anal* 2011;**3**(7–8):454–463. https://doi.org/10.1002/dta.312

211. Benzie F, Hekman K, Cameron L, et al. Emergency department visits after use of a drug sold as 'bath salts' – Michigan, November 13, 2010–March 31, 2011. *Morb Mort Wkly Rep* 2011;60(19):624–627.

212. Wood DM, Dargan PI. Understanding how data triangulation identifies acute toxicity of novel psychoactive drugs. *J Med Toxicol* 2012;**8**:300–303. https://doi.org/10.1007/s13181-012-0241-3

213. Dybdal-Hargreaves N, Holder N, Ottoson P, Sweeney M, Williams T. Mephedrone: public health risk, mechanisms of action and behaviorial effects. *Eur J Pharmacol* 2013; **714**:32–40.

214. Zawilska J, Wojcieszak J. Designer cathinone: an emerging class of novel recreational drugs. *Forensic Sci Int* 2013; **231**:42–53.

215. Wood D, Davies S, Puchnarewicz M, et al. Recreational use of mephedrone (4-methylmethcathinone, 4-MMC) with associated sympathomimetic toxicity. *J Med Toxicol* 2010; **6**:327–330.

216. Kolli V, Sharma A, Amani M, Bestha D, Chaturvedi R. 'Meow meow' (mephedrone) and catatonia. *Innov Clin Neurosci* 2013;**10**(2):11–12.

217. Prosser JM, Nelson LS. The toxicology of bath salts: a review of synthetic cathinones. *J Med Toxicol* 2012;**8**(1):33–42.

218. Szily E., Bitter I. Designer drugs in psychiatric practise – a review of the literature and recent situation in Hungary. *Neuropsychopharmacol Hung* 2013;**5**(4): 223–231.

219. Segrec N, Kastelic A, Pregelj P. Pentedrone-induced acute psychosis in a patient with opioid addiction: a case report. *Case Rep Heroin Addict Relat Clin Probl* 2016;**18** (3):53–56.

220. Weinstein AM, Rosca P, Fattore L. London ED. Synthetic cathinone and cannabinoid designer drugs pose a major risk for public health. *Front Psychiatry* 2017;8:156.

221. Prosser JM, Nelson LS. The toxicology of bath salts: a review of synthetic cathinones. *JMed Toxicol* 2012;**8**(1):33–42.

222. Szily E, Bitter I. Designer drugs in psychiatric practise – a review of the literature and recent situation in Hungary. *Neuropsychopharmacol* 2013;**5**(4):223–231.

223. Segrec N, Kastelic A, Pregelj P. Pentedrone-induced acute psychosis in a patient with opioid addiction: a case report. *Heroin Addict Relat Clin Probl* 2016;**18**(3):53–56.

224. Antonowicz JL, Metzger AK, Ramanujam SL. Paranoid psychosis induced by consumption of methylenedioxypyrovalerone: two cases. *Gen Hosp Psychiatry* 2011;**33**(6):640.

225. Farkas K, Sirály E, Szily E, Csukly G, Réthelyi J. Clinical characteristics of 5 hospitalized 3,4-methylenedioxypyrovalerone (MDPV) users. *Psychiatr Hung* 2013;**28**(4):431–439.

226. Stiles BM, Fish AF, Cook CA, Silva V. Bath salt-induced psychosis: nursing assessment, diagnosis, treatment, and outcomes. *Perspect Psychiatr Care* 2015;**52**(1):68–78.

227. Thornton SL, Gerona RR, Tomaszewski CA. Psychosis from a bath salt product containing flephedrone and MDPV with serum, urine, and product quantification. *J Med Toxicol* 2012;**8** (3):310–313.

228. Segrec N, Kastelic A, Pregelj P. Pentedrone-induced acute psychosis in a patient with opioid addiction: a case report. *Case Rep Heroin Addict Relat Clin Probl* 2016;**18**(3):53–56.

229. Tekulve K, Alexander A, Tormoehlen L. Seizures associated with synthetic cathinone exposures in the pediatric population. *Pediatr Neurol* 2014;**51**(1):67–70. https://doi.org/10.1016/j.pediatrneurol.2014.03.003

230. European Monitoring Centre for Drugs and Drug Addiction. Annex 2. Technical Report on 1-(1,3-benzodioxol-5-yl)-2-(pyrrolidin-1-yl)pentan-1-one (3,4-methylenedioxypyrovalerone, MDPV). Prepared by Ms Alison M Dines, Dr David M Wood and Dr Paul I Dargan.

231. Baumann MH, Partilla JS. Lehner KR, et al. Powerful cocaine-like actions of 3,4-methylenedioxypyrovalerone (MDPV), a principal constituent of psychoactive 'bath salts' products. *Neuropsychopharmcology* 2013;**38**:552–562.

232. European Monitoring Centre for Drugs and Drug Addiction. Annex 2. Technical Report on 1-(1,3-benzodioxol-5-yl)-2-(pyrrolidin-1-yl)pentan-1-one (3,4-methylenedioxypyrovalerone, MDPV). Prepared by Ms Alison M Dines, Dr David M Wood and Dr Paul I Dargan.

233. Beck O, Franzen L, Bäckberg M, Signell P, Helander A. Intoxications involving MDPV in Sweden during 2010–2014: results from the STRIDA project. *Clin Toxicol* 2015;**53** (9):865–873. https://doi.org/10.3109/15563650.2015.1089576

234. Lindeman E, Hulten P, Strom S, Enlund M, Al-Saffar Y, Helander A. Increased abuse of the Internet drug MDPV in Vastmanland. Severe cases of poisoning have given health care major problems. *Lakartidningen* 2012;109:1954–1957.

235. Beck O, Franzen L, Bäckberg M, Signell P, Helander A. Intoxications involving MDPV in Sweden during 2010–2014: results from the STRIDA project. *Clin Toxicol* 2015;**53** (9):865–873. https://doi.org/10.3109/15563650.2015.1089576

236. Coppola M, Mondola R. 3,4-Methylenedioxypyrovalerone (MDPV): chemistry, pharmacology and toxicology of a new designer drug of abuse marketed online. *Toxicol Lett* 2012;208:12–15.

237. Simonsen KW, Edvardsen HME, Thelander G, et al. Fatal poisoning in drug addicts in the Nordic countries in 2012. *Forensic Sci Int* 2015;248:172–180.

238. European Monitoring Centre for Drugs and Drug Addiction. Risk assessments of MDPV. Available at: www.emcdda.europa. eu/attachements.cfm/ att_228256_EN_TDAK14003ENN.pdf [last accessed 18 March 2022].

239. Karila L, Lafay G, Scocard A, Cottencin O, Benyamins A. MDPV and α-PVP use in humans: the twisted sisters. *Neuropharmacology* 2018;134(Part A):65–72.

240. Csák R, Demetrovics Z, Rácz J. Transition to injecting 3,4-methylene-dioxy-pyrovalerone (MDPV) among needle exchange program participants in Hungary. *J Psychopharmacol* 2013;27(6):559–563. doi.org/10.1177/0269881113480987

241. Antonowicz JL, Metzger AK, Ramanujam SL. Paranoid psychosis induced by consumption of methylenedioxypyrovalerone: two cases. *Gen Hosp Psych* 2011;33(640):e5.

242. Boulanger-Gobeil C, St-Onge M, Laliberte M, Auger PL. Seizures and hyponatremia related to ethcathinone and methylone poisoning. *J Med Toxicol* 2012;8(1):59–61.

243. European Monitoring Centre for Drugs and Drug Addiction. Drug profiles. Synthetic cathinones, 2012. Available at: www.emcdda.europa.eu/publications/drug-profiles/synthetic-cathinones_en [last accessed 18 March 2022].

244. Derungs A, Schietzel S, Meyer MR, Maurer HH, Kr€ahenb€uhl S, Liechti ME. Sympathomimetic toxicity in a case of analytically confirmed recreational use of naphyrone (naphthylpyrovalerone). *Clin Toxicol* 2011;49(7):691–693.

245. Winder GS, Stern N, Hosanagar A. Are 'bath salts' the next generation of stimulant abuse? *J Subst Abuse Treat* 2013;44(1):42–45.

246. Spiller HA, Ryan ML, Weston RG, Jansen J. Clinical experience with and analytical confirmation of 'bath salts' and 'legal highs' (synthetic cathinones) in the United States. *Clin Toxicol* 2011;49(6):499–505.

247. Centers for Disease Control and Prevention (CDC). Emergency department visits after use of a drug sold as bath salts – Michigan, November 13, 2010 to March 31, 2011. *Morb Mort Wkly Rep* 2011;60(19):624–627.

248. Zawilska JB, Słomiak K, Wasiak M, et al. Beta-cathinone derivatives: a new generation of dangerous psychostimulant 'designer drugs'. *Przegl Lek* 2013;70(6):386–391.

249. Kelly JP. Cathinone derivatives: a review of their chemistry, pharmacology and toxicology. *Drug Test Anal* 2011;3(7-8):43953.

250. Thornton SL, Gerona RR, Tomaszewski CA. Psychosis from a bath salt product containing flephedrone and MDPV with serum, urine, and product quantification. *J Med Toxicol* 2012;8(3):310–313.

251. Péterfi A, Tarján A, Csaba Horváth G, Csesztregib T, Nyírády A. Changes in patterns of injecting drug use in Hungary: a shift to synthetic cathinones. *Drug Test Anal* 2014;6(7–8):825–831.

252. Botescu A, Abagiu A, Mardarescu M, Ursan M. HIV/AIDS among injecting drug users in Romania – report of a recent outbreak and initial response policies. EMCDDA, Lisbon, 2012. Available at: www.emcdda.europa.eu/publications/ad-hoc/2012/romania-hiv-update [last accessed 18 March 2022].

253. European Monitoring Centre for Drugs and Drug Addiction. Report on the risk assessment of mephedrone in the framework of the Council Decision on new psychoactive substances. EMCDDA, Lisbon, 2011.

254. Van Hout MC, Bingham T. 'A costly turn on': patterns of use and perceived consequences of mephedrone-based head shop products amongst Irish injectors. *Int J Drug Policy* 2012;23:188.

255. European Monitoring Centre for Drugs and Drug Addiction. High-risk drug use and new psychoactive substances. EMCDDA Rapid Communication. Luxembourg, Publications Office of the European Union.

256. Schifano F, Corkery C, Ghodse AH. Background: suspected and confirmed fatalities associated with mephedrone (4-methylmethcathinone, 'meow meow') in the United Kingdom. *J Clin Psychopharmacol* 2012;32(5):710–714. https://doi.org/10.1097/JCP.0b013e318266c70c

257. Pacifici R, Zuccaro P, Farre M, et al. Cell-mediated immune response in MDMA users after repeated dose administration: studies in controlled versus noncontrolled settings. *Ann N Y Acad Sci* 2002;965:421–433.

258. Schifano F, Oyefeso A, Corkery J, et al. Death rates from ecstasy (MDMA, MDA) and polydrug use in England and Wales 1996–2002. *Hum Psychopharmacol Clin Exp* 2003;18:519–524.

259. McGaw C, Kankam O. The co-ingestion of alcohol and mephedrone – an emerging cause of acute medical admissions in young adults and a potential cause of tachyarrhythmias. *West London Med J* 2010;2:9–13.

260. Angoa-Perez M, Kane M, Briggs D, et al. Mephedrone does not damage dopamine nerve endings of the striatum, but enhances the neurotoxicity of methamphetamine, amphetamine and MDMA. *J Neurochem* 2013;125:102–110.

261. Aromatario M, Bottoni E, Santoni M, Ciallella C. New 'lethal highs': a case of a deadly cocktail of GHB and mephedrone. *Forensic Sci Int* 2012;223(1–3):e38–e41.

262. Potocka-Banas B, Janus T, Majdanik S, Banas T, Dembinska T, Borowiak K. Fatal intoxication with a-PVP, a synthetic cathinone derivative. *J Forensic Sci* 2016 (online). https://doi.org/10.1111/1556-4029.13326

263. Zaami S, Giorgetti R, Pichini S, Pantano F, Marinelli E, Busardò FP. *Synthetic cathinones related fatalities: an update. Eur Rev Med Pharmacol Sci* 2018;22:268–274.

264. European Monitoring Centre for Drugs and Drug Addiction. Annex 2. Technical Report on 1-(1,3-benzodioxol-5-yl)-2-(pyrrolidin-1-yl)pentan-1-one (3,4-methylenedioxypyrovalerone, MDPV). Prepared by Ms Alison M Dines, Dr David M Wood and Dr Paul I Dargan.

265. Potocka-Banas B, Janus T, Majdanik S, Banas T, Dembinska T, Borowiak K. Fatal intoxication with a-PVP, a synthetic cathinone derivative. *J Forensic Sci* 2016 (online). https://doi.org/10.1111/1556-4029.13326

266. Ikeji C, Sittambalam CD, Camire LM, Weisman DS. Fatal intoxication with N-ethylpentylone: a case report. *J Community Hosp Int Med Perspect* 2018;8(5):307–310. doi.org/10.1080/20009666.2018.1510711

267. Majchrzak M, Celiński R, Kowalska T, Sajewicz M. Fatal case of poisoning with a new cathinone derivative: α-propylaminopentiophenone (N-PP). *Forensic Toxicol* 2018;36(2):525–533. doi.org/10.1007/s11419-018-0417-x

268. Atherton D, Dye D, Robinson CA, Beck R. n-Ethyl pentylone-related deaths in Alabama. *J Forensic Sci* 2019;64(1);304–308. doi.org/10.1111/1556-4029.13823

269. Pieprzyca E, Skowronek R, Korczyńska M, Kulikowska J, Chowaniec MA. Two fatal cases of poisoning involving new cathinone derivative PV8. *Leg Med* 2018;33;42–47. doi.org/10.1016/j.legalmed.2018.05.002

270. Sykutera M, Cychowska M, Bloch-Boguslawska E. A fatal case of pentedrone and a-pyrrolidinovalerophenone poisoning. *Anal Toxicol* 2015;39:324–329. https://doi.org/10.1093/jat/bkv011

271. Shah AD, Wood DM, Dargan PI. Survey of ICD-10 coding of hospital admissions in the UK due to recreational drug toxicity. *QJM* 2011;104(9):779–784. https://doi.org/10.1093/qjmed/hcr074

272. Regan L, Mitchelson M, Macdonald C. Mephedrone toxicity in a Scottish emergency department. *Emerg Med J* 2011;28:1055–1058.

273. Atreya RV, Sun J, Zhao Z. Exploring drug-target interaction networks of illicit drugs. *BMC Genom* 2013;14(Suppl. 4):S1. https://doi. org/10.1186/1471-2164-14-S4-S1

274. Spiller HA, Ryan ML, Weston RG, Jansen J. Clinical experience with and analytical confirmation of 'bath salts' and 'legal highs' (synthetic cathinones) in the United States. *Clin Toxicol* 2011;49(6):499–505. https://doi.org/10.3109/15563650.2011.590812

275. Woo TM, Hanley J. 'How do they look?' Identification and treatment of common ingestions in adolescents. *J Pediatr Health Care* 2013;27(2):135–144. https://doi.org/10.1016/j.pedhc.2012.12.002

276. Beck O, Franzen L, Bäckberg M, Signell P, Helander A. Intoxications involving MDPV in Sweden during 2010–2014: results from the STRIDA project. *Clin Toxicol* 2015;53(9):865–873. https://doi.org/10.3109/15563650.2015.1089576

277. Baumann MH, Ayestas MA Jr, Partilla JS, et al. The designer methcathinone analogs, mephedrone and methylone, are substrates for monoamine transporters in brain tissue. *Neuropsychopharmacology* 2012;37(5):1192–1203. https://doi.org/10.1038/npp.2011.304

278. Bajaj N, Mullen D, Wylie S. Dependence and psychosis with 4-methylmethcathinone (mephedrone) use. *BMJ Case Rep* 2010;2010:bcr0220102780. https://doi.org/10.1136/bcr.02.2010.2780

279. Simmler LD, Buser TA, Donzelli M, et al. Pharmacological characterization of designer cathinones in vitro. *Br J Pharmacol* 2013;168:458–470.

280. European Monitoring Centre for Drugs and Drug Addiction. Annex 2. Technical Report on 1-(1,3-benzodioxol-5-yl)-2-(pyrrolidin-1-yl)pentan-1-one (3,4-methylenedioxypyrovalerone, MDPV). Prepared by Ms Alison M Dines, Dr David M Wood and Dr Paul I Dargan.

281. Antonowicz JL, Metzger AK, Ramanujam SL. Paranoid psychosis induced by consumption of methylenedioxypyrovalerone: two cases. *Gen Hosp Psych* 2011;33(640):e5.

282. Boulanger-Gobeil C, St-Onge M, Laliberte M, Auger PL. Seizures and hyponatremia related to ethcathinone and methylone poisoning. *J Med Toxicol* 2012;8(1):59–61.

283. European Monitoring Centre for Drugs and Drug Addiction. Drug profiles. Synthetic cathinones, 2012. Available at: www.emcdda.europa.eu/publications/drug-profiles/synthetic-cathinones_en [last accessed 18 March 2022].

284. Derungs A, Schietzel S, Meyer MR, Maurer HH, Krähenbühl S, Liechti ME. Sympathomimetic toxicity in a case of analytically confirmed recreational use of naphyrone (naphthylpyrovalerone). *Clin Toxicol* 2011;49(7):691–693.

285. Winder GS, Stern N, Hosanagar A. Are 'bath salts' the next generation of stimulant abuse? *J Subst Abuse Treat* 2013;44(1):42–45.

286. Spiller HA, Ryan ML, Weston RG, Jansen J. Clinical experience with and analytical confirmation of 'bath salts' and 'legal highs' (synthetic cathinones) in the United States. *Clin Toxicol* 2011;49(6):499–505.

287. Centers for Disease Control and Prevention (CDC). Emergency department visits after use of a drug sold as bath salts – Michigan, November 13, 2010 to March 31, 2011. *Morb Mort Wkly Rep* 2011;60(19):624–627.

288. Zawilska JB, Słomiak K, Wasiak M, et al. Beta-cathinone derivatives – a new generation of dangerous psychostimulant 'designer drugs'. *Przegl Lek* 2013;70(6):386–391.

289. Kelly JP. Cathinone derivatives: a review of their chemistry, pharmacology and toxicology. *Drug Test Anal* 2011;3(7–8):43953.

290. Thornton SL, Gerona RR, Tomaszewski CA. Psychosis from a bath salt product containing flephedrone and MDPV with serum, urine, and product quantification. *J Med Toxicol* 2012;8(3):310–313.

291. European Monitoring Centre for Drugs and Drug Addiction. Report on the risk assessment of 1-phenyl-2-(pyrrolidin-1-yl) pentan-1-one (αpyrrolidinovalerophenone, α-PVP). Luxembourg, Publications Office of the European Union, 2016. https://doi.org/10.2810/71700. ISBN 978-92-9168-931-6. Available at: www.emcdda.europa.eu/system/files/publications/2934/TDAK16001ENN.pdf[last accessed 18 March 2022].

292. International Classification of Disorders (ICD-11). Synthetic cathinone dependence. Available at: https://icd .who.int/browse11/l-m/en#http%3a%2f%2fid.who.int%2ficd %2fentity%2f2070676103 [last accessed 18 March 2022].

293. Hill SL, Thomas SH. Clinical toxicology of newer recreational drugs. *Clin Toxicol* 2011;**49**:705–719.

294. Sande M. Characteristics of the use of 3-MMC and other new psychoactive drugs in Slovenia, and the perceived problems experienced by users. *Int J Drug Policy* 2016;27:65–73.

295. Winstock A, Mitcheson L, Ramsey J, Davies S, Puchnarewics M, Marsden J. Mephedrone: subjective effects and health risks. *Addiction* 2011;**106**:1991–1996.

296. Corkery JM, Guirguis A, Papanti DG, Orsolini L, Schifano F. Synthetic cathinones: prevalence and motivations for use. In: J Zawilska (ed.), *Synthetic Cathinones. Current Topics in Neurotoxicity*, vol. 12. Cham, Springer. https://doi.org/10.1007 /978-3-319-78707-7_9

297. Van Hout MC. An internet study of user's experiences of the synthetic cathinone 4- methylethcathinone (4-MEC).

298. Winder GS, Stern N, Hosanagar A. Are 'bath salts' the next generation of stimulant abuse? *J Subst Abuse Treat* 2013;**44** (1):42–45. https://doi.org/10.1016/j.jsat.2012.02.003

299. Coppola M, Mondola R. Synthetic cathinones: chemistry, pharmacology and toxicology of a new class of designer drugs of abuse marketed as 'bath salts' or 'plant food'. *Toxicol Lett* 2012;**211**(2):144–149. https://doi.org/10.1016/j .toxlet.2012.03.009

300. Lev-Ran S. A case of treating cathinone dependence and comorbid depression using bupropion. *J Psychoactive Drugs.* 2012;**44**(5):434–436.

301. Antonowicz JL, Metzger AK, Ramanujam SL. Paranoid psychosis induced by consumption of methylenedioxypyrovalerone: two cases. *Gen Hosp Psychiatry* 2011;**33**(6):640.e5–6. https://doi.org/10.1016/j .genhosppsych.2011.04.010

302. Sande M, Paš M, Nahtigal K, Šabić S. Patterns of NPS use and risk reduction in Slovenia. *Subst Use Misuse* 2018;**53**(9):1424–1432. doi.org/10.1080/10826084 .2017.1411366

303. Burch HJ, Clarke EJ, Hubbard AM, Scott-Ham M. Concentrations of drugs determined in blood samples collected from suspected drugged drivers in England and Wales. *J Forensic Leg Med* 2013;**20**(4):278–289. https://doi.org /10.1016/j.jflm.2012.10.005

J Psychoactive Drugs 2014;**46**(4):273–286. https://doi.org/10 .1080/02791072.2014.934979

Hallucinogenic Drugs

12

12.1 Introduction

Hallucinogens are drugs that distort the way a user perceives time, motion, colour, sounds and self.

The varied perceptual distortions caused by such drugs do not strictly correspond to clinical definitions of 'hallucinations' (perceptions in the absence of external stimuli that are experienced as if they were real, as seen in psychoses and delirium).[1,2] Therefore, alternative terms, such as 'illusions', 'pseudo-hallucinations' and 'perceptual distortions' have also been employed.[3]

Some authors have suggested that the term 'psychedelic' should replace terms like 'classical hallucinogen' to describe drugs such as LSD and psilocybin,[4] but it has also been argued that this term carries disadvantages because of its cultural connotations of a style of music and art associated with Western counter-culture in the 1960s.

Other terms used for drugs with hallucinogenic effects include 'psychomimetic', a term previously used to emphasise effects that resemble the symptoms of psychosis, and the term 'entheogen', which emphasises the mystical-type experiences the drugs are said to promote. However, these terms have also been criticised, as they highlight only a single aspect of a much broader range of hallucinogenic effects.[5]

Based on their mechanism of action in the human central nervous system, hallucinogenic drugs in general can be divided into two main groups: classic hallucinogens and dissociative or anaesthetic hallucinogens,[6] with the latter including ketamine and its analogues discussed in Chapter 6.

This chapter will use the term 'hallucinogen' to refer only to the classic hallucinogens: drugs with a mechanism of action mediated primarily by agonism of the 5HT2A serotonin receptor. LSD (N, N-diethyl-D-lysergamide) and psilocybin are the prototypical and most prevalent drugs of this class.

Classic or serotonergic hallucinogens fall into several chemically related groups. They act as serotonin receptor agonists, and therefore ultimately produce altered perceptions of reality and synaesthesia.[7,8] They have been traditionally classified by either their primary mechanism of action or by chemical groups, including:

- tryptamines (e.g., psilocin and N, N-dimethyltryptamine/ DMT);
- ergolines (lysergic acid diethylamide/LSD); and
- phenethylamines (e.g., mescaline, 2CB series).[9]

In recent years, new drugs with primarily hallucinogenic effects from all of these chemical groups have been synthesised and have emerged in the recreational drug market, with claims to be the next-generation designer drugs, or with claims to replace or to be the 'legal' alternatives of existing hallucinogenic drugs such as LSD, for example.

These include, for example, the tryptamines alpha-methyltryptamine (AMT); 5-methoxy-N, N-dimethyltryptamine (5-MeO-DMT) and 5-methoxy-N,N-diisopropyltryptamine (5-MeO-DIPT)[10] and new phenethylamines, including the 2C-series and its structural analogues, such as N-benzylphenethylamines (NBOMes).[11] For more information see Table 12.1.

As with other novel psychoactive substances (NPS), new generations of hallucinogenics have emerged over time,[12] in some cases exhibiting much potency and potentially increased adverse effects. For example, 2C-B appeared on the drug market in the mid-1980s and its more recent derivative 2-(4-bromo-2,5-dimethoxyphenyl)- N-(2-methoxybenzyl)ethanamine (25B-NBOMe) is highly potent even at microgram-level doses.[13] Similarly, other NPS such as bromo-dragonfly are particularly potent and long-lasting.[14]

12.2 Legal Status

The status of control for different hallucinogens, including NPS with hallucinogenic effects, varies: most of the common hallucinogens are controlled

Table 12.1 Hallucinogenic drugs used for recreational purposes

Lysergamides

- (6aR,9 R)-N,N-diethyl-7-methyl4,6,6a,7,8,9-hexahydroindolo-[4,3-fg]quinoline-9-carboxamide (N,N-diethyl-D-lysergamide) **LSD**[27]
- (8β)-9,10-didehydro-6-methylergoline-8-carboxamide **LSA (ergine)**
- (6aR,9 R)-4-acetyl-N,Ndiethyl-7-methyl-4,6,6a,7,8,9-hexahydroindolo[4,3-fg]quinoline-9-carboxamide9 (1-acetyl-N, N-diethyllysergamide) **ALD-52**[28]
- (6aR,9 R)-N,N-diethyl-7-ethyl4,6,6a,7,8,9-hexahydroindolo-[4,3-fg]quinoline-9-carboxamide (6-ethyl-6-nor-lysergic aciddiethylamide) **ETH-LAD**[28]
- (8β)-N,N-Diethyl-6-propyl-9,10-didehydroergoline-8-carboxamide(6-propyl- 6-nor- Lysergic acid diethylamide) **PRO-LAD**[28]
- 6-allyl-6-nor-lysergic acid diethylamide **AL-LAD**[28]
- (8β)-8-{[(2S,4S)-2,4-Dimethylazetidin-1-yl]carbonyl}-6-methyl-9,10-didehydroergoline (lysergic acid 2,4-dimethylazetidide) **LSZ**[28]

Lysergamide NPS Summary

Some novel LSD derivatives have recently reached the market, such as those listed above. They produce effects resembling those of LSD, having similar pharmacological action at 5-HT2A-receptors, but possessing different potencies, onset and duration of effects.[29]

For example, LSZ was synthesised as an analogue of LSD. We know little about it, but it was found that the S isomer of LSZ was slightly more potent than LSD itself and showed greater binding affinity to 5-HTA receptors in rats.[30]

A more recent NPS is 1-P-LSD (1-propionyl-d-lysergic acid diethylamide hemitartrate),[31] which seems to have been developed as an alternative to LSZ, after it was banned. 1PLSD is also believed to be slightly more potent than its parent drug and more potent than LSZ.[32]

Tryptamines

Tryptamine NPS include

- O-phosphoryl-4-hydroxy-N,Ndimethyltryptamine 4-hydroxy-N,N-dimethyltryptamine **Psilocybin**
- N,N-dimethyltryptamine **DMT**
- alpha-methyltryptamine **αMT 'AMT'**[28]
- N,N-diallyl-5-methoxytryptamine **5-MeO-DALT**
- N,N-diisopropyltryptamine **DiPT** (sometimes known as'Foxy')
- 5-methoxy-N,N-diisopropyltryptamine **5-MeO-DiPT** (sometimes known as'Foxy Methoxy')

Tryptamine NPS Summary

Tryptamines are hallucinogenic drugs that act primarily as agonists of the serotonergic receptor 5-HT2A, but their action may also be modulated by interactions with other targets, including other 5-HT receptors, monoamine transporters, and trace amine-associated receptors.[33]

Tryptamines require low doses to produce changes in perception, mood, and thought. The effects of tryptamine NPS are expected to be similar to those of the legally controlled tryptamines, such as psilocybin or DMT. However, information available suggests that there may be significant differences with traditional drugs as well as among the various tryptamine NPS.

For example, 5-methoxy group, such as in 5-MeOAMT, 5-MeO-AMT and α-MT seem to have d increased potency, compared to psilocybin and DMT which produce hallucinogenic effects with relatively low potency.[34]

A study of the receptor interaction profiles of the tryptamine NPS (DiPT, 4-OH-DiPT, 4-OH-MET, 5-MeO-AMT, and 5-MeO-MiPT) also suggested that hallucinogenic effects are similar to classic serotonergic hallucinogens, but that they also possessed MDMA-like psychoactive properties.[35]

Some NPS, such as 5-MeO-AMT, also have structural similarity to the amphetamines. 5-MeO-AMT produces a strong binding activity at 5-HT1A and 5- HT2A receptors, whilst inhibiting monoamines' reuptake. It is associated with a range of sympathomimetic effects.[36] AMT and AET have also been found to possess central stimulant as well as hallucinogenic properties.[37]

Phenethylamines

The classic hallucinogenic phenethylamine is 3,4,5-trimethoxyphenethylamine, which is also known as Mescaline.
Phenethylamine NPS include:

- 2C Series, and their derivatives 2C-B has various close analogues; bk-2C-B, and 25B-NBOMe. The same selection of analogues may exist for the rest of the 2C series, e.g. 2C-E, 2C-I, 2C-T-7.
- Hallucinogenic amphetamines, DOx series and their derivatives DOM, DOI, DOB, TMA-2.
- Tetrahydrodifranyl compounds 10 2C-B-FLY, 'bromodragonfly'. They are called 'FLY' because their molecular structure resembles the insect.[17]

Phenethylamines Summary

Phenethylamines include a wide range of natural or synthetic substances which have psychostimulant, empathogenic and hallucinogenic effects. They include several potent hallucinogenics that exert their effects through interactions with the serotonergic 5- hydroxytryptamine 2 (5-HT2) receptor site.

Table 12.1 (cont.)

Benzofurans, which are phenethylamines structurally related to MDMA and MDA (3,4-methylenedioxyamphetamine), include several compounds, e.g.: 6- APB (6-(2-aminopropyl) benzofuran; aka 'BenzoFury'); 5-APB (s (5-(2- aminopropyl)benzofuran; 6-APDB (6-(2-Aminopropyl)-2,3-dihydrobenzofuran; aka '4-Desoxy-MDA'); 5-APDB (5-(2-Aminopropyl)-2,3-dihydrobenzofuran; aka '3-Desoxy-MDA'); etc. They are typically ingested, since nasal insufflation may be painful.[38]

Phenethylamine NPS derivatives include 'Bromodragonfly', NBOMe derivatives; indanes; benzofurans; and the class of 2C- molecules such (2C-B), (2C-I); (2C-E).

It has been shown that substances such as Bromo-Dragonfly (aka 'DOB-Dragonfly'/'3C-Bromo-Dragonfly' displays a high affinity for 5-HT2A, 5-HT2B, and 5-HT2C receptors and effects include long-standing hallucinations, mood elevation, paranoid ideation, confusion, anxiety and flashbacks.[39]

The 2C-series, 2C drugs are a subfamily of substituted phenethylamines, with hallucinogenic and psychostimulant properties.[40] Over the last decade 2C-B has gained popularity among electronic music party goers as the replacement of choice for MDMA and LSD, either alone or combined.[41,42,43]

Preclinical studies have demonstrated that 2C-drugs inhibit the norepinephrine (NE) and serotonin transporters (NET and SERT, respectively) with very low potency in comparison to amphetamines.

Like other hallucinogenic phenethylamines, 2C-series is a partial agonist of 5HT2A, 5HT2B, and 5HT2C receptors, although some studies have reported it may act as a 5HT2A full antagonist.[44] They also display low-affinity binding to D2 receptors and a low inhibitory activity to monoamine transporters.[45] In addition to 5-HT2A effects, some 2C agents can inhibit the reuptake of dopamine, norepinephrine, and serotonin.[46]

All 2C compounds are capable of producing clinical effects at doses as low as 50 µg. Affinity for these receptors generally correlates with the hallucinogenic properties of the drug.[47]

It appears that NBOMe compounds, which are derivatives of the 2C series, exhibit even higher 5-HT2A potency than the parent 2C class, and there is some evidence from *in-vitro* receptor studies that NBOMe compounds act as potent full agonists at the 5-HT2A and 5-HT2C receptors.[48,49] Their higher 5-HT2A receptor affinity, compared to the 2C- derivatives, is associated with hallucinations and delusions.[50]

NBOMe are pharmacologically active at very low, sub-milligram, doses.[51,52] It has been suggested that NBOMe are similar to classic hallucinogens like LSD, although they do not possess LSD's affinity for 5-HT1A receptors.[53] Their potency is reportedly in the same range as that for LSD.[54]

NBOMEs also possess sympathomimetic properties, which may be linked to their activity at adrenergic receptors.[55] They also have affinity for dopaminergic, and histaminergic receptors, as well as monoamine transporters.[56,57]

under the Convention on Psychotropic Substances of 1971, although some NPS synthetic hallucinogens are not currently under international control.[15]

12.3 Quality of Research Evidence

The international evidence on the clinical management of the harms related to the use of hallucinogens remains limited. The bulk of it focuses on LSD and psilocybin, although research on the clinical management of harms of even these substances is limited. Very little has been published about other hallucinogenic drugs, with evidence limited to case reports and series of patients with acute toxicity.

12.4 Brief Summary of Pharmacology

Structurally, most hallucinogens can be roughly divided into tryptamines, phenethylamines and lysergamides (LSD-like structures), as shown in table 12.1 below.[2,16] LSD and other lysergamides share a complex molecular structure with both tryptamine and phenethylamine backbones. However, lysergamide structures are sufficiently elaborated from

these skeletons for them to be more usefully considered a distinct class of hallucinogenic.[2] Some hallucinogenic NPS, such as the 'Fly' series, are less easy to classify, because they are fairly distant structural analogues of their phenethylamine parent compound.[17]

The common denominator in the pharmacology of true hallucinogenic drugs is agonism or partial agonism of 5-HT2 serotonin receptors,[2] particularly 5-HT2A and/or other 5-HT2 receptors.[18] This activity is of central importance to their characteristic hallucinogenic effects.[18] Hallucinogenic drugs interact with an array of other sites too, contributing to the psychopharmacological and behavioural effects.[18,19,20] A recent study looking at the hallucinogenic drug DMT, a tryptamine, suggests that it may be an endogenous ligand for the sigma-1 receptor in humans. This suggests the need to look beyond the serotonin system for a complete understanding of the pharmacology of tryptamines.[21]

Understanding of hallucinogenic drugs is still very limited. It is assumed that qualitative differences in the subjective phenomenology of the drugs may relate to their individual affinity profiles.[19] In a recent study, psilocybin, the prototypical hallucinogenic tryptamine, has been shown to reduce apparent activity in hub regions, and to uncouple synchronised activity in the posterior cingulate cortex and the medial prefrontal cortex.[22] This suppression of orderly and regulated patterns of activity between different brain areas has been interpreted as allowing for the relatively unconstrained patterns of cognition, with abnormal integration of sensory information, that seem to characterise the 'psychedelic state'.[22] More research is needed.

The structure–activity relationships of hallucinogens are complex, and differ between the various drugs. This means that hallucinogen NPS appearing on the market may be structurally similar to other NPS, or to other well-known hallucinogenic drugs, but may have different levels of potency, effects, duration of effects and risks.

For example, the phenethylamines 2C-B and bk-2C-B 28 differ only by the addition of a ketone group, but some reports suggest that the latter drug has a significantly longer duration of effect, with the peak lasting in some instances for 10 to 14 hours.[23] The duration of the effects of 5-methoxy-N,N-diisopropyltryptamine (5-MeO-DiPT, foxy methoxy) is seven times greater than that for N,N-diisopropyltryptamine (DiPT or 'Foxy').[24]

Bromo-dragonfly is a distant derivative from the core phenethylamine structure, with a potency similar to that of LSD, but has a far longer duration of effect (1–3 days) and apparently has greater toxicity.[17] In terms of acute toxicity, within the 2C family, 2-CB has not been associated with any fatalities, whereas there are reports from the US of deaths in which 2C-T-7 has been implicated.[25]

Some hallucinogens have strong stimulant effects. For example, αMT is a tryptamine, with a methyl group in the alpha position, just like an amphetamine, and has marked stimulant effects, seen in clinical observations.[26] On the other hand, some phenethylamines, which are amphetamine-type substances, are also hallucinogenic drugs. These include ring-substituted substances, such as the '2C series' and the 'D series' (e.g. DOI, DOC), and benzodifurans (e.g. bromo-dragonfly, 2C-B-Fly). Similarly, the phenethylamines DOB(2,5-dimethoxy-4-bromoamphetamine)

and MEM are highly selective for 5-HT2 receptors.[19]

12.5 Clinical Uses

There are currently no hallucinogenic drugs that are licensed for clinical use, and many of the compounds, including LSD and psilocybin, are restricted as Schedule 1 substances.

Some research on the clinical use of hallucinogens was carried out in the 1950s, 1960s and 1970s. A meta-analysis of early randomised controlled trials of LSD for alcoholism showed that a single application of LSD in a variety of treatment modalities reduced alcohol intake or maintained abstinence at rates which compare favourably to mainstream treatment with naltrexone and acamprosate.[58]

Some clinical research involving the administration of classical hallucinogens is currently taking place.[59,60,61,62] This includes small pilot studies looking at the utility of LSD[63] and psilocybin[64] for treating anxiety associated with life-threatening diseases. Psilocybin has also been trialled in nine people with obsessive-compulsive disorder, all of whom experienced improvement in symptoms, mostly short-lived, but with one experiencing full, lasting remission.[65] Another trial has been approved for testing psilocybin in treatment-resistant depression.

There is increasing interest in, and studies of, therapeutic use of hallucinogens in a controlled setting,[59–62,66] including for treatment-resistant depression[67,68,69,70,71] anxiety and depression in life-threatening illnesses[4,72,73,74,75,76] and in palliative care[77] and as a treatment for alcohol dependence,[78] smoking cessation.[79] The need for more research on the role of classic hallucinogens in the treatment of addictions has been emphasised.[80,81] It is argued that clinical research has shown them to be safe when appropriate precautions are taken.[82] Research is at an early stage and more evidence is needed before recommendations can be made.

12.6 Prevalence and Patterns of Use

At a global level, the 2019 World Drug Report has suggested that the quantities of substances with hallucinogenic properties (other than ketamine) seized globally have been fluctuating over time, but have shown an upward trend in recent years. This is in line with some information suggesting an increase in use of such substances in recent years.[83]

In Europe, information on the prevalence of the use of hallucinogens relates mainly to 'traditional' rather than NPS hallucinogens. Available data suggest that the overall prevalence of LSD and hallucinogenic mushroom use has been generally low and stable for a number of years. Among young adults (15–34 years), national surveys report last year prevalence estimates of less than 1% for both substances in 2017 or the most recent year the survey was conducted. Exceptions are prevalence estimates of Finland (1.9%) and the Netherlands (1.6%) for hallucinogenic mushrooms, and Norway (1.1%) and Finland (1.3%) for LSD.[84]

Although limited, there is some increasing interest among some people in 'micro-dosing' hallucinogen. This is discussed in Box 12.1.

Box 12.1 Micro-dosing

'Micro-dosing' is a term used for a pattern of using hallucinogens that has been growing in popularity and visibility.[85] It refers to the use of a dose of hallucinogenic drug that is too small to cause intoxication or significant alteration of consciousness. The intention is that micro-dosing affects mood, health and cognition in positive ways, while allowing the user to carry on with everyday activities.[86]

People involved in miro-dosing argue that taking small amounts of psilocybin mushrooms, LSD or mescaline enhances cognitive function, perception and creativity and adds a new dimension to what could be considered 'illegal cognitive enhancement'. This reflects a new desired effect of hallucinogenic drugs.[87]

There is currently little evidence to draw upon regarding the benefits and harms of micro-dosing, although studies are proposed.[88]

The micro-dosing phenomenon has been spread most recently by the Internet, where discussion fora enable users to share experiences and exchange information in ways that make new practices accessible for others. Its growing visibility has been reflected in substantial recent media coverage.[89]

12.7 Routes of Ingestion and Frequency of Dosing

There are very marked differences between the various hallucinogenic drugs in terms of potency and type, onset and duration of effects.

12.7.1 Potency

The potency of a hallucinogenic substance appears to be broadly, but not entirely, a function of its affinity for the 5-HT2A receptor.[2,18] Substances with lower affinity for the receptor, and lower potency, include mescaline[2] (typical oral dose approximately 0.25 g). LSD has a high affinity, and is the most commonly used potent hallucinogenic substance (a typical dose may be 75–150 µg[90]).

Over the years, very potent new hallucinogenic substances have emerged on the recreational market, such as the NBOMe series and bromo-dragonfly.[91] The latter, for example, has been described by users (on drug user websites) as 'just too powerful', due to its duration as well as potency.[17] This may have contributed to the fact that some new drugs, such as bromo-dragonfly, appeared on the market but then disappeared quickly.[17]

For more information on NPS properties and differences see Table 12.1.

12.7.2 Onset of Effects and Duration

There are significant differences between hallucinogenic substances in terms of the speed of the onset of effects after ingestion, ranging from a few moments to hours.

The duration of the effect of hallucinogens also differs widely and can range from between minutes and days, depending on the substance used.

- **Very short effects** (e.g. DMT).[92,93] Vaporised DMT is an example of a very short-acting drug with rapid onset.[94] DMT's effects appear in under a minute and may peak within 5 minutes, with minimal adverse after-effects (come-down).[93,95] Similarly, 5-MeO-DMT is associated with experiences similar in intensity to those caused by psilocybin, but with a much shorter duration of action (half-life 12–19 minutes).[96]
- **Intermediate duration of effects**, (e.g. 2C-B, with effects lasting 2–3 hours[97])
- **Long duration of effects** (e.g. LSD and mescaline are longer-acting hallucinogens and a duration of 8–12 hours is common.[98] LSZ has a duration of

action lasting from 7–10 hours. After effects can be felt for up to 3 hours.[99,100]

- **Very long duration of effects**. Including DOM and others in the DOx series, ibogaine, 2C-P and bromo-dragonfly, have effects which have been reported to last a day or longer, and in some cases can lead to exhaustion.[17,98,101,102,103] AMT's desired effects peak in 3–4 hours and last up to 12–24 hours,[104] 1-P-LSD duration of action lasts up to 12 hours, with after-effects lasting up to 24 hours.[105] Bromo-dragonfly is a distant derivative from the core phenethylamine structure, with a potency similar to that of LSD, but has a far longer duration of effect (1–3 days) and apparently has greater toxicity.[17]

There are also differences between the onset of the effect of the various hallucinogenic drugs, including NPS. For example, onset of action of the tryptamine DMT occur almost immediately whereas in the case of the NPS, AET occurs within 30–90 minutes.[106] User reports suggest that maximal effects following ingestion of bromo-dragonfly may not be reached for up to 6 hours after ingestion,[107] posing a risk that users re-dose because of a mistaken belief that the first dose has had no effect.

The purity and quantity of the active compounds in a single dose and the reliability of hallucinogenic drugs (in terms of being the drug users think they are buying) varies between product and batches, contributing risk to dose estimation. As with other drugs, users will not know the strength of the product they are taking, or may not be ingesting the substance they intended to use, or think they are taking. Hallucinogen NPS have, on some occasions, been sold as LSD.[108]

Some drugs can be more 'reliable' than others at particular times and in different locations. For example, in a Spanish study, 99% of samples purporting to be 2C-B actually contained 2C-B (average for the four-year study period), a high reliability compared with 66.8% for MDMA, 86.3% for amphetamines, 87.4% for cocaine, and 92.2% for ketamine.[97] Similarly, there are differences between different batches for the same product; for example, bromo-dragonfly appears to come in batches of different potency.[17]

Changes in the drugs' strength and potency over time have also been documented. LSD 'tabs' in 2003 contained significantly less LSD on average than in the early years of use, in the 1960s and 1970s; doses of above 100 μg/tab were then typical, but, by 2003, 30–40 μg/tab was more usual.[109]

12.7.3 Modes of Ingestion

Hallucinogens are typically ingested orally, or sublingually/buccally, often through small blotter paper portions or 'tabs', which are held in the mouth to allow absorption through the oral mucosa. Other less common routes of administration include insufflation, smoking, rectally and by injection[26] (see also Boxes 12.2, 12.3 and 12.4).

As with other drugs, the route of administration of hallucinogens may have an impact on effects, their onset and duration. User reports suggest, for example, that the effects of 25I-NBOMe last 6–8 hours when the drug is taken sublingually or buccally, but only 4–6 hours when it is insufflated.

12.7.4 Frequency of Use

Overall, bingeing is not reported with hallucinogen drugs, partly because once the effects begin to fade, subsequent doses usually do not produce further psychoactive effects (tachyphylaxis)[2] (see Section 12.13.1 on dependence).

Box 12.2 Tryptamines

Tryptamine derivatives are usually available as capsules, tablets, powder and liquid formulations and may be ingested, snorted, smoked or injected.[110]

NBOMe-containing products are usually available as tablets, capsules, powder, liquid, spray, and blotters. They are usually taken sublingually/orally or via nasal insufflation.[111] Injection (intravenous and intramuscular), rectal and smoking routes have also been reported.[112,113]

Salvia extracts and DMT are usually vaporised or smoked. As DMT is inactive after oral administration unless combined with monoamine oxidase inhibitors (MAOIs), it is usually smoked, snorted, or injected.[114] However, it is interesting to note that capsules, known as *pharmahuasca*, have become available containing DMT together with some MAOIs, such as synthetic harmaline, or plant-based MAOIs such as Harmala alkaloids. The MAOIs inhibit the otherwise rapid metabolisation of DMT and, thus, allow for the hallucinogenic effects when the drug is taken orally.[115]

Box 12.3 Ergoline NPS

LSZ and 1P-LSD have been marketed in the form of blotters containing usually 150 micrograms of the substance which is placed under the tongue in a similar fashion to LSD. 1P-LSD is also available in tablet or ampoule forms.[116]

Box 12.4 Phenethylamines

2CB was in some countries, such as Spain for example, initially sold as powder, but tablets (including small pills) were later developed.[117]

In the US, drugs of the 2C family first appeared on the US market in 2010 and are frequently sold as 'LSD' on blotter paper, although tablets and liquid preparations are also available.[118]

12.7.5 Poly-drug Use

Hallucinogens are sometimes combined with other drugs, in poly-drug repertoires, particularly with stimulant drugs.[119] In a Spanish study of 52 users of 2C-B, 83% reported that they had taken it simultaneously with other drugs, most commonly with MDMA (69%), alcohol (43%) or cannabis (40%).[97] Reported combinations with bromo-dragonfly include: alcohol, prescribed drugs such as alprazolam, cannabis, cocaine, amphetamine, LSD, and legal highs, including salvia and kratom.[17,120]

Some combinations have their own user names. For instance, LSD or magic mushrooms taken with ecstasy is called candyflipping and hippyflipping respectively.[121] It has even been suggested that the popularity of these combinations may have contributed to a resurgence of LSD use, following the increasing popularity and use of MDMA.[122]

12.8 Desired Effects of Recreational Use

Hallucinogens are a diverse group of drugs that alter and distort perception, producing sensory distortions, most notably visual, and also modify thought and mood.[123] DiPT is atypical because (at least according to anecdotal reports) it produces predominately auditory perceptual changes.[124,125,126,127,128,129]

The use of hallucinogens was strongly linked with higher expansion motive and lower degree of coping, social and conformity motives by Benschop et al. 2020.[130] Desired effects of hallucinogens include euphoria, mild stimulation, enhanced appreciation of music and lights, visually appealing distortions, intensification of sensual or sexual feelings, altered sense of time and place, and a sense of shared and heightened significance of the situation. In a survey where 22,000 people in different parts of the world ranked drugs in terms of pleasure and pain, drug-using respondents placed LSD and magic mushrooms as the second and third most pleasurable drugs, following MDMA.[131]

A study that developed a cross-culturally valid standardised tool to identify the reasons of NPS use in six European countries reported that the use of psychedelics (hallucinogenics) was linked with a high score on the expansion motive. The author argued that this result may be explained by the pharmacodynamical properties and subjective effects of psychedelics.[132]

Reports from users and the work of researchers, such as the Shulgins, strongly suggest that each drug has distinct characteristics, and that there are qualitative differences between the different drugs, with variability in multiple sensory and emotional dimensions.[101,129]

Overall, the effects of hallucinogenic phenethylamines include euphoria, increased sociability, visual/auditory/olfactory/tactile perceptual disturbances, empathy, depersonalisation, dissociation and derealisation.[133]

It has been reported for example that 2C-B produces constellations of psychedelic-psychostimulant-like effects.[134] 2C-B has been described as inducing 'perceptual enhancement' and euphoria, but these are milder than those of classical hallucinogens such as LSD and the drug lacks the potent hallucinogenic effects of LSD.[135] This has contributed to its association with 'clubbing'. While it elicits perceptual modifications that are similar to other hallucinogens, the lower impairment and higher pleasurable effects make it comparable with MDMA.[136] 2C-B has proved popular as a dance drug, and has sometimes appeared in tablets sold as ecstasy.[137] In the Spanish study of 52 users of 2C-B, 60% reported that typical settings of 2C-B use were recreational environments (clubs, parties, raves), followed by home use with friends (54%), at home with partner (37%) or in the countryside (20%).[97]

The main clinical effects of tryptamines in general are visual hallucinations, alterations in sensory perception, intensification of colours, distortion of body image, depersonalisation, marked mood lability, euphoria, relaxation, entactogenic properties, and anxiety.[138] For example, AMT possesses central stimulant and hallucinogenic properties. Its effects include euphoria, distortion of colour/shapes and visual hallucinations.[139]

Users have also reported a variety of moderate-to-strong mystical experiences associated with tryptamines (e.g. awe or awesomeness, amazement, loss of time and space, and difficulty putting experience into words), with fewer experiencing more challenging experiences (e.g. fear, anxiousness).[140,141,142,143]

Some tryptamines, such as DMT, produce strong hallucinogenic LSD-like effects, powerful entheogenic or 'spiritual' experiences, euphoria and intense visual hallucinations, especially when DMT is ingested at high concentrations.[144,145] A recent small study on DMT reported significant increases in phenomenological features associated with near death experience following DMT administration compared to placebo.[146]

People who use ergoline or LSD-like NPS, such as of LSZ or 1P-LSD, reported mostly similar effects to those of LSD, with experiences such as internal–external visual hallucinations, loss of ego, empathy, euphoria, increased tactile sensation and perception alteration. Users also sometimes reported 'self-realisation' or 'spiritual' experiences whilst tripping. Overall, most reports of LSZ or 1P-LSD are positive, with users often reporting a more positive outlook on life afterwards and an agreeable experience they are willing to repeat.[147]

Self-described 'psychonauts' use a wide range of hallucinogens and may experiment with newly emerging psychoactive substances, potent substances and with drug combinations. The emphasis of use is on seeking novelty and extremes of experience and sometimes a spiritual experience. Users may push boundaries in terms of potency of the substance and dose. The Internet plays an important role in providing a platform for sharing experience and information.

However, as with other substances, the effects of hallucinogens are dose-dependent. For example, at lower doses, 2CB is described by users on discussion fora as an energetic experience similar to that produced by MDMA. At higher doses the experience is more similar to that of LSD. In addition, and even when the same substance is used at similar doses, any two experiences by the same individual user may be strikingly dissimilar qualitatively.[148]

Unlike most other drugs, the effects of hallucinogens are highly variable, producing different effects in different people at different times. Non-pharmacological variables such as expectations, personality, environment and emotional state appear to have a much greater influence on the effects of hallucinogens than with other drugs.[149] Compared with the more predictable and replicable effects of stimulants and depressants, the desired and actual effects of hallucinogenic drugs are highly context-dependent and user-specific.[20,48]

The use of hallucinogenic drugs for self-medication has been reported. The 'therapeutic' effects of hallucinogens have been noted by people who use them, with a study showing that a large proportion of respondents reported that 5-MeO-DMT use contributed to improvements in symptoms related to several psychiatric conditions, including anxiety, depression, substance use problems, and post-traumatic stress disorder, suggesting that 5-MeO-DMT may have psychotherapeutic effects under optimal conditions.[150] It has been argued that the therapeutic potential of tryptamines appears to be due, at least in part, to their ability to occasion mystical experiences, which has been demonstrated to have lasting beneficial effects.[151]

LSD and psilocybin are both reportedly used by some sufferers of cluster headaches,[152] and are anecdotally effective in aborting clusters and also reducing headache frequency in the long term.[153] A non-hallucinogenic analogue of LSD has been tested on a small number of people with apparent success, although the trial was neither blinded nor randomised.[154]

12.9 Unwanted Acute Effects

The hallucinogenic experience, even when positive, is often experienced as emotionally and physically draining.[155] Unwanted psychological effects are common to many hallucinogens and include what is referred to as a 'bad trip', characterised by anxiety, fear/panic, dysphoria and/or paranoia.

Distressing effects can be sensory (e.g. frightening perceptions), somatic (e.g. distressing awareness of physiological processes), personal (e.g. troubling thoughts or feelings) or even metaphysical (e.g. feelings about evil forces).[5,156,157,158,159] In very rare cases, this may escalate to dangerous behaviour; for example, fear and paranoid delusions may lead to erratic behaviour and potential aggression against self and others.[5,158]

Adverse psychological reactions can occur at typical doses, and may feature feelings of loss of control, disturbing perceptions and attacks of anxiety, agitation and panic, which can be severe.[123] A patient's mental state may switch rapidly between severe anxiety and relative normality and back again.[160]

Even when a user is not experiencing a 'bad trip', unwanted effects can include confusion, disorientation, anxiety and unwanted thoughts, emotions and memories.[161] Other unwanted physical effects can include nausea, diarrhoea or non-specific gastric discomfort,[148] heaviness or tingling, feelings of heat and cold, trembling and weakness.[129,101,161] They also include dizziness, weakness, tremors, drowsiness, paraesthesia, blurred vision, dilated pupils and increased tendon reflexes.[5] Sub-acute effects may include headache, which for psilocybin has been shown by an experimental study to be dose-dependent.[162] Hallucinogens can also moderately increase pulse rate and systolic and diastolic blood pressure.[5] However, it has been noted that physical effects vary and are 'unimpressive even at doses yielding powerful psychological effects'.[5]

Adverse effects related to hallucinogen NPS are in some cases linked to the fact that they are mis-sold to people on the illicit markets as 'traditional' substances such as LDS, or as so-called legal alternatives for these traditional substances. For example, people in a series of ten cases in New Zealand were sold or given 25BNBOMe as 'Synthetic LSD', 'synthetic speed' and '2C-B'. Other studies also show that NBOMes also appear to be commonly sold as LSD,[163,164] substituting LSD with a more potent and potentially lethal drug.

If people who use these substances think they are using a less potent drug, then the risk of inadvertently overdosing is compounded. As the minimum psychoactive dose of NBOMes is very small in comparison to LSD, the risk of measurement error is high.[165] The very long duration of some hallucinogen NPS, discussed in Section 12.4, also poses a risk, especially when the user assumes that s/he has taken LSD and that the effects should have dissipated.

12.10 Acute Harms

It is common to see psychological effects of hallucinogens without marked physiological symptoms, especially from the use of LSD and magic mushrooms, which are of low intrinsic toxicity, unless a very large dose is ingested.[166]

However, this is not true of all hallucinogenic NPS. Among hallucinogenic NPS, the patterns of systemic toxicity vary across the drug class and type. Some hallucinogens will have a potential to cause toxicity with stimulant features (e.g. αMT88); others drugs may more typically evoke symptoms of serotonin syndrome (e.g 5-MeO-DiPT30).

For example, the highly potent phenethylamine hallucinogens, 'NBOMes', were found to be toxic and have been associated with several fatalities.[167] Similarly, other hallucinogenic NPS, such as bromo-dragonfly and other 'Fly' drugs, the DOx family, the NBOMe series and AMT, have much narrower therapeutic ratios and a very different safety ratio, and so carry greater risk of acute toxicity and death.[108,168]

12.10.1 Features of Toxicity

Reported overall features of acute toxicity linked mainly to the use of controlled hallucinogenic drugs are listed in Box 12.5. For specific information on NPS hallucinogens harms by group see Boxes12.2 to 12.4.

Box 12.5 Reported Features of Acute Toxicity Linked to the Use of Hallucinogenic Drugs

CNS, Neurobehavioural and Psychiatric

Dilated pupils, mydriasis (common, psilocybin[169])

Sensory distortions, visual hallucinations, auditory illusions, synaesthesia,[27,170] tactile hallucinations, e.g. formication[171]

Affect lability, euphoria[172]

Dysphoria[158]

Acute panic[27]

Paranoia, ideas of reference[27,170]

De-personalisation[27,170,173]

Anxiety[27,170]

Disorientation[174]

Dissociation[174]

Box 12.5 (cont.)

Agitation[24,48]

Aggression, combativeness[24]

Delirium, depression, suicidal ideation, attempted suicide[175]

Psychosis, delusions, hallucinations[176,177]

Seizures[26]

Confusion[58,178]

Ataxia[27,170]

'Bizarre behaviour'[58]

Lightheadedness[27,173]

Headaches[27]

Paraethesias,[174] abnormal sensations of heat and cold, chills[27]

Restlessness, excitement[24,178]

Cardiovascular

Tachycardia[24,27]

Hypertension[27]

Musculoskeletal

Myalgias[27]

Twitching[173]

Muscle tension and jaw clenching[24]

Shaking[179]

Respiratory tachypnoea[24,173]

Metabolic acidosis[24]

Gastrointestinal/Urological

Gastrointestinal symptoms may be more common after consumption of natural unrefined products containing hallucinogens such as ayahuasca,[148] mushrooms and cacti, in comparison with refined chemical substances such as LSD Nausea, vomiting[58,174] (psilocybin common)[169]

Diarrhoea[148,174]

Renal

Acute kidney injury/acute kidney failure[27]

Other Symptoms

Hyperthermia,[24,27] pyrexia[174]

Hypoglycaemia

Rhabdomyolysis[24]

Flushing,[173] sweating[179]

12.10.2 Physiological Adverse Effects

The adverse effects of hallucinogenic NPS are listed in Boxes 12.6, 12.7 and 12.8.

Box 12.6 Ergoline NPS

Overdose with LSD is rare, but may cause collapse, coma, vomiting, respiratory arrest and hyperthermia. Platelet dysfunction may occur causing mild, generalised bleeding tendency and polymorph leukocytosis.[159,180] Rhabdomyolysis has been reported.[181] Sympathomimetic toxicity has been reported after ingestion of LSD.[182]

Tachycardia, tachypnoea, agitation, hyperpyrexia and hypertension have been reported following ingestion of bromo-dragonfly, a drug with a potency similar to LSD, but a far longer duration (1–3 days) and apparently greater toxicity.[17] The vasoconstriction that has been observed in cases of bromo-dragonfly toxicity has appeared resistant to treatment with ACE inhibitors, nitroprusside, prostacyclin analogues, glyceryltrinitrate or calcium channel blockers.[91]

LSD has a safety ratio (the ratio of the typical effective dose to the lethal dose) of around 1:1000, making accidental overdoses rare.[183]

There is little evidence that the NPS LSZ and 1P-LSD are linked with cases of acute toxicity cases or hospitalisation.[184] An overview of harms that looked at the views of users on Internet forums reported that both LSZ and 1P-LSD were deemed by users to have no addictive potential and very low toxicity.[185] More research is needed.

Box 12.7 Hallucinogenic Phenethylamine NPS Harms

Although classic 2C drugs are considered physiologically relatively safe, several incidences, including sympathomimetic toxicity, psychosis, and death, have been reported.[186,187,188] Severe and life-threatening effects have been associated with the ingestion of NBOMes[189,190] and bromo-dragonfly.[17]

Their adverse effects may include nausea, vomiting, headache, panic/severe agitation, aggressiveness, seizures, insomnia, muscle rigidity/rhabdomyolysis with renal failure, tremors and cardiopulmonary arrest. Several fatalities have been reported following the intake of NBOMe compounds.[191]

Adverse effects of substances in the 2C family include headache, dysphoria, hallucinations, mydriasis, seizures, severe agitation, and apnoea.[192] Clinical symptoms of patients with 2C or NBOMe toxicity are typically those of serotonergic and

Box 12.7 (cont.)

sympathomimetic excess. These include tachycardia, hypertension, nausea, vomiting, dizziness, hallucination, agitation, and confusion. Hyperthermia and seizures may occur and acute kidney injury and rhabdomyolysis have been reported. NBOMe in particular has been associated with a high level of toxicity.

It has been suggested that the diagnosis of NBOMe intoxication can be difficult.[193] Associated clinical features include internal preoccupation, violent agitation and hallucinations. Serotonergic effects such as mydriasis, sweating, agitation, tachycardia hypertension, hyperreflexia, increased muscle tone and clonus can be present but difficult to distinguish from sympathomimetic excess.[194,195,196] The most common adverse clinical effects reported to a poison centre by users were tachycardia, agitation, hallucinations, hypertension and confusion.[197]

A higher incidence of hallucination and delirium has been reported for the NBOMe drugs compared with the parent 2C compounds.[198,199,200] Symptoms of NBOMe toxicity include nausea, vomiting, headache, panic/severe agitation, aggressiveness, seizures, insomnia, muscle rigidity/rhabdomyolysis with renal failure, tremors and cardiopulmonary arrest.[201]

A review of 51 cases of NBOMe toxicity showed that rhabdomyolysis is a relatively common complication of severe NBOMe toxicity, an effect that may be linked to NBOMe-induced seizures, hyperthermia and vasoconstriction.[202]

In a case series of ten patients, 25B-NBOMe intoxication caused hallucinations with violent agitation. Serotonergic and sympathetic signs were observed; mydriasis, tachycardia, hypertension and hyperthermia. These effects were also similar to those described in other reports involving other analogues in the class; 25I-NBOMe and 25CNBOMe.[203] 25B-NBOMe appears to cause similar physiological and psychoactive effects compared to 25I and 25C NBOMe analogues.[204,205,206,207]

Seizures are frequently reported after 25I-NBOMe and 25BNBOMe use. In a retrospective review of 148 cases of NBOMe use (mostly 25I-NBOMe), 8.8% had associated seizures.[208] Poklis et al. reported a case of 25B-NBOMe intoxication that went into status epilepticus. Lorazepam IV and a phenytoin infusion were required to terminate seizure activity.[209]

Benzofurans, are phenethylamines structurally related to MDMA and MDA (3,4-methylenedioxyamphetamine) and include several compounds, 6-APB (aka 'BenzoFury');

Box 12.7 (cont.)

5-APB 6-APDB ('4-Desoxy-MDA'); 5-APDB; aka '3-Desoxy-MDA').[210] Their intake may be associated with stimulant, empathogenic and hallucinogenic effects. Adverse effects may include: dry mouth, nausea, jaw/teeth clenching, insomnia, diarrhoea, light hypersensitivity, hot flushes, headache, drowsiness, panic attacks/ anxiety, depression, severe paranoia and psychosis. An unpleasant 'come-down', lasting several days, has been reported. Several deaths related to 5- and 6-APB have been identified.[211]

Benzofurans have been associated with stimulant, entactogenic and hallucinogenic effects.[212] Adverse effects may include: dry mouth, nausea, jaw/teeth clenching, insomnia, diarrhoea, light hypersensitivity, hot flushes, headache, drowsiness, panic attacks/anxiety, depression, severe paranoia and psychosis. The use of benzofuran has been associated with an unpleasant 'come-down', lasting several days.[213] Several deaths related to 5- and 6-APB have been reported.[214]

Bromo-dragonfly has also been linked to a number of related acute intoxications with convulsions, respiratory problems, liver and kidney failure and severe vasoconstriction. Fatalities have been described.[215] It has been shown that substances such as 'DOB-Dragonfly'/'3C-Bromo-Dragonfly' displays a high affinity for 5-HT2A, 5-HT2B, and 5-HT2C receptors and effects include long-standing hallucinations, mood elevation, paranoid ideation, confusion, anxiety and flashbacks.[216]

Box 12.8 Tryptamine NPS

Hallucinogens, particularly when taken in combination with other serotonergic drugs such as MDMA and SSRI antidepressants, may contribute to serotonin syndrome, which may be life-threatening (see Chapter 8 and Section 9.14.3). Drugs with the potential to cause serotonin toxicity, for example 5-MeO-DiPT, may mimic the toxicity profile of MDMA.[24]

Other adverse effects of tryptamine include agitation, tachyarrhythmias, hyperpyrexia, serotoninergic and neurotoxicity. Deaths have been reported.[217,218] Our knowledge of the adverse effects of the specific drugs remains limited, but research has shown the following for example:

Box 12.8 (cont.)

- AET adverse effects may include: facial flushing, headache, gastrointestinal disorders, irritability, insomnia and at times, hyperthermia and agitated delirium.[219]
- DET adverse effects include anxiety, tremors, nausea/vomiting, mydriasis, disinhibition, visual distortions and increased blood pressure.[220]
- 5-MeO-AMT presents with a range of sympathomimetic effects.[221,222]
- 5-MeODIPT (aka 'foxy'/'foxy methoxy'/5MEO), adverse effects include disinhibition, nausea, vomiting, mydriasis, auditory and visual hallucinations, formication, tachycardia, hypertension, echolalia, paranoia, restlessness/agitation and muscle tension, colour/shapes, auditory and visual hallucinations, muscle tension and tremors.[223,224]

12.10.3 Psychological and Psychiatric Effects

As mentioned previously, the most common cause of hospital presentations related to hallucinogens[27,225] is what people sometimes refer to as 'bad trips'.[27]

A typical distressing hallucinogenic experience is distinct from delirious or dissociative states. On typical recreational doses, it is usual for people to maintain insight into the cause of their experiences, but the dread of permanent madness or of death is not unusual.[226] Hallucinogenic drugs may provoke distressing thoughts and reflection on personal problems and past experiences and traumas.[5] They can profoundly exaggerate existing or underlying negative moods.[225] Some studies have identified factors that may contribute to the onset of paranoid delusions and psychosis, which include depressed emotional state at the time of taking the drug and doing so among strangers.[177]

12.10.3.1 Psychosis

As mentioned above, the term 'psychosis' has been used in the literature to describe typical hallucinogenic intoxications.[227]

A study using data from the large representative sample of the US National Survey on Drug Use and Health found that the use of hallucinogenic drugs appears not to be causally linked to the de novo development of chronic disorders of mental health such as schizophrenia or depression.[228]

Hallucinogens are rarely a cause of substance-induced psychosis, where the drug triggers a psychotic episode that may persist hours, days or even weeks after the acute intoxication should have run its course.[229] Nonetheless, psychotic symptoms in the context of LSD use have been reported, as well as in the context of hallucinogenic NPS, for example 2C-T-4.[230] It has been suggested that salvia[231] can trigger psychosis in people with existing psychotic illnesses or predispositions,[20] although there are also reports of the appearance of psychosis de novo.[232] There are a few case reports of psilocybin mushrooms causing an exacerbation of psychosis.[233] Similarly, it was also reported that there was greater psychotic response to LSD in persons with a genetic predisposition to schizophrenia.[234]

Overall, the evidence suggests that individuals who suffer from prolonged hallucinogen-induced psychosis may have pre-morbid mental illness. It is not known whether the onset of psychosis in these individuals represents a psychotic reaction that would not have occurred in the absence of use of hallucinogens, or whether it represents an earlier onset of psychosis that would have occurred anyway.[5,158]

Psychoses, apparently triggered by hallucinogens, have been reported in a small number of cases associated with violence and homicide. However, these have also been reported in subjects with pre-existing psychiatric conditions.[177,232]

12.10.3.2 Excited Delirium

LSD has been involved in a small number of fatalities attributed to 'excited delirium', more commonly associated with cocaine.[235] Excited delirium has also been associated with 5-MeO-DALT[236] and αMT.[179] It has been argued that, in some instances, fatalities attributed to excited delirium may reflect underlying serotonergic and/or sympathomimetic toxicity.[237] Excited delirium is often associated with the use of force and restraint, including cases where hallucinogens were implicated; the mechanism of death can be positional asphyxia or sudden cardiac arrest.[235,238]

12.10.4 Trauma and Self-injury

Intoxication with hallucinogenic drugs can lead to accidental injury and death, including from traffic accidents, falls or hypothermia.[235,239] There are a few case reports of self-injury associated with the use of hallucinogenic NPS and a case report of a fatality following AMT consumption.[179] Unusual self-injurious acts have also been recorded following hallucinogen use with or without co-intoxicants.[240] These include at least two cases of severe ocular self-injury,[240] a case of self-castration after LSD consumption,[241] and two cases of self-inflicted stab wounds following consumption of magic mushrooms.[242]

Hallucinogen NPS can also be associated with trauma and accidents. For example, the effects of LSZ or 1P-LSD have been reported to significantly alter cognitive functions enough to endanger the user if in a potentially unsafe situation in that state, such as walking on roads.[243]

12.11 Mortality

Deaths directly attributed to acute toxicity linked to the use of the most prevalent drugs (LSD and magic mushrooms) are uncommon, but some have been reported.[158,244]

Hallucinogenic drugs have been implicated with accidents secondary to intoxication, such as traffic accidents and falls.[245] There are also several reports of suicides during or following LSD intoxication, although studies have not necessarily implied causality.[158,180] There are also reports of fatalities following ingestion of ibogaine, or products containing mixed iboga alkaloids.[246]

Hallucinogen NPS have also been associated with a small number of deaths. αMT has been linked to reported tryptamine-related deaths.[28] 5-MeO-DALT,[247] DOC,[248] 25C-NBOMe and 25H-NBOMe consumption have also been implicated.[249,250]

12.12 Clinical Management of Acute Toxicity

The management of acute toxicity resulting from the use of hallucinogens will in part depend on the hallucinogenic substance consumed. It has been suggested that monitoring and supportive treatment is all that is required for the majority of patients,[123] including airway management. TOXBASE® recommends that all patients be observed for at least 4 hours after exposure. Asymptomatic patients can then be discharged with advice to return if symptoms develop.

Some products sold as LSD may in fact contain potent hallucinogens with far narrower therapeutic ratios,[108] such as NBOMes, with a greater potential to cause acute toxicity. It has therefore been suggested that emergency room staff monitor patients presenting following ingestion of 'LSD' with the greater intensity and supportive care necessary for the management of NBOMe intoxications.[251]

The management of phenethylamine derivatives, such as 2-CB, which acts as a serotonin agonist, will need to consider the effects and harms relating to the use of amphetamine-type substances, as well as the potential risks of serotonin syndrome. As with other stimulants, some recommend that in the event of cardiac arrest, CPR should be continued for at least 1 hour and stopped only after discussion with a senior clinician. Prolonged resuscitation for cardiac arrest is recommended following poisoning, as recovery with good neurological outcome may occur.

It has been recommended, for example, that the management of 2C intoxication is supportive and should focus on control of agitation and a close monitoring of the patient's core temperature is prudent, as serotonergic and sympathomimetic effects can lead to hyperthermia. It is suggested that benzodiazepines and IV fluids can be used to successfully treat tachycardia, agitation, hypertension, and hyperthermia in most cases of phenylethylamine toxicity, although active cooling measures should be considered if hyperthermia is severe or unresponsive to other measures.[252,253,254]

The literature on NBOMe intoxication management is limited, but suggests symptomatic management with intravenous fluids, benzodiazepines and mechanical ventilator support when indicated.[255,256,257] The clinician should also keep in mind that a patient presenting with hallucinatory symptoms after ingesting what is thought to be LSD or drugs in the 2C family may, in fact, suffer from NBOMe poisoning.

The management of patients with mild to moderate NBOMe intoxication is often focused on controlling agitation and preventing physical harm.[258] Many users get injuries arising from their agitation.[259,260,261] Patients with only minor agitation may be managed without pharmaceutical intervention, by providing a quiet, non-stimulating environment and close monitoring. More severely agitated patients require physical restraints to prevent self-harm; rapid pharmacological sedation with benzodiazepines should be commenced concurrently.[262]

In Gee et al.'s case series (ten patients) it is suggested that large doses of benzodiazepines may be required to overcome agitation, tachycardia and hypertension. Hyperthermia may be present due to serotonergic and adrenergic excess. Fuelled by agitation, core temperature may rise precipitously. Large doses of benzodiazepines have generally been reported as first line treatment, with additional early paralysis and active cooling if required.[263]

For up-to-date information consult local protocol, national guidance and national and regional poisons information services.

12.12.1 Management of Adverse Psychological Effects, Agitation and Drug-induced Psychosis

A number of studies have looked at the management of adverse reactions and the following have been shown to be beneficial:

- Attempts to 'talk the patient down'. Sympathetic,[27] non-judgemental[264] reassurance, support and observation were often sufficient.[5] Where possible, the patient should be placed in a well-lit room with minimal disturbance.[20,27] Patients may be prone to mistrust and paranoid ideation, and early efforts in empathising, expressing understanding of their fears and establishing confidence have been shown to be beneficial.[27,160] Finding a more peaceful corner or room may prove worthwhile,[123] as the typical clinical environment (with medical equipment and white coats) has been shown to be a predictor of adverse anxious reactions in participants in psychedelic research.[149]
- Benzodiazepines, particularly diazepam or lorazepam,[27,123] have been reported by some studies to be first-line choice if pharmacological interventions are needed and in cases of agitation.[5,20,265]
- Antipsychotics should be considered as a second line if benzodiazepines do not produce adequate sedation.[264]
- In cases of severe agitation or 'excited delirium', physical restraint should be avoided, as this is associated with sudden cardiovascular collapse.[266]

12.13 Harms Associated with Chronic Use

There is no evidence that 'classical' hallucinogens such as LSD or psilocybin have potential neurotoxic effects, as for example MDMA does in high doses.[5] A brain imaging study comparing hallucinogen users with ecstasy users found evidence for serotonergic neurotoxicity only among the latter.[267]

12.13.1 Dependence

The use of LSD or other classic hallucinogens does not appear to lead to dependence. Typically, there is no persistent and compulsive pattern of use[20,268] and the use of hallucinogens is not associated with any recognised withdrawal syndrome. There are currently no reports of hallucinogen NPS causing physiological dependence.[61,265,269,270,271]

Hallucinogens do not appear to show classic patterns of tolerance,[270] but, on the contrary, are associated with tachyphylaxis.[2] This means that sensitivity to the effects of LSD and other hallucinogens appears to be strongly attenuated for a period after use. It may therefore prove difficult for a user to achieve desired effects from LSD if taken two days in a row, or indeed to get a desired effect from other hallucinogens.[1,2]

DMT consumed by vaporisation (usually called 'smoking' by users) appears to be an exception to this rule, having both an unusually brief duration of action and a proportionately brief duration of tachyphylaxis.[272] Anecdotal evidence confirms that this enables users to have the desired effects multiple times a day if they want to.[273] According to the authors of one survey, this, added to DMT's fewer unwanted effects and less of a 'come-down' than LSD or mushrooms, gives it a higher potential for misuse.[93] However, the same survey did not find an increased desire to use.[93]

12.13.2 Hallucinogen Persisting Perceptual Disorder (HPPD)

'Flashbacks' and hallucinogen persisting perception disorder (HPPD) have been associated with use of classic hallucinogens in particular, but also with other substances ranging from cannabis to MDMA. Hallucinogen NPS may also be linked to HPPD,[274,275,276,277,278,279,280,281,282,283] as well as other types of NPS, including synthetic cannabinoids.[284,285]

It has been argued that HPPD is a poorly understood aspect of hallucinogen consumption and is the total or partial recurrence of perceptual disturbances that appeared during previous hallucinogenic 'trips' or intoxications and re-emerged without recent use.[286] Some have argued that it is an understudied mental disorder that has a complex and unpredictable nature with overlapping psychiatric, psychological, and neurological symptoms.[287] It is also frequently unrecognised in clinical practice.[288]

Although knowledge of HPPD remains very limited, symptoms of this disorder can persist for months or years after the use of hallucinogens.[289] For some, this long-term change to vision and hearing is much less problematic than for others,[290,291] for whom it can cause substantial morbidity.[289]

The concept of HPPD remains contested. It is described in DSM-5 (F16.983), but is not identified as such nor mentioned in ICD-11. ICD-11 also does not mention the concept of 'flashbacks' as associated with hallucinogenic drugs, in contrast to ICD-10, which does.

A number of people have challenged the value of the concept of 'flashbacks'.[289] Indeed, it has been argued that the distinction between 'flashback' and HPPD remains unclear and requires further investigation. Some have even argued that the concept of 'flashback' is not a useful diagnostic entity, has been defined in very many different ways and is 'essentially valueless'.[289] In the literature, there is sometimes a distinction between the two, with 'flashbacks' generally used to describe intermittent, infrequent experiences, in contrast to the more persistent experiences of HPPD.[292] 'Flashbacks' are generally transient and often pleasant, in contrast to HPPD, which is chronic and can be highly debilitating.[293]

Transient 'flashback' phenomena appear largely absent from the more recent clinical literature, in which the chronic visual distortions critical for a diagnosis of HPPD predominate. These are commonly associated with co-morbid psychiatric symptoms, particularly anxiety, somatisation, panic and affective disorders.[228,289,293]

In fact, the notion of HPPD itself has been contested. It been suggested that there may not be a common aetiology to the diverse phenomena described as HPPD and 'flashbacks' in the literature,[289,294] with diverse interpretations having been made. It has been suggested that some cases may be explained in terms of a heightened awareness of and concern about ordinary visual phenomena,[289] which is supported by the high rates of anxiety, obsessive compulsive disorder, somatisation, hypochondria and paranoia seen in many such patients. Visual symptoms like 'visual snow', 'floaters', palinopsia (after-images) and trails are all common in the healthy general population,[228,289] may not depend on the effect of psychotropic substances on the brain,[295] or may be symptoms of psychosis, seizure disorders, persistent migraine aura without headache,

or stroke,[292] and is often associated with migraine and tinnitus.[296]

Others attribute a directly causal effect through neurotoxicity caused by the drug (e.g. 'destruction of inhibitory serotonergic interneurons'[123]). Some have argued that serotonergic neurological damage underlies HPPD, resulting in imbalances of excitation and inhibition in brain regions responsible for early visual processing.[297] However, these models based on neurological disorders have also been questioned in light of reports of HPPD involving a single use of a typical dose of a hallucinogen, while many users with a much higher frequency and dose of use do not present with these symptoms.[289]

12.13.2.1 HPPD Definitions

Halpern et al. (2016) have described HPPD as a re-experiencing of some perceptual distortions induced while intoxicated and suggested that this can cause functional impairment and anxiety.[298] HPPD is described in the *Diagnostic and Statistical Manual of Mental Disorders* (DSM-V), as discussed in Box 12.9.

Box 12.9 HPPD in DSM-5

The concept of HPPD was first introduced in DSM-3, based on the work of Abraham on habitual LSD users.[299] More recently, the diagnostic criteria of HPPD as defined by DSM-5 (292.89 F16.983) are as follows:

- Following cessation of use of a hallucinogen, the re-experiencing of one or more of the perceptual symptoms that were experienced while intoxicated with the hallucinogen (e.g. geometric hallucinations, false perceptions of movement in the peripheral visual fields, flashes of colours, intensified colours, trails of images of moving objects, positive afterimages, halos around objects, macropsia, and micropsia).

- The symptoms listed in the previous criterion cause clinically significant distress or impairment in social, occupational, or other important areas of functioning.

- The symptoms are not due to a general medical condition (e.g. anatomical lesions and infections of the brain, visual epilepsies) and are not better accounted for by another mental disorder (e.g. delirium, dementia, schizophrenia) or hypnopompic hallucinations.

In contrast with genuine psychosis, there is no paranoid misinterpretation of the perceptions in people who suffer from HPPD.[293] Studies on HPPD have recommended that other conditions be ruled out before a diagnosis of HPPD is made, including post-traumatic stress disorder (PTSD), depersonalisation and derealisation associated with severe anxiety and depression, as well as other hallucinogen-induced disorders recognised by DSM, such as hallucinogen-induced psychosis and mood or anxiety disorders.[289]

HPPD is both rare and unpredictable.[292] Estimates of the proportion of users who have experienced flashbacks on one or more occasions after hallucinogen use vary widely, from 5% to 50%.[300,301] However, many of these studies were conducted before the development of the DSM-3 diagnostic criteria for HPPD and are therefore difficult to interpret.[289] More recently, a 2003 review of the literature concluded that 'it seems inescapable that at least some individuals who have used LSD, in particular, experience persistent perceptual abnormalities reminiscent of acute intoxication, not better attributable to another medical or psychiatric condition, and persisting for weeks or months after last hallucinogen exposure'.[289] Current prevalence estimates are unknown, but DSM-5 suggests 4.2%.[302]

The exact causes of HPPD are not known. The condition is more often seen in individuals with a history of psychological problems or substance misuse,[303] but can arise in anyone, even after a single exposure.[304] HPPD is mainly associated with LSD use, but it has also been reported after use of other psychedelic drugs, including mushrooms,[305] mescaline[289] and 5-MeO-DIPT.[306] Other substances may trigger HPPD, including cannabis,[307] alcohol and MDMA.[308] HPPD or flashbacks have also been reported in people who have taken pharmaceutical drugs such as risperidone,[309] topiramate,[310] trazodone, mirtazapine, nefazodone[293] and SSRIs[311] and it has been suggested recently that hallucinogen use is not actually a necessary condition for this multifactorial syndrome.[293]

It has also been suggested that HPPD is in most cases due to a subtle over-activation of predominantly neural visual pathways after the use of hallucinogens. Factors that may predict vulnerability to HPPD include individual or family histories of anxiety, pre-drug use complaints of tinnitus, eye floaters, and concentration problems.[312]

HPPD also appears to be associated with the co-occurrence of depressive and anxiety traits and with severe mental illnesses such as major depressive disorder, bipolar disorder and schizophrenia spectrum disorders. However, onset of HPPD is not necessarily accompanied by any prominent additional psychiatric disorder, and is an independent condition.

Although not fully understood, reported triggers include existing mental disorders such as anxiety, mood and sleep disturbance, entering a dark environment, pregnancy and post-partum states, flashing car or neon lights, exposure to noise, and exercise.[313,314] Triggers including emotional (e.g. tension and anxiety), environmental (e.g. flickering lights), behavioural (e.g. sexual activity) and biological (e.g. use of other substances) triggers.[315,316,317] Among the many triggers able to precipitate the symptoms of those with existing HPPD, the use of natural and synthetic cannabinoids appears to be frequent.[318]

The analysis of the literature on HPPD suggests classification into two major subtypes of hallucinogenic substance-use related to recurring perceptual disturbances have been identified and reported: HPPD type I, also described and named as benign Flashback, or Flashback type I; and HPPD type II.[319,320]

It has been noted that the distinction between HPPD type I and HPPD type II has not yet been made in DSM-5 and is still debated. HPPD type I is consistent with the diagnostic definition in ICD-10, while HPPD type II better matches the DMS-5 criteria.[321]

- **HPPD type I** or brief flashbacks. HPPD type I is short-term, reversible and benign. HPPD type I is typically associated with 'auras', minor feelings of self-detachment, mild bewilderment, and mild depersonalisation and derealisation. Although it can provoke unpleasant feelings, it is not associated with significant concern, distress, and impairment in individual, familial, social, occupational, or other important areas of functioning.[20,21] The impairment is mild and the prognosis is usually good.[322,323,324,325,326,327]

- **HPPD type II** is suggested to have a chronic, relapsing and remitting course with fluctuating symptoms lasting months or even years, while HPPD type II visual disturbances are generally unpleasant, long-term, slowly reversible or irreversible, intruding, distressing, disabling, and pervasive reoccurrences.[328] It has a long-term, irreversible or slowly reversible and pervasive course The impairment of HPPD type II is severe with visual distortions and dissociative effects causing significant distress and the prognosis is worse than for HPPD type I. Significant impairment in social, occupational, or other important areas of functioning is usually observed in HPPD type II, but not HPPD type I.[329,330] Some of the patients fail to adapt and live with these long-lasting recurrent 'trips', and may require long-term support.[331,332,333, 334,335]

A study explored differences in triggers between individuals with HPPD type I and HPPD type II perceptual disturbances following LSD use and found that individuals in the HPPD type II group initiated LSD use at an earlier age in comparison to those in the HPPD type I group and used it more frequently than those with HPPD type I. In addition, in this sample, the mean age of subjects with HPPD type II was younger than among those with HPPD type I.[336] Individuals in the HPPD type II group reported significantly higher rates of lifetime use of synthetic cannabinoids, inhalants, and stimulants.[337]

12.13.2.2 Features, Symptoms and Increased Risks from HPPD

The symptoms of HPPD can include a range of ongoing disturbances, although visual disturbances appear most common. In contrast with psychosis, there is rarely persecutory misinterpretation of the perceptions in people who suffer from HPPD.[338,339,340,341,342,343,344,345,346,347,348]

Visual disturbances, which tend to be more prominent in HPPD, may be episodic or nearly continuous and must cause significant distress or impairment as specified in DSM-V type II, described in Section 12.13.2.1. There seems to be no strong correlation between HPPD and frequency of use of hallucinogens, with reported instances of HPPD in individuals with minimal exposure to hallucinogens.[349]

Common visual features include geometrical hallucinations, flashes or intensification of colour, movements, particularly in the peripheral vision, after images (palinopsia), visual trails and haloes.[350] Intensification of colour, flashing colours, geometric imagery and visual 'snow' appear to be common and resistant symptoms. Other visual symptoms can include teleopsia, pelopsia, macropsia, micropsia and false perception of movement of images in the peripheral field. Dissociative symptoms including depersonalisation and derealisation are also consistently associated with HPPD.[351] Moreover, some HPPD subjects report that

adaptation to the dark takes significantly longer compared with the general population.[352,353,354]

12.13.2.3 Treatment of HPPD

A survey using a web-based questionnaire reported that although symptoms of HPPD were common, only a few found them distressing enough or impairing enough to consider treatment, with constant symptoms increasing the likelihood of seeking treatment. Even when these symptoms were constant, they were not always considered problematic.[292]

Another study has found similarly that individuals in the HPPD type I group reported longer overall persistence of perceptual disorders than those in type II. However, this may be partially due to postponing psychiatric treatment, as flashback-type perceptual disorders commonly do not cause psychological distress and impaired function.[355]

There is no established treatment for HPPD and research is very limited. Some cases of HPPD are reported to have improved with the use of sunglasses,[299] psychotherapy[299] and behaviour modification.[356]

It has been argued that the fact that distinct substances, with completely different mechanisms of action, might lead or precipitate the genesis of HPPD, therefore suggesting a multifaceted aetiology. Thus, it is accordingly conceivable that different medications could be useful and helpful in the treatment of different subtypes of HPPD.[357]

Treatment outcomes have been reported from a number of pharmacological interventions, but the multifactorial nature of the disorder, and the prominence of co-morbidities, suggest the need for highly individualised treatment, with stress reduction, reduction of or abstinence from substance use (including alcohol and perhaps caffeine) and treatment of co-morbid disorders.[293]

Pharmacological interventions for HPPD have been used but many of the studies (especially older ones) had methodological limitations. These interventions have included several classes of antidepressants, anxiolytics and antipsychotics, a COMT inhibitor, naltrexone, levodopa, clonidine, lamotrigine[293] and citalopram.[358]

Over the years, there have been reports of treatment and positive outcomes using haloperidol,[359] diphenylhydantoin,[360] trifluoperazine,[361] barbiturates,[299] benzodiazepines,[299,362,363] carbamazepine,[364] sertraline,[365] naltrexone,[366], clonidine,[367,368], a combination of olanzapine and fluoxetine,[369] sertraline,[370] clonazepam,[371,372] reboxetine,[373,374] risperidone,[375,376,377] and lamotrigine.[378,379] Hermle et al. have suggested that the anti-epileptic lamotrigine may be a promising new medication for HPPD.[293,380]

Whereas some case reports described improvements in patients receiving these medications, there are also reports of worsening of HPPD in patients receiving for example phenothiazines,[299] risperidone[381,382,383] or serotonin-selective reuptake inhibitors.[384]

12.14 Psychosocial Interventions

See also Chapter 2.

References

1. Halpern JH, Suzuki J, Huertas PE, Passie T. Hallucinogens. In: *Addiction Medicine*, pp. 1083–1098. Cham, Springer, 2011.

2. Fantegrossi WE, Murnane KS, Reissig CJ. The behavioral pharmacology of hallucinogens. *Biochem Pharmacol* 2008;**75** (1):17–33.

3. Sinke C, Halpern JH, Zedler M, Neufeld J, Emrich HM, Passie T. Genuine and drug-induced synesthesia: a comparison. *Conscious Cogn* 2012;**21**(3):1419–1434.

4. Jacob P III, Shulgin AT. Structure-activity relationships of classic hallucinogens and their analogs. *NIDA Res Monogr* 1994;**146**:74–91.

5. Johnson M, Richards W, Griffiths R. Human hallucinogen research: guidelines for safety. *J Psychopharmacol* 2008;**22**(6):603–620. https://doi.org/10.1177 /0269881108093587

6. World Drug Report 2019 (United Nations publication, Sales No. E.19.XI.8).

7. World Drug Report 2019 (United Nations publication, Sales No. E.19.XI.8).

8. World Drug Report 2019 (United Nations publication, Sales No. E.19.XI.8).

9. Rickli A, Moning OD, Hoener MC, Liechti ME. Receptor interaction profiles of novel psychoactive tryptamines compared with classic hallucinogens. *Eur Neuropsychopharmacol* 2016;26(8):1327–1337. https://doi.org /10.1016/j.euroneuro.2016.05.001

10. Araújo AM, Carvalho F, de Lourdes Bastos M, Guedes de Pinho P, Carvalho M. The hallucinogenic world of tryptamines: an updated review. *Arch Toxicol* 2015 (online). https://doi.org/10.1007/s00204-015-1513-x

11. Tracy DK, Wood DM, Baumeister D. Novel psychoactive substances: types, mechanisms of action, and effects. *Br Med J* 2017;**356**:i6848. https://doi.org/10.1136/bmj.i6848

12. Araújo AM, Carvalho F, de Lourdes Bastos M, Guedes de Pinho P, Carvalho M. The hallucinogenic world of tryptamines: an updated review. *Arch Toxicol* 2015 (online). https://doi.org/10.1007/s00204-015-1513-x

13. Papoutsis I, Nikolaou P, Stefanidou M, Spiliopoulou C, Athanaselis S. 25B-NBOMe and its precursor 2C-B: modern trends and hidden dangers. *Forensic Toxicol* 2015;**33**:1–11. https://doi.org/10.1007/s11419-014-0242-9

14. Corazza O, Schifano F, Farre M, et al. Designer drugs on the Internet: a phenomenon out-of-control? The emergence of hallucinogenic drug Bromo-Dragonfly. *Curr Clin Pharmacol* 2011;**6**(2):125–129.

15. World Drug Report 2019 (United Nations publication, Sales No. E.19.XI.8).

16. Winter JC. Hallucinogens as discriminative stimuli in animals: LSD, phenethylamines, and tryptamines. *Psychopharmacology* 2009;**203**(2):251–263. https://doi.org/10.1007/s00213-008-1356-8

17. Corazza O, Schifano F, Farre M, et al. Designer drugs on the Internet: a phenomenon out-of-control? The emergence of hallucinogenic drug Bromo-Dragonfly. *Curr Clin Pharmacol* 2011;**6**(2):125–129.

18. Halberstadt AL, Geyer MA. Multiple receptors contribute to the behavioral effects of indoleamine hallucinogens. *Neuropharmacology* 2011;**61**(3):364–381.

19. Ray TS. Psychedelics and the human receptorome. *PLoS ONE* 2010;**5**(2):e9019.

20. Nichols DE. Hallucinogens. *Pharmacol Ther* 2004;**101** (2):131–181.

21. Frecska E, Szabo A, Winkelman MJ, Luna LE, McKenna DJ. A possibly sigma-1 receptor mediated role of dimethyltryptamine in tissue protection, regeneration, and immunity. *J Neural Transm* 2013;**120**(9):1295–1303.

22. Carhart-Harris RL, Erritzoe D, Williams T, et al. Neural correlates of the psychedelic state as determined by fMRI studies with psilocybin. *Proc Natl Acad Sci U S A* 2012;**109**(6):2138–2143. https://doi.org/10.1073/pnas .1119598109

23. Psychonaut Wiki Experience: BK-2C-B: Various experiences. https://psychonautwiki.org/wiki/Experience:BK-2C-B_-_Various_experiences

24. Alatrash G, Majhail NS, Pile JC. Rhabdomyolysis after ingestion of 'foxy', a hallucinogenic tryptaminederivative. *Mayo Clin Proc* 2006;**81**(4):550–551.

25. Curtis B, Kemp P, Harty L, Choi C, Christensen D. Postmortem identification and quantitation of 2,5-dimethoxy-4-n-propylthiophenethylamine using GC-MSD and GC-NPD. *J Anal Toxicol* 2003;**27**(7):493–498.

26. Kamour A, James D, Spears R, et al. Patterns of presentation and clinical toxicity after reported use of alpha methyltryptamine in the United Kingdom. A report from the UK National Poisons Information Service. *Clin Toxicol* 2014;**52**(3):192–197. https://doi.org/10.3109/15563650 .2014.885983

27. Meehan TJ, Bryant SM, Aks SE. Drugs of abuse: the highs and lows of altered mental states in the emergency department. *Emerg Med Clin North Am* 2010;**28**(3):663–682. https://doi.org /10.1016/j. emc.2010.03.012

28. Advisory Council on the Misuse of Drugs (ACMD). Update of the Generic Definition for Tryptamines. Published June 2014. Available at: www.gov.uk/government/uploads/system/uploa ds/attachment_data/file/318693/UpdateGenericDefinitionTry ptamines.pdf [last accessed 21 March 2022].

29. European Monitoring Centre for Drugs and Drug Addiction. New psychoactive substances in Europe: an update from the EU Early Warning System. Luxembourg, Publications Office of the European Union, 2015.

30. Gibbons S, Beharry S. An overview of emerging and new psychoactive substances in the United Kingdom. *Forensic Sci Int* 2016;**267**:25–34.

31. Schifano F, Duccio Papanti G, Orsolini L, Corkery JM. Novel psychoactive substances: the pharmacology of stimulants and hallucinogens. *Exp Rev Clin Pharmacol* 2016;**9**(7):943–954.

32. Gibbons S, Beharry S. An overview of emerging and new psychoactive substances in the United Kingdom. *Forensic Sci Int* 2016;**267**:25–34.

33. Rickli A, Moning OD, Hoener MC, Liechti ME. Receptor interaction profiles of novel psychoactive tryptamines compared with classic hallucinogens. *Eur Neuropsychopharmacol* 2016;**26**(8):1327–1337. https://doi.org /10.1016/j.euroneuro.2016.05.001

34. Palma-Conesa AJ, Ventura M, Galindo L, et al. Something new about something old: a 10-year follow-up on classical and new psychoactive tryptamines and results of analysis. *J Psychoactive Drugs* 2017 (online). https://doi.org/10.1080/02791072 .2017.1320732

35. Rickli A, Moning OD, Hoener MC, Liechti ME. Receptor interaction profiles of novel psychoactive tryptamines compared with classic hallucinogens. *Eur Neuropsychopharmacol* 2016;**26**(8):1327–1337. https://doi.org /10.1016/j.euroneuro.2016.05.001

36. Schifano F, Duccio Papanti G, Orsolini L, Corkery JM. Novel psychoactive substances: the pharmacology of stimulants and hallucinogens. *Exp Rev Clin Pharmacol* 2016;**9**(7):943–954.

37. Schifano F, Duccio Papanti G, Orsolini L, Corkery JM. Novel psychoactive substances: the pharmacology of stimulants and hallucinogens. *Exp Rev Clin Pharmacol* 2016;**9**(7):943–954.

38. Schifano F, Duccio Papanti G, Orsolini L, Corkery JM. Novel psychoactive substances: the pharmacology of stimulants and hallucinogens. *Exp Rev Clin Pharmacol* 2016;**9**(7):943–954.

39. Schifano F, Duccio Papanti G, Orsolini L, Corkery JM. Novel psychoactive substances: the pharmacology of stimulants and hallucinogens. *Exp Rev Clin Pharmacol* 2016;**9**(7):943–954.

40. Papaseit E, Farré M, Pérez-Mañá C, et al. Acute pharmacological effects of 2C-B in humans: an observational study. *Front Pharmacol* 2018;**9**:206.

41. González D, Torrens M, Farré M. Acute effects of the novel psychoactive drug 2C-B on emotions. *Biomed Res Int* 2015;**2015**:643878. https://doi.org/10.1155/2015/643878

42. González D, Ventura M, Caudevilla F, Torrens M, Farre M. Consumption of new psychoactive substances in a Spanish sample of research chemical users. *Hum Psychopharmacol* 2013;**28**:332–340. https://doi.org/10.1002/hup.2323

43. Fernández-Calderón F, Cleland CM, Palamar JJ. Polysubstance use profiles among electronic dance music party attendees in New York City and their relation to use of new psychoactive substances. *Addict Behav* 2017;**78**:85–93. https:// doi.org/10.1016/j.addbeh.2017.11.004

44. Papaseit E, Farré M, Pérez-Mañá C, et al. Acute pharmacological effects of 2C-B in humans: an observational study. *Front Pharmacol* 2018;**9**:206.

45. Schifano F, Duccio Papanti G, Orsolini L, Corkery JM. Novel psychoactive substances: the pharmacology of stimulants and hallucinogens. *Exp Rev Clin Pharmacol* 2016;**9**(7):943–954.

46. Nagai F, Nonaka R, Satoh Hasashi Kamimura K. The effects of non-medically used psychoactive drugs on monoamine neurotransmission in rat brain. *Eur J Pharmacol* 2007;**559**:132–137.

47. Rickli A, Luethi D, Reinisch J, et al. Receptor interaction profiles of novel N-2-methoxybenzyl (NBOMe) derivatives of 2,5-dimethoxy-substituted phenethylamines (2C drugs). *Neuropharmacology* 2015;**99**:546–553.

48. Braden MR, Parrish JC, Naylor JC, Nichols DE. Molecular interaction of serotonin 5-HT2A receptor residues Phe339 (6.51) and Phe340(6.52) with superpotent N-benzyl phenethylamine agonists. *Mol Pharmacol* 2006;**70**:1956–1964.

49. Schifano F, Duccio Papanti G, Orsolini L, Corkery JM. Novel psychoactive substances: the pharmacology of stimulants and hallucinogens. *Exp Rev Clin Pharmacol* 2016;**9**(7):943–954.

50. Schifano F, Duccio Papanti G, Orsolini L, Corkery JM. Novel psychoactive substances: the pharmacology of stimulants and hallucinogens. *Exp Rev Clin Pharmacol* 2016;**9**(7):943–954.

51. Schifano F, Duccio Papanti G, Orsolini L, Corkery JM. Novel psychoactive substances: the pharmacology of stimulants and hallucinogens. *Exp Rev Clin Pharmacol* 2016;**9**(7):943–954.

52. European Monitoring Centre for Drugs and Drug Addiction. EMCDDA–Europol Joint Report on a new psychoactive substance: 25I-NBOMe (4-iodo-2,5-dimethoxy-N-(2-methoxybenzyl)phenethylamine). Joint Reports, Luxembourg, Publications Office of the European Union, 2014. Available at: www.emcdda.europa.eu/system/files/publi cations/817/TDAS14003ENN_466654.pdf [last accessed 26 April 2022].

53. Rickli A, Luethi D, Reinisch J, et al. Receptor interaction profiles of novel N-2-methoxybenzyl (NBOMe) derivatives of 2,5-dimethoxy-substituted phenethylamines (2C drugs). *Neuropharmacology* 2015;**99**:546–553.

54. European Monitoring Centre for Drugs and Drug Addiction. EMCDDA–Europol Joint Report on a new psychoactive substance: 25I-NBOMe (4-iodo-2,5-dimethoxy-N-(2- methoxybenzyl)phenethylamine). Joint Reports, Luxembourg, Publications Office of the European Union, 2014. Available at: www.emcdda.europa.eu/system/files/pub lications/817/TDAS14003ENN_466654.pdf [last accessed 26 April 2022].

55. Rickli A, Luethi D, Reinisch J, et al. Receptor interaction profiles of novel N-2-methoxybenzyl (NBOMe) derivatives of 2,5-dimethoxy-substituted phenethylamines (2C drugs). *Neuropharmacology* 2015;**99**:546–553.

56. Rickli A, Hoener MC, Liechti ME. Monoamine transporter and receptor interaction profiles of novel psychoactive substances: para-halogenated amphetamines and pyrovalerone cathinones. *Eur Neuropsychopharmacol* 2015;**25**:365–376.

57. Rickli A, Luethi D, Reinisch J, et al. Receptor interaction profiles of novel N-2-methoxybenzyl (NBOMe) derivatives of 2,5-dimethoxy-substituted phenethylamines (2C drugs). *Neuropharmacology* 2015;**99**:546–553.

58. Krebs TS, Johansen P-Ø. Lysergic acid diethylamide (LSD) for alcoholism: meta-analysis of randomized controlled trials. *J Psychopharmacol* 2012;**26**(7):994–1002.

59. Lancet. Reviving research into psychedelic drugs (editorial). *Lancet* 2006;**367**:1214.

60. Sessa B. Can psychedelics have a role in psychiatry once again. *Br J Psychiatry* 2005;**186**:457–458.

61. Frecska E, Luna LE. The adverse effects of hallucinogens from intramural perspective. *Neuropsychopharmacol* 2006;**8**:189–200.

62. Morris K. Hallucinogen research inspires 'neurotheology'. *Lancet Neurol* 2006;**5**:732.

63. Gasser P, Holstein D, Michel Y, Doblin R, Passie T, Brenneisen R. Safety and efficacy of lysergic acid diethylamide-assisted psychotherapy for anxiety associated with life-threatening diseases. *J Nerv Ment Dis* 2014;**202** (7):513–520. https://doi.org/10.1097/NMD .0000000000000113

64. Grob CS, Danforth AL, Chopra GS, et al. Pilot study of psilocybin treatment for anxiety in patients with advanced-stage cancer. *Arch Gen Psychiatry* 2011;**68** (1):71–78. https://doi.org/10.1001/archgenpsychiatry .2010.116

65. Moreno FA, Wiegand CB, Taitano EK, Delgado PL. Safety, tolerability, and efficacy of psilocybin in 9 patients with obsessive-compulsive disorder. *J Clin Psychiatry* 2006;**67** (11):1735–1740.

66. Carhart-Harris RL, Goodwin GM. The therapeutic potential of psychedelic drugs: past, present, and future. *Neuropsychopharmacology* 2017;**42**:2105–2113.

67. Garcia-Romeu A, Kersgaard B, Addy PH. Clinical applications of hallucinogens: a review. *Exp Clin Psychopharmacol* 2016;**24**:229–268.

68. Carhart-Harris RL, Murphy K, Leech R, et al. The effects of acutely administered 3,4-methylenedioxymethamphetamine on spontaneous brain function in healthy volunteers measured with arterial spin labeling and blood oxygen level-dependent resting state functional connectivity. *Biol Psychiatry* 2015;**78**:554–562.

69. Carhart-Harris RL, Wall MB, Erritzoe D, et al. The effect of acutely administered MDMA on subjective and BOLD-fMRI responses to favourite and worst autobiographical memories. *Int J Neuropsychopharmacol* 2014;**17**:527–540.

70. Carhart-Harris RL, Bolstridge M, Rucker J, et al. Psilocybin with psychological support for treatment-resistant depression: an open-label feasibility study. *Lancet Psychiatry* 2016;**3**:619–627.

71. Davis AK, So S, Lancelotta R, Barsuglia JP, Griffiths RR. Methoxy-N,N-dimethyltryptamine (5-MeO-DMT) used in a naturalistic group setting is associated with unintended improvements in depression and anxiety.*Am J Drug Alcohol Abuse* 2019;**45**(2):161–169. doi.org/10.1080/00952990 .2018.1545024

72. Griffiths RR, Johnson MW, Carducci MA, et al. Psilocybin produces substantial and sustained decreases in depression and anxiety in patients with life-threatening cancer: a randomized double-blind trial. *J Psychopharmacol* 2016;**30**:1181–1197.

73. Ross S, Bossis A, Guss J, et al. Rapid and sustained symptom reduction following psilocybin treatment for anxiety and depression in patients with life-threatening cancer: a randomized controlled trial. *J Psychopharmacol* 2016;**30**:1165–1180.

74. Gasser P, Holstein D, Michel Y, et al. Safety and efficacy of lysergic acid diethylamide-assisted psychotherapy for anxiety associated with life-threatening diseases. *J Nerv Ment Dis* 2014;**202**:513–520.

75. Nutt D. Psilocybin for anxiety and depression in cancer care? Lessons from the past and prospects for the future. *J Psychopharmacol* 2016;30(12):1163–1164. https://doi.org/10 .1177/0269881116675754

76. Griffiths RR, Johnson MW, Carducci MA, et al. Psilocybin produces substantial and sustained decreases in depression and anxiety in patients with life-threatening cancer: a randomized double-blind trial. *J Psychopharmacol* 2016;**30**:1181–1197.

77. Byock I. Taking psychedelics seriously. *J Palliat Med* 2018;**21** (4):417–421.

78. Bogenschutz MP, Forcehimes AA, Pommy JA, Wilcox CE, Barbosa PC, Strassman RJ. Psilocybin-assisted treatment for alcohol dependence: a proof-of-concept study. *J Psychopharmacol* 2015;**29**:289–299.

79. Johnson MW, Garcia-Romeu A, Griffiths RR. Long-term follow-up of psilocybin-facilitated smoking cessation. *Am J Drug Alcohol Abuse* 2017;**43**:55–60.

80. Bogenschutz MP, Johnson MW. Classic hallucinogens in the treatment of addictions. *Prog Neuropsychopharmacol*2016;**64**:250–258.

81. Bogenschutz MP, Johnson MW. Classic hallucinogens in the treatment of addictions. *Prog Neuropsychopharmacol*2016;**64**:250–258.

82. Bogenschutz MP, Johnson MW. Classic hallucinogens in the treatment of addictions. *Prog Neuropsychopharmacol*2016;**64**:250–258.

83. World Drug Report 2019 (United Nations publication, Sales No. E.19.XI.8).

84. European Monitoring Centre for Drugs and Drug Addiction. European Drug Report 2019: Trends and Developments. Luxembourg, Publications Office of the European Union, 2019.

85. See for example www.bbc.co.uk/news/health-39516345 [last accessed 21 March 2022].

86. Johnstad PG. Powerful substances in tiny amounts: an interview study of psychedelic microdosing. *Nordic Studies on Alcohol and Drugs* 2018;**35**(1):39–51.

87. Savulich G, Piercy T, Bruhl AB, et al. Focusing the neuroscience and societal implications of cognitive enhancers. *Clin Pharmacol Ther* 2017;**101**(2):170–172.

88. d'Angelo L-SC, Savulich G, Sahakian BJ. Lifestyle use of drugs by healthy people for enhancing cognition, creativity, motivation and pleasure. *Br J Pharmacol* 2017;**174**:3257–3267.

89. Johnstad PG. Powerful substances in tiny amounts: an interview study of psychedelic microdosing. *Nordic Studies on Alcohol and Drugs* 2018;**35**(1):39–51.

90. Passie T, Halpern JH, Stichtenoth DO, Emrich HM, Hintzen A. The pharmacology of lysergic acid diethylamide: a review. *CNS Neurosci Ther* 2008;**14**(4):295–314.

91. Coppola M, Mondola R. Bromo-Dragon Fly: chemistry, pharmacology and toxicology of a benzodifuran derivative producing LSD-like effects. *J Addict Res Ther* 2012;**3**(133):2.

92. Schifano F, Duccio Papanti G, Orsolini L, Corkery JM. Novel psychoactive substances: the pharmacology of stimulants and hallucinogens. *Exp Rev Clin Pharmacol* 2016;**9**(7):943–954.

93. Winstock AR, Kaar S, Borschmann R. Dimethyltryptamine (DMT): prevalence, user characteristics and abuse liability in a large global sample. *J Psychopharmacol* 2014;**28**(1):49–54. https://doi.org/10.1177/0269881113513852

94. Schifano F, Duccio Papanti G, Orsolini L, Corkery JM. Novel psychoactive substances: the pharmacology of stimulants and hallucinogens. *Exp Rev Clin Pharmacol* 2016;**9**(7):943–954.

95. Winstock AR, Kaar S, Borschmann R. Dimethyltryptamine (DMT): prevalence, user characteristics and abuse liability in a large global sample. *J Psychopharmacol* 2014;**28**(1):49–54. https://doi.org/10.1177/0269881113513852

96. Barsuglia J, Davis AK, Palmer R, et al. Intensity of mystical experiences occasioned by 5-MeO-DMT and comparison with a prior psilocybin.*Study Front Psychol* 2018;**9**:2459. doi.org/10.3389/fpsyg.2018.02459

97. Caudevilla-Gálligo F, Riba J, Ventura M, et al. 4-bromo-2,5-dimethoxyphenethylamine (2C-B): presence in the recreational drug market in Spain, pattern of use and subjective effects. *J Psychopharmacol* 2012;**26**(7):1026–1035. https://doi.org/10.1177/0269881111431752

98. Strassman R. Human psychopharmacology of LSD, dimethyltryptamine and related compounds. In: A Pletscher, D Ladewig, (eds.), *Fifty Years of LSD: Current Status and Perspectives of Hallucinogens*, pp. 145–174. New York, Parthenon, 1994.

99. Gibbons S, Beharry S. An overview of emerging and new psychoactive substances in the United Kingdom. *Forensic Sci Int* 2016;**267**:25–34.

100. Schifano F, Duccio Papanti G, Orsolini L, Corkery JM. Novel psychoactive substances: the pharmacology of stimulants and hallucinogens. *Exp Rev Clin Pharmacol* 2016;**9**(7):943–954.

101. Shulgin A, Shulgin A. *PIHKAL: A Chemical Love Story*. Berkeley, CA, Transform Press, 1991.

102. Corazza O, Schifano F, Farre M, et al. Designer drugs on the Internet: a phenomenon out-of-control? The emergence of hallucinogenic drug Bromo-Dragonfly. *Curr Clin Pharmacol* 2011;**6**(2):125–129.

103. Strassman R. Human psychopharmacology of LSD, dimethyltryptamine and related compounds. In: A Pletscher, D Ladewig, (eds.), *Fifty Years of LSD: Current Status and Perspectives of Hallucinogens*, pp. 145–174. New York, Parthenon, 1994.

104. Schifano F, Duccio Papanti G, Orsolini L, Corkery JM. Novel psychoactive substances: the pharmacology of stimulants and hallucinogens. *Exp Rev Clin Pharmacol* 2016;**9**(7):943–954.

105. Gibbons S, Beharry S. An overview of emerging and new psychoactive substances in the United Kingdom. *Forensic Sci Int* 2016;**267**:25–34.

106. Schifano F, Duccio Papanti G, Orsolini L, Corkery JM. Novel psychoactive substances: the pharmacology of stimulants and hallucinogens. *Exp Rev Clin Pharmacol* 2016;**9**(7):943–954.

107. Corazza O, Schifano F, Farre M, et al. Designer drugs on the Internet: a phenomenon out-of-control? The emergence of hallucinogenic drug Bromo-Dragonfly. *Curr Clin Pharmacol* 2011;6(2):125–129.

108. Caldicott DG, Bright SJ, Barratt MJ. NBOMe – a very different kettle of fish. . . . *Med J Aust* 2013;**199**(5):322–323.

109. Laing RR, Beyerstein BL. Forms of the drug. In: JA Siegel, (ed.), *Hallucinogens: A Forensic Drug Handbook*, pp. 39–41. Washington DC, Academic Press, 2003.

110. Schifano F, Duccio Papanti G, Orsolini L, Corkery JM. Novel psychoactive substances: the pharmacology of stimulants and hallucinogens. *Exp Rev Clin Pharmacol* 2016;**9**(7):943–954.

111. Rickli A, Hoener MC, Liechti ME. Monoamine transporter and receptor interaction profiles of novel psychoactive substances: para-halogenated amphetamines and pyrovalerone cathinones. *Eur Neuropsychopharmacol* 2015;**25**:365–376

112. Lawn W, Barratt M, Williams M, Horne A, Winstock A. The NBOMe hallucinogenic drug series: patterns of use,

characteristics of users and self-reported effects in a large international sample. *J Psychopharmacol* 2014;**28**(8):780–788.

113. Bersani FS, Corazza O, Albano G, et al. 25C-NBOme: preliminary data on pharmacology, psychoactive effects, and toxicity of a new potent and dangerous hallucinogenic drug. *Biomed Res Int* 2014;**2014**:734749. https://doi.org/10.1155/2014/734749

114. Schifano F, Duccio Papanti G, Orsolini L, Corkery JM. Novel psychoactive substances: the pharmacology of stimulants and hallucinogens. *Exp Rev Clin Pharmacol* 2016;**9**(7):943–954.

115. Hassan Z, Bosch OG, Singh D, et al. Novel psychoactive substances: recent progress on neuropharmacological mechanisms of action for selected drugs. *Front Psychiatry* 2017 (online). https://doi.org/10.3389/fpsyt.2017.00152

116. Gibbons S, Beharry S. An overview of emerging and new psychoactive substances in the United Kingdom. *Forensic Sci Int* 2016;**267**:25–34.

117. Caudevilla-Gálligo F, Riba J, Ventura M, et al. 4-Bromo-2,5-dimethoxyphenethylamine (2C-B): presence in the recreational drug market in Spain, pattern of use and subjective effects. *J Psychopharmacol* 2012;26(7):1026–1035. https://doi.org/10.1177/0269881111431752

118. Valento M, Lebin J. Emerging drugs of abuse: synthetic cannabinoids, phenylethylamines (2C drugs), and synthetic cathinones. *Clin Pediatr Emerg Med* 2017;**18**(3):203–211. https://doi.org/10.1016/j.cpem.2017.07.009

119. Buffin J, Roy A, Williams H, Winter A. Part of the Picture: Lesbian, Gay and Bisexual People's Alcohol and Drug Use in England (2009–2011). Manchester, Lesbian and Gay Foundation, 2012.

120. Andreasen MF, Telving R, Birkler RI, Schumacher B, Johannsen M. A fatal poisoning involving BromoDragonfly. *Forensic Sci Int* 2009;**183**(1–3):91–96. https://doi.org/10.1016/j.forsciint.2008.11.001

121. Lheureux P, Penaloza A, Gris M. Club drugs: a new challenge in clinical toxicology. In: *Intensive Care Medicine*, pp. 811–820. Cham, Springer, 2003.

122. McCambridge J, Winstock A, Hunt N, Mitcheson L. 5-year trends in use of hallucinogens and other adjunct drugs among UK dance drug users. *Eur Addict Res* 2006;**13**(1):57–64.

123. Williams RH, Erickson T. Evaluating hallucinogenic or psychedelic drug intoxication in an emergency setting. *Lab Med* 2000;**31**(7):394–401.

124. World Drug Report 2019 (United Nations publication, Sales No. E.19.XI.8).

125. World Drug Report 2019 (United Nations publication, Sales No. E.19.XI.8).

126. World Drug Report 2019 (United Nations publication, Sales No. E.19.XI.8).

127. World Drug Report 2019 (United Nations publication, Sales No. E.19.XI.8).

128. Schifano F, Duccio Papanti G, Orsolini L, Corkery JM. Novel psychoactive substances: the pharmacology of stimulants and hallucinogens. *Exp Rev Clin Pharmacol* 2016;**9**(7):943–954.

129. Shulgin A, Shulgin A. *TIHKAL: The Continuation.* Washington, DC, Transform Press, 1997.

130. Benschop A, Urbán R, Kapitány-Fövény M, et al. Why do people use new psychoactive substances? Development of a new measurement tool in six European countries. *J Psychopharmacol* 2020;**34**(6):600–611. https://doi.org/10.1177/0269881120904951

131. Global Drug Survey. Drug Pleasure Ratings. Available at: www.globaldrugsurvey.com/past-findings/the-net-pleasure-index-results/ [last accessed 26 April 2022].

132. Benschop A, Urbán R, Kapitány-Fövény M, et al. Why do people use new psychoactive substances? Development of a new measurement tool in six European countries. *J Psychopharmacol* 2020;**34**(6):600–611. https://doi.org/10.1177/0269881120904951

133. Schifano F, Duccio Papanti G, Orsolini L, Corkery JM. Novel psychoactive substances: the pharmacology of stimulants and hallucinogens. *Exp Rev Clin Pharmacol* 2016;**9**(7):943–954.

134. Papaseit E, Farré M, Pérez-Mañá C, et al. Acute pharmacological effects of 2C-B in humans: an observational study. *Front Pharmacol* 2018;9:206.

135. Shulgin AT, Carter MF. Centrally active phenethylamines. *Psychopharm Commun* 1975;**1**:93–98.

136. C audevilla-Gálligo F, Riba J, Ventura M, et al. 4-Bromo-2,5-dimethoxyphenethylamine (2C-B): presence in the recreational drug market in Spain, pattern of use and subjective effects. *J Psychopharmacol* 2012;**26**(7):1026–1035. https://doi.org/10.1177/0269881111431752

137. De Boer D, Gijzels MJ, Bosman IJ, Maes RAA. More data about the new psychoactive drug 2C-B. *J Analytic Toxicol* 1999;**23**(3):227–228.

138. Schifano F, Duccio Papanti G, Orsolini L, Corkery JM. Novel psychoactive substances: the pharmacology of stimulants and hallucinogens. *Exp Rev Clin Pharmacol* 2016;**9**(7):943–954.

139. Schifano F, Duccio Papanti G, Orsolini L, Corkery JM. Novel psychoactive substances: the pharmacology of stimulants and hallucinogens. *Exp Rev Clin Pharmacol* 2016;**9**(7):943–954.

140. Davis AK, Barsuglia JP, Lancelotta R, Grant RM, Renn E. The epidemiology of 5-methoxy-N,N-dimethyltryptamine (5-MeODMT) use: benefits, consequences, patterns of use, subjective effects, and reasons for consumption. *Psychopharmacology* 2018;**32**(7):779–792. https://doi.org/10.1177/0269881118769063

141. Griffiths RR, Richards WA, McCann U, et al. Psilocybin can occasion mystical-type experiences having substantial and sustained personal meaning and spiritual significance. *Psychopharmacology* 2006;**187**(3):268–283; discussion 284–292. https://doi.org/10.1007/s00213-006-0457-5

142. Maclean KA, Leoutsakos J-MS, Johnson MW, et al. Factor analysis of the mystical experience questionnaire: a study of experiences occasioned by the hallucinogen psilocybin. *JSSR* 2012;**51**(4): 721–737. https://doi.org/10.1111/j.1468-5906.2012.01685.x

143. Barrett FS, Bradstreet MP, Leoutsakos J-MS, et al. The Challenging Experience Questionnaire: characterization of challenging experiences with psilocybin mushrooms. *J Psychopharmacol* 2016;**30**(12):1279–1295. https://doi.org/10.1177/0269881116678781

144. Schifano F, Duccio Papanti G, Orsolini L, Corkery JM. Novel psychoactive substances: the pharmacology of stimulants and hallucinogens. *Exp Rev Clin Pharmacol* 2016;**9**(7):943–954.

145. Hassan Z, Bosch OG, Singh D, et al. Novel psychoactive substances: recent progress on neuropharmacological mechanisms of action for selected drugs. *Front Psychiatry* 2017 (online). https://doi.org/10.3389/fpsyt.2017.00152

146. Timmermann C, Roseman L, Williams L, et al. DMT models the near-death experience. *Front Psychol* 2018;**9**:1424.

147. Gibbons S, Beharry S. An overview of emerging and new psychoactive substances in the United Kingdom. *Forensic Sci Int* 2016;**267**:25–34.

148. Gable RS. Risk assessment of ritual use of oral dimethyltryptamine (DMT) and harmala alkaloids. *Addiction* 2007;**102**(1):24–34.

149. Studerus EA. Prediction of psilocybin response in healthy volunteers. *PloS ONE* 2012;**7**(2):e30800.

150. Davis AK, Barsuglia JP, Lancelotta R, Grant RM, Renn E. The epidemiology of 5-methoxy-N,N-dimethyltryptamine (5-MeODMT) use: benefits, consequences, patterns of use, subjective effects, and reasons for consumption. *Psychopharmacology* 2018;**32**(7):779–792. https://doi.org/10.1177/0269881118769063

151. Garcia-Romeu A, Griffiths RR, Johnson MW. Psilocybin-occasioned mystical experiences in the treatment of tobacco addiction. *Curr Drug Abuse Rev* 2015;**7**(3):157–164.

152. McGeeney BE. Cannabinoids and hallucinogens for headache. *Headache* 2013;**53**:447–458. https://doi.org/10.1111/head.12025

153. Sewell RA, Halpern JH, Pope HG. Response of cluster headache to psilocybin and LSD. *Neurology* 2006;**66**(12):1920–1922

154. Karst M, Halpern JH, Bernateck M, Passie T. The non-hallucinogen 2-bromo-lysergic acid diethylamide as preventative treatment for cluster headache: an open, non-randomized case series. *Cephalalgia* 2010;**30**(9):1140–1144.

155. Kast EC, Collins VJ. Study of lysergic acid diethylamide as an analgesic agent. *Anesth Analg* 1964;**43**(3):285–291.

156. McCabe OL. Psychedelic drug crises: toxicity and therapeutics. *J Psychedelic Drugs* 1977;**9**:107–121.

157. Grinspoon L, Bakalar JB. *Psychedelic Drugs Reconsidered.* New York, Basic Books, 1979.

158. Strassman RJ. Adverse reactions to psychedelic drugs: a review of the literature. *J Nerv Ment Dis* 1984;**172**:577–595.

159. Klock JC, Boerner U, Becker CE. Coma, hyperthermia and bleeding associated with massive LSD overdose. A report of eight cases. *West J Med* 1974;**120**(3):183–188.

160. Solursh LP, Clement WR. Hallucinogenic drug abuse: manifestations and management. *Can Med Assoc J* 1968;**98**(8):407.

161. Riba J, Barbanoj MJ. Bringing ayahuasca to the clinical research laboratory. *J Psychoactive Drugs* 2005;**37**(2):219–230.

162. Johnson MW, Sewell RA, Griffiths RR. Psilocybin dose-dependently causes delayed, transient headaches in healthy volunteers. *Drug Alcohol Depend* 2012;**123**(1):132–140.

163. Lawn W, Barratt M, Williams M, et al. The NBOMe hallucinogenic drug series: patterns of use, characteristics of users and self-reported effects in a large international sample. *J Psychopharmacol* 2014;**28**:780–788.

164. Caldicott DG, Bright SJ, Barratt MJ. NBOMe – a very different kettle of fish. *Med J Aust* 2013;**199**:322–323.

165. Gee P, Schep LJ, Jensen BP, Moore G, Barrington S. Case series: toxicity from 25B-NBOMe – a cluster of N-bomb cases. *Clin Toxicol* 2016;**54**(2):141–146. https://doi.org/10.3109/15563650.2015.1115056

166. Gable RS. Comparison of acute lethal toxicity of commonly abused psychoactive substances. *Addiction* 2004;**99**(6):686–696.

167. Luethi D, Trachsel D, Hoener MC, Liechti ME. Monoamine receptor interaction profiles of 4-thio-substituted phenethylamines (2C-T drugs). *Neuropharmacology* 2018;**134**(Part A):141–148. https://doi.org/10.1016/j.neuropharm.2017.07.012

168. Wood DM. Delayed onset of seizures and toxicity associated with recreational use of Bromo-dragon Fly. *J Med Toxicol* 2009;**5**(4):226–229.

169. Peden NR, Pringle SD, Crooks J. The problem of psilocybin mushroom abuse. *Hum Exp Toxicol* 1982;**1**(4):417–424.

170. Kaufman KR. Anxiety and panic. In: AB Ettinger, DM Weisbrot, (eds.), *Neurologic Differential Diagnosis: A Case-Based Approach*, pp. 22–33. Cambridge, Cambridge University Press, 2014.

171. Wilson JM, McGeorge F, Smolinske S, Meatherall R. A foxy intoxication. *Forensic Sci Int* 2005;**148**(1):31–36.

172. Cooles P. Abuse of the mushroom *Panaeolus foenisecii. Br Med J* 1980;**280**(6212):446.

173. TOXBASE®. LSD. www.toxbase.org

174. TOXBASE®. Ayahuasca. www.toxbase.org

175. Hinkelbein J, Gabel A, Volz M, Ellinger K. Suicide attempt with high-dose ecstasy. *Der Anaesthesist* 2003;**52**(1):51–54.

176. Nielen RJ, van der Heijden FM, Tuinier S, Verhoeven WM. Khat and mushrooms associated with psychosis. *World J Biol Psychiatry* 2004;**5**(1):49–53.

177. Reich P, Hepps RB. Homicide during a psychosis induced by LSD. *JAMA* 1972;**219**(7):869–871.

178. Itokawa M, Iwata K, Takahashi M et al. Acute confusional state after designer tryptamine abuse. *Psychiatry Clin Neurosci* 2007;**61**(2):196–199.

179. Boland DM, Andollo W, Hime GW, Hearn WL. Fatality due to acute α-methyltryptamine intoxication. *J Analytic Toxicol* 2005;**29**(5):394–397.

180. Fysh RR, Oon MCH, Robinson KN, Smith RN, White PC, Whitehouse MJ. A fatal poisoning with LSD. *Forensic Sci Int* 1985;**8**(2):109–113.

181. Berrens Z, Lammers J, White C. Rhabdomyolysis after LSD ingestion. *Psychosomatics* 2010;**51**(4):356. https://doi.org/10.1176/appi.psy.51.4.356

182. Goforth HW, Fernandez F. Acute neurologic effects of alcohol and drugs. *Neurol Clin* 2012;**30**(1):277–284.

183. Gable RS. Acute toxic effects of club drugs. *J Psychoactive Drugs* 2004;**36**(3):303–313.

184. Gibbons S, Beharry S. An overview of emerging and new psychoactive substances in the United Kingdom. *Forensic Sci Int* 2016;**267**:25–34.

185. Gibbons S, Beharry S. An overview of emerging and new psychoactive substances in the United Kingdom. *Forensic Sci Int* 2016;**267**:25–34.

186. Luethi D, Trachsel D, Hoener MC, Liechti ME. Monoamine receptor interaction profiles of 4-thio-substituted phenethylamines (2C-T drugs). *Neuropharmacology* 2018;**134** (Part A):141–148. https://doi.org/10.1016/j.neuropharm.2017.07.012

187. Schifano F, Duccio Papanti G, Orsolini L, Corkery JM. Novel psychoactive substances: the pharmacology of stimulants and hallucinogens. *Exp Rev Clin Pharmacol* 2016;**9**(7):943–954.

188. Dean BV, Stellpflug SJ, Burnett AM, Engebretsen KM. 2C or not 2C: phenethylamine designer drug review. *J Med Toxicol* 2013;**9**(2):172–178. https://doi.org/10.1007/s13181-013-0295-x

189. Tang MH, Ching CK, Tsui MS, Chu FK, Mak TW. Two cases of severe intoxication associated with analytically confirmed use of the novel psychoactive substances 25B-NBOMe and 25C-NBOMe. *Clin Toxicol* 2014;**52**(5):561–565. https://doi.org/10.3109/15563650.2014.909932

190. Armenian P, Gerona RR. The electric Kool-Aid NBOMe test: LC-TOF/MS confirmed 2C-C-NBOMe (25C) intoxication at Burning Man. *Am J Emerg Med* 2014;**32**(11):1444.e3–5. https://doi.org/10.1016/j.ajem.2014.04.047

191. Schifano F, Duccio Papanti G, Orsolini L, Corkery JM. Novel psychoactive substances: the pharmacology of stimulants and hallucinogens. *Exp Rev Clin Pharmacol* 2016;**9**(7):943–954.

192. Schifano F, Duccio Papanti G, Orsolini L, Corkery JM. Novel psychoactive substances: the pharmacology of stimulants and hallucinogens. *Exp Rev Clin Pharmacol* 2016;**9**(7):943–954.

193. Gee P, Schep LJ, Jensen BP, Moore G, Barrington S. Case series: toxicity from 25B-NBOMe – a cluster of N-bomb cases. *Clin Toxicol* 2016;**54**(2):141–146. https://doi.org/10.3109/15563650.2015.1115056

194. Kelly A, Eisenga B, Riley B, et al. Case series of 25I-NBOMe exposures with laboratory confirmation. *Clin Toxicol* 2012;**50**:702.

195. Rose SR, Poklis JL, Poklis A. A case of 25I-NBOMe (25-I) intoxication: a new potent 5-HT2A agonist designer drug. *Clin Toxicol* 2013;**51**:174.

196. Hill SL, Doris T, Gurung S, et al. Severe clinical toxicity associated with analytically confirmed recreational use of 25I-NBOMe: case series. *Clin Toxicol* 2013;**51**:487.

197. Srisuma S, Bronstein AC, Hoyte CO. NBOMe and 2C substitute phenylethylamine exposures reported to the National Poison Data System. *Clin Toxicol* 2015;**11**:1–5.
    Forrester MB. NBOMe designer drug exposures reported to Texas poison centers. *J Addict Dis* 2014;**33**:196–201.

198. Valento M, Lebin J. Emerging drugs of abuse: synthetic cannabinoids, phenylethylamines (2C drugs), and synthetic cathinones. *Clin Pediatr Emerg Med* 2017;**18**(3):203–211. https://doi.org/10.1016/j.cpem.2017.07.009

199. Gee P, Schep LJ, Jensen BP, et al. Case series: toxicity from 25B-NBOMe: a cluster of N-bomb cases. *Clin Toxicol* 2016;**54**:141–146.

200. Wood DM, Sedefov R, Cunningham A, Dargan PI. Prevalence of use and acute toxicity associated with the use of NBOMe drugs. *Clin Toxicol* 2015;**53**:85–92.

201. Schifano F, Duccio Papanti G, Orsolini L, Corkery JM. Novel psychoactive substances: the pharmacology of stimulants and hallucinogens. *Exp Rev Clin Pharmacol* 2016;**9**(7):943–954.

202. Halberstadt AL. Pharmacology and toxicology of N-Benzylphenethylamine ('NBOMe') Hallucinogens. In: M Baumann, R Glennon, J Wiley (eds.), *Neuropharmacology of New Psychoactive Substances (NPS). Current Topics in Behavioral Neurosciences*, **vol. 32**. Cham, Springer, 2017.

203. Gee P, Schep LJ, Jensen BP, et al. Case series: toxicity from 25B-NBOMe: a cluster of N-bomb cases. *Clin Toxicol* 2016;**54**:141–146.

204. Gee P, Schep LJ, Jensen BP, et al. Case series: toxicity from 25B-NBOMe: a cluster of N-bomb cases. *Clin Toxicol* 2016;**54**:141–146.

205. Forrester MB. NBOMe designer drug exposures reported to Texas poison centers. *J Addict Dis* 2014;**33**:196–201.

206. Suzuki J, Dekker MA, Valenti ES, et al. Toxicities associated with NBOMe ingestion: a novel class of potent hallucinogens: a review of the literature. *Psychosomatics*. 2014;**56**:129–139.

207. Wood DM, Sedefov R, Cunningham A, et al. Prevalence of use and acute toxicity associated with the use of NBOMe drugs. *Clin Toxicol* 2015;**53**:85–92.

208. Srisuma S, Bronstein AC, Hoyte CO. NBOMe and 2C substitute phenylethylamine exposures reported to the National Poison Data System. *Clin Toxicol* 2015;**11**:1–5.

209. Poklis JL, Nanco CR, Troendle MM, et al. Determination of 4-bromo2,5-dimethoxy-N-[(2-methoxyphenyl)methyl]-benzeneethanamine (25B-NBOMe) in serum and urine by high performance liquid chromatography with tandem mass spectrometry in a case of severe intoxication. *Drug Test Anal* 2014;**6**:764–769.

210. Schifano F, Duccio Papanti G, Orsolini L, Corkery JM. Novel psychoactive substances: the pharmacology of stimulants and hallucinogens. *Exp Rev Clin Pharmacol* 2016;**9**(7):943–954.

211. Schifano F, Duccio Papanti G, Orsolini L, Corkery JM. Novel psychoactive substances: the pharmacology of stimulants and hallucinogens. *Exp Rev Clin Pharmacol* 2016;**9**(7):943–954.

212. Schifano F, Duccio Papanti G, Orsolini L, Corkery JM. Novel psychoactive substances: the pharmacology of stimulants and hallucinogens. *Exp Rev Clin Pharmacol* 2016;**9**(7):943–954.

213. Jebadurai J, Schifano F, Deluca P. Recreational use of 1-(2-naphthyl)-2-(1- pyrrolidinyl)-1-pentanone hydrochloride (NRG-1), 6-(2-aminopropyl) benzofuran (benzofury/6-APB) and NRG-2 with review of available evidence-based literature. *Hum Psychopharmacol* 2013;**28**:356–364.

214. Schifano F, Duccio Papanti G, Orsolini L, Corkery JM. Novel psychoactive substances: the pharmacology of stimulants and hallucinogens. *Exp Rev Clin Pharmacol* 2016;**9**(7):943–954.

215. Corazza O, Schifano F, Farre M, et al. Designer drugs on the Internet: a phenomenon out-of-control? The emergence of hallucinogenic drug Bromo-Dragonfly. *Curr Clin Pharmacol* 2011;**6**:125–129.

216. Schifano F, Duccio Papanti G, Orsolini L, Corkery JM. Novel psychoactive substances: the pharmacology of stimulants and hallucinogens. *Exp Rev Clin Pharmacol* 2016;**9**(7):943–954.

217. Schifano F, Duccio Papanti G, Orsolini L, Corkery JM. Novel psychoactive substances: the pharmacology of stimulants and hallucinogens. *Exp Rev Clin Pharmacol* 2016;**9**(7):943–954.

218. Dargan PI, Wood DM. *Novel Psychoactive Substances: Classification, Pharmacology and Toxicology*. London, Academic Press/Elsevier, 2013.

219. Schifano F, Duccio Papanti G, Orsolini L, Corkery JM. Novel psychoactive substances: the pharmacology of stimulants and hallucinogens. *Exp Rev Clin Pharmacol* 2016;**9**(7):943–954.

220. Schifano F, Duccio Papanti G, Orsolini L, Corkery JM. Novel psychoactive substances: the pharmacology of stimulants and hallucinogens. *Exp Rev Clin Pharmacol* 2016;**9**(7):943–954.

221. Schifano F, Duccio Papanti G, Orsolini L, Corkery JM. Novel psychoactive substances: the pharmacology of stimulants and hallucinogens. *Exp Rev Clin Pharmacol* 2016;**9**(7):943–954.

222. Dargan PI, Wood DM. *Novel Psychoactive Substances: Classification, Pharmacology and Toxicology*. London, Academic Press/Elsevier, 2013.

223. Schifano F, Duccio Papanti G, Orsolini L, Corkery JM. Novel psychoactive substances: the pharmacology of stimulants and hallucinogens. *Exp Rev Clin Pharmacol* 2016;**9**(7):943–954.

224. Dargan PI, Wood DM. *Novel Psychoactive Substances: Classification, Pharmacology and Toxicology*. London, Academic Press/Elsevier, 2013.

225. Abraham HD, Aldridge AM, Gogia P. The psychopharmacology of hallucinogens. *Neuropsychopharmacology* 1996;**14**(4):285–298.

226. Twemlow SW, Bowen WT. Psychedelic drug-induced psychological crises: attitudes of the 'crisis therapist'. *J Psychoactive Drugs* 1979;**11**(4):331–335.

227. Vollenweider FX, Vollenweider-Scherpenhuyzen MF, Bäbler A, Vogel H, Hell D. Psilocybin induces schizophrenia-like psychosis in humans via a serotonin-2 agonist action. *Neuroreport* 1998;**9**(17):3897–3902.

228. Krebs TS, Johansen P-Ø. Psychedelics and mental health: a population study. *PloS ONE* 2013;**8**(8):e63972.

229. Keshavan MS, Kaneko Y. Secondary psychoses: an update. *World Psychiatry* 2013;**12**(1):4–15.

230. Miyajima M, Matsumoto T, Ito S. 2C-T-4 intoxication: acute psychosis caused by a designer drug. *Psychiatry Clin Neurosci* 2008;**62**(2):243.

231. Przekop P, Lee T. Persistent psychosis associated with Salvia divinorum use. *Am J Psychiatry* 2009;**166**(7):832.

232. Matsumoto T, Okada T. Designer drugs as a cause of homicide. *Addiction* 2006;**101**(11):1666–1667.

233. van Amsterdam J, Opperhuizen A, van den Brink W. Harm potential of magic mushroom use: a review. *Regul Toxicol Pharmacol* 2011;**59**(3):423–429. https://doi.org/10.1016/j.yrtph.2011.01.006

234. Vardy MM, Kay SR. LSD psychosis or LSD-induced schizophrenia? A multimethod inquiry. *Arch Gen Psychiatry* 1983;**40**:877–883.

235. O'Halloran RL, Lewman LV. Restraint asphyxiation in excited delirium. *Am J Forensic Med Pathol* 1993;**14**(4):289–295.

236. Jovel A, Felthous A, Bhattacharyya A. Delirium due to intoxication from the novel synthetic tryptamine 5-MeO-DALT. *J Forensic Sci* 2014;**59**(3):844–846.

237. Dean BV, Stellpflug SJ, Burnett AM, Engebretsen KM. 2C or not 2C: phenethylamine designer drug review. *J Med Toxicol* 2013;**9**(2):172–178. https://doi.org/10.1007/s13181-013-0295-x

238. Vilke GM, DeBard ML, Chan TC, et al. Excited delirium syndrome (ExDS): defining based on a review of the literature. *J Emerg Med* 2012;**43**(5):897–905. https://doi.org/10.1016/j.jemermed.2011.02.017

239. Gonmori KYN. Fatal ingestion of magic mushrooms: a case report. *Ann Toxicol Anal* 2002;**14**(3):350.

240. Gahr M, Plener PL, Kölle MA, Freudenmann RW, Schönfeldt-Lecuona C. Self-mutilation induced by psychotropic substances: a systematic review. *Psychiatry Res* 2012;**200**(2–3):977–983. https://doi.org/10.1016/j.psychres.2012.06.028

241. Blacha C, Schmid MM, Gahr M, et al. Self-inflicted testicular amputation in first lysergic acid diethylamide use. *J Addict*

Med 2013;7(1):83–84. https://doi.org/10.1097/ADM
.0b013e318279737b

242. Attema-de Jonge ME, Portier CB, Franssen EJ. Automutilation after consumption of hallucinogenic mushrooms. *Nederlands Tijdschrift voor Geneeskunde* 2007;**151**(52):2869–2872.

243. Beharry S, Gibbons S. An overview of emerging and new psychoactive substances in the United Kingdom. *Forensic Sci Int* 2016; **267**:25–34.

244. Malleson N. Acute adverse reactions to LSD in clinical and experimental use in the United Kingdom. *Br J Psychiatry* 1971;**118**(543):229–230.

245. Arunotayanun W, Dalley JW, Huang XP, et al. An analysis of the synthetic tryptamines AMT and 5-MeO-DALT: emerging 'novel psychoactive drugs'. *Bioorg Med Chem Lett* 2013;**23**(11):3411–3415. https://doi.org/10.1016/j.bmcl.2013.03.066

246. Alper KR, Stajic M, Gill JR. Fatalities temporally associated with the ingestion of ibogaine. *J Forensic Sci* 2012;**57**(2):398–412.

247. Corkery J, Durkin E, Elliott S, Schifano F, Ghodse AH. The recreational tryptamine 5-MeO-DALT (N, Ndiallyl-5-methoxytryptamine): a brief review. Prog Neuropsychopharmacol Biol Psychiatry. 2012;**39**(2):259–62.

248. Corkery J, Claridge H, Loi B, Goodair C, Schifano F. Drug-Related Deaths in the UK: January–December 2012: Annual Report 2013. London, NPSAD, 2014. Available at: www.sgul.ac.uk/about/our-institutes/population-health/documents/NPSAD-Drug-Related-Deaths-January-December-2012.pdf [last accessed 26 April 2022].

249. Morini L, Bernini M, Vezzoli S, et al. Death after 25C-NBOMe and 25H-NBOMe consumption. *Forensic Sci Int* 2017;**279**:e1–6. https://doi.org/10.1016/j.forsciint.2017.08.028

250. Schifano F, Duccio Papanti G, Orsolini L, Corkery JM. Novel psychoactive substances: the pharmacology of stimulants and hallucinogens. *Exp Rev Clin Pharmacol* 2016;**9**(7):943–954.

251. Ninnemann A, Stuart GL. The NBOMe series: a novel, dangerous group of hallucinogenic drugs. *J Studies Alcohol Drugs* 2013;**74**(6):977.

252. Gillman PK. The serotonin syndrome and its treatment. *J Psychopharmacol* 1999;**13**:100–109.

253. Boyer EW, Shannon M. The serotonin syndrome. *New Engl J Med* 2005;**352**:1112–1120.

254. Valento M, Lebin J. Emerging drugs of abuse: synthetic cannabinoids, phenylethylamines (2C drugs), and synthetic cathinones. *Clin Pediatr Emerg Med* 2017;**18**(3):203–211. https://doi.org/10.1016/j.cpem.2017.07.00

255. Madsen GR, Petersen TS, Dalhoff KP. NBOMe hallucinogenic drug exposures reported to the Danish Poison Information Centre. *Dan Med J* 2017;**64**(6):A5386.

256. Suzuki J, Dekker MA, Valenti ES, et al. Toxicities associated with NBOMe ingestion – a novel class of potent hallucinogens: a review of the literature. *Psychosomatics* 2015;**56**:129–139.

257. Andrabi S, Greene S, Moukkadam N, et al. New drugs of abuse and withdrawal syndromes. *Emerg Med Clin North Am* 2015;**33**:779–795.

258. Gee P, Schep LJ, Jensen BP, et al. Case series: toxicity from 25B-NBOMe: a cluster of N-bomb cases. *Clin Toxicol* 2016;**54**:141–146.

259. Gee P, Schep LJ, Jensen BP, et al. Case series: toxicity from 25B-NBOMe: a cluster of N-bomb cases. *Clin Toxicol* 2016;**54**:141–146.

260. Wood DM, Sedefov R, Cunningham A, et al. Prevalence of use and acute toxicity associated with the use of NBOMe drugs. *Clin Toxicol* 2015;**53**:85–92.

261. Suzuki J, Poklis JL, Poklis A. "My friend said it was good LSD": a suicide attempt following analytically confirmed 25I-NBOMe ingestion. *J Psychoactive Drugs*. 2014;**46**:379–382.

262. Gee P, Schep LJ, Jensen BP, et al. Case series: toxicity from 25B-NBOMe: a cluster of N-bomb cases. *Clin Toxicol* 2016;**54**:141–146.

263. Gee P, Schep LJ, Jensen BP, et al. Case series: toxicity from 25B-NBOMe: a cluster of N-bomb cases. *Clin Toxicol* 2016;**54**:141–146.

264. Miller PL, Gay GR, Ferris KC, Anderson S. Treatment of acute, adverse psychedelic reactions: 'I've tripped and I can't get down'. *J Psychoactive Drugs* 1992;**24**(3):277–279.

265. O'Brien CP. Drug addiction and drug abuse. In: LL Brunton, JS Lazo, KL Parker, (eds.), *Goodman & Gilman's The Pharmacological Basis of Therapeutics*, 11th ed., pp. 607–627. New York, McGraw-Hill, 2006.

266. Huesgen K. Towards evidence-based emergency medicine: best BETs from the Manchester Royal Infirmary. BET 1: excited delirium syndrome and sudden death. *Emerg Med J* 2013;**30**(11):958–960. https://doi.org/10.1136/emermed-2013-203139.1

267. Erritzoe D, Frokjaer VG, Holst KK, et al. In vivo imaging of cerebral serotonin transporter and serotonin2a receptor binding in 3,4-methylenedioxymethamphetamine (MDMA or 'ecstasy') and hallucinogen users. *Arch Gen Psychiatry* 2011;**68**(6):562–576. https://doi.org/10.1001/archgenpsychiatry.2011.56

268. Griffiths RR, Johnson MW, Richards WA, Richards BD, McCann U, Jesse R. Psilocybin occasioned mystical-type experiences: immediate and persisting dose-related effects. *Psychopharmacology* 2011;**218**(4):649–665. https://doi.org/10.1007/s00213-011-2358-5

269. Nichols DE. Hallucinogens. *Pharmacol Ther* 2004;**101**(2):131–181.

270. Gillespie NA, Neale MC, Prescott CA, Aggen SH, Kendler KS. Factor and item-response analysis DSM-IV criteria for abuse of and dependence on cannabis, cocaine, hallucinogens, sedatives, stimulants and opioids. *Addiction* 2007;**102**(6):920–930.

271. Griffiths RR, Johnson MW, Richards WA, Richards BD, McCann U, Jesse R. Psilocybin occasioned mystical-type

experiences: immediate and persisting dose-related effects. *Psychopharmacology* 2011;**218**(4):649–665. https://doi .org10.1007/s00213-011-2358-5

272. Strassman RJ, Qualls CR, Berg LM. Differential tolerance to biological and subjective effects of four closely spaced doses of N,N-dimethyltryptamine in humans. Biol Psychiatry 1996;**39** (9):784–795.

273. Drugs-Forum (various authors). Smoking – DMT tolerance? 2012. Available at: https://drugs-forum.com/threads/dmt-tolerance.176077/ [last accessed 26 April 2022].

274. Halpern JH, Pope HG Jr. Hallucinogen persisting perception disorder: what do we know after 50 years? *Drug Alcohol Depend* 2003;**69**(2):109–119.

275. Carhart-Harris RL, Nutt DJ. User perceptions of the benefits and harms of hallucinogenic drug use: a web-based questionnaire study. *J Substance Use* 2010;**15** (4):283–300.

276. Baggott MJ, Coyle JR, Erowid E, Erowid F, Robertson LC. Abnormal visual experiences in individuals with histories of hallucinogen use: a web-based questionnaire. *Drug Alcohol Depend* 2011;**114**(1):61–67. https://doi.org/10.1016/j .drugalcdep.2010.09.006

277. Abraham H. Visual phenomenology of the LSD flashback. *Arch Gen Psychiatry* 1983;**40**:884–889.

278. Hermle L, Simon M, Ruchsow M, Batra A, Geppert M. Hallucinogen persisting perception disorder (HPPD) and flashback – are they identical? *J Alcoholism Drug Depend* 2013;**1**:121. https://doi.org/10.4172/ jaldd.1000121

279. National Institute on Drug Abuse (NIDA). Hallucinogens and Dissociative Drugs, Including LSD, PCP, Ketamine, Psilocybin, Salvia, Peyote, and Dextromethorphan. NIDA, 2014. Available at: https://nida.nih.gov/sites/default/files/rrha lluc.pdf [last accessed 26 April 2022].

280. Kilpatrick ZP, Ermentrout GB. Hallucinogen persisting perception disorder in neuronal networks with adaptation. *J Computational Neurosci* 2012;**32**(1):25–53.

281. Alacorn RD, Dickinson WA Dohn HH. Flashback phenomena: clinical and diagnostic dilemma. *J Nerv Ment Dis* 1982;**170**:217–223.

282. McGee R. Flashbacks and memory phenomena. A comment on 'Flashback phenomena: clinical and diagnostic dilemmas. *J Nerv Ment Dis* 1984;**172**:273–278.

283. Stanciu CN, Penders TM. Hallucinogen persistent perception disorder induced by new psychoactive substituted phenethylamines; a review with illustrative case. *Curr Psychiatry Rev* 2016;**12**(2):221–223. https://doi.org/10.2174/ 1573400512999160803102947

284. Martinotti G, Santacroce R, Pettorruso M, et al. Hallucinogen persisting perception disorder: etiology, clinical features, and therapeutic perspectives. *Brain Sci* 2018;**8**:47. https://doi.org/ 10.3390/brainsci8030047

285. Orsolini L, Papanti GD, De Berardis D, et al. The 'endless trip' among the NPS users: psychopathology and psychopharmacology in the hallucinogen-persisting

perception disorder. A systematic review. *Front Psychiatry* 2017;**8**:240. https://doi.org/10.3389/fpsyt.2017.00240

286. Martinotti G, Santacroce R, Pettorruso M, et al. Hallucinogen persisting perception disorder: etiology, clinical features, and therapeutic perspectives. *Brain Sci* 2018;**8**:47. https://doi.org/ 10.3390/brainsci8030047

287. Lewis D. Faces of HPPD: hallucinogen persisting perception disorder patient survey results and a descriptive analysis of patient demographics, medical background, drug use history, symptoms, and treatments. *Addict DisTreat* 2020;**19**(1):36–51. https://doi.org/10.1097/ADT.0000000000000178

288. Lerner AG, Gelkopf M, Skladman I, Oyffe I. Flashback and hallucinogen persisting perception disorder: clinical aspects and pharmacological treatment approach. *Isr J Psychiatry Relat Sci* 2002;**39**:92–99.2

289. Halpern JH, Pope HG Jr. Hallucinogen persisting perception disorder: what do we know after 50 years? *Drug Alcohol Depend* 2003;**69**(2):109–119.

290. Carhart-Harris RL, Nutt DJ. User perceptions of the benefits and harms of hallucinogenic drug use: a web-based questionnaire study. *J Subst Use* 2010;**15**(4):283–300.

291. Baggott MJ, Coyle JR, Erowid E, Erowid F, Robertson LC. Abnormal visual experiences in individuals with histories of hallucinogen use: a web-based questionnaire. *Drug Alcohol Depend* 2011;**114**(1):61–67. https://doi.org/10.1016/j .drugalcdep.2010.09.006

292. Baggott MJ, Coyle JR, Erowid E, Erowid F, Robertson LC. Abnormal visual experiences in individuals with histories of hallucinogen use: a web-based questionnaire. *Drug Alcohol Depend* 2011;**114**(1):61–67. https://doi.org/10.1016/j .drugalcdep.2010.09.006

293. Hermle L, Simon M, Ruchsow M, Batra A, Geppert M. Hallucinogen persisting perception disorder (HPPD) and flashback – are they identical? *J Alcoholism Drug Depend* 2013;**1**:121. https://doi.org/10.4172/jaldd.1000121

294. Frankel FH. The concept of flashbacks in historical perspective. *Int J Clin Exp Hypn* 1994;**42**(4):321–336.

295. Puledda F, Schankin C, Goadsby PJ. Visual snow syndrome: a clinical and phenotypical description of 1,100 cases. *Neurology* 2020;**94**(6):e564–e574. https://doi.org/10.1212/W NL.0000000000008909

296. Puledda F, Schankin C, Goadsby PJ. Visual snow syndrome: a clinical and phenotypical description of 1,100 cases. *Neurology* 2020;**94**(6):e564–e574. https://doi.org/10.1212/W NL.0000000000008909

297. Litjens RPW, Brunt TM, Alderliefste G-J, Westerink RHS. Hallucinogen persisting perception disorder and the serotonergic system: a comprehensive review including new MDMA-related clinical cases. *Eur Neuropsychopharmacol* 2014;**24**(8):1309–1323. https://doi.org/10.1016/j .euroneuro.2014.05.008

298. Halpern JH, Lerner AG, Passie T. A review of hallucinogen persisting perception disorder (HPPD) and an exploratory study of subjects claiming symptoms of HPPD. In: AL Halberstadt, FX Vollenweider, DE Nichols (eds.), *Behavioral*

Neurobiology of Psychedelic Drugs. Current Topics in Behavioral Neurosciences, vol. **36**. Berlin, Heidelberg, Springer, 2016.

299. Abraham H. Visual phenomenology of the LSD flashback. *Arch Gen Psychiatry* 1983;**40**:884–889.

300. Alacorn RD, Dickinson WA, Dohn HH. Flashback phenomena: clinical and diagnostic dilemma. *J Nerv Ment Dis* 1982;**170**:217–223.

301. McGee R. Flashbacks and memory phenomena. A comment on flashback phenomena: clinical and diagnostic dilemmas. *J Nerv Ment Dis* 1984;**172**:273–278.

302. American Psychiatric Association. *Diagnostic and Statistical Manual of Mental Disorders*, 5th ed. Arlington, VA, American Psychiatric Publishing, 2013.

303. Baggott MJ, Coyle JR, Erowid E, Erowid F, Robertson LC. Abnormal visual experiences in individuals with histories of hallucinogen use: a web-based questionnaire. *Drug Alcohol Depend* 2011;114:61–67.

304. National Institute on Drug Abuse (NIDA). How do hallucinogens (LSD and psilocybin) affect the brain and body? Available at: https://nida.nih.gov/publications/research-reports/hallucinogens-dissociative-drugs/how-do-hallucinogens-lsd-psilocybin-peyote-dmt-ayahuasca-affect-brain-body [last accessed 26 April 2022].

305. Espiard ML, Lecardeur L, Abadie P, Halbecq I, Dollfus S. Hallucinogen persisting perception disorder after psilocybin consumption: a case study. *Eur Psychiatry* 2005; **20**(5–6):458–460.

306. Ikeda A, Sekiguchi K, Fujita K, Yamadera H, Koga Y. 5-methoxy-N, N-diisopropyltryptamine-induced flashbacks. *Am J Psychiatry* 2005;**162**(4):815.

307. Lerner AG, Goodman C, Rudinski D, Bleich A. Benign and time-limited visual disturbances (flashbacks) in recent abstinent high-potency heavy cannabis smokers: a case series study. *Isr J Psychiatry Relat Sci* 2010;**48**(1):25–29.

308. Litjens RPW, Brunt TM, Alderliefste G-J, Westerink RHS. Hallucinogen persisting perception disorder and the serotonergic system: a comprehensive review including new MDMA-related clinical cases. *Eur Neuropsychopharmacol* 2014;**24**(8):1309–1323. https://doi.org/10.1016/j.euroneuro.2014.05.008

309. Lauterbach E, Abdelhamid A, Annandale JB. Posthallucinogen-like visual illusions (palinopsia) with risperidone in a patient without previous hallucinogen exposure: possible relation to serotonin 5HT2a receptor blockade. *Pharmacopsychiatry* 2000;**33**(1):38–41.

310. Evans RW. Reversible palinopsia and the Alice in Wonderland syndrome associated with topiramate use in migraineurs. *Headache* 2006;**46**:815–818.

311. Goldman S, Galarneau D, Friedman R. New onset LSD flashback syndrome triggered by the initiation of SSRIs. *Ochsner J* 2007;**7**(1):37–39.

312. Halpern JH, Lerner AG, Passie T. A review of hallucinogen persisting perception disorder (HPPD) and an exploratory study of subjects claiming symptoms of HPPD. In: AL Halberstadt, FX Vollenweider, DE Nichols (eds.), *Behavioral Neurobiology of Psychedelic Drugs. Current Topics in Behavioral Neurosciences*, **vol. 36**. Berlin, Heidelberg, Springer, 2016.

313. Anderson L, Lake H, Walterfang M. The trip of a lifetime: hallucinogen persisting perceptual disorder. *Australas Psychiatry* 2018;**26**(1):11–12. https://doi.org/10.1177/1039856217726694

314. Lerner AG, Rudinski D, Bor O, et al. Flashbacks and HPPD: a clinical-oriented concise review. *Isr J Psychiatry Relat Sci* 2014;**51**:296–301.

315. Shaul L-R, Feingold D, Goodman C, Lerner AG. Brief report: comparing triggers to visual disturbances among individuals with positive versus negative experiences of hallucinogen-persisting perception disorder (HPPD) following use of LSD. *Am J Addict* 2017;**26**:568–571. https://doi.org/10.1111/ajad.12577

316. Lerner AG, Rudinski D, Bor O, et al. Flashbacks and HPPD: a clinical-oriented concise review. *Isr J Psychiatry Relat Sci* 2014;**51**:296–301.

317. Shaul L-R, Feingold D, Goodman C, Lerner AG. Brief report: comparing triggers to visual disturbances among individuals with positive versus negative experiences of hallucinogen-persisting perception disorder (HPPD) following use of LSD. *Am J Addict* 2017;**26**:568–571. https://doi.org/10.1111/ajad.12577

318. Shaul L-R, Feingold D, Goodman C, Lerner AG. Brief report: comparing triggers to visual disturbances among individuals with positive versus negative experiences of hallucinogen-persisting perception disorder (HPPD) following use of LSD. *Am J Addict* 2017;**26**:568–571. https://doi.org/10.1111/ajad.12577

319. Halpern JH, Lerner AG, Passie T. A review of hallucinogen persisting perception disorder (HPPD) and an exploratory study of subjects claiming symptoms of HPPD. In: AL Halberstadt, FX Vollenweider, DE Nichols (eds.), *Behavioral Neurobiology of Psychedelic Drugs. Current Topics in Behavioral Neurosciences*, vol. **36**. Berlin, Heidelberg, Springer, 2016.

320. Martinotti G, Santacroce R, Pettorruso M, et al. Hallucinogen persisting perception disorder: etiology, clinical features, and therapeutic perspectives. *Brain Sci* 2018;**8**:47. https://doi.org/10.3390/brainsci8030047

321. Martinotti G, Santacroce R, Pettorruso M, et al. Hallucinogen persisting perception disorder: etiology, clinical features, and therapeutic perspectives. *Brain Sci* 2018;**8**:47. https://doi.org/10.3390/brainsci8030047

322. Halpern JH, Lerner AG, Passie T. A review of hallucinogen persisting perception disorder (HPPD) and an exploratory study of subjects claiming symptoms of HPPD. In: AL Halberstadt, FX Vollenweider, DE Nichols (eds.), *Behavioral Neurobiology of Psychedelic Drugs. Current Topics in Behavioral Neurosciences*, vol. **36**. Berlin, Heidelberg, Springer, 2016.

323. Lerner AG, Gelkopf M, Skladman I, Oyffe I. Flashback and hallucinogen persisting perception disorder: Clinical aspects and pharmacological treatment approach. *Isr J Psychiatry Relat Sci* 2002;**39**:92–99.

324. Lerner AG, Rudinski D, Bor O, Goodman C. Flashbacks and HPPD: a clinical-oriented concise review. *Isr J Psychiatry Relat Sci* 2014;**51**:296–302.

325. Martinotti G, Santacroce R, Pettorruso M, et al. Hallucinogen persisting perception disorder: etiology, clinical features, and therapeutic perspectives. *Brain Sci* 2018;**8**:47. https://doi.org/10.3390/brainsci8030047

326. Lerner AG, Goodman C, Rudinski D, Lev-Ran S. LSD flashbacks—the appearance of new visual imagery not experienced during initial intoxication: two case reports. *Isr J Psychiatry Relat Sci* 2014;**51**:307–309.

327. Lerner AG, Shufman E, Kodesh A, Kretzmer G, Sigal M. LSD-induced hallucinogen persisting perception disorder with depressive features treatment with reboxetine. *Isr J Psychiatry Relat Sci* 2002;**39**:100–103.

328. Lerner AG, Lev-Ran S. LSD-associated 'Alice in Wonderland Syndrome' (AIWS): a hallucinogen persisting perception disorder (HPPD) case report. *Isr J Psychiatry Relat Sci* 2015;**52**:67–68.

329. Shaul L-R, Feingold D, Goodman C, Lerner AG. Brief report: comparing triggers to visual disturbances among individuals with positive versus negative experiences of hallucinogen-persisting perception disorder (HPPD) following use of LSD. *Am J Addict* 2017;**26**:568–571. https://doi.org/10.1111/ajad.12577

330. Lerner AG, Rudinski D, Bor O, et al. Flashbacks and HPPD: a clinical oriented concise review. *Isr J Psychiatry Relat Sci* 2014;**51**:296–301.

331. Martinotti G, Santacroce R, Pettorruso M, et al. Hallucinogen persisting perception disorder: etiology, clinical features, and therapeutic perspectives. *Brain Sci* 2018;**8**:47. https://doi.org/10.3390/brainsci8030047

332. Lerner AG, Gelkopf M, Skladman I, Oyffe I. Flashback and hallucinogen persisting perception disorder: clinical aspects and pharmacological treatment approach. *Isr J Psychiatry Relat Sci* 2002;**39**:92–99.

333. Lerner AG, Rudinski D, Bor O, Goodman C. Flashbacks and HPPD: a clinical-oriented concise review. *Isr J Psychiatry Relat Sci* 2014;**51**:296–302.

334. Lerner AG, Goodman C, Rudinski D, Lev-Ran S. LSD flashbacks: the appearance of new visual imagery not experienced during initial intoxication: two case reports. *Isr J Psychiatry Relat Sci* 2014;**51**:307–309.

335. Lerner AG, Shufman E, Kodesh A, Kretzmer G, Sigal M. LSD-induced hallucinogen persisting perception disorder with depressive features treatment with reboxetine. *Isr J Psychiatry Relat Sci* 2002;**39**:100–103.

336. Shaul L-R, Feingold D, Goodman C, Lerner AG. Brief report: comparing triggers to visual disturbances among individuals with positive versus negative experiences of hallucinogen-persisting perception disorder (HPPD) following use of LSD. *Am J Addict* 2017;**26**:568–571. https://doi.org/10.1111/ajad.12577

337. Shaul L-R, Feingold D, Goodman C, Lerner AG. Brief report: comparing triggers to visual disturbances among individuals with positive versus negative experiences of hallucinogen-persisting perception disorder (HPPD) following use of LSD. *Am J Addict* 2017;**26**:568–571. https://doi.org/10.1111/ajad.12577

338. Halpern JH, Pope HG Jr. Hallucinogen persisting perception disorder: what do we know after 50 years? *Drug Alcohol Depend* 2003;**69**(2):109–119.

339. Carhart-Harris RL, Nutt DJ. User perceptions of the benefits and harms of hallucinogenic drug use: a web-based questionnaire study. *J Subst Use* 2010;**15**(4):283–300.

340. Baggott MJ, Coyle JR, Erowid E, Erowid F, Robertson LC. Abnormal visual experiences in individuals with histories of hallucinogen use: a web-based questionnaire. *Drug Alcohol Depend* 2011;**114**(1):61–67. https://doi.org/10.1016/j.drugalcdep.2010.09.006

341. Abraham H. Visual phenomenology of the LSD flashback. *Arch Gen Psychiatry.* 1983;**40**:884–889.

342. Hermle L, Simon M, Ruchsow M, Batra A, Geppert M. Hallucinogen persisting perception disorder (HPPD) and flashback – are they identical? *J Alcoholism Drug Depend* 2013;**1**:121. https://doi.org/10.4172/ jaldd.1000121

343. National Institute on Drug Abuse (NIDA). Hallucinogens and Dissociative Drugs, Including LSD, PCP, Ketamine, Psilocybin, Salvia, Peyote, and Dextromethorphan. New South Wales, NIDA, 2014. Available at: https://nida.nih.gov/sites/default/files/rrhalluc.pdf [last accessed 24 March 2022].

344. Kilpatrick ZP, Ermentrout GB. Hallucinogen persisting perception disorder in neuronal networks with adaptation. *J Computational Neurosci* 2012;**32**(1):25–53.

345. Espiard ML, Lecardeur L, Abadie P, Halbecq I, Dollfus S. Hallucinogen persisting perception disorder after psilocybin consumption: a case study. *Eur Psychiatry* 2005;**20**(5–6):458–460.

346. Ikeda A, Sekiguchi K, Fujita K, Yamadera H, Koga Y. 5-methoxy-N, N-diisopropyltryptamine-induced flashbacks. *Am J Psychiatry* 2005;**162**(4):815.

347. Lerner AG, Goodman C, Rudinski D, Bleich A. Benign and time-limited visual disturbances (flashbacks) in recent abstinent high-potency heavy cannabis smokers: a case series study. *Isr J Psychiatry Relat Sci* 2010;**48**(1):25–29.

348. Litjens RPW, Brunt TM, Alderliefste G-J, Westerink RHS. Hallucinogen persisting perception disorder and the serotonergic system: a comprehensive review including new MDMA-related clinical cases. *Eur Neuropsychopharmacol* 2014;**24**(8):1309–1323. https://doi.org/0.1016/j.euroneuro.2014.05.008

349. National Institute on Drug Abuse (NIDA). Hallucinogens and Dissociative Drugs, Including LSD, PCP, Ketamine, Psilocybin, Salvia, Peyote, and Dextromethorphan. New South Wales, NIDA, 2014. Available at: https://nida.nih.gov/sites/default/files/rrhalluc.pdf [last accessed 24 March 2022].

350. Kilpatrick ZP, Ermentrout GB. Hallucinogen persisting perception disorder in neuronal networks with adaptation. *J Comput Neurosci* 2012;**32**(1):25–53.

351. Orsolini L, Duccio Papanti G, De Berardis D, Guirguis A, Corkery JM, Schifano F. The 'endless trip' among the NPS users: psychopathology and psychopharmacology in the hallucinogen-persisting perception disorder. A systematic review. *Front Psychiatry* 2017;8:240. https://doi.org/10.3389/fpsyt.2017.00240

352. Orsolini L, Duccio Papanti G, De Berardis D, Guirguis A, Corkery JM, Schifano F. The 'endless trip' among the NPS users: psychopathology and psychopharmacology in the hallucinogen-persisting perception disorder. A systematic review. *Front Psychiatry* 2017;8:240. https://doi.org/10.3389/fpsyt.2017.00240

353. Anderson L, Lake H, Walterfang M. The trip of a lifetime: hallucinogen persisting perceptual disorder. Australas Psychiatry 2018;**26**(1):11–12. https://doi.org/10.1177/1039856217726694

354. Lerner AG, Rudinski D, Bor O, et al. Flashbacks and HPPD: a clinical-oriented concise review. *Isr J Psychiatry Relat Sci* 2014;**51**:296–301.

355. Shaul L-R, Feingold D, Goodman C, Lerner AG. Brief report: comparing triggers to visual disturbances among individuals with positive versus negative experiences of hallucinogen-persisting perception disorder (HPPD) following use of LSD. *Am J Addict* 2017;**26**:568–571. https://doi.org/10.1111/ajad.12577

356. Matefy RE. Behavior therapy to extinguish spontaneous recurrences of LSD effects: a case study. *J Nerv Ment Dis* 1973;**156**:226–231.

357. Martinotti G, Santacroce R, Pettorruso M, et al. Hallucinogen persisting perception disorder: etiology, clinical features, and therapeutic perspectives. *Brain Sci* 2018;**8**:47. https://doi.org/10.3390/brainsci8030047

358. Hanck AL, Scellenken AF. Hallucinogen persistent perceptive disorder after ecstasy use. *Ned Tijdschr Geneeskd* 2013;**157** (24):A5649.

359. Moskowitz D. Use of haloperidol to reduce LSD flashbacks. *Mil Med* 1971;**136**:754–756.

360. Thurlow HJ, Girvin JP. Use of antiepileptic medication in treating 'flashbacks' from hallucinogenic drugs. *Can Med Assoc J* 1971;**105**(9):947–948.

361. Anderson W, O'Malley J. Trifluoperazine for the trailing phenomenon. *JAMA* 1972;**220**:1244–1245.

362. Lerner AG, Skladman I, Kodesh A, Sigal M, Shufman E. LSD-induced hallucinogen persisting perception disorder treated with clonazepam: two case reports. *Isr J Psychiatry Relat Sci* 2001;**38**(2):133–136.

363. Abraham HD. Visual phenomenology of the LSD flashback. *Arch Gen Psychiatry* 1983;**40**:884–889. https://doi.org/10.1001/archpsyc.1983.01790070074009

364. Abraham HD. LSD flashbacks (Letters to the editor/In reply). *Arch Gen Psychiatry* 1984;**41**:632.

365. Young CR. Sertraline treatment of hallucinogen persisting perception disorder. *J Clin Psychiatry* 1997;**58**:85.

366. Lerner AG, Oyffe I, Issacs G, Mircea M. Naltrexone treatment of hallucinogen persisting perception disorder. *Am J Psychiatry* 1997;**154**:437.

367. Lerner AG, Finkel B, Oyffe I, Merenzon I, Sigal M. Clonidine treatment for hallucinogen persisting perception disorder. *Am J Psychiatry* 1998;**155**:1460.

368. Lerner AG, Gelkopf M, Oyffe I, et al. LSD-induced hallucinogen persisting perception disorder treatment with clonidine: an open pilot study. *Int Clin Psychopharmacol* 2000;**15**:35–37.

369. Aldurra G, Crayton JW. Improvement of hallucinogen persisting perception disorder by treatment with a combination of fluoxetine and olanzapine: case report. *J Clin Psychopharmacol* 2001;**2**:343–344.

370. Young CR. Sertraline treatment of hallucinogen persisting perception disorder. *J Clin Psychiatry* 1997;**58**:85. https://doi.org/10.4088/JCP.v58n0206a

371. Lerner AG, Skladman I, Kodesh A, Sigal M, Shufman E. LSD-induced hallucinogen persisting perception disorder treated with clonazepam: two case reports. *Isr J Psychiatry Relat Sci* 2001;**38**(2):133–136.

372. Lerner AG, Gelkopf M, Skladman I, Rudinski D, Nachshon H, Bleich A. Clonazepam treatment of lysergic acid diethylamide-induced hallucinogen persisting perception disorder with anxiety features. *Int Clin Psychopharmacol* 2003;**18**(2):101–105. https://doi.org10.1097/00004850-200303000-00007

373. Lerner AG, Shufman E, Kodesh A, Kretzmer G, Sigal M. LSD-induced hallucinogen persisting perception disorder with depressive features treated with reboxetine: case report. *Isr J Psychiatry Relat Sci* (2002) 39(2):100–3.

374. Feeney K. Revisiting Wasson's soma: exploring the effects of preparation on the chemistry of Amanita muscaria. *J Psychoactive Drugs* 2010;**42**(4):499–506.

375. Subramanian N, Doran M. Improvement of hallucinogen persisting perception disorder (HPPD) with oral risperidone: case report. *Ir J Psychol Med* 2013;**31**(1):47–49. https://doi.org/10.1017/ipm.2013.59

376. Orsolini L, Duccio Papanti G, De Berardis D, Guirguis A, Corkery JM, Schifano F. The 'endless trip' among the NPS users: psychopathology and psychopharmacology in the hallucinogen-persisting perception disorder. A systematic review. *Front Psychiatry* 2017;8:240. https://doi.org/10.3389/fpsyt.2017.00240

377. Subramanian N, Doran M. Improvement of hallucinogen persisting perception disorder (HPPD) with oral risperidone: case report. *Ir J Psychol Med* 2013;**31**(1):47–49. https://doi.org/10.1017/ipm.2013.59

378. Hermle L, Simon M, Ruchsow M, Geppert M. Hallucinogen-persisting perception disorder. *Ther Adv Psychopharmacol* 2012;**2**(5):199–205. https://doi.org/10.1177/2045125312451270

379. Hermle L, Simon M, Ruchsow M, Batra A, Geppert M. Hallucinogen persisting perception disorder (HPPD) and flashback are they identical? *J Alcohol Drug Depend* 2013;1:4. https://doi.org/10.4172/1000121

380. Hermle L, Simon M, Ruchsow M, Batra A, Geppert M. Hallucinogen persisting perception disorder (HPPD) and flashback are they identical? *J Alcohol Drug Depend* 2013;1:4. https://doi.org/10.4172/1000121

381. Hermle L, Simon M, Ruchsow M, Geppert M. Hallucinogen-persisting perception disorder. *Ther Adv Psychopharmacol* 2012;2(5):199–205. https://doi.org/10.1177/2045125312451270

382. Abraham HD, Mamen A. LSD-like panic from risperidone in post-LSD visual disorder. *J Clin Psychopharmacol* 1996;**16**

(3):238–241. https://doi.org/10.1097/00004714-199606000-00008

383. Morehead DB. Exacerbation of hallucinogen-persisting perception disorder with risperidone. *J Clin Psychopharmacol* 1997;**17**:327–328.

384. Markel H, Lee A, Holmes RD, Domino EF. LSD flashback syndrome exacerbated by selective serotonin reuptake inhibitor antidepressants in adolescents. *J Pediatr* 1994;**125**:817–819.

Chapter 13

Synthetic Cannabinoid Receptor Agonists

13.1 Introduction to Synthetic Cannabinoid Receptor Agonists

Synthetic cannabinoid receptor agonists (SCRAs), also referred to as synthetic cannabinoids, or synthetic cannabimimetics, are a large group of smokeable drugs initially sold as legal alternatives to cannabis. They have a strong effect on the endocannabinoid system. More than 200 different SCRA compounds were available in Europe at the end of 2020.

Synthetic cannabinoid receptors play an important part in the novel psychoactive substances (NPS) market. Although the number of newly synthesised SCRA has decreased in comparison to previous years, SCRAs (and synthetic stimulants) continue to be the largest total number of substances reported to EMCDDA and UNODC.[1,2] Although they first appeared in Europe, they are now part of the drugs market throughout the world.[3] It has been argued that the number of synthetic cannabinoids, their chemical diversity and the speed of their emergence make this group of compounds particularly challenging in terms of detection, monitoring, and responding.[4]

13.2 Street Names

A variety of street names are used for SCRAs. The term 'Spice', which is the brand name of one the most common SCRA products sold in Europe, is often used as a generic term for all synthetic cannabinoids. They are often referred to as 'K2' in the US, and 'Kronic' in Australia and New Zealand.[5]

A wide range of branded herbal products containing synthetic cannabinoids has been available on the market, containing different SCRAs, with different levels of potency (see also Box 3.1). Herbal products are often marked 'not for human consumption' and sometimes presented in attractive and colourful packaging. Where they have been controlled, SCRAs are increasingly being sold in plain plastic packets by street dealers, similar to those used for natural cannabis.

Brands names appear and disappear and include, but are not limited to, Spice, Black Mamba or K2. Products of the same 'brand' do not necessarily contain the same type of SCRA. What particular brands contain is likely to vary, and certainly brand names are not reliable indicators of what is consumed. Analytical tests have shown that the cannabinoid constituents and dosage can vary greatly both between products and between batches of the same brand. There may even be differences within the same package, if for example the SCRA has been sprayed unevenly on the herbal product. There is also evidence that some products contain a combination of different SCRA compounds.

13.3 Legal Status

Synthetic cannabinoid receptor agonists (SCRAs) are not under international control through UN drug control conventions.

However, in Europe, SCRAs are controlled in Denmark, Germany, Estonia, France, Ireland, Italy, Latvia, Lithuania, Luxembourg, Austria, Poland, Romania, Sweden and the UK.[6]

13.4 Quality of the Research Evidence

Although it is increasing, the research evidence on SCRAs, especially on clinical harms and their management, continues to be limited to case reports and case series, as well as retrospective studies, human and animal laboratory studies, surveys and interviews with SCRA users. Longitudinal studies and randomised controlled trials are rare.

13.5 Brief Summary of Pharmacology

Synthetic cannabinoid receptor agonists have been developed since the discovery of delta-9-tetrahydrocannabinol (Δ9-THC or THC) cannabinoids. They are a large and chemically diverse group of molecules with some functional similarity to THC and other phytocannabinoids, with 14 recognisable chemical families of synthetic cannabinoids.[7]

Overall, SCRAs produce effects that have similarities to THC, although they are not the same.[8,9,10] Both SCRAs and phytocannabinoids (natural cannabis) bind CB1 and CB2 receptors.[11] However, SCRAs can range from those with potency similar to THC to those that are significantly greater.[12] And in general, SCRAs have a much higher affinity for those receptors than natural cannabinoids and produce a stronger effect.[13] Structure–activity relationship analyses reveal that SCRA compounds may indeed exhibit higher potency. In fact, SCRAs are full agonists on the endocannabinoid system, while THC is only a partial agonist.[14,15]

The second most prevalent cannabinoid in natural-grown cannabis is cannabidiol (CBD). This is absent in SCRAs.[16] CBD seems to possess anxiolytic, antipsychotic and anti-craving properties.[17,18] These effects of CBD in cannabis cannot be found in SCRAs.[16] It has been suggested that the presence of CBD reduces the risk of THC-induced psychosis in natural cannabis. As SCRAs do not contain CBD, their risk of causing psychosis is argued to be greater.[19]

Synthetic cannabinoid receptor agonists were initially synthesised for biomedical research purposes,[20] by scientists investigating the mode of action of cannabinoids on signalling pathways in the body or as therapeutic agents.[21] This includes the analogues to THC (the classical cannabinoid) which were developed by Raphael Mechoulam at the Hebrew University (the 'HU' compounds) in the 1960s and include HU-210, which is structurally similar to Δ9-THC, but more potent, and difficult to synthesise.

The cyclohexylphenols ('CPs'), referred to as nonclassical cannabinoids, were developed by Pfizer in the 1970s. In the 1990s, John W. Huffman developed the 'JWH' series of synthetic cannabinoids which evolved from a computational melding of the chemical structural features of Δ9-THC with previously developed aminoalkylindoles.[22] Other indole-derived cannabinoids detected in products for recreational use are those synthesised by Alexandros Makriyannis (the 'AM' compounds).[9]

Today, products derived from these and other more recently synthetised SCRAs are sold on the drugs market. There are currently over 200 cannabinoid receptor agonists that have been detected globally. A total of 209 new synthetic cannabinoids have been detected in Europe since 2008, including 11 reported for the first time in 2020. SCRAs fall into seven major structural groups: naphthoylindoles (e.g. JWH-018, JWH-073 and JWH-398); naphthylmethylindoles; naphthoylpyrroles; naphthylmethylindenes; phenylacetylindoles (i.e. benzoylindoles, e.g. JWH-250); cyclohexylphenols (e.g. CP 47,497 and homologues of CP 47,497) and classical cannabinoids (e.g. HU-210).

Synthetic cannabinoid receptor agonists overall have a complex molecular structure, consisting of four pharmacophore components which are referred to as the 'core', 'tail', 'linker' and 'linked' groups. It is suggested that this structural complexity offers multiple opportunities for chemical modification to evade drug control legislation based on chemical structure, and this explains the large numbers of individual products that have been detected.[23]

The large structural heterogeneity of the different SCRA compounds means that some are more potent than others. There are differences in terms of metabolism, toxicity and duration of effects. Generally speaking, the greater the affinity to the CB1 receptor, the higher is the pharmacological activity and psychoactive effect of the agonist compound.

The JWH series of SCRAs were at first the most commonly used in Europe.[24,25] Their chemical structure is markedly different from THC. In comparison with THC, the JWH class has a much greater affinity for and full agonism on cannabinoid receptors.[26,27] The CP compounds are another commonly used group of cannabinoid receptor agonists and also lack the classical cannabinoid structure. CP-47,497, often found in herbal products, is up to 28 times more potent than THC.[28,29] The HU compounds are structurally similar to THC but are 100–800 times more potent.[30] Benzoylindoles are a fourth group and they include AM-694 and RCS-4, which have also been detected in herbal blends.[31,32]

As mentioned in Chapter 1, with time, new generations and formulations of drugs were developed as NPS. Often, they were more potent than earlier forms and may be associated with greater harms. There is evidence that the evolution of the synthetic cannabinoid drug market may be focused toward compounds with increased potency.[33] In January 2009, Germany banned the production, sale, acquisition and possession of the two specific psychoactive synthetic chemicals (CP 47,497-C8 and

JWH-018). Within 4 weeks of this legal control, samples of 'Spice' obtained throughout Germany demonstrated replacement of those two recently banned compounds with JWH-073, a then unregulated chemical homologue.[26,34] A study by the Poisons Information Centre in Freiburg, Germany, undertaken between September 2008 and February 2011, reported that, after January 2010, when JWH-073 and JWH-019 were added to the list of scheduled substances, there was an increase in emergency presentations associated with the extremely potent synthetic cannabinoids JWH-122 and JWH-210. The authors commented that in early cases (i.e. patients presenting after taking JWH-018), symptoms were generally mild, but later presentations, mainly due to the highly potent agonists JWH-081, JWH-122 or JWH-210, involved much more severe symptoms.[35]

Elsewhere too, producers of these products have been quick to adapt to changes in legislation by using similar compounds that are yet to be controlled.[3] Slight modifications are made to banned compounds and new derivatives continue to emerge as older ones are regulated. Chemists have synthesised similar compounds easily by the addition of a halogen, alkyl, alkoxy or other substitutes to one of the aromatic ring systems, or by making small changes in the length and configuration of the alkyl chain, for example.[3]

New formulations belonging to chemically diverse families, such as for example naphthoylpyrroles (including JWH-307 and JWH-030), the adamantyl-indoles/indazoles (e.g. APICA and APINACA), and the dicarboxamide-indazoles (e.g. AB-PINACA and AB-FUBINACA) have been developed.[36]

The so-called third generation SCRAs, such as MDMB-CHMICA, FUBIMINA, FUBIMINA analogues, AB-PINACA and 5F-ADB, for example, have been particularly associated with altered mental states, including what was described as 'zombie-like' behaviours.[37] They have also been associated with adverse effects, which can be severe and life-threatening.[38]

People who have used MDMB-CHMICA, for example, have described a spectrum of effects that are consistent with other synthetic cannabinoids, but there was a high prevalence of adverse effects; users and even suppliers have warned of its high potency.[39]

Similarly, a qualitative analysis of Norwegian web forum data showed how the opinion of forum users gradually changed from an 'initial attractiveness' in late 2007, to 'ambivalent opinion' in late 2008/early 2009, to finally becoming thereafter what the authors refer to as 'communal rejection', mainly because the number of negative effects overweighed the number of positive effects over time.[40] More recently, another study of posts by users on Internet forums suggests that the proportion of negative effects linked to SCRAs mentioned has increased over time, suggesting that recent generations of SCRAs generate more harms.[41]

13.6 What Are Synthetic Cannabinoid Products?

In the pure state, SCRAs are either solids or oils. Most synthetic cannabinoids are produced in China and exported, usually in powder form, using wrong declarations, such as 'polyphosphate', 'maleic acid', 'fluorescent whitening agent' or 'ethyl vanillin'[3]. See also Box 13.1.

Box 13.1 Production of SCRA products

Once in Europe, the retail products are assembled by lacing inert herbal products with synthetic cannabinoids. Commonly used herbal bases for the active chemical ingredients are damiana (Turnera diffusa) and lamiaceae herbs, such as Mellissa, Mentha and Thymus. The synthetic chemicals are mixed with or sprayed onto the herbs, typically on an industrial scale, often using equipment like cement mixers and liquid solvents, such as acetone or methanol, to dissolve the powders. They are then dried and packaged for sale.[21]

Pure compounds (not sprayed on inert herbal products) are also available for sale on websites, which users can mix with their own herbal mixture.[42,43] This practice of selling products as pure powders may increase the risk of overdose, in comparison to the ready-to-use herbal smoking mixtures.[44] There are reports from countries such as the UK that SCRAs are sometimes sprayed on letters or photos and smuggled into prisons for use by inmates.[45,46]

It has also been reported that SCRAs have been found in products that look like cannabis resin, as well as in samples of herbal cannabis. This may be to strengthen the potency of weak cannabis or to reduce the 'harvest time' and increase production rates by improving the poor potency of immature plants.

Box 13.1 (cont.)

The unpredictability of the content and of the potency of a SCRA product compounds to their potential harms. SCRA composition and dose within a single SCRA package, or in a production lot of SCRA products, are often unpredictable and variable, and place SCRA users at a significant health risk.[47,48,49]

For instance, in one analysis, the JWH-018 content ranged from 6.8 mg/g to 44.4 mg/g within a single product.[50] Another study looked at the purity of JWH-018 and JWH-073 from three online suppliers. Purity was determined using high-performance liquid chromatography with ultraviolet detection, and compared against validated standards obtained from a traditional research chemical supplier. The study found that products bought online were of comparable purity to validated standards, even though the products varied from each other in colour, texture and odour.[51] On the other hand, other studies found that the cannabinoid constituents and dosage vary greatly between products and batches.[52,53,54,55] Even within the same package, the uneven spraying of the inert herb may give rise to what are known as 'hot spots', with some of the product being stronger than the rest.[56]

In addition, one of the factors associated with SCRA-related harms is that SCRA products often contain multiple SCRA compounds.[57,58,59] In Japan, Kikura-Hanajiri et al.[60] detected an average of 2.6 different SCRAs per product. The most detected in one mixture by the authors was ten different SCRAs. Some SCRAs (JWH-018, JWH073, AM-2201, APICA and ADB-PINACA) have active metabolites that possess high affinity and full agonist effect on both the CB1 and CB2 receptor. These metabolites may predispose users to severe adverse effects when combined with other SCRAs.[61]

Synthetic cannabinoid receptor agonists have also been detected in mixtures containing other NPS, such as stimulants, hallucinogens and sedatives/hypnotics or have been detected in what appear to be 'ecstasy' tablets or capsules. It has been reported that SCRAs have been detected in mixtures containing other psychoactive herbs and plants,[62] but also in medications including benzodiazepines, such as phenazepam, opioid analgesics,[63] benzocaine,[64] and diphenidine,[21,65,66] as well as other drugs including tryptamines,[65,67] phenethylamines/NBOMe compounds,[68] cathinones, benzocaine[64] and diphenidine.[21,65,66]

Other substances identified in SCRA products include fatty acids and their esters (linoleic acid, palmitic acid), amide fatty acids (oleamide, palmitoylethanolamide), plant-derived substances (eugenol, thymol and flavours like acetyl vanillin), preservatives (benzyl benzoate) and additives (alpha-tocopherol).[69,70] SCRA products may also contain high quantities of tocopherol (vitamin E), possibly to mask analysis of the active cannabinoids.[71] They are often contaminated with the beta2 -adrenergic agonist clenbuterol,[72] thus providing a basis for sympathomimetic-like effects (tremor, tachycardia, anxiety) often described in intoxicated patients presenting to emergency departments.[73,74]

Although the herbal blend that contains the SCRA is most likely to be an inert product, the pharmacology and toxicology of the plant material in these blends is unclear.[75] The herbal material, which is used as a basis for the smoking of these mixtures, may contain toxicologically relevant substances like pesticides.[58]

13.7 Clinical and Other Legitimate Uses of Synthetic Cannabinoids

Synthetic cannabinoids have been developed for the past 40 years as potential pharmaceutical agents, often for pain management[76] or nausea. Those currently used include nabilone (Cesamet®), for the treatment of anorexia and for its antiemetic properties in cancer patients. Dronabinol (Marinol®) and nabiximol (Sativex®) and the cannabidiol Epidiolex® are used in the management of multiple sclerosis and pain[3,77] and the treatment of seizures associated with two rare and severe forms of epilepsy.

SCRA products are different from medicinal cannabis products, which are derived from natural products. They are not synthetic versions of natural cannabis.

13.8 Prevalence and Patterns of Use

Herbal products containing SCRA first appeared around 2004.[75] The first SCRA detected in Europe as a so-called legal high was JWH-018, which was detected in Germany and Austria in late 2008.[21] It has been noted that the popularity of these drugs increased significantly around 2008, as a result of numerous media reports that called them a 'legal' alternative to cannabis.[3]

Although SCRA are one of the largest groups of NPS,[78,79,80] their overall prevalence of use by the general population in Europe is relatively low.[81,82] For example, in their most recent surveys, last year estimates of the use of synthetic cannabinoids among 15- to 34-year-olds ranged from 0.1% in the Netherlands to 1.5% in Latvia.[83]

Although the prevalence of SCRA use is generally low in Europe, it has gained popularity among more marginalised social groups, such as homeless and prison populations.[84] Use in these populations has been identified as a concern.[85] For example, a UK survey of eight prisons reported the prevalence of 'spice' use within the previous month had increased from 10% in 2015 to 33% in 2016, with 46% of those users using almost daily.[86,87] In the US, a study found that people who reported using SCRAs were more likely to have experienced past-12-month homelessness, higher rates of probation/parole involvement and incarceration.[88]

It also appears that people who have used synthetic cannabinoids were more likely to have also used natural cannabis. A study of college students in the Netherlands has shown that people who have used natural cannabis were more than seven times more likely than those who had not to have used SCRAs.[89]

Overall, there is evidence that poly-drug use is common among SCRA users. A study of young people in treatment for SCRA use found that those using these drugs were also more likely to use a range of other substances.[76] Similarly, among non-treatment-seekers, an Internet survey of 168 users in 13 countries found that lifetime use included: alcohol (92%), cannabis (84%), tobacco (66%), hallucinogens (37%), prescription opioids (34%), MDMA (29%), benzodiazepines (23%), amphetamines (22%), cocaine (17%), Salvia divinorum (17%), heroin (7%), inhalants (7%), dissociative anaesthetics (6%), methamphetamine (3%) and miscellaneous other drugs (mephedrone, dextromethorphan, kratom; 12%).[90] Poly-substance use with SCRAs, especially alcohol and cannabis, has been described in case reports and series, online surveys and toxicology retrospective reviews.[91,92,93,94,95,96] Poly-drug use of other NPS together with SCRAs has been described too.[97,98]

13.9 Routes of Ingestion and Frequency of Dosing

Based on user reports and on the dosage forms of products, the primary route of administration of SCRAs is inhalation, either by smoking the 'herbal mixture' as a joint, or by utilising a vaporiser, 'bong' or pipe.[58] Both oral consumption and snorting of the compounds have

also been described.[64] There are also reports that SCRAs can be ingested as an infusion, although this is rare.[3]

The onset of the action of SCRAs is usually within minutes of smoking, like cannabis, because of the instant absorption via the lungs and redistribution into the brain and other organs, within minutes of use. This seems to be true for the new generation SCRAs, whereby for example the onset of effect of 5F-AKB-48 is reported to be between 2 and 15 minutes when smoked.[99] There is a delay of absorption following oral consumption.[3]

The length of the effect of SCRAs varies. It has been reported that within 10 minutes of inhaling a 0.3 g dose, users demonstrate mild to moderate cognitive impairment, as well as changes in perception and mood. Effects gradually diminish over 6 hours.[28] Although there are no controlled studies in humans, there are reports that the duration of action for JWH-018 is 1–2 hours, that the effects of 5F-AKB-48 last 1–2 hours,[100] and for CP 47,497 it is 6–8 hours.[28] Compared with THC, the effects seem to be shorter for JWH-018 and longer for CP-47,497 (and its C8 homologues, the effects of which last 5–6 hours).

As many of the SCRA products are much more potent than THC, it has been postulated that the psychoactive dose may be less than 1 mg.[76,101] Apart from high potency, some of these substances could have long half-lives and active metabolites,[102] potentially leading to a prolonged psychoactive effect.[21] It has been noted that naive users in particular mistakenly equate the safety and dosing profile of natural cannabis to that of SCRA herbal products.[75]

13.10 Desired and Undesired Effects for Recreational SCRA Use

One of the main reasons for the misuse of SCRAs is the difficulty detecting consumption by analysis of biological samples for THC, such as clinic-based urine drug testing kits. The non-detectability of SCRAs makes them attractive for persons undergoing regular drug tests (e.g. patients of forensic or withdrawal clinics, people obliged to undergo workplace drug testing, and driving license re-granting candidates, those working in law enforcement, fire-fighting, the armed forces,[103] prisoners or clients on probation, mining workers, and athletes).[16] Laboratory techniques have been developed to detect an increasing number of SCRA compounds, but these are currently not widely available to frontline clinical staff. They will also not detect every newly emerging compound.

Other reported motivations to use SCRAs centre on their availability, low pricing and in some cases a perception of safety.[104] SCRA are also popular in some countries among homeless people and particularly rough sleepers, as well as prison inmates because of their sedating effects and high potency, as seen in box 13.2 below

The desired effects of SCRAs are similar to those of cannabis intoxication[90]: relaxation, altered consciousness, disinhibition, a state of 'being energised' and euphoric[90,92, 105] and other factors mentioned previously, such as availability, affordability and the fact that it is not detected by many commonly used urine drug tests.[8,106,107]

An Australian survey of 316 SCRA users reported reasons for first use include curiosity (50%), legal status (before its control) (39%), availability (23%), recreational effects (20%), therapeutic effects (9%), non-detection in standard drug screening assays (8%) and to aid the reduction or cessation of cannabis use (5%).[91]

Box 13.2 SCRA Use among Homeless People and Prisoners

In some European countries, there is a relatively high use of SCRAs among vulnerable populations including the street homeless and among prisoners.

The appeal of SCRAs to vulnerable groups appears to be that they are cheap and potent intoxicants.[108] SCRAs are sought by homeless people and rough sleepers for their ability to detach those under the drug's influence from reality and their environment. However, because they frequently result in rapid intoxication, individuals under the influence of SCRAs are vulnerable to crime, particularly theft, robbery and exploitation.[109]

Research carried out in British prisons has shown that SCRAs are very widely available and that prevalence of SCRA use is significantly higher than among the general population despite being sold at much higher value inside custodial settings than on the street.[110] Similar findings have been reported in prison and probation services in Sweden.[101]

The most commonly reported motives for SCRA use in prison were boredom and escapism; other reasons include relaxation and addiction and less detectable smell compared to cannabis.[111] It has been reported that prisoners use SCRA to 'clear their mind', 'manipulate time', and 'escape the basic confines of prison life,'[112] and that 'boredom' is a reason for consumption and that Spice 'kills time' and 'makes prison life more bearable.'[113]

Castellanos et al. suggested that the effects cluster in four areas: cognitive impairment; behavioural disturbances; changes in mood; and sensory and perceptual changes.[76] Although they are related to THC (found in natural cannabis), SCRAs are five times more likely to be associated with hallucinations.[114]

In one Internet survey of 168 SCRA adult users from a number of countries, the majority of respondents (87%) reported having a positive experience after the use of Spice, although 40% also reported negative or unwanted effects. The quantities of SCRA products consumed did not vary significantly between those who had negative effects and those who did not. In addition, 11% reported that multiple use of the same brand of SCRA product results in variable and unpredictable effects.[90]

A study of 11 adolescents aged 15–19 who had used SCRA found that all the subjects reported a feeling of euphoria but nine (82%) also reported negative mood changes, four irritability and three anxiety. All 11 respondents reported difficulties with memory, one described auditory perceptual disorders, five visual perceptual disorders and two described paranoid thoughts.[92]

Reported subjective and physiological effects of SCRA products can vary greatly.[10,115] There are some reports of sedation, while other users have reported agitation, sickness, hot flushes, burning eyes, mydriasis and xerostomia (dryness in the mouth). The most commonly reported unwanted physical effects are nausea and vomiting.[28,116] There are some reports that the frequency of hallucinations is greater than for cannabis. For example, in a survey of 168 users by Vandrey et al., 28% reported hallucinations following SCRA use, which the authors describe as greater than what would be expected for cannabis consumption.[90]

In a study of university students in the US, common reasons for use were legality, not appearing on drug tests, and availability, not that students enjoyed using synthetic cannabinoids or thought they were safe to use.[117]

In the Australian survey of 316 SCRA users, more than two-thirds (68%) reported at least one side-effect during their last session of use, including decreased motor coordination (39%), fast or irregular heartbeat (33%), dissociation (22%), dizziness (20%), paranoia (18%) and psychosis (4%). Four respondents reported seeking help. More side-effects were reported by males, respondents aged 18–25 years, those who had used water pipes and those who had concurrently used alcohol.[91]

Despite indicating that the effects of SCRAs are broadly similar to those of cannabis, 54% of respondents to an Internet survey reported that SCRAs produce subjective effects unique and discernible from other licit or illicit drugs.[90] Similarly, findings from the Global Drug Survey also suggest that, when products are smoked, users are able to differentiate between the effects of natural versus synthetic cannabis.[5]

Respondents to the Global Drug Survey reported a strong preference for natural over synthetic cannabis (it was preferred by 93% of users), with natural cannabis rated as giving greater pleasurable effects while leaving the user able to function better. SCRAs were given significantly higher scores for self-reported hangover effects and other negative effects compared to scores given for natural cannabis. The survey also found that natural cannabis was used more frequently and more recently than SCRAs. Only a small minority of users seem to have fully substituted natural for synthetic cannabis.[5]

Similarly, in a US study of 500 clients enrolled in a residential drug recovery programme, almost two-thirds (68.4%) of clients reported lifetime SCRA use. Individuals reporting SCRA use also showed extensive substance use histories and favoured heroin, opioids, and amphetamines compared with SCRAs. Only 5.2% of the SCRA-using group stated that SCRAs were a preferred substance, and only 11.8% reported that they would try SCRAs again, indicating that SCRAs are not a preferred drug.[118]

13.11 Mortality

A number of deaths have been related to SCRA ingestion, either on their own or in combination, in analytically confirmed reports.[119–127] and include but are not limited to completed suicides following a SCRA intake.[120,128,129] Death associated with newer generations of SCRAs have been documented in a number of countries (including 5F-ADB 5F-AMB, AMB-FUBINACA and AB-CHMINACA).[130,131,132,133,134]

In a recent Australian study of 55 SCRA-related deaths, the mean age of the deceased was 37.2 years and 91.1% were male. Causes of death comprised of accidental toxicity (38.2%), accidental toxicity/cardiovascular disease (9.1%), natural disease (20.0%), suicide (10.9%) and traumatic accident (10.9%). The most common clinical presentation was sudden collapse (25.5%). Cardiovascular disease was prominent, including severe atherosclerosis (20.0%), myocardial replacement fibrosis (18.0%), cardiomegaly (12.0%).[135]

13.12 Acute Harms

13.12.1 Acute Toxicity

It has been suggested that synthetic cannabinoid intoxication appears to be a distinct and novel clinical entity[136], with differences between SCRA and natural cannabis discussed in Box 13.3. Overall, SCRAs are

---

Box 13.3 SCRA: Differences with Natural Cannabis and THC

Synthetic cannabinoids receptor agonists are not synthetic versions of the substances occurring in herbal cannabis (THC). Both SCRAs and natural cannabis bind CB1 and CB2 receptors. However, SCRAs have a much higher affinity for CB1 receptors than natural cannabinoids, produce a stronger effect and may have higher potency.

Overall, the adverse side effects induced by SCRAs in general may be more severe and occur more frequently than those induced by natural cannabis.[142,143,144,145,146,147] Unlike natural cannabis, SCRAs are associated with serious adverse effects, including cardiotoxicity, nephrotoxicity and death.[148] SCRA overdoses appear to be associated with significantly pronounced neurotoxicity and cardiotoxicity, compared with natural cannabis.[149]

Similarly, studies have shown that SCRA use is associated with increased mental health symptoms compared to natural cannabis use[150] and that the severity of psychiatric symptoms has been observed to be greater for SCRA users than that of natural cannabis user.[151] Similarly, in a clinical population, differences between natural cannabis and SCRA users were observed, which indicated an association of SCRA use with increased psychotic problems, agitation, and longer hospitalisations.[152,153]

It seems that the risk of requiring medical attention following use of SCRA is greater than that for natural cannabis consumption. For example, a study carried out among Dutch students showed that approximately 17% of those who had ever used SCRAs said they considered or did go to the emergency room while using synthetic cannabinoids.[154] Similarly, a number of other user surveys also suggest higher need for emergency medical care by those using SCRAs in comparison to natural cannabis.[155,156]

However, there is also evidence that these episodes of medical care appeared to largely require only symptomatic or supportive care[157] and were of short duration.[158,159] A systematic review of adverse events found

Box 13.3 (cont.)

that typically events requiring hospitalisation were not severe, only required symptomatic or supportive care and were of short duration. Nonetheless, the review also reported that a number of deaths have been attributed either directly or indirectly to SCRA consumption, as well as a number of other adverse effects, including a significant number with persistent effects such as new onset psychosis with no family history of psychosis.[160]

It is important to remember that SCRAs are not a single drug as discussed previously (see Section 13.5). There are over 200 different SCRA molecules which can produce a wide range of physiological and psychiatric adverse effects that can vary in duration and severity.[161] More recent formulations and new generations of SCRAs are typically more potent that earlier SCRAs and seem to be associated with greater harms.[66,162,163]

It has been suggested that early reports on SCRA acute harms noted a similar pattern of toxicity to cannabis. These include typical neuropsychiatric and cardiovascular effects – drowsiness, paranoia, delusion, hallucination, impaired cognition/memory as well as tachycardia and hypotension.[164,165] Later reports have suggested that SCRAs have additional toxicity including acute kidney injury, sympathomimetic (stimulant) toxicity and seizures.[166,167]

An analysis of US National Poison System data showed that with new generations of SCRAs appearing, clinical toxicity from SCRA use changed significantly between 2010 and 2015, with an increasing proportion of patients experiencing prolonged adverse effects each year, leading to increasing hospitalisation.[168]

It seems that even in the case of new generation SCRA acute intoxication and hospitalisation, most of the single-substance SCRAs were associated with self-limited symptoms and required supportive care. Nonetheless, the study also found that SCRA-associated clinical toxicity had changing since 2010. Each year, larger proportions of patients experienced more severe and prolonged adverse effects resulting in higher utilisation of healthcare resources (e.g. emergency department presentation, hospitalisation and therapeutic interventions),[169] and although SCRA toxicity only rarely results in death, the number of deaths increased each year. The authors argue that it is possible to speculate that this trend may be due to the higher potency of new SCRAs.[170]

During 2015, US poison control centres fielded 1,501 cases regarding SCRAs and reported that 11% of cases were noted to have a major adverse event. Males or those more than 30 years old were more likely to have a severe outcome. In these case clusters, intensive care unit (ICU) admission rates were from 8% to 27%.[171]

New generations and new formulations of SCRAs brought with them new harms. For example, acute kidney injury (AKI) related to synthetic cannabinoid use was first described in the US in 2012, even though SCRAs have been on the market since the 2000s. It was therefore argued that a new SCRA metabolite, likely introduced in 2012, seemed to be associated with AKI,[172] leading to the identification of XLR-11.[173] Similarly, ADB-FUBINACA and AB-CHMINACA were also identified through outbreak investigations of severe delirium in some US states.[174,175,176]

Report of 'zombie-like' features of ABM-FUBINACA exposure suggest that the clinical effects of SCRA exposure appears to be changing with the introduction of new SCRA compounds.[177] Some SCRAs have specific effects which have not been reported for others. For example, 5F-AKB-48 has been associated with paranoia, intense anxiety and an unpalatable taste in the mouth like 'burned plastic'.[178]

more potent, unpredictable and toxic than natural cannabis. It is agreed that it cannot be assumed that the risks associated with the use of SCRAs will be comparable to those of THC, as SCRAs appear to have greater potential to cause harm.

There is a wide range of adverse health effects reported following the consumption of SCRAs, with unpredictable effects ranging from profound sedation to intense agitation and psychosis.[137] As mentioned above, like the users of other NPS and illicit drugs, people who use SCRAs are not able to know exactly what it is they are consuming. The lack of quality control leads to batch-to-batch differences in SCRA concentrations in different products.[3] The amount and type of SCRA may vary, within and between products,[76] and some may contain more than intended.[11,34,69]

A major health problem arises from the fact that mixtures differ with regard to their active ingredients.[58] As a consequence, it is not possible for the consumer to estimate the dose at all accurately. Two cigarettes or 'joints', prepared from the same mixture, could contain significantly different amounts of the drug, and this raises the risk of harm.

In addition, SCRA products also often contain more than one form or type of SCRA and these can interact in unpredictable ways.[138,139,140]

Furthermore, variability is due to the differences between the particular SCRA compounds, but could also be related to individual susceptibility to the effect of the drug or the dose, or it may be multifactorial.[141] It has been suggested that the effects of SCRAs are greater in individuals with less previous exposure to cannabis, and especially those who are drug naïve.[35]

Harms associated with adulterants found in SCRAs have also been reported. It has been noted that the rationale for using adulterants, such as brodifacoum (BDF), in SCRA products may be associated with attempts to enhance the psychoactive effects of the drug, keeping the user high for a longer period of time because of lipid storage, hepatic metabolism and slow release.[179]

Studies have reported a range of symptoms associated with the various adulterants in SCRAs. This includes suggestions that superwarfarin adulterants of synthetic cannabinoids can lead to clinically significant coagulopathy,[180] or that rat poison adulterants in SCRAs may be linked to haematuria.[181,182,183]

13.12.2 Features of Acute Intoxication

Adverse effects of intoxication have been reported.[184] Overall, SCRAs can cause minor and moderate adverse effects similar to those of cannabis intoxication, including tachycardia, nausea, somnolence, hallucinations, paranoia, xerostomia, and injected conjunctivae (hyperaemia).

SCRAs are, also associated with more severe adverse effects and complications, such as renal injuries, aggressiveness, cerebral ischaemia and myocardial infarction.[185] The use of SCRAs has been associated with sympathomimetic effects such as mydriasis, hypertension and tachycardia.[186]

Common symptoms reported in outbreak clusters of adverse effects of SCRAs reported by the literature include lethargy, agitation, intermittent lethargy and agitation, aggressive behaviour, confusion, tachycardia, hypokalaemia, hyperglycaemia, vomiting and tonic-clonic seizures.[187,188,189,190,191]

A UK study of a series of 179 people with acute recreational drug toxicity presenting to hospital emergency departments identified synthetic cannabinoids in 18 (10%) patients. The most frequently observed clinical features were cardiovascular (tachycardia, (n=5, 28%), chest pain, (n=1, 6%)); neurological (seizures, (n=4, 22%), coma, (n=1, 6%)); and neuro-psychiatric (agitation, (n=4, 22%), psychosis, (n=1, 6%)); there was one case of elevated body temperature (n=1, 6%) that was also associated with the co-ingestion of serotonergic agents. The fluorinated analogues of the SCRAnAKB-48 and PB-22 were most commonly seen in this study and the authors argue that the data are reflective of the increasing concern in the UK

regarding the emergence of 'third generation' synthetic cannabinoids and their increasing market availability.[192]

Similarly, a case series of seven male patients with analytically confirmed MDMB-CHMICA toxicity also found that clinical features common to all seven presentations were heart rate disturbances (tachycardia/bradycardia), as well as reduced level of consciousness and mydriasis. Tonic–clonic seizures and agitation were reported in one individual with no other co-ingestants. Respiratory depression was reported with all three presentations of lone MDMB-CHMICA intoxication.[193] Analytically confirmed exposure to MDMB-CHMICA was associated with acidosis (often of respiratory origin), reduced level of consciousness, mydriasis, heart rate disturbances and convulsions.[194] PB-22 has also been associated with seizures.[195] The overall features of acute SCRA toxicity are listed in Box 13.4.

13.12.2.1 Cognitive Effects and Effects on Mental Health

A number of studies have reported cognitive changes associated with SCRA use, including difficulty in thinking clearly, confusion, sedation and somnolence, disorganisation, thought blocking, or nonsensical speech or alogia, memory changes/problems, increased focus and internal unrest.[74,90,92,107,229,230,231,232,233] Studies have also reported a variety of behavioural disturbances, including a change of activity from decreased activity to excitability, agitation and restlessness. Aggression has been reported in a small number of subjects.[74,92,94,107,234,235,239,240] Psychomotor retardation and nightmares were reported in one study.[93,238]

A study has suggested impaired cognitive function in chronic users of SCRAs compared with recreational users of cannabis and non-users. Impairments in working and long-term memories and response inhibition were observed among SCRA users compared with recreational cannabis and non-cannabis users. No difference was found in cognitive performance between recreational cannabis and non-cannabis users. Additionally, synthetic cannabis users showed higher depressive and anxiety symptoms than the users of natural cannabis and non-users.[236]

A controlled study found that acute SCRA intoxication can potentially result in impaired motor functioning, attention and response inhibition, but does

Box 13.4 Features of SCRA Toxicity

SCRA overdoses have significantly pronounced neurotoxicity and cardiotoxicity compared with natural cannabis.[196] Unlike their predecessors, some novel SCRAs may be associated with significant central nervous system depression and bradycardia. Commonly identified compounds such as CID and alkyl SCRA derivatives, such as INACA compounds and XLR-11, tend to be full agonists at the cannabinoid receptor and are presumably more potent.[197] At least some SCRAs could lead to severe or even life-threatening intoxication when taken in sufficiently larger doses, particularly so in the case of compounds that act as full agonists at the CB1 receptor, such as HU-210, CP-55,940 or WIN-55,212–2.[198,199]

- SCRAs have been linked to **sympathomimetic effects** such as mydriasis, hypertension, tachycardia[200] seizures, diaphoresis, agitation and combativeness.
- **Serotonin syndrome** – SCRAs fall into the major structural groups, based on their chemical structure.[3,201] Many of the compounds incorporate indole-derived moieties, as components of the structure or as substituents.[202] Indoles are groups structurally similar to serotonin, and so are active on 5-HT receptors.[203] It has been argued that ingestion of indole SCRA compounds may be associated with particularly high levels of activation of serotonin receptors.[204,205] Furthermore, it has been suggested that, at high doses, SCRA compounds may also possess some monoamine oxidase inhibitory properties.[206] This element may further increase the risk of serotonin syndrome in SCRA users (for serotonin syndrome see Chapter 8 and Section 9.14).

SCRA toxicity is characterised by the following features, listed in Box 13.5.

Box 13.5 Features of SCRA Toxicity

Features of SCRA toxicity include[35,106,207,208,209,210,211,212,213,214,215,216,217,218,219,220,221,222,223,224,225,226,227,228]

Neurological, cognitive and psychiatric effects

- Severe anxiety, agitation, aggressiveness, mood disturbance and suicidal thoughts, thought disorganisation, perceptual changes, persecutory thinking, delusions, auditory and visual hallucinations.
- Numbness, tingling, light-headedness, dizziness, pallor, tinnitus, diaphoresis, tremor, impaired motor performance, somnolence, syncope, nystagmus and convulsions, reduced levels of consciousness, catatonia, coma.
- Short-term memory and cognitive deficits, confusion, amnesia.

Cardiovascular and cerebral effects

- Tachycardia, hypertension, hypotension, hypokalaemia, chest pain, palpitations, myocardial ischaemia, myocardial infarction, ischaemic stroke.

Neuromuscular and musculoskeletal effects

- Hypertonia, myoclonus, tonic-clonic seizures, myalgia, rhabdomyolysis.

Renal effects

- Acute kidney injury (aetiology unknown)

Other effects

- Hyperglycaemia, hypoglycaemia, respiratory acidosis, cold extremities, dyspnoea, mydriasis, nausea, vomiting, loss of sight and speech

Serotonin syndrome

- Some SCRAs have been linked to serotonin syndrome.

not have an effect on other executive functions such as spatial memory and information processing.[237]

SCRAs are also associated with adverse effects on mental health and are linked to psychotic symptoms. Studies have reported changes in mood and affect associated with SCRAs. There are reports of subjective feelings of euphoric mood associated with intoxication,[90,92] but reports of users experiencing negative mood changes are more common and typify intoxication associated with SCRA rather than cannabis use.[76] There are also reports of inappropriate or uncontrollable laughter,[90,238] anger and sadness,[92] with an odd/flat affect.[93]

Sensory and perceptual changes include paranoid thinking,[90,92,94,107,241,242,239] delusions[93,94,107,240,240] and auditory and visual hallucinations.[90,93,107,242–244,241] Other problems associated with SCRA use include combativeness, irritability,[92,239,249] thought disorganisation,[241,248] anxiety and panic attacks,[92,239,249] depression and suicidal thoughts,[93,94,140,242,243] as well as self-harm, agitation and aggressive behaviour.[244] In addition, SCRA use has been associated with increased levels of violence.[245]

It has been argued that there has been an increase of case reports of individuals with no pre-existing mental health conditions experiencing acute psychotic reactions, as well as anxiety,[244] suicidality, and other adverse psychological reactions resulting from SCRA use[246,247,248,249] and compared to natural cannabis users and non-users.[250,251] In some cases, these have resolved quickly with minimal intervention, but in others, there have been persistent difficulties.[252,253,254,255,256]

13.12.3 Psychotic Symptoms and SCRA-induced Psychosis

The use of SCRA has been associated with psychosis and psychosis linked to SCRA has been associated with more agitation than would be expected from cannabis alone.[73,247,249,257] It has also been argued by some that there is a greater risk of psychosis with SCRA than with cannabis.[258] This is due to a combination of factors which may include the absence of cannabidiol (CBD), a naturally occurring product in cannabis which may have antipsychotic properties.[249] The impact of the absence of CBD has been described in relation to natural cannabis with low cannabidiol content, such as 'skunk'.[259]

Studies have shown that SCRA use is significantly associated with psychotic symptoms and there is an association between SCRA use with a wide range of positive and negative psychotic symptoms and higher levels of positive psychotic symptoms than natural cannabis users.[260,261,262]

There is some evidence that SCRAs may precipitate psychosis in vulnerable individuals,[35,73,240,241,247,249] including those with a history of psychosis.[93,94,240–243, 249,252] There is also some evidence of new-onset psychosis in otherwise healthy people with no history of psychosis. This will be discussed in Section 13.13, on the harms of chronic SCRA use.

SCRA use may lead to psychotic symptoms in individuals with no past psychiatric history, or in the absence of a personal or family history of psychosis.

There are reports of SCRA-associated acute transient psychosis,[35,95,243] as well as reports that some individuals may experience psychosis that persists for weeks after the acute intoxication.[93,248,249,252]

A small number of reports has described the association between the use of SCRAs and hallucinogen persisting perception disorder (HPPD).[263,264,265] There is also some evidence that one of the triggers able to precipitate the symptoms of those with existing HPPD, is the use of natural and synthetic cannabinoids.[266]

13.12.4 Physiological Effects

13.12.4.1 Cardiovascular

SCRAs have been reported to be two or three times more likely to be associated with sympathomimetic effects such as tachycardia and hypertension than natural cannabis.[73,74,267]

SCRAs are cardio-toxic, with increased risks posed by new generations of SCRAs. MDMB-CHMICA for example has also been associated with serious cardiovascular toxicity, particularly sudden cardiac deaths in young people.[268,269,270,271,272,273]

SCRAs can be linked to severe cardiovascular events and pathologies.[274] The consumption of SCRAs increases the risk of myocardial infarction.[237,275] Case reports and case series have described a range of cardiovascular problems, including bradycardia, chest pain and cardiac ischaemia,[74,247,250,276] and cerebrovascular accident (CVA) associated with the use of synthetic cannabinoid.[277]

13.12.4.2 Neurological

SCRAs have neurotoxic properties. Some neurological and neuromuscular effects linked to the use of SCRAs have also been reported and include tremors,[238,239,244] numbness,[92,238,244] tingling,[244] lightheadedness,[90,250] and dizziness.[90] Also reported are pallor,[239,244] tinnitus,[90] excessive sweating,[238] diaphoresis,[242] and unresponsiveness.[73]

SCRAs may be associated with lowering the seizure threshold in susceptible individuals.[278] Although seizures or convulsions associated with the use of (natural) cannabis seem to be unusual, there are some reports associated with SCRA use. These include a case report which describes a patient presenting to hospital with seizures after consuming a large quantity of analytically confirmed SCRA powder and alcohol, and reports of generalised convulsions occurring after SCRA use.[279,280,281,282,283]

Out of the 1,898 exposures to SCRA reported to the US National Poison Data System between January 2010 and October 2010, 52 cases of seizures were reported; the majority (43) were single episodes, although two patients developed status epilepticus. The majority of all 1,898 patients had minimal symptoms but the study identified 34 cases in which there were life-threatening effects associated with exposure, and more than half of these involved seizures.[284]

In a study on toxicity linked to MDMB-CHMICA, the development of seizures and deep unconsciousness were common features.[285] Similarly, some new generation SCRAs have been associated with delayed onset seizures.[286]

A prospective observational study of patients with suspected synthetic cannabinoids toxicity treated in emergency departments in Germany reported analytically confirmed intake of AB-CHMINACA or MDMB-CHMICA in 45 patients (age range: 12–48 years), of which the majority were male (40) and in 21 presentations more than one synthetic cannabinoid was present. The majority of the clinical features described were neurological/neuro-psychiatric, with reporting of somnolence (25 patients), disorientation (19), hallucinations (16), generalised seizures (13), aggressive behaviour (11), psychosis (6), syncope (6), muscle weakness/loss of control (5), amnesia (5) and dysarthria (2).[287]

13.12.4.3 Renal and Gastrointestinal

Gastrointestinal effects of SCRAs include nausea[90,238] and vomiting.[90,238,244] Acute kidney injury (AKI) associated with SCRA use has also been described.[106,288,289,290,291,292] Even without prolonged agitation, AKI has been noted with some specific compounds, such as the 16 cases of AKI from XLR-11.[293] SCRAs have also been linked to thrombotic microangiopathy (TMA) secondary to synthetic cannabinoids.[294] A recent case series has reported a case of SCRA-associated acute liver failure requiring organ transplantation.[295]

13.12.4.4 Other

Xerostomia, hyperglycaemia and hypokalaemia have been described in case reports.[28,74,247] Nystagmus, conjunctival injection and mydriasis were reported in a small number of cases.[28,247] The loss of eyesight and speech has been reported.[296]

Other reported harms linked to the use of SCRAs include case reports of hyperthermia,[297] diffuse alveolar haemorrhage,[298] and hypokalaemia.[21]

Delirium, severe rhabdomyolysis, acute kidney injury, and hyperthermia are common in patients with synthetic cannabinoid intoxication.[299]

13.12.5 Multi-organ Failure

Reports of multiple organ failure and hepatic failure in particular, associated with SCRA toxicity are rare. A recent case series described six patients displaying similar symptoms and sequelae resulting from multiple organ failure secondary to SCRA use.[300] In this series the majority or 5/6 patients presented with acute kidney injury; 4/6 required continuous renal replacement therapy. Five of six patients experienced fever and myocardial injury, as evidenced by a troponin elevation (3/6Seizures occurred in half of patients (3/6 patients). Two patients required emergent fasciotomies of the bilateral lower extremities for acute compartment syndrome. Two patients developed fulminant hepatic failure that necessitated liver transplant evaluation, one requiring Molecular Adsorbent Recirculating System (MARS) therapy as a bridge to successful transplant, while the patient without it did not survive.

13.12.6 Presentations for Treatment for Acute Intoxication

Although the prevalence of use of SCRA is generally low at population levels, it has been noted that the risk of requiring medical attention following use of SCRA appears to be greater than that for natural cannabis consumption.[301]

A systematic review of adverse events found that typically events associated with acute SCRA toxicity were not severe. They generally only required symptomatic or supportive care and were of short duration.[302] Similarly, in a study of 1,898 exposures to SCRA reported to the US National Poison Data System between January and October 2010, the majority of cases had self-limited signs and symptoms. Only 7.3% of symptomatic exposures were coded by a poison centre specialist as potentially life-threatening.[286]

Overall, the most frequently reported effects were tachycardia (37.7%), hypertension (8.1%), chest pain (4.7%), syncope (2.1%), hypotension (1.3%) and bradycardia (1.3%). Reported central nervous system effects included agitation/irritability (23.4%), drowsiness/lethargy (13.5%), confusion (12%), hallucinations or delusions (9.4%), dizziness (7.3%) and respiratory depression (>1%). Although the majority of cases had self-limiting symptoms, the study identified 34 cases in which there were life-threatening effects associated with exposure; more than half were seizures, which were reported in 3.8% of cases.[286] As shown above, some people will present to hospitals with harms which can be severe and a number of deaths have been attributed either directly or indirectly to SCRA consumption.[303]

In the US, the rise in the use of SCRA was mirrored by a rise in the incidence of SCRA-related health problems. For example, a report on monthly calls to all poison centres, which are tracked by the National Poison Data System, reported that adverse health effects or concerns about possible adverse health effects related to synthetic cannabinoid use increased 330%, from 349 cases in January 2015 to 1,501 cases in April 2015.[3,304]

A study of consecutive patients presenting to hospital emergency departments with SCRA toxicity reported that the most common clinical features at presentation were seizures and agitation.[305] Others also reported that the most commonly reported adverse health effects reported by this study during this period were agitation (35.3%), tachycardia (29.0%), drowsiness or lethargy (26.3%), vomiting (16.4%), and confusion (4.2%). Among 2,961 calls for which a medical outcome was reported, 11.3% of callers had a major adverse effect; 47.5% had a moderate effect). Just over one-third (37.0%) had a minor effect and (3.7%) had no effect. A total of 15 (0.5%) deaths were reported.[306]

A case report of 21 patients presenting to an emergency department with analytically confirmed SCRA use presents a broadly similar picture. The most frequent clinical symptoms were tachycardia (12 cases), nausea/vomiting (11), somnolence (9) and hyperglycaemia (9). Less frequent symptoms were hypokalaemia (4), syncope (4), dyspnoea (3), aggressive behaviour (3), amnesia (2), diplopia (2) and seizures (2). Acute psychosis in one individual lasted for 5 days. One patient with diabetes mellitus developed pronounced hyperglycaemia.[307]

A retrospective review of cases presenting to an emergency department during a three-month period, with chief complaint of SCRA use before arrival, reported that most such patients can be discharged after a period of observation (an average of 2.8 hours).[140]

The psychotomimetic effects of synthetic cannabinoids, even following a moderate dose, have been reported.[308] The use of SCRAs has been linked to major adverse consequences, including a significant number with persistent effects including new on-set psychosis with no family history of psychosis.[309]

An Australian study of patients hospitalised in an acute psychiatric ward for problems associated with SCRA use found that they represented 13% of all admissions on the ward (17 patients with 21 admissions). For four patients, this was their first hospitalisation and these patients presented with new psychotic symptoms; nine had a recurrence of a pre-existing disorder. Symptoms included psychotic symptoms, affective symptoms, disturbances and/or intense suicidal ideation/behaviour. The mean length of admission was 8.5 days, with significantly longer duration for those presenting with psychotic symptoms (13.1 days versus 4.4 days).[310]

It has also been noted that among patients with psychiatric illness, the use of SCRAs may increase the number of nights spent in hospital and the need to ask specifically about SCRAs has been highlighted.[311]

13.12.7 Increasing SCRA Harms with New Generations

The evolution of clinical effects appears to be linked to the identification of new SCRA compounds,[312] such as increased risk of nephrotoxicity, for example (discussed in the following). It also appeared that in comparison to older generation SCRAs, such as JWH-018, newer generations, for example AB-CHMINACA MDMB-CHMICA, were associated with a higher prevalence of certain neuropsychiatric symptoms, more severe poisoning and duration of symptoms.[313] This was reflected in an increase in hospitalisation. US study of hospitalisation resulting from toxicity from synthetic cannabinoid receptor agonist exposure in the US increased significantly between 2010 and 2015.[314] The study also identified that SCRA-associated clinical toxicity has been changing since 2010. Each year, larger proportions of patients experienced more severe and prolonged adverse effects resulting in higher utilisation of healthcare resources (e.g. emergency department presentation, hospitalisation and therapeutic interventions).

Data from this study has shown that SCRA toxicity rarely results in death; however, the number of deaths increased each year. The authors speculate that this trend may be due to the higher potency of new SCRAs. With increasing occurrence of bradycardia, hypotension, coma and respiratory depression, SCRA toxicity may lead to higher fatality in the future, especially in the setting of polysubstance abuse.[315]

Distribution of new SCRAs has been associated with outbreaks of severe adverse effects. For example, in the US in 2012, an outbreak of acute kidney injury in Wyoming and Oregon led to the discovery of XLR-11, a previously unreported SCRA.[316] ADB-FUBINACA and AB-CHMINACA were also identified through outbreak investigations of severe delirium in Georgia and Florida.[317,318]

Similarly, very low concentration MDMB-CHMICA have been reported in fatal cases and severely ill patients.[319,320,321,322,323] Other new generation drugs were associated with significant analytically confirmed toxicity include 5F-AKB-48 and 5F-PB-22.[324]

13.12.8 Acute Withdrawal

For withdrawal, see Section 13.14.

13.13 Management of Acute Harms

13.13.1 Identification and Assessment

SCRAs cannot be detected by the screening tests for phytocannabinoid delta-9-transtetrahydrocannabinol (THC). Although laboratory techniques have been developed to detect some compounds,[116,325,326,327] there are currently no widely available tests. In addition, more than one SCRA can be found within the same mixture or product, and the regular appearance of new compounds poses another challenge.[16]

It has therefore been recommended that clinicians need to rely on clinical skills to detect SCRA use. This includes specifically asking about SCRA use, being aware of the physiological effects, such as conjunctival injection, and having a high index of suspicion in the context of unexplained deterioration despite a negative urine screen.[248]

13.13.2 Clinical Management of Acute Toxicity

Synthetic cannabinoid receptor agonists do not give a positive result on routine urine screening tests for metabolites of delta-9-tetrahydrocannabinol (THC).[247,328] Although there are currently specific mass spectrometry tests for a number of SCRAs, these are currently not widely available to frontline clinical staff. Moreover, the forensic chemical detection of SCRA remains complex,[71] not least because of continuously emerging compounds and the lack of reference samples in laboratories to identify them.

It has been argued that given the diversity of available SCRA compounds, the constantly changing composition even within brands, difficulties with detection and the limited available evidence, making specific clinical recommendations is currently problematic.[329]

It is suggested that people present to emergency departments as a result of behavioural issues (agitation, psychosis, anxiety) or symptoms associated with acute critical illness. These can include seizure, (themselves potentially associated with rhabdomyolysis and hyperthermia), acute kidney injury and myocardial ischaemia and infarction.[330,331]

Symptoms of SCRA intoxication may be self-limiting and resolve spontaneously.[76,286] Case reports suggest that, in emergency departments, hydration and monitoring may be enough for patients with mild to moderate intoxication.[74,239,241,243,332]

It seems that the majority of the single-substance SCRA exposures resulted in self-limited symptoms and required supportive care.[333] The majority of mild intoxications may only require symptomatic treatment and generally do not require hospital admission. For example, a nine-month study of the National Poison Data System that reported 1,898 SCRA exposures found that the majority had self-limited signs and symptoms and received only symptomatic treatment.[286]

SCRAs can have sedating effects on users, but Armenian at al. (2017) have argued that clinically it is best to characterise SCRAs as stimulants, since they lead to tachycardia, hypertension, hyperthermia, diaphoresis, generalised tonic-clonic seizures, agitation, and delirium, similar to other CNS stimulant drugs.[334] If agitation and seizures are uncontrolled they can lead to hyperthermia and rhabdomyolysis, which can cause end-organ damage to the brain, kidneys, liver and coagulation system.[335,336,337]

The management of SCRA toxicity is symptomatic and supportive, as no antidotes exist.[106] Supportive treatment is dependent on a patient's specific presentation. Treatment is primarily symptomatic, with airway protection and control of agitated delirium being the key initial steps in caring for the intoxicated patient.[338] Intravenous fluids may be required to treat electrolyte and fluid disturbances.[339]

It is argued that severe intoxications, involving seizures, severe agitation or mental health disturbances, arrhythmias and significant chest pain, should be admitted to hospital for further investigation.[340] In cases of acute SCRA intoxication, it has been suggested that an electrocardiogram should be performed, because misusers may present with vomiting and associated hypokalaemia.[341]

In a small case series of patients with psychosis presentations to acute psychiatric settings, the clinical presentations were characterised by an acute onset of agitation and aggressive behaviour. The symptoms decreased in intensity and frequency in no less than 72 hours. The management of acute intoxications included treating the symptoms with benzodiazepines and antipsychotic medications. In addition, vital parameters were monitored and nursing observations were increased. These measures led to rapid and successful resolutions of symptoms and reduced the need for transfer to more intensive care settings. Furthermore, they promoted more rapid step-down and recovery in the community.[342]

Benzodiazepines may be of benefit to patients who present with symptoms of anxiety, panic and agitation.[74,94,107,239] Antipsychotic medication may be indicated for some patients, especially those who present with agitation or aggression, when the patient has a history of psychotic disorders, and when the psychotic symptoms do not remit spontaneously or with supportive care.[93,94,249,252]

Only a few specific interventions have been described. Intravenous benzodiazepines have been reported for the management of seizures and monitored observation for cases of SCRA-related psychosis.[73] One study reported that the most common intervention for patients with a single-agent SCRA exposure was the administration of intravenous fluids (25.3%), followed by benzodiazepine (16%), supplemental oxygen (5.8%) and anti-emetics (4.7%). The duration of clinical effect was recorded in 907 cases. Out of those, clinical effect lasted less than 8 hours in 78.4% of cases, between 8 and 24 hours in 16.6% and more than 24 hours in 4.9% of cases.[286]

> For up-to-date information and clinical guidance please also refer to national and regional poison information services as well as national guidance and local protocols.

13.14 Harms Associated with Chronic Use

13.14.1 Dependence, Tolerance and Withdrawal Symptoms

The evidence remains limited, but it seems that SCRAs have the potential for misuse and dependence.[343] There is increasing evidence that the chronic use of SCRAs may be associated with tolerance.[76] Tolerance may develop more quickly for SCRAs than for natural cannabis and the quicker development of tolerance may contribute to the higher dependence potential in comparison to natural cannabis.[238,344]

Although the evidence is currently limited, SCRAs may have greater dependence liability than natural cannabis and this may develop more quickly. Withdrawal symptoms have been reported to be the primary reason given by daily users for their continued use.[345]

Abrupt discontinuation of prolonged daily SCRA use is associated with withdrawal symptoms, which can be severe and prolonged. Symptoms include craving, lack of appetite, irritability, sleep disruptions, drug craving, insomnia, nocturnal nightmares, profuse diaphoresis, headache, severe anxiety, nausea and vomiting, diarrhoea and loss of appetite. They can also include in severe cases tremor and reoccurring seizures and cardiovascular and respiratory risks (tachycardia, chest pain, palpitations, dyspnoea) and suicidal ideation.[238,248,346-356] It has been suggested that the magnitude of withdrawal may correspond to quantity of use.

There may be a link between the severity of withdrawal symptoms and the quantity of SCRA used daily. A study found for example a link between amount smoked and whether the patient required outpatient care, inpatient care or complex care, with intensity of care increasing with amount of SCRA used daily.[357]

13.14.2 Other Harms of Chronic Use

Knowledge of the long-term effects of the use of SCRAs is still limited. Although no experimental data are available, it is expected that these SCRAs, as lipophilic compounds, have high volumes of distribution. It is therefore likely that chronic use of them can lead to accumulation of the substances themselves and/or their metabolites in fat-containing compartments in the body.[3] There is also speculation that some of these products, and particularly the aminoalkylindoles carrying a naphthyl moiety, may have carcinogenic potential.[358]

There may also be gastrointestinal effects, which range from mild symptoms, such as abdominal pain and vomiting, to more severe ones such as intestinal ischaemia. One case report suggests that frequent habitual smoking of SCRAs can cause cannabinoid hyperemesis syndrome, which is mediated by cannabinoid receptors.[359] Xerostomia[28,90] has been reported, as well as lactic or metabolic acidosis.[28,247]

Case reports have described multiple-organ-failure-associated symptoms of acute SCRA toxicity.[360] There is one case report of pulmonary infiltrates associated with chronic SCRA use.[361]

Psychosis has also been reported among frequent users. One study describes new-onset psychosis in otherwise healthy young men.[93] A case series reported on ten patients admitted in the context of SCRA use, none of whom had a history of psychosis. All of the patients reported smoking SCRAs on more than one occasion (ranging from four uses over a three-week period to daily use for a year and a half). The onset of psychotic symptoms varied from after the fourth use to after more than a year of use. Presentations were characterised by paranoid delusions, ideas of reference and a disorganised, confused mental state. It was noted that a distinct, though waxing and waning, stuporous appearance was often present for weeks after last SCRA use. The mood of patients was described as generally flat, with most patients reporting significant depressive symptoms and 40% describing suicidal ideation. Hospitalisation generally lasted 6–10 days. Although psychotic symptoms did remit in most patients, 30% were noted to have persistent psychosis at eight-month follow-up.[93]

For example, three patients who presented to an emergency department with persistent psychosis, which did not resolve within 24–48 hours, required at least 2 weeks of hospitalisation. Two of the patients were treated with haloperidol and one with risperidone and although the patients demonstrated improvements, in no cases had symptoms resolved completely upon discharge.[94]

13.15 Management of Harms Related to Chronic Use

It has been argued the onset and severity of SCRA withdrawal symptoms reflect greater CB1 receptor efficacy and pharmacokinetic differences relative to THC. As such, it has been argued that managing and treating SCRA withdrawal poses a unique clinical challenge. Withdrawal symptoms range from mild, requiring only outpatient care, to severe, warranting inpatient care and continuous monitoring.[362]

It has been suggested that many adverse effects associated with acute intoxication are identical to some withdrawal symptoms and consequently, they are treated similarly.

Patients who present with irritability, agitation, anxiety, and seizures associated with intoxication or withdrawal[363,364,365] are generally administered benzodiazepines as a firstline treatment. In cases where patients did not respond to benzodiazepines, there are reports of neuroleptics being administered for acute psychosis and agitation[366,367] and psychotic symptoms.[368] Some have argued that the use of second-generation antipsychotics may be a rational approach as they may present with lower risk of increase in cravings[369] and a more significant antagonism at 5-HT2A receptors.[370] There are reports of the prescribing of quetiapine[371,372] for example. The administration of antipsychotics with antidepressants has also been described in cases of concurrent depression.[233]

One case report has described the use of naltrexone, which appeared to reduce SCRA cravings associated with detoxification.[373]

Anti-emetics have been administered for hyperemesis although are not always effective.[374,375]

13.15.1 Clinical Management of Dependence and Chronic Use

In comparison with natural cannabis, SCRAs show a potential need for more intensive management.[376]

Patients with SCRA withdrawal symptoms often require intense medical support and admission to inpatient detoxification.[377,378,379]

Psychosocial interventions remain the most effective treatment for the management of harmful patterns of SCRA use and dependence. No pharmacological interventions for SCRA withdrawal are indicated.

See Chapter 2 on psychosocial interventions.

13.15.2 Aftercare and Support

See Chapter 2 on psychosocial interventions.

Psychotherapeutic strategies to reduce use and/ or harm related to SCRAs are recommended.[380]

13.15.3 Harm Reduction and Public Safety

A study focusing on analytical results and signs of impairment documented by the police or the physicians who had taken the blood sample from suspects driving under the influence of SCRAs reported that the use of SCRAs can lead to impairment similar to typical performance deficits caused by cannabis use.[381]

A study of drivers found that officers or drug recognition experts (DREs) reported that drivers suspected of using SCRAs were more confused and disoriented, and were involved in more motor vehicle crashes than those suspected of using natural cannabis. DREs documented significantly more confusion (6/10) or disorientation (5/10) in the 'Spice' group versus those in the marijuana group (0/25). A significantly larger proportion of cannabis users had tremors (25/25) than those in the 'Spice' group (8/13).[382]

One study has reported that concentrations of SCRA in the range below 1 ng/mL may cause significant impairment for operating a vehicle.[383]

References

1. United Nations Office on Drugs and Crime. World Drug Report 2019. New York, United Nations Office on Drugs and Crime, 2019.

2. European Monitoring Centre for Drugs and Drug Addiction. European Drug Report 2019: Trends and Developments. Luxembourg, Publications Office of the European Union, 2019.

3. United Nations Office on Drugs and Crime (UNODC). Synthetic Cannabinoids in Herbal Products. New York, United Nations Office on Drugs and Crime, 2011. Available at: www.unodc.org/documents/scientific/Synthetic_Cannabinoids.pdf [last accessed 24 March 2022].

4. European Monitoring Centre for Drugs and Drug Addiction. Perspectives on Drugs. Synthetic Cannabinoids in Europe. Update 6 June 2017. Available at: www.emcdda.europa.eu/system/files/publications/2753/POD_Synthetic%20cannabinoids_0.pdf [last accessed 26 April 2022].

5. Winstock AR, Barratt MJ. Synthetic cannabis: a comparison of patterns of use and effect profile with natural cannabis in a large global sample. *Drug Alcohol Depend* 2013;**131**(1–3):106–111. https://doi.org/10.1016/j.drugalcdep.2012.12.011

6. European Monitoring Centre for Drugs and Drug Addiction. Synthetic Cannabinoids and 'Spice' Drug Profile. Available at: www.emcdda.europa.eu/publications/drug-profiles/synthetic-cannabinoids [last accessed 24 March 2022].

7. European Monitoring Centre for Drugs and Drug Addiction. Perspectives on Drugs. Synthetic Cannabinoids in Europe. Update 6 June 2017. Available at: https://www.emcdda.europa.eu/system/files/publications/2753/POD_Synthetic%20cannabinoids_0.pdf [last accessed 26 April 2022].

8. Fattore L, Fratta W. Beyond THC: the new generation of cannabinoid designer drugs. *Front Behav Neurosci* 2011;**5**:60. https://doi.org/10.3389/fnbeh.2011.00060

9. Hudson S, Ramsey J. The emergence and analysis of synthetic cannabinoids. *Drug Test Anal* 2011;**3**:466–478.

10. Vardakou I, Pistos C, Spiliopoulou C. Spice drugs as a new trend: mode of action, identification and legislation. *Toxicol Lett* 2010;**197**:157–162.

11. Loeffler G, Hurst D, Penn A, Yung K. Spice, bath salts, and the US military: the emergence of synthetic cannabinoid receptor agonists and cathinones in the US Armed Forces. *Mil Med* 2012;**177**(9):1041–1048.

12. Bonaccorso S, Metastasio A, Ricciardi A, et al. Synthetic cannabinoid use in a case series of patients with psychosis presenting to acute psychiatric settings: clinical presentation and management issues. *Brain Sci* 2018;**8**:133. https://doi.org/10.3390/brainsci8070133

13. Hudson S, Ramsey J, King L, et al. Use of high-resolution accurate mass spectrometry to detect reported and previously unreported cannabinomimetics in 'herbal high' products. *J Anal Toxicol* 2010;**34**(5):252–260.

14. Huffman JW, Padgett LW. Recent developments in the medicinal chemistry of cannabinomimetic indoles, pyrroles and indenes. *Curr Med Chem* 2005;**12**:1395–1411.

15. D'Souza DC, Perry E, MacDougall L, et al. The psychotomimetic effects of intravenous delta-9-tetrahydrocannabinol in healthy individuals: implications for psychosis. *Neuropsychopharmacology* 2004;**29**(8):1558–1572.

16. Papanti D, Orsolini L, Francesconi G, Schifano F. 'Noids' in a nutshell: everything you (don't) want to know about synthetic cannabimimetics. *Adv Dual Diagn* 2014;**7**(3):1–13.

17. Zuardi AW, Crippa JA, Hallak JE, Moreira FA, Guimarães FS. Cannabidiol, a cannabis sativa constituent, as an antipsychotic drug. *Braz J Med Biol Res* 2006;**39**(4):421–429.

18. Morgan CJ, Das RK, Joye A, Curran HV, Kamboj SK. Cannabidiol reduces cigarette consumption in tobacco smokers: preliminary findings. *Addict Behav* 2013;**38**(9):2433–2436. https://doi.org/10.1016/j.addbeh.2013.03.011

19. Murray RM, Quigley H, Quattrone D, Englund A, Di Forti M. Traditional marijuana, high potency cannabis and synthetic cannabinoids: increasing risk for psychosis. *World Psychiatry* 2016;**15**:195–204.

20. Seely KA, Prather PL, James LP, Moran JH. Marijuana-based drugs: innovative therapeutics or designer drugs of abuse? *Mol Interv* 2011;**11**:36–51.

21. European Monitoring Centre for Drugs and Drug Addiction (EMCDDA). Synthetic Cannabinoids in Europe (updated 28 May 2013) (Perspectives on Drugs series). EMCDDA, 2013. Available at: www.emcdda.europa.eu/topics/pods/synthetic-cannabinoids [last accessed 24 March 2022].

22. Huffman JW, Dai D, Martin BR, Compton DR. Design, synthesis and pharmacology of cannabimimetic indoles. *Bioorg Med Chem Lett* 1994;**4**:563–566.

23. Potts AJ, Cano C, Thomas SHL, Hill SL. Synthetic cannabinoid receptor agonists: classification and nomenclature. *Clin Toxicol* 2020;**58**(2):82–98. https://doi.org/10.1080/15563650 .2019.1661425

24. Carroll FI, Lewin AH, Mascarella SW, Seltzman HH, Reddy PA. Designer drugs: a medicinal chemistry perspective. *Ann NY Acad Sci* 2012;**1248**:18–38.

25. Uchiyama N, Kawamura M, Kikura-Hanajiri R, Goda Y. Identification and quantitative analyses of two cannabimimetic phenylacetylindoles, JWH-251 and JWH-250, and four cannabimimetic naphthoylindoles, JWH-081, JWH-015, JWH-200 and JWH-073, as designer drugs in illegal products. *Forensic Toxicol* 2011;**29**:25–37.

26. Huffman J. Cannabimimetic indoles, pyrroles, and indenes: structure–activity relationships and receptor interactions. In: PH Reggio, (ed.), *The Cannabinoid Receptors*, pp. 49–94. New York, Humana Press, 2009.

27. Huffman JW, Mabon R, Wu MJ, et al. 3-indolyl1-naphthylmethanes: new cannabimimetic indoles provide evidence for aromatic stacking interactions with the CB(1) cannabinoid receptor. *Bioorg Med Chem* 2003;**11**:539–549.

28. Auwärter V, Dresen S, Weinmann W, Müller M, Pütz M, Ferreirós N. 'Spice' and other herbal blends: harmless incense or cannabinoid designer drugs? *J Mass Spectrom* 2009;**44** (5):832–837. https://doi.org/10.1002/jms.1558

29. Weissman A, Milne GM, Melvin LS Jr. Cannabimimetic activity from CP-47,497, a derivative of 3-phenylcyclohexanol. *J Pharmacol Exp Ther* 1982;**223**:516–523.

30. Devane WA, Breuer A, Sheskin T, Järbe TU, Eisen MS, Mechoulam R. A novel probe for the cannabinoid receptor. *J Med Chem* 1992;**35**(11):2065–2069.

31. Gottardo R, Chiarini A, Dal Prà I, et al. Direct screening of herbal blends for new synthetic cannabinoids by MALDI-TOF MS. *J Mass Spectrom* 2012;**47**(1):141–146. https://doi.org/10 .1002/jms.2036

32. Hutter M, Broecker S, Kneisel S, Auwärter V. Identification of the major urinary metabolites in man of seven synthetic cannabinoids of the aminoalkylindole type present as adulterants in 'herbal mixtures' using LC-MS/MS techniques. *J Mass Spectrom* 2012;**47**(1):54–65. https://doi.org/10.1002/jms.2026

33. Marusich JA, Wiley JL, Lefever TW, Patel PR, Thomas BF. Finding order in chemical chaos – continuing characterization of synthetic cannabinoid receptor agonists. *Neuropharmacology* 2018;**134**(Pt A):73–81. https://doi.org/10 .1016/j.neuropharm.2017.10.041

34. Lindigkeit R, Boehme A, Eiserloh I, et al. Spice: a never-ending story? *Forensic Sci Int* 2009;**191**:58–63.

35. Hermanns-Clausen M, Kneisel S, Szabo B, Auwärter V. Acute toxicity due to the confirmed consumption of synthetic cannabinoids: clinical and laboratory findings. *Addiction* 2013;**108**(3):534–544. https://doi.org/10.1111/j.1360-0443 .2012.04078.x

36. Uchiyama N, Matsuda S, Kawamura M, Kikura-Hanajiri R, Goda Y. Two new-type cannabimimetic quinolinyl carboxylates, QUPIC and QUCHIC, two new cannabimimetic carboxamide derivatives, ADB-FUBINACA and ADBICA, and five synthetic cannabinoids detected with a thiophene derivative a-PVT and an opioid receptor agonist AH-7921 identified in illegal products. *Forensic Toxicol* 2013;**31**:223–240. https://doi.org/10.1007/s11419-013–0182-9

37. Adams AJ, Banister SD, Irizarry L, Trecki J, Schwartz M, Gerona R. 'Zombie' outbreak caused by the synthetic cannabinoid AMB-FUBINACA in New York. *N Engl J Med* 2017;**376**:235–242. https://doi.org/10.1056 /NEJMoa1610300

38. McCain KR, Jones JO, Chilbert KT, Patton AL, James LP, Moran JH. Impaired driving associated with the synthetic cannabinoid 5fAdb. *J Forensic Sci Criminol* 2018;**6**(1). https:// doi.org/10.15744/2348-9804.6.105

39. Haden M, Archer JRH, Dargan PI, Wood DM. MDMB-CHMICA: availability, patterns of use, and toxicity associated with this novel psychoactive substance. *Subst Use Misuse* 2017;**52**(2):223–232. https://doi.org/10.1080/10826084 .2016.1223692

40. Bilgrei OR. From 'herbal highs' to the 'heroin of cannabis': Exploring the evolving discourse on synthetic cannabinoid use in a Norwegian Internet drug forum. *Int J Drug Policy* 2016;**29**:1–8.

41. Lamy FR, Daniulaityte R, Nahhas RW, et al. Increases in synthetic cannabinoid-related harms: results from a longitudinal web-based content analysis. *Int J Drug Policy* 2017;**44**:121–129. https://doi.org/10.1016/j .drugpo.2017.05.007

42. Bäckberg M, Tworek L, Beck O, et al. Analytically confirmed intoxications involving MDMB-CHMICA from the STRIDA Project. *J Med Toxicol* 2017;**13**:52–60. https://doi.org/10.1007 /s13181-016-0584-2

43. Advisory Council on the Misuse of Drugs (ACMD). Further Consideration of the Synthetic Cannabinoids. ACMD, October 2012. Available at: https://assets .publishing.service.gov.uk/government/uploads/system/uploa ds/attachment_data/file/929909/FOR_PUBLICATION_-_AC MD_SCRA_report_final.pdf [last accessed 26 April 2022].

44. Bäckberg M, Tworek L, Beck O, et al. Analytically confirmed intoxications involving MDMB-CHMICA from the STRIDA Project. *J Med Toxicol* 2017;**13**:52–60. https://doi.org/10.1007/s13181-016-0584-2

45. See for example www.telegraph.co.uk/news/2017/09/22/letters-sent-prison-photocopied-amid-fears-soaked-drugs/ [last accessed 24 March 2022].

46. Ford LT, Berg JD. Analytical evidence to show letters impregnated with novel psychoactive substances are a means of getting drugs to inmates within the UK prison service. *Ann Clin Biochem* 2018;**55**(6):673–678. https://doi.org/10.1177/0004563218767462

47. Moosmann B, Angerer V, Auwärter V. Inhomogeneities in herbal mixtures: a serious risk for consumers. *Forensic Toxicol* 2014;**33**:54–60.

48. Choi H, Heo S, Choe S, et al. Simultaneous analysis of synthetic cannabinoids in the materials seized during drug trafficking using GC-MS. *Anal Bioanal Chem* 2013;**405**:3937–3944.

49. Frinculescu A, Lyall CL, Ramsey J, Miserez B. Variation in commercial smoking mixtures containing third generation synthetic cannabinoids. *Drug Test Anal* 2017;**9**:327–333.

50. Choi H, Heo S, Choe S, et al. Simultaneous analysis of synthetic cannabinoids in the materials seized during drug trafficking using GC-MS. *Anal Bioanal Chem* 2013;**405**(12):3937–3944. https://doi.org/10.1007/s00216-012-6560-z

51. Ginsburg BC, McMahon LR, Sanchez JJ, Javors MA. Purity of synthetic cannabinoids sold online for recreational use. *J Anal Toxicol* 2012;**36**(1):66–68. https://doi.org/10.1093/jat/bkr018

52. Brandt SD, Sumnall HR, Measham F, Cole J. Analyses of second-generation 'legal highs' in the UK: initial findings. *Drug Test Anal* 2010;**2**:377–382.

53. Brandt SD, Sumnall HR, Measham, F, Cole J. Second generation mephedrone: the confusing case of NRG-1. *Br Med J* 2010;**341**:c3564.

54. Davies S, Wood DM, Smith G, et al. Purchasing 'legal highs' on the Internet – is there consistency in what you get? *QJM* 2010;**103**:489–493.

55. Ramsey J, Dargan PI, Smyllie M, et al. Buying 'legal' recreational drugs does not mean that you are not breaking the law. *QJM* 2010;**103**:777–783.

56. Hillebrand J, Olszewski D, Sedefov R. Legal highs on the Internet. *Subst Use Misuse* 2010;**45**:330–340.

57. Pintori N, Loi B, Mereu M. Synthetic cannabinoids: the hidden side of spice drugs. *Behav Pharmacol* 2017;**28**:409–419.

58. World Health Organization (WHO). JWH-018. Critical Review Report Agenda Item 4.5. Expert Committee on Drug Dependence 36th Meeting, Geneva, 16–20 June 2014.

59. Abouchedid R, Hudson S, Thurtle N, et al. Analytical confirmation of synthetic cannabinoids in a cohort of 179 presentations with acute recreational drug toxicity to an emergency department in London, UK in the first half of 2015. *Clin Toxicol* 2017;**55**:338–345.

60. Kikura-Hanajiri R, Uchiyama N, Kawamura M, et al. Changes in the prevalence of synthetic cannabinoids and cathinone derivatives in Japan until early 2012. *Forensic Toxicol* 2013;**31**:44–53.

61. Cordeiro SK, Daro RC, Seung H, Klein-Schwartz W, Kim HK. Evolution of clinical characteristics and outcomes of synthetic cannabinoid receptor agonist exposure in the United States: analysis of National Poison Data System data from 2010 to 2015. *Addiction* 2018;**113**:1850–1861.

62. Ogata J, Uchiyama N, Kikura-Hanajiri R, Goda Y. DNA sequence analyses of blended herbal products including synthetic cannabinoids as designer drugs. *Forensic Sci Int* 2013;**227**(1–3):33–41.

63. Uchiyama N, Matsuda S, Kawamura M, Kikura-Hanajiri R, Goda Y. Two new-type cannabimimetic quinolinyl carboxylates, QUPIC and QUCHIC, two new cannabimimetic carboxamide derivatives, ADB-FUBINACA and ADBICA, and five synthetic cannabinoids detected with a thiophene derivative a-PVT and an opioid receptor agonist AH-7921 identified in illegal products. *Forensic Toxicol* 2013;**31**:223–240.

64. Lonati D, Buscaglia E, Papa P, et al. MAM-2201 (analytically confirmed) intoxication after 'Synthacaine' consumption. *Ann Emerg Med* 2014;**64**(6):629–632. https://doi.org/10.1016/j.annemergmed.2014.01.007

65. Uchiyama N, Kawamura M, Kikura-Hanajiri R, Goda Y. URB-754: a new class of designer drug and 12 synthetic cannabinoids detected in illegal products. *Forensic Sci Int* 2013;**227**(1–3):21–32.

66. Wurita A, Hasegawa K, Minakata K, Watanabe K, Suzuki O. A large amount of new designer drug diphenidine coexisting with a synthetic cannabinoid 5-fluoro-AB-PINACA found in a dubious herbal product. *Forensic Toxicol* 2014;**32**(2):331–337.

67. Park Y, Lee C, Lee H, et al. Identification of a new synthetic cannabinoid in a herbal mixture: 1-butyl-3-(2-ethoxybenzoyl) indole. *Forensic Toxicol* 2013;**31**:187–196.

68. Uchiyama N, Shimokawa Y, Matsuda S, Kawamura M, Kikura-Hanajiri R, Goda Y. Two new synthetic cannabinoids, AM-2201 benzimidazole analog (FUBIMINA) and (4-methylpiperazin1-yl)(1-pentyl-1H-indol-3-yl)methanone (MEPIRAPIM), and three phenethylamine derivatives, 25H-NBOMe 3,4,5-trimethoxybenzyl analog, 25B-NBOMe, and 2C-N-NBOMe, identified in illegal products. *Forensic Toxicol* 2014;**32**(1):105–115.

69. Uchiyama N, Kikura-Hanajiri R, Ogata J, Goda Y. Chemical analysis of synthetic cannabinoids as designer drugs in herbal products. *Forensic Sci Int* 2010;**198**:31–38.

70. Zuba D, Byrska B, Maciow M. Comparison of 'herbal highs' composition. *Anal Bioanal Chem* 2011;**400**:119–126.

71. European Monitoring Centre for Drugs and Drug Addiction (EMCDDA). Synthetic Cannabinoids and 'Spice' Drug Profile. Available at: www.emcdda.europa.eu/publications/drug-profiles/synthetic-cannabinoids [last accessed 24 March 2022].

72. Dresen S, Ferreirós N, Pütz M, Westphal F, Zimmermann R, Auwärter V. Monitoring of herbal mixtures potentially containing synthetic cannabinoids as psychoactive compounds. *J Mass Spectrom* 2010;**45**(10):1186–1194. https://doi.org/10.1002/jms.1811

73. Simmons J, Cookman L, Kang C, Skinner C. Three cases of 'spice' exposure. *Clin Toxicol* 2011;**49**:431–433.

74. Simmons JR, Skinner CG, Williams J, Kang CS, Schwartz MD, Wills BK. Intoxication from smoking 'Spice'. *Ann Emerg Med* 2011;**57**:187–188.

75. Seely KA, Lapoint J, Moran JH, Fattore L. Spice drugs are more than harmless herbal blends: a review of the pharmacology and toxicology of synthetic cannabinoids. *Prog Neuropsychopharmacol Biol Psychiatry* 2012;**39**(2):234–243. https://doi.org/10.1016/j.pnpbp.2012.04.017

76. Castellanos D, Thornton G. Synthetic cannabinoid use: recognition and management. *J Psychiatr Pract* 2012;**18**(2):86–93. https://doi.org/10.1097/01.pra.0000413274.09305.9c

77. Dargan PI, Hudson S, Ramsey J, Wood DM. The impact of changes in UK classification of the synthetic cannabinoid receptor agonists in 'Spice'. *Int J Drug Policy* 2011;**22**(4):274–277. https://doi.org/10.1016/j.drugpo.2011.02.006

78. Adams AJ, Banister SD, Irizarry L, Trecki J, Schwartz M, Gerona R. 'Zombie' outbreak caused by the synthetic cannabinoid AMB-FUBINACA in New York. *N Engl J Med* 2017;**376**:235–242.

79. European Monitoring Centre for Drugs and Drug Addiction. New Psychoactive Substances in Europe: An Update from the EU Early Warning System. 2015. Available at: www.emcdda.europa.eu/system/files/publications/2753/POD_Synthetic%20cannabinoids_0.pdf [last accessed 26 April 2022].

80. United Nations Office on Drugs and Crime. World Drug Report 2016. Available at: https://www.unodc.org/LSS/Home/BothAreas [last accessed 26 April 2022].

81. Van Amsterdam J, Nutt D, van den Brink W. Generic legislation of new psychoactive drugs. *J Psychopharmacol* 2013;**27**(3):317–324.

82. European Monitoring Centre for Drugs and Drug Addiction. Perspectives on Drugs. Synthetic Cannabinoids in Europe. Available at: www.emcdda.europa.eu/system/files/publications/2753/POD_Synthetic%20cannabinoids_0.pdf [last accessed 26 March 2022].

83. European Monitoring Centre for Drugs and Drug Addiction. European Drug Report 2019: Trends and Developments. Luxembourg, Publications Office of the European Union, 2019.

84. HM Inspectorate of Prisons. HM Chief Inspector of Prisons for England and Wales: Annual Report 2013-2014.

85. European Monitoring Centre for Drugs and Drug Addiction. European Drug Report: Trends and Developments. Luxembourg, Publications Office of the European Union, 2018.

86. European Monitoring Centre for Drugs and Drug Addiction. Perspective on Drugs: Synthetic Cannabinoids in Europe. Luxembourg, Publications Office of the European Union, 2017.

87. Akram H, Mokrysz C, Curran HV. What are the psychological effects of using synthetic cannabinoids? A systematic review. *J Psychopharmacol* 2019;**33**(3):271–283. https://doi.org/10.1177/0269881119826592

88. Smith KE, Staton M. Synthetic cannabinoid use among a sample of individuals enrolled in community-based recovery programs: are synthetic cannabinoids actually preferred to other drugs? *Subst Abuse* 2018;**40**(2):1–10. https://doi.org/10.1080/08897077.2018.1528495

89. Mathews EM, Jeffries E, Hsieh C, Jones G, Buckner JD. Synthetic cannabinoid use among college students. *Addict Behav* 2019;**93**:219–224. https://doi.org/10.1016/j.addbeh.2019.02.009

90. Vandrey R, Dunn KE, Fry JA, Girling ER. A survey study to characterize use of Spice products (synthetic cannabinoids). *Drug Alcohol Depend* 2012;**120**(1–3):238–241. https://doi.org/10.1016/j.drugalcdep.2011.07.011

91. Barratt MJ, Cakic V, Lenton S. Patterns of synthetic cannabinoid use in Australia. *Drug Alcohol Rev* 2013;**32**(2):141–146. https://doi.org/10.1111/j.1465-3362.2012.00519.x

92. Castellanos D, Singh S, Thornton G, Avila M, Moreno A. Synthetic cannabinoid use: a case series of adolescents. *J Adolesc Health* 2011;**49**(4):347–349.

93. Hurst D, Loeffler G, McLay R. Synthetic cannabinoid agonist induced psychosis: a case series. APA poster. San Diego, Naval Medical Centre, 2011. Abstract in *Am J Psychiatry* 2011;**168**(10):1119. https://doi.org/10.1176/appi.ajp.2011.11010176).

94. Van Der Veer N, Friday J. Persistent psychosis following the use of Spice. *Schizophrenia Res* 2011;**130**:285–286.

95. Peglow S, Buchner J, Briscoe G. Synthetic cannabinoid-induced psychosis in a previously nonpsychotic patient. *Am J Addict* 2012;**21**:287–288.

96. Tung CK, Chiang TP, Lam M. Acute mental disturbance caused by synthetic cannabinoid: a potential emerging substance of abuse in Hong Kong. *East Asian Arch Psychiatry* 2012;**22**(1):31–33.

97. Chan WL, Wood DM, Hudson S, Dargan PI. Acute psychosis associated with recreational use of benzofuran 6-(2 aminopropyl)benzofuran (6-APB) and cannabis. *J Med Toxicol* 2013;**9**(3):278–281. https://doi.org/10.1007/s13181-013-0306-y

98. Thornton SL, Lo J, Clark RF, Wu AH, Gerona RR. Simultaneous detection of multiple designer drugs in serum, urine, and CSF in a patient with prolonged psychosis. *Clin Toxicol* 2012;**50**(10):1165–1168. https://doi.org/10.3109/15563650.2012.744996

99. Abouchedid R, Ho JH, Hudson S, et al. Acute toxicity associated with use of 5F-derivations of synthetic cannabinoid receptor agonists with analytical confirmation. *J Med Toxicol* 2016;**12**(4):396–401. https://doi.org/10.1007/s13181-016-0571-7

100. Abouchedid R, Ho JH, Hudson S, et al. Acute toxicity associated with use of 5F-derivations of synthetic cannabinoid receptor agonists with analytical confirmation. *J Med Toxicol* 2016;**12**(4):396–401. https://doi.org/10.1007/s13181-016-0571-7

101. European Monitoring Centre for Drugs and Drug Addiction (EMCDDA). Understanding the Spice Phenomenon. EMCDDA, 2009.

102. Brents LK, Prather PL. The K2/Spice phenomenon: emergence, identification, legislation and metabolic characterization of synthetic cannabinoids in herbal incense products. *Drug Metab Rev* 2014;**46**(1):72–85. https://doi.org/10.3109/03602532.2013.839700

103. Johnson LA, Johnson RL, Portier RB. Current 'legal highs'. *J Emerg Med* 2013;**44**(6):1108–1115. https://doi.org/10.1016/j.jemermed.2012.09.147

104. Van Hout MC, Hearne E. User experiences of development of dependence on the synthetic cannabinoids, 5f-AKB48 and 5F-PB-22, and subsequent withdrawal syndromes. *Int J Ment Health Addict* 2017;**15**(3):565–579.

105. Schifano F, Corazza O, Deluca P, et al. Psychoactive drug or mystical incense? Overview of the online available information on spice products. *Int J Cult Ment Health* 2009;**2**:137–144.

106. Centers for Disease Control and Prevention (CDC). Acute kidney injury associated with synthetic cannabinoid use: multiple states. *Morb Mort Wkly Rep* 2013;**62**(6):93–98.

107. Bebarta VS, Ramirez S, Varney SM. Spice: a new 'legal' herbal mixture abused by young active-duty military personnel. *Subst Abuse* 2012;**33**:191–194.

108. European Monitoring Centre for Drugs and Drug Addiction. European Drug Report 2019: Trends and Developments. Luxembourg, Publications Office of the European Union, 2019.

109. Ellsworth JT. Spice, vulnerability, and victimization: synthetic cannabinoids and interpersonal crime victimization among homeless adults [published online ahead of print, 7 November 2019]. *Subst Abus* 2019;**2019**:1–7. https://doi.org/10.1080/08897077.2019.1686725

110. Advisory Council on the Misuse of Drugs (ACMD). Benzofurans: A Review of the Evidence of Use and Harm. ACMD, November 2013.

111. Ralphs R, Williams L, Askew R, Norton A. Adding Spice to the Porridge: the development of a synthetic cannabinoid market in an English prison. *Int J Drug Policy* 2017;**40**:57–69.

112. Walker, DF. The informal economy in prison. *Crim Justice Matters* 2015;**99**(1):18–19.

113. User Voice: Spice: The Bird Killer. What Prisoners Think about the Use of Spice and Other Legal Highs in Prison. Published May 2016. Available at: www.uservoice.org/wp-content/uploads/2020/07/User-Voice-Spice-The-Bird-Killer-Report-compressed.pdf [last accessed 26 April 2022].

114. Forrester M, Kleinschmidt K, Schwarz E, Young A. Synthetic cannabinoid and marijuana exposures reported to poison centers. *Hum Exp Toxicol* 2012;**31**:1006–1011.

115. Schifano F, Deluca P, Baldacchino A, et al. Drugs on the web; the Psychonaut 2002 EU project. *Prog Neuropsychopharmacol Biol Psychiatry* 2006;**30**:640–646.

116. Teske J, Weller JP, Fieguth A, Rothämel T, Schulz Y, Tröger HD. Sensitive and rapid quantification of the cannabinoid receptor agonist naphthalen-1-yl-(1-pentylindol-3-yl) methanone (JWH-018) in human serum by liquid chromatography–tandem mass spectrometry. *J Chromatogr B Analyt Technol Biomed Life Sci* 2010;**878**:2659–2663.

117. Mathews EM, Jeffries E, Hsieh C, Jones G, Buckner JD. Synthetic cannabinoid use among college students. *Addict Behav* 2019;**93**:219–224. https://doi.org/10.1016/j.addbeh.2019.02.009

118. Smith KElin, Staton M. Synthetic cannabinoid use among a sample of individuals enrolled in community-based recovery programs: are synthetic cannabinoids actually preferred to other drugs? *Subst Abuse* 2018;**2018**:1–10. https://doi.org/10.1080/08897077.2018.1528495

119. Shanks KG, Dahn T, Terrell AR. Detection of JWH-018 and JWH-073 by UPLC–MS-MS in postmortem whole blood casework. *J Analytical Toxicol* 2012;**36**:145–152.

120. Saito T, Namera A, Miura N, et al. A fatal case of MAM-2201 poisoning. *Forensic Toxicol* 2013;**31**:333–337.

121. Kronstrand R, Roman M, Andersson M, Eklund A. Toxicological findings of synthetic cannabinoids in recreational users. *J Analytical Toxicol* 2013;**37**(8):534–541.

122. Schaefer N, Peters B, Bregel D, et al. A fatal case involving several synthetic cannabinoids. *Toxichem Krimtech* 2013;**80** (special issue):248.

123. Behonick G, Shanks KG, Firchau DJ, et al. Four postmortem case reports with quantitative detection of the synthetic cannabinoid, 5F-PB-22. *J Anal Toxicol* 2014;**38**(8):559–562. https://doi.org/10.1093/jat/bku048

124. Savasman CM, Peterson DC, Pietak BR, Dudley MH, Clinton Frazee III C, Garg U. Two fatalities due to the use of synthetic cannabinoids alone. In: Proceedings of the 66th Annual Scientific Meeting of the American Academy of Forensic Sciences, Seattle, WA 17–22 February, 2014, p. 316. Denver, CO, Publication Printers, 2014.

125. Corkery J, Claridge H, Loi B, Goodair C, Schifano F. NPSAD Annual Report 2013 – Drug-Related Deaths in the UK: January–December 2012. National Programme on Substance Abuse Deaths (NPSAD), 2014.

126. Elliott S, Evans J. A 3-year review of new psychoactive substances in casework. *Forensic Sci Int* 2014;**243**:55–60.

127. Wikstrom M, Thelander G, Dahlgren M, Kronstrand R. An accidental fatal intoxication with methoxetamine. *J Analytic Toxicol* 2013;**37**(1):43–46.

128. Rosenbaum CD, Scalzo AJ, Long C, et al. K2 and Spice abusers: a case series of clinical and laboratory findings. Paper presented at the North American Congress of Clinical Toxicology (NACCT), 21–26 September, Washington, DC, 2011.

129. Patton AL, Chimalakonda KC, Moran CL, et al. K2 toxicity: fatal case of psychiatric complications following AM2201

exposure. *J Forensic Sci* 2013;**58**(6):1676–1680. https://doi.org/10.1111/1556-4029.12216

130. Reports to PHE's Drug Alerts, March 2018.

131. Report to PHE by Manchester Local Drug Information System 'Spice Warning,' August 2018.

132. Shanks KG, Behonick GS. Death after use of the synthetic cannabinoid 5F-AMB. *Forensic Sci Int* 2016;**262**:e21–e24.

133. Somerville RF, Hassan VR, Kolbe E, et al. The identification and quantification of synthetic cannabinoids seized in New Zealand in 2017. *Forensic Sci Int* 2019;**300**:19–27.

134. Darke S, Duflou J, Farrell M, Peacock A, Lappin J. Characteristics and circumstances of synthetic cannabinoid-related death. *Clin Toxicol* 2019 (online). https://doi.org/10.1080/15563650.2019.1647344

135. Darke S, Duflou J, Farrell M, Peacock A, Lappin J. Characteristics and circumstances of synthetic cannabinoid-related death. *Clin Toxicol* 2019 (online). https://doi.org/10.1080/15563650.2019.1647344

136. Tait RJ, Caldicott D, Mountain D, Hill SL, Lenton S. A systematic review of adverse events arising from the use of synthetic cannabinoids and their associated treatment. *Clin Toxicol* 2016;**54**(1):1–13.

137. European Monitoring Centre for Drugs and Drug Addiction. Fentanils and synthetic cannabinoids: driving greater complexity into the drug situation. An update from the EU Early Warning System (June 2018). Luxembourg, Publications Office of the European Union, 2018.

138. Fattore L, Fratta W. Beyond THC: the new generation of cannabinoid designer drugs. *Front Behav Neurosci* 2011;**5**:60.

139. Seely KA, Prather PL, James LP, et al. Marijuana-based drugs: innovative therapeutics or designer drugs of abuse? *Mol Interv* 2011;**11**:36–51.

140. Mills B, Yepes A, Nugent K. Synthetic cannabinoids. *Am J Med Sci* 2015;**350**(1): 59–62.

141. Harris CR, Brown A. Synthetic cannabinoid intoxication: a case series and review. *J Emerg Med* 2013;**44**(2):360–366. https://doi.org/10.1016/j.jemermed.2012.07.061

142. Akram H, Mokrysz C, Curran HV. What are the psychological effects of using synthetic cannabinoids? A systematic review. *J Psychopharmacol* 2019;**33**(3):271–283. https://doi.org/10.1177/0269881119826592

143. Albertson TE, Chenoweth JA, Colby DK, et al. The changing drug culture: medical and recreational marijuana. FP Essent 2016;**441**:11–17.

144. D'Souza DC, Radhakrishnan R, Sherif M, et al. Cannabinoids and psychosis. *Curr Pharm Des* 2016;**22**(42):6380–6391.

145. Gray R, Bressington D, Hughes E, et al. A systematic review of the effects of novel psychoactive substances 'legal highs' on people with severe mental illness. *J Psychiatr Ment Health Nurs* 2016;**23**(5):267–281.

146. Van Amsterdam J, Brunt T, van den Brink W. The adverse health effects of synthetic cannabinoids with emphasis on psychosis-like effects. *J Psychopharmacol* 2015;**29**(3): 254–263.

147. White CM. The pharmacologic and clinical effects of illicit synthetic cannabinoids. *J Clin Pharmacol* 2017;**57**(3):297–304.

148. Banister SD, Connor M. The chemistry and pharmacology of synthetic cannabinoid receptor agonists as new psychoactive substances: origins. *Handb Exp Pharmacol* 2018;**252**:165–190. https://doi.org/10.1007/164_2018_143

149. Zaurova M, Hoffman RS, Vlahov D, Manini AF. Clinical effects of synthetic cannabinoid receptor agonists compared with marijuana in emergency department patients with acute drug overdose. *J Med Toxicol* 2016;**12**(4):335–340. https://doi.org/10.1007/s13181-016-0558-4

150. Mensen VT, Vreeker A, Nordgren J, et al. Psychopathological symptoms associated with synthetic cannabinoid use: a comparison with natural cannabis. *Psychopharmacology* 2019;**236**:2677–2685. https://doi.org/10.1007/s00213-019-05238-8

151. Bassir Nia A, Medrano B, Perkel C, et al. Psychiatric comorbidity associated with synthetic cannabinoid use compared to cannabis. *J Psychopharmacol* 2016;**30**(12):1321–1330.

152. Bassir Nia A, Medrano B, Perkel C, et al. Psychiatric comorbidity associated with synthetic cannabinoid use compared to cannabis. *J Psychopharmacol* 2016;**30**(12):1321–1330.

153. Shalit N, Barzilay R, Shoval G, et al. Characteristics of synthetic cannabinoid and cannabis users admitted to a psychiatric hospital: a comparative study. *J Clin Psychiatry* 2016;**77**(8): e989–e995. https://doi.org/10.4088/JCP.15m09938

154. Mathews EM, Jeffries E, Hsieh C, Jones G, Buckner JD. Synthetic cannabinoid use among college students. *Addict Behav* 2019;**93**:219–224. https://doi.org/10.1016/j.addbeh.2019.02.009

155. Winstock AR, Barratt MJ. Synthetic cannabis: a comparison of patterns of use and effect profile with natural cannabis in a large global sample. *Drug Alcohol Depend* 2013;**131**(1–3):106–111. https://doi.org/10.1016/j.drugalcdep.2012.12.011

156. Winstock AR, Barratt MJ. The 12-month prevalence and nature of adverse experiences resulting in emergency medical presentations associated with the use of synthetic cannabinoid products. *Hum Psychopharmacol* 2013;**28**(4):390–393. https://doi.org/10.1002/hup.2292

157. Hoyte CO, Jacob J, Monte AA, Al-Jumaan M, Bronstein AC, Heard KJ. A characterization of synthetic cannabinoid exposures reported to the National Poison Data System in 2010. *Ann Emerg Med* 2012;**60**:435–438.

158. Winstock AR, Barratt MJ. Synthetic cannabis: a comparison of patterns of use and effect profile with natural cannabis in a large global sample. *Drug Alcohol Depend* 2013;**131**(1–3):106–111. https://doi.org/10.1016/j.drugalcdep.2012.12.011

159. Winstock AR, Barratt MJ. The 12-month prevalence and nature of adverse experiences resulting in emergency medical presentations associated with the use of synthetic cannabinoid products. *Hum Psychopharmacol* 2013;**28**(4):390–393. https://doi.org/10.1002/hup.2292

160. Tait RJ, Caldicott D, Mountain D, Hill SL, Lenton S. A systematic review of adverse events arising from the use of synthetic cannabinoids and their associated treatment. *Clin Toxicol* 2016;**54**(1):1–13.

161. Cooper ZD. Adverse effects of synthetic cannabinoids: management of acute toxicity and withdrawal. *Curr Psychiatry Rep* 2016;**18**:52. https://doi.org/10.1007/s11920-016-0694-11

162. Advisory Council on the Misuse of Drugs. 'Third Generation' Synthetic Cannabinoids. ACMD, 2014.

163. Tait RJ, Caldicott D, Mountain D, Hill SL, Lenton S. A systematic review of adverse events arising from the use of synthetic cannabinoids and their associated treatment. *Clin Toxicol* 2016;**54**(1):1–13.

164. Karila L, Roux P, Rolland B, et al. Acute and long-term effects of cannabis use: a review. *Curr Pharm Des* 2014;**20**:4112–4118.

165. Schneir AB, Cullen J, Ly BT. 'Spice' girls: synthetic cannabinoid intoxication. *J Emerg Med* 2011;**40**:296–299.

166. Tait RJ, Caldicott D, Mountain D, Hill SL, Lenton S. A systematic review of adverse events arising from the use of synthetic cannabinoids and their associated treatment. *Clin Toxicol* 2016;**54**(1):1–13.

167. Lovett C, Wood DM, Dargan PI. Pharmacology and toxicology of the synthetic cannabinoid receptor agonists. *Réanimation* 2015;**24**:527–541.

168. Cordeiro SK, Daro RC, Seung H, Klein-Schwartz W, Kim HK. Evolution of clinical characteristics and outcomes of synthetic cannabinoid receptor agonist exposure in the United States: analysis of National Poison Data System data from 2010 to 2015. *Addiction* 2018;**113**:1850–1861.

169. Cordeiro SK, Daro RC, Seung H, Klein-Schwartz W, Kim HK. Evolution of clinical characteristics and outcomes of synthetic cannabinoid receptor agonist exposure in the United States: analysis of National Poison Data System data from 2010 to 2015. *Addiction* **2018**;113:1850–1861.

170. Cordeiro SK, Daro RC, Seung H, Klein-Schwartz W, Kim HK. Evolution of clinical characteristics and outcomes of synthetic cannabinoid receptor agonist exposure in the United States: analysis of National Poison Data System data from 2010 to 2015. *Addiction* **2018**;113:1850–1861.

171. Law R, Schier J, Martin C, et al. Notes from the field: increase in reported adverse health effects related to synthetic cannabinoid use in the United States, January to May 2015. *Morb Mort Wkly Rep* 2015;**64**(22):618e619.

172. Centers for Disease Control and Prevention (CDC). Acute kidney injury associated with synthetic cannabinoid use: multiple states, 2012. *Morb Mort Wkly Rep* 2013;**62**(6):93–98.

173. Murphy TD, Weidenbach KN, Houten CV, et al. Acute kidney injury associated with synthetic cannabinoid use: multiple states, 2012. *Morb Mort Wkly Rep* 2013;**62**:93–98.

174. Schwartz MD, Trecki J, Edison LA, Steck AR, Arnold JK, Gerona RR. A common source outbreak of severe delirium associated with exposure to the novel synthetic cannabinoid ADB-PINACA. *J Emerg Med* 2015;**48**:573–580.

175. Tyndall JA, Gerona R, De Portu G, et al. An outbreak of acute delirium from exposure to the synthetic cannabinoid AB-CHMINACA. *Clin Toxicol* 2015;**53**:950–956.

176. Cordeiro SK, Daro RC, Seung H, Klein-Schwartz W, Kim HK. Evolution of clinical characteristics and outcomes of synthetic cannabinoid receptor agonist exposure in the United States: analysis of National Poison Data System data from 2010 to 2015. *Addiction* 2018;**113**:1850–1861.

177. Adams AJ, Banister SD, Irizarry L, Trecki J, Schwartz M, Gerona R. 'Zombie' outbreak caused by the synthetic cannabinoid AMB-FUBINACA in New York. *N Engl J Med* 2017;**376**:235–242.

178. Abouchedid R, Ho JH, Hudson S, et al. Acute toxicity associated with use of 5F-derivations of synthetic cannabinoid receptor agonists with analytical confirmation. *J Med Toxicol* 2016;**12**(4):396–401. https://doi.org/10.1007/s13181-0 16-0571-7

179. Ross CH, Singh P, Simon EL. Hemorrhagic soft tissue upper airway obstruction from brodifacoum-contaminated synthetic cannabinoid. *J Emerg Med* 2019;**57**(1):47–50.

180. Kelkar AH, Smith NA, Martial A, Moole H, Tarantino MD, Roberts JC. An outbreak of synthetic cannabinoid–associated coagulopathy in Illinois. *N Engl J Med* 2018;**379**:1216–1223. https://doi.org/10.1056/NEJMoa1807652

181. See for example, Hasan O, Patel AA, Siegert JJ. A new differential diagnosis: synthetic cannabinoid-associated gross hematuria. *Case Rep Med* 2019;2019:6327819. https://doi.org/ 10.1155/2019/6327819

182. Riley SB, Sochat M, Moser K, et al. Case of brodifacoum-contaminated synthetic cannabinoid. *Clin Toxicol* 2019;**57**(2):143–144. https://doi.org/10.1080/15563650 .2018.1502444

183. Chan A, Adashek M, Kang J, Medinab AJ. Disseminated intravascular coagulopathy secondary to unintentional brodifacoum poisoning via synthetic marijuana. *Hematol* 2019;**8**(1):40–43.

184. Cooper ZD. Adverse effects of synthetic cannabinoids: management of acute toxicity and withdrawal. *Curr Psychiatry Rep* 2016;18:52. https://doi.org/10.1007/s11920-016-0694-1

185. Tournebize J, Gibaja V, Kahn JP. Acute effects of synthetic cannabinoids: update 2015. *Subst Abuse* 2017;**38** (3):344–366. https://doi.org/10.1080/08897077.2016.1219438

186. Sud P, Gordon M, Tortora L, et al. Retrospective chart review of synthetic cannabinoid intoxication with toxicologic analysis. *West J Emerg Med* 2018;**19**(3):567–572. https://doi .org/10.5811/westjem.2017.12.36968

187. Centers for Disease Control and Prevention (CDC). Notes from the field: severe illness associated with reported use of synthetic marijuana – Colorado, August to September 2013. *Morb Mort Wkly Rep* 2013;**62**(49):1016e1017.

188. Drenzek C, Geller RJ, Steck A. Notes from the field: severe illness associated with synthetic cannabinoid use –Brunswick, Georgia, 2013. *Morb Mort Wkly Rep* 2013;**62**(46):939.

189. Kasper AM, Ridpath AD, Arnold JK, et al. Notes from the field: severe illness associated with reported use of synthetic cannabinoids –Mississippi, April 2015. *Morb Mort Wkly Rep* 2015;**64**(39):1121–1122.

190. Law R, Schier J, Martin C, et al. Notes from the field: increase in reported adverse health effects related to synthetic cannabinoid use – United States, January–May 2015. *Morb Mort Wkly Rep* 2015;**64**(22):618–619.

191. Springer YP, Gerona R, Scheunemann E, et al. Increase in adverse reactions associated with use of synthetic cannabinoids – Anchorage, Alaska, 2015–2016. *Morb Mortal Wkly Rep* 2016;65:1108e1111.

192. Abouchedid R, Hudson S, Thurtle N, et al. Analytical confirmation of synthetic cannabinoids in a cohort of 179 presentations with acute recreational drug toxicity to an emergency department in London, UK in the first half of 2015. *Clin Toxicol* 2017;**55**(5):338–345. https://doi.org/10.1080/15563650.2017.1287373

193. Hill SL, Najafi J, Dunn M, et al. Clinical toxicity following analytically confirmed use of the synthetic cannabinoids MDMBCHMICA. A report from the Identification Of Novel psychoActive substances (IONA) study. *Clin Toxicol* 2016;**54**:638–643.

194. Hill SL, Najafi J, Dunn M, et al. Clinical toxicity following analytically confirmed use of the synthetic cannabinoids MDMBCHMICA. A report from the Identification Of Novel psychoActive substances (IONA) study. *Clin Toxicol* 2016;**54**:638–643.

195. Gugelmann H, Gerona R, Li C, et al. 'Crazy Monkey' poisons man and dog: human and canine seizures due to PB-22, a novel synthetic cannabinoid. *Clin Toxicol* 2014;**52**:635–638.

196. Zaurova M, Hoffman RS, Vlahov D, Manini AF. clinical effects of synthetic cannabinoid receptor agonists compared with marijuana in emergency department patients with acute drug overdose. *J Med Toxicol* 2016;**12**(4):335–340. https://doi.org/10.1007/s13181-016-0558-4

197. Sud P, Gordon M, Tortora L, et al. Retrospective chart review of synthetic cannabinoid intoxication with toxicologic analysis. *West J Emerg Med* 2018;**19**(3):567–572. https://doi.org/10.5811/westjem.2017.12.36968

198. Compton DR, Johnson MR, Melvin LS, Martin BR. Pharmacological profile of a series of bicyclic cannabinoid analogs: classification as cannabimimetic agents. *J Pharmacol Exp Ther* 1992;**260**(1):201–209.

199. D'Ambra TE, Estep KG, Bell MR, et al. Conformationally restrained analogues of pravadoline: nanomolar potent, enantioselective, (aminoalkyl)indole agonists of the cannabinoid receptor. *J Med Chem* 1992;**35**(1):124–135.

200. Sud P, Gordon M, Tortora L, et al. Retrospective chart review of synthetic cannabinoid intoxication with toxicologic analysis. *West J Emerg Med* 2018;**19**(3):567–572. https://doi.org/10.5811/westjem.2017.12.36968

201. De Brabanter N, Deventer K, Stove V, Van Eenoo P. Synthetic cannabinoids: general considerations. *P Belg Roy Acad Med* 2013;2:209–225.

202. Wiley JL, Marusich JA, Huffman JW. Moving around the molecule: relationship between chemical structure and in vivo activity of synthetic cannabinoids. *Life Sci* 2014;**97**(1):55–63. https://doi.org/10.1016/j.lfs.2013.09.011

203. Halberstadt AL, Geyer MA. Multiple receptors contribute to the behavioral effects of indoleamine hallucinogens. *Neuropharmacology* 2011;**61**(3):364–381.

204. Wells DL, Ott CA. The new marijuana. *Ann Pharmacother* 2011;**45**(3):414–417.

205. Yip L, Dart RC. Is there something more about synthetic cannabinoids? *Forensic Toxicol* 2014;**32**(2):340–341.

206. Fisar Z. Inhibition of monoamine oxidase activity by cannabinoids. *Naunyn Schmiedebergs Arch Pharmacol* 2010;**381** (6):563–572. https://doi.org/10.1007/s00210-010-0517-6

207. Bonaccorso S, Metastasio A, Ricciardi A, et al. Synthetic cannabinoid use in a case series of patients with psychosis presenting to acute psychiatric settings: clinical presentation and management issues. *Brain Sci* 2018;**8**:133. https://doi.org/10.3390/brainsci8070133

208. Zarifi C, Vyas S. Spice-y kidney failure: a case report and systematic review of acute kidney injury attributable to the use of synthetic cannabis. *Perm J* 2017;**21**:16–160. https://doi.org/10.7812/TPP/16-160

209. Tournebize J, Gibaja V, Kahn JP. Acute effects of synthetic cannabinoids: update 2015. *Subst Abuse* 2017;**38** (3):344–366. https://doi.org/10.1080/08897077.2016.1219438

210. Sud P, Gordon M, Tortora L, et al. Retrospective chart review of synthetic cannabinoid intoxication with toxicologic analysis. *West J Emerg Med* 2018;**19**(3):567–572. https://doi.org/10.5811/westjem.2017.12.36968

211. Centers for Disease Control and Prevention (CDC). Notes from the field: severe illness associated with reported use of synthetic marijuana – Colorado, August–September 2013. *Morb Mort Wkly Rep* 2013;62(49):1016e1017.

212. Drenzek C, Geller RJ, Steck A. Notes from the field: severe illness associated with synthetic cannabinoid use – Brunswick, Georgia, 2013. *Morb Mort Wkly Rep* 2013;**62**(46):939.

213. Kasper AM, Ridpath AD, Arnold JK, et al. Notes from the field: severe illness associated with reported use of synthetic cannabinoids – Mississippi, April 2015. *Morb Mort Wkly Rep* 2015;**64**(39):1121e1122.

214. Law R, Schier J, Martin C, et al. Notes from the field: increase in reported adverse health effects related to synthetic cannabinoid use – United States, January–May 2015. *Morb Mort Wkly Rep* 2015;**64**(22):618e619.

215. Springer YP, Gerona R, Scheunemann E, et al. Increase in adverse reactions associated with use of synthetic cannabinoids – Anchorage, Alaska, 2015e2016. *Morb Mort Wkly Rep* 2016;**65**:1108e1111.

216. Hill SL, Najafi J, Dunn M, et al. Clinical toxicity following analytically confirmed use of the synthetic cannabinoids MDMBCHMICA. A report from the Identification Of Novel psychoActive substances (IONA) study. *Clin Toxicol* 2016;**54**:638–643.

217. Gugelmann H, Gerona R, Li C, et al. 'Crazy Monkey' poisons man and dog: human and canine seizures due to PB-22, a novel synthetic cannabinoid. *Clin Toxicol* 2014;**52**:635–638.

218. Karila L, Roux P, Rolland B, et al. Acute and long-term effects of cannabis use: a review. *Curr Pharm Des* 2014;**20**:4112–4118.

219. Abouchedid R, Hudson S, Thurtle N, et al. Analytical confirmation of synthetic cannabinoids in a cohort of 179 presentations with acute recreational drug toxicity to an emergency department in London, UK in the first half of 2015. *Clin Toxicol* 2017;**55**(5):338–345. https://doi.org/10.1080/155 63650.2017.1287373

220. Schneir AB, Cullen J, Ly BT . 'Spice' girls: synthetic cannabinoid intoxication. *J Emerg Med* 2011;**40**:296–299.

221. Tait RJ, Caldicott D, Mountain D, Hill SL, Lenton S. A systematic review of adverse events arising from the use of synthetic cannabinoids and their associated treatment. *Clin Toxicol* 2015;**15**:1–13.

222. Lovett C, Wood DM, Dargan PI. Pharmacology and toxicology of the synthetic cannabinoid receptor agonists. *Réanimation* 2015;**24**:527–541.

223. McQuade D, Hudson S, Dargan PI, Wood DM. First European case of convulsions related to analytically confirmed use of the synthetic cannabinoid receptor agonist AM-2201. *Eur J Clin Pharmacol* 2013;**69**:373–376. https://doi.org/10.1007/s00228-01 2-1379-2

224. Papanti D, Schifano F, Botteon G, et al. 'Spiceophrenia': a systematic overview of 'spice'-related psychopathological issues and a case report. *Hum Psychopharmacol* 2013;**28**(4):379–389. https://doi.org/10.1002/hup.2312

225. Spaderna M, Addy P, D'Souza DC. Spicing things up: synthetic cannabinoids. *Psychopharmacology* 2013;**228**(4):525–540.

226. Winstock AR, Barratt MJ. The 12-month prevalence and nature of adverse experiences resulting in emergency medical presentations associated with the use of synthetic cannabinoid products. *Hum Psychopharmacol* 2013;**28**(4):390–393. https:// doi.org/10.1002/hup.2292

227. Freeman MJ, Rose DZ, Myers MA, Gooch CL, Bozeman AC, Burgin WS. Ischemic stroke after use of the synthetic marijuana 'spice'. *Neurology* 2013;**81**(24):2090–2093.

228. Mir A, Obafemi A, Young A, Kane C. Myocardial infarction associated with use of the synthetic cannabinoid K2. *Pediatrics* 2011;**128**(6):e1622–1627.

229. Zimmermann US, Winkelmann PR, Pilhatsch M, Nees JA, Spanagel R, Schulz K. Withdrawal phenomena and dependence syndrome after the consumption of 'Spice Gold'. *Dtsch Arztebl Int* 2009;**106**(27):464–467. https://doi.org/10 .3238/arztebl.2009.0464

230. Banerji S, Deutsch CM, Bronstein AC. Spice ain't so nice. *Clin Toxicol* 2010;**48**:632(abstract 137). Available at: http://infor mahealthcare.com/doi/pdf/10.3109/15563650.2010.493290 [last accessed 27 March 2022].

231. Every-Palmer S. Warning: legal synthetic cannabinoid receptor agonists such as JWH-018 may precipitate psychosis in vulnerable individuals. *Addiction* 2010;**105**:1959–1960.

232. Johnson LA, Johnson RL, Alfonzo C. Spice: a legal marijuana equivalent. *Mil Med* 2011;**176**:718–720.

233. Benford DM, Caplan JP. Psychiatric sequelae of spice, K2, and synthetic cannabinoid receptor agonists. *Psychosomatics* 2011;**52**:295.

234. Vearrier D, Osterhoudt KC. A teenager with agitation: higher than she should have climbed. *Pediatr Emerg Care* 2010;**26**:462–465.

235. Donnelly MT. Health Advisory: K2 Synthetic Marijuana Use Among Teenagers and Young Adults in Missouri. Missouri Department of Health and Senior Services, 5 March 2010. Available at: http://health.mo.gov /emergencies/ert/ alertsadvisories/pdf/HAd3-5-2010.pdf [last accessed 27 March 2022].

236. Cohen K, Kapitány-Fövény M, Mama Y, et al. The effects of synthetic cannabinoids on executive function. *Psychopharmacology* 2017;**234**(7):1121–1134. https://doi.org/ 10.1007/s00213-017-4546-4

237. Theunissen EL, Hutten NR, Mason NL, et al. Neurocognition and subjective experience following acute doses of the synthetic cannabinoid JWH-018: a phase 1, placebo-controlled, pilot study. *Br J Pharmacol* 2018;**175**(1):18–28.

238. Schneir AB, Cullen J, Ly BT. 'Spice' girls: synthetic cannabinoid intoxication. *J Emerg Med* 2011;**40**(3):296–299. https://doi.org/10.1016/j.jemermed.2010.10.014

239. Every-Palmer S. Synthetic cannabinoid JWH-018 and psychosis: an explorative study. *Drug Alcohol Depend* 2011;**117**:152–157.

240. Müller H, Sperling W, Köhrmann M, et al. The synthetic cannabinoid Spice as a trigger for an acute exacerbation of cannabis-induced recurrent psychotic episodes. *Schizophr Res* 2010;**118**:309–310.

241. Young AC, Schwarz E, Medina G, et al. Cardiotoxicity associated with the synthetic cannabinoid, K9, with laboratory confirmation. *Am J Emerg Med* 2012;**30**(7):1320.e5–7. https:// doi.org/10.1016/j.ajem.2011.05.013

242. Thomas S, Bliss S, Malik M. Suicidal ideation and self-harm following K2 use. *J Okla State Med Assoc* 2012;**105** (11):430–433.

243. Pierre JM. Cannabis, synthetic cannabinoids, and psychosis risk: what the evidence says. *Curr Psychiatr* 2011;**10**:49–58.

244. Hobbs M, Kalk NJ, Morrison PD, Stone J. Spicing it up: synthetic cannabinoid receptor agonists and psychosis: a systematic review. *Eur Neuropsychopharmacol* 2018;**28** (12):1289–1304. https://doi.org/10.1016/j.euroneuro.2018.10 .004

245. Shafi A, Gallagher P, Stewart N, Martinotti G, Corazza O. The risk of violence associated with novel psychoactive substance misuse in patients presenting to acute mental health services. *Hum Psychopharmacol* 2017;**32**:3.

246. Akram H, Mokrysz C, Curran HV. What are the psychological effects of using synthetic cannabinoids? A systematic review. *J Psychopharmacol* 2019;**33**(3):271–283. https://doi.org/10 .1177/0269881119826592

247. Cohen K, Weinstein AM. Synthetic and non-synthetic cannabinoid drugs and their adverse effects: a review from a public health perspective. *Front Public Health* 2018;7(6):162.

248. Papanti D, Schifano F, Botteon G, et al. 'Spiceophrenia': a systematic overview of 'Spice'-related psychopathological issues and a case report. *Hum Psychopharmacol Clin Exp* 2013;28(4):379–389.

249. Karila L, Benyamina A, Blecha L, Cottencin O, Billieux J. The synthetic cannabinoids phenomenon. *Curr Pharm Des* 2016;22(42):6420–6425.

250. Cohen K, Kapitány-Fövény M, Mama Y, et al. The effects of synthetic cannabinoids on executive function. *Psychopharmacology* 2017;234(7):1121–1134. https://doi.org/10.1007/s00213-017-4546-4

251. Clayton HB, Lowry R, Ashley C, et al. Health risk behaviors with synthetic cannabinoids versus marijuana. *Pediatrics* 2017;139(4):e20162675.

252. Müller HH, Kornhuber J, Sperling W. The behavioral profile of spice and synthetic cannabinoids in humans. *Brain Res Bull* 2016;126:3–7.

253. Van Der Veer N, Friday J. Persistent psychosis following the use of Spice. *Schizophr Res* 2011;130(1):285–286.

254. Pereira LE, Toteja N, Khizar A, et al.Effect of synthetic cannabinoids and natural cannabis on severity of psychotic symptoms and aggression in adolescents and young adults with psychosis in an inpatient setting. *J Am Acad Child Adolesc Psychiatry* 2016;55(10):235–236.

255. Shalit N, Barzilay R, Shoval G, et al. Characteristics of synthetic cannabinoid and cannabis users admitted to a psychiatric hospital: a comparative study. *J Clin Psychiatry* 2016;77 (8):989–995.

256. Wilkinson ST, Radhakrishnan R, D'Souza DC. Impact of cannabis use on the development of psychotic disorders. *Curr Addict Rep* 2014;1(2):115–128.

257. Brakoulias V. Products containing synthetic cannabinoids and psychosis. *Aust NZ J Psychiatry* 2012;46(3):281–282. https://doi.org/10.1177/0004867411433974

258. Hobbs M, Kalk NJ, Morrison PD, Stone JM. Spicing it up – synthetic cannabinoid receptor agonists and psychosis – a systematic review. *Eur Neuropsychopharmacol* 2018;28 (12):1289–1304. https://doi.org/10.1016/j.euroneuro.2018.10.004

259. Morgan CJ, Schafer G, Freeman TP, Curran HV. Impact of cannabidiol on the acute memory and psychotomimetic effects of smoked cannabis: naturalistic study. *Br J Psychiatry* 2010;197(4):285–290. https://doi.org/10.1192/bjp.bp.110.077503

260. Hobbs M, Kalk NJ, Morrison PD, Stone JM. Spicing it up – synthetic cannabinoid receptor agonists and psychosis – a systematic review. *Eur Neuropsychopharmacol* 2018;28 (12):1289–1304. https://doi.org/10.1016/j.euroneuro.2018.10.004

261. Pereira LE, Toteja N, Khizar A, et al.Effect of synthetic cannabinoids and natural cannabis on severity of psychotic

symptoms and aggression in adolescents and young adults with psychosis in an inpatient setting. *J Am Acad Child Adolesc Psychiatry* 2016;55(10):235–236.

262. Shalit N, Barzilay R, Shoval G, et al. Characteristics of synthetic cannabinoid and cannabis users admitted to a psychiatric hospital: a comparative study. *J Clin Psychiatry* 2016;77 (8):989–995.

263. Coppola M, Mondola R. JWH-122 Consumption adverse effects: a case of hallucinogen persisting perception disorder five-year follow-up. *J Psychoactive Drugs* 2017;49 (3):262–265. https://doi.org/10.1080/02791072.2017.1316431

264. Martinotti G, Santacroce R, Pettorruso M, et al. Hallucinogen persisting perception disorder: etiology, clinical features, and therapeutic perspectives. *Brain Sci* 2018;8:47. https://doi.org/10.3390/brainsci8030047

265. Orsolini L, Papanti GD, De Berardis D, et al. The 'endless trip' among the NPS users: psychopathology and psychopharmacology in the hallucinogen-persisting perception disorder. A systematic review. *Front Psychiatry* 2017;8:240. https://doi.org/10.3389/fpsyt.2017.00240

266. Lev-Ran D, Feingold D, Goodman C, Lerner AG. Brief report: comparing triggers to visual disturbances among individuals with positive versus negative experiences of hallucinogen-persisting perception disorder (HPPD) following use of LSD. *Am J Addict* 2017;26:568–571. https://doi.org/10.1111/ajad.12577

267. Forrester MB, Kleinschmidt K, Schwarz E, Young A. Synthetic cannabinoid exposures reported to Texas poison centers. *J Addict Dis* 2011;30:351–358.

268. Haden M, Dargan PI, Archer JRH, et al. MDMB-CHMICA: availability, patterns of use and toxicity associated with this novel psychoactive substance. *Subst Use Misuse* 2017;52:223–232.

269. Westin AA, Frost J, Brede WR, et al. Sudden cardiac death following use of the synthetic cannabinoid MDMB-CHMICA. *J Anal Toxicol* 2016;40:86–87.

270. Adamowicz P. Fatal intoxication with synthetic cannabinoid MDMB-CHMICA. *Forensic Sci Int* 2016;261:e5–10.

271. European Monitoring Centre for Drugs and Drug Addiction [Internet]. EMCDDA–Europol Joint Report on a new psychoactive substance: methyl 2-[[1-(cyclohexylmethyl)indole-3-carbonyl]amino]-3,3-dimethylbutanoate (MDMB-CHMICA), Joint Reports. Luxembourg, Publications Office of the European Union, 2016.

272. Hill SL, Najafi J, Dunn M, et al.Clinical toxicity following analytically confirmed use of the synthetic cannabinoids MDMBCHMICA. A report from the Identification Of Novel psychoActive substances (IONA) study. *Clin Toxicol* 2016;54:638–643.

273. Angerer V, Franz F, Schwarze B, et al. Reply to 'Sudden cardiac death following use of the synthetic cannabinoid MDMBCHMICA'. *J Anal Toxicol* 2016;40:240–242.

274. Pacher P, Steffens S, Haskó G, Schindler TH, Kunos G. Cardiovascular effects of marijuana and synthetic

cannabinoids: the good, the bad, and the ugly. *Nat Rev Cardiol* 2018;**15**(3):151–166. https://doi.org/10.1038/nrcardio.2017.130

275. Tait RJ, Caldicott D, Mountain D, Hill SL, Lenton S. A systematic review of adverse events arising from the use of synthetic cannabinoids and their associated treatment. *Clin Toxicol* 2015;**15**:1–13.

276. Canning J, Ruha A, Pierce R, Torrey M, Reinhart S. Severe GI distress after smoking JWH-018. *Clin Toxicol* 2010;**48**:618.

277. Yen M, Berger RE, Roberts J, Ganetsky M. Middle cerebral artery stroke associated with use of synthetic cannabinoid K2. *Clin Toxicol* 2012;**50**(7):673–674.

278. Gunderson EW, Haughey HM, Ait-Daoud N, et al. A survey of synthetic cannabinoid consumption by current cannabis users. *Subst Abus* 2014;**35**:184–189.

279. Lapoint J, Nelson LS. Synthetic cannabinoids: the newest, almost illicit drug of abuse. *Emerg Med* 2011;**43**(2):26–28.

280. Ng SK, Brust JC, Hauser WA, Susser M. Illicit drug use and the risk of new-onset seizures. *Am J Epidemiol* 1990;**132**:47–57.

281. Gordon E, Devinsky O. Alcohol and marijuana: effects on epilepsy and use by patients with epilepsy. *Epilepsia* 2001;**42**:1266–1272.

282. Keeler MH, Reifler CB. Grand mal convulsions subsequent to marijuana use. Case report. *Dis Nerv Syst* 1967;**28**:474–475.

283. Schneir A, Baumbacher T. Convulsions as a complication of synthetic cannabinoid use. *Clin Toxicol* 2011;**49**(6):526.

284. Hoyte CO, Jacob J, Monte AA, Al-Jumaan M, Bronstein AC, Heard KJ. A characterization of synthetic cannabinoid exposures reported to the National Poison Data System in 2010. *Ann Emerg Med* 2012;**60**:435–438.

285. Bäckberg M, Tworek L, Beck O, et al. Analytically confirmed intoxications involving MDMB-CHMICA from the STRIDA Project. *J Med Toxicol* 2017;**13**:52–60. https://doi.org/10.1007/s13181-016-0584-2

286. Schep LJ, Slaughter RJ, Hudson S, et al.Delayed seizure-like activity following analytically confirmed use of previously unreported synthetic cannabinoid analogues. *Hum Exp Toxicol* 2015;**34**:557–560.

287. Hermanns-Clausen M, Muller D, Kithinji J, et al. Acute side effects after consumption of the novel synthetic cannabinoids ABCHMINACA and MDMB-CHMICA. 36th International Congress of the European Association of Poisons Centres and Clinical Toxicologists (EAPCCT), 24–27 May, 2016, Madrid, Spain. *Clin Toxicol* 2016;**54**:344–519 (Abstract 17).

288. Zarifi C, Vyas S. Spice-y kidney failure: a case report and systematic review of acute kidney injury attributable to the use of synthetic cannabis. *Perm J* 2017;**21**:16–160.

289. Seifert SA, Brazwell EM, Smeltzer C, Gibb J, Logan BK. Seizure and acute kidney injury associated with synthetic cannabinoid use. *Clin Toxicol* 2013;**51**(7):667.

290. Kazory A, Aiyer R. Synthetic marijuana and acute kidney injury: an unforeseen association. *Clin Kidney J* 2013;**6**(3):330–333.

291. Bhanushali GK, Jain G, Fatima H, Leisch LJ, Thornley-Brown D. AKI associated with synthetic cannabinoids: a case series. *Clin J Am Soc Nephrol* 2013;**8**(4):523–526. https://doi.org/10.2215/CJN.05690612

292. Coca SG, Singanamala S, Parikh CR. Chronic kidney disease after kidney injury: a systemic review and meta-analysis. *Kid Int* 2012;**81**:442–448.

293. Murphy TD, Weidenbach KN, Houten CV, et al. Acute kidney injury associated with synthetic cannabinoid use: multiple states, 2012. *Morb Mort Wkly Rep* 2013;**62**:93–98.

294. Karass M, Chugh S, Andries G, et al. Thrombotic microangiopathy associated with synthetic cannabinoid receptor agonists. Stem Cell Investig 2017;**4**:43. https://doi.org/10.21037/sci.2017.05.05

295. Armstrong F, McCurdy MT, Heavner MS. Synthetic cannabinoid-associated multiple organ failure: case series and literature review. *Pharmacotherapy* 2019;**39**(4):508–513. https://doi.org/10.1002/phar.2241

296. Westerbergh J, Hulten P. Novel synthetic cannabinoids, CRA13, JWH-015, JWH-081 and JWH-210 – detected in a case series. (Abstracts of the 2011 International Congress of the European Association of Poisons Centres and Clinical Toxicologists, 24–27 May 2011, Dubrovnik, Croatia.) *Clin Toxicol* 2011;**49**(3):199.

297. Su M, Laskowski L, Hoffman RS. Hyperthermia and severe rhabdomyolysis from synthetic cannabinoids. *Am J Emerg Med* 2016;**34**:121.e1–2. https://doi.org/10.1016/j.Ajem.2015.05.052. Epub 12 June 2015. *Am J Emerg Med* 2016;34(8):1690. https://doi.org/10.1016/j.ajem.2016.05.015

298. March R, Guentert P, Kloska-Kearney E, et al. Utilization of extracorporeal membrane oxygenation for pulmonary toxicity caused by inhaled synthetic cannabinoid. a harbinger of future complications associated with inhaled cannabinoid products. *Int J Clin Med* 2020;**11**:53–61. https://doi.org/10.4236/ijcm.2020.112006

299. Armstrong F, McCurdy MT, Heavner MS. Synthetic cannabinoid-associated multiple organ failure: case series and literature review. *Pharmacotherapy* 2019;**39**(4):508–513.

300. Armstrong F, McCurdy MT, Heavner MS. Synthetic cannabinoid-associated multiple organ failure: case series and literature review. *Pharmacotherapy* 2019;**39**(4):508–513.

301. Winstock AR, Barratt MJ. The 12-month prevalence and nature of adverse experiences resulting in emergency medical presentations associated with the use of synthetic cannabinoid products. *Hum Psychopharmacol* 2013;**28**:390–393.

302. Tait RJ, Caldicott D, Mountain D, Hill SL, Lenton S. A systematic review of adverse events arising from the use of synthetic cannabinoids and their associated treatment. *Clin Toxicol* 2015;**15**:1–13.

303. Tait RJ, Caldicott D, Mountain D, Hill SL, Lenton S. A systematic review of adverse events arising from the use of synthetic cannabinoids and their associated treatment. *Clin Toxicol* 2015;**15**:1–13.

304. Smith K, Flatley J, (eds.). Drug Misuse Declared: Findings from the 2010/11 British Crime Survey. England and Wales (Home Office Statistical Bulletin). London, Home Office, 2011.

305. Abouchedid R, Hudson S, Thurtle N, et al. Analytical confirmation of synthetic cannabinoids in a cohort of 179 presentations with acute recreational drug toxicity to an emergency department in London, UK in the first half of 2015. *Clin Toxicol* 2017;**55**:338–345.

306. Law RK, Schier J, Martin C, Chang A, Wolkin A. Increase in reported adverse health effects related to synthetic cannabinoid use – United States, January–May 2015. *Morb Mort Wkly Rep* 2016;**64**(22).

307. Hermanns-Clausen M, Kneisel S, Szabo B, Auwärter V. Intoxications by synthetic cannabinoids – current trends. (Abstracts of the 2011 International Congress of the European Association of Poisons Centres and Clinical Toxicologists, 24–27 May 2011, Dubrovnik, Croatia.) *Clin Toxicol* 2011;**49**(3).

308. Theunissen EL, Reckweg JT, Hutten NRPW, et al. Psychotomimetic symptoms after a moderate dose of a synthetic cannabinoid (JWH-018): implications for psychosis. *Psychopharmacology* 2021 (online). https://doi.org/10.1007/s00213-021-05768-0

309. Tait RJ, Caldicott D, Mountain D, Hill SL, Lenton S. A systematic review of adverse events arising from the use of synthetic cannabinoids and their associated treatment. *Clin Toxicol* 2015;**15**:1–13.

310. Glue P, Al-Shaqsi S, Hancock D, Gale C, Strong B, Schep L. Hospitalisation associated with use of the synthetic cannabinoid K2. *NZ Med J* 2013;**126**(1377):18–22.

311. Hobbs M, Patel R, Morrison PD, Kalk N, Stone JM. Synthetic cannabinoid use in psychiatric patients and relationship to hospitalisation: a retrospective electronic case register study. *J Psychopharmacol* 2020;**34**(6):648–653.

312. Cordeiro SK, Daro RC, Seung H, Klein-Schwartz W, Kim HK. Evolution of clinical characteristics and outcomes of synthetic cannabinoid receptor agonist exposure in the United States: analysis of National Poison Data System data from 2010 to 2015. *Addiction* 2018;**113**:1850–1861.

313. Hermanns-Clausen M, Müller D, Kithinji J, et al. Acute side effects after consumption of the new synthetic cannabinoids AB-CHMINACA and MDMB-CHMICA. *Clin Toxicol* 2018;**56**(6):404–411. https://doi.org/10.1080/15563650.2017.1393082

314. Cordeiro SK, Daro RC, Seung H, Klein-Schwartz W, Kim HK. Evolution of clinical characteristics and outcomes of synthetic cannabinoid receptor agonist exposure in the United States: analysis of National Poison Data System data from 2010 to 2015. *Addiction* **2018**;113:1850–1861.

315. Cordeiro SK, Daro RC, Seung H, Klein-Schwartz W, Kim HK. Evolution of clinical characteristics and outcomes of synthetic cannabinoid receptor agonist exposure in the United States: analysis of National Poison Data System data from 2010 to 2015. *Addiction* **2018**;113:1850–1861.

316. Cordeiro SK, Daro RC, Seung H, Klein-Schwartz W, Kim HK. Evolution of clinical characteristics and outcomes of synthetic cannabinoid receptor agonist exposure in the United States:

analysis of National Poison Data System data from 2010 to 2015. *Addiction* **2018**;113:1850–1861.

317. Schwartz MD, Trecki J, Edison LA, et al. A common source outbreak of severe delirium associated with exposure to the novel synthetic cannabinoid ADB-PINACA. *J Emerg Med* 2015;**48**:573–580.

318. Tyndall JA, Gerona R, De Portu G, et al. An outbreak of acute delirium from exposure to the synthetic cannabinoid AB-CHMINACA. *Clin Toxicol* 2015;**53**:950–956.

319. Bäckberg M, Tworek L, Beck O, et al. Analytically confirmed intoxications involving MDMB-CHMICA from the STRIDA Project. *J Med Toxicol* 2017;**13**:52–60. https://doi.org/10.1007/s13181-016-0584-2

320. Adamowicz P. Fatal intoxication with synthetic cannabinoid MDMB-CHMICA. *Forensic Sci Int* 2016;**261**:e5–10.

321. Angerer V, Franz F, Schwarze B, Moosmann B, Auwarter V. Reply to 'Sudden cardiac death following use of the synthetic cannabinoid MDMB-CHMICA'. *J Anal Toxicol* 2016;**40**:240–242.

322. Westin AA, Frost J, Brede WR, et al. Sudden cardiac death following use of the synthetic cannabinoid MDMB-CHMICA. *J Anal Toxicol* 2016;**40**:86–87.

323. Abouchedid R, Thurtle N, Yamamoto T, et al. (eds.). Analytical confirmation of the synthetic cannabinoid receptor agonists (SCRAs) present in a cohort of presentations with acute recreational drug toxicity to an Emergency Department (ED) in London, UK. 36th International Congress of the European Association of Poisons Centres and Clinical Toxicologists (EAPCCT), Madrid, Spain, 2016. *Clin Toxicol* 2016;**54**(4):344–519. https://doi.org/10.3109/1556365020161165952

324. Abouchedid R, Ho JH, Hudson S, et al. Acute toxicity associated with use of 5F-derivations of synthetic cannabinoid receptor agonists with analytical confirmation. *J Med Toxicol* 2016;**12**(4):396–401. https://doi.org/10.1007/s13181-016-0571-7

325. Sobolevsky T, Prasolov I, Rodchenkov G. Detection of JWH-018 metabolites in smoking mixture post-administration urine. *Forensic Sci Int* 2010;**200**:141–147.

326. Emerson B, Durham B, Gidden J, Lay JO Jr. Gas chromatography–mass spectrometry of JWH-018 metabolites in urine samples with direct comparison to analytical standards. *Forensic Sci Int* 2013;**229**(1–3):1–6. https://doi.org/10.1016/j.forsciint.2013.03.006

327. Lovett DP, Yanes EG, Herbelin TW, Knoerzer TA, Levisky JA. Structure elucidation and identification of a common metabolite for naphthoylindole-based synthetic cannabinoids using LC-TOF and comparison to a synthetic reference standard. *Forensic Sci Int* 2013;**226**(1–3):81–87. https://doi.org/10.1016/j.forsciint.2012.12.012

328. Schneir AB, Cullen J, Ly BT. 'Spice' girls: synthetic cannabinoid intoxication. *J Emerg Med* 2011;**40**(3):296–299. https://doi.org/10.1016/j.jemermed.2010.10.014

329. Coppola M, Mondola R. JWH-122 Consumption adverse effects: a case of hallucinogen persisting perception disorder

five-year follow-up. *J Psychoactive Drugs* 2017;**49** (3):262–265. https://doi.org/10.1080/02791072.2017.1316431

330. Tait RJ, Caldicott D, Mountain D, Hill SL, Lenton S. A systematic review of adverse events arising from the use of synthetic cannabinoids and their associated treatment. *Clin Toxicol* 2015;**15**:1–13.

331. Zhao A, Tan M, Maung A, Salifu M, Mallappallil M. Case rhabdomyolysis and acute kidney injury requiring dialysis as a result of concomitant use of atypical neuroleptics and synthetic cannabinoids. *Rep Nephrol* 2015;2015:235982. https://doi.org/ doi.org/10.1155/2015/235982

332. Rodgman C, Kinzie E, Leimbach E. Bad mojo: use of the new marijuana substitute leads to more and more ED visits for acute psychosis. *Am J Emerg Med* 2011;**29**:232.

333. Cordeiro SK, Daro RC, Seung H, Klein-Schwartz W, Kim HK. Evolution of clinical characteristics and outcomes of synthetic cannabinoid receptor agonist exposure in the United States: analysis of National Poison Data System data from 2010 to 2015. *Addiction* **2018**;113:1850–1861.

334. Armenian P, Darracq M, Gevorkyan J, et al. Intoxication from the novel synthetic cannabinoids AB-PINACA and ADB-PINACA: a case series and review of the literature. *Neuropharmacology* 2017 (online). https://doi.org/10.1016/j.neuropharm.2017.10.017

335. Tait RJ, Caldicott D, Mountain D, Hill SL, Lenton S. A systematic review of adverse events arising from the use of synthetic cannabinoids and their associated treatment. *Clin Toxicol* 2015;**15**:1–13.

336. Castaneto MS, Gorelick DA, Desrosiers NA, et al.2014. Synthetic cannabinoids: epidemiology, pharmacodynamics, and clinical implications. *Drug Alcohol Depend* **2014**;144:12e41.

337. Armenian P, Darracq M, Gevorkyan J, et al. Intoxication from the novel synthetic cannabinoids AB-PINACA and ADB-PINACA: a case series and review of the literature. *Neuropharmacology* 2017 (online). https://doi.org/10.1016/j.neuropharm.2017.10.017

338. Armenian P, Darracq M, Gevorkyan J, et al. Intoxication from the novel synthetic cannabinoids AB-PINACA and ADB-PINACA: a case series and review of the literature. *Neuropharmacology* 2017 (online). https://doi.org/10.1016/j.neuropharm.2017.10.017

339. Hermanns-Clausen M, Kneisel S, Szabo B, Auwärter V. Acute toxicity due to the confirmed consumption of synthetic cannabinoids: clinical and laboratory findings. *Addiction* 2013;**108**:534–544.

340. Tait RJ, Caldicott D, Mountain D, Hill SL, Lenton S. A systematic review of adverse events arising from the use of synthetic cannabinoids and their associated treatment. *Clin Toxicol* 2015;**15**:1–13.

341. Monte AA, Bronstein AC, Dahze JC, et al. Supplementary appendix to an outbreak of exposure to a novel synthetic cannabinoid. *New Engl J Med* 2014;**370**(4):389–390. Available at: www.nejm.org/doi/suppl/10.1056/NEJMc1313655/suppl_file/nejmc1313655_appendix.pdf [last accessed 28 March 2022].

342. Bonaccorso S, Metastasio A, Ricciardi A, et al. Synthetic cannabinoid use in a case series of patients with psychosis presenting to acute psychiatric settings: clinical presentation and management issues. *Brain Sci* 2018;8:133. https://doi.org/10.3390/brainsci8070133

343. Zimmermann US, Winkelmann PR, Pilhatsch M, Nees JA, Spanagel R, Schulz K. Withdrawal phenomena and dependence syndrome after the consumption of 'Spice Gold'. *Dtsch Arztebl Int* 2009;**106**:464–467.

344. Atwood BK, Huffman J, Straiker A, Mackie K. JWH018, a common constituent of 'Spice' herbal blends, is a potent and efficacious cannabinoid CB receptor agonist. *Br J Pharmacol* 2010;**160**(3):585–593.

345. Macfarlane V, Christie G. Synthetic cannabinoid withdrawal: a new demand on detoxification services. *Drug Alcohol Rev* 2015;**34**:147–153.

346. Rodgman CJ, Verrico CD, Worthy RB, Lewis EE. Inpatient detoxification from a synthetic cannabinoid and control of postdetoxification cravings with naltrexone. *Prim Care Companion CNS* 2014;**16**:4.

347. Nacca N, Vatti D, Sullivan R, Sud P, Su M, Marraffa J. The synthetic cannabinoid withdrawal syndrome. *J Addict Med* 2013;**7**(4):296–298. https://doi.org/10.1097/ADM.0b013e31828e1881

348. Cooper ZD, Haney M. Cannabis reinforcement and dependence: role of the cannabinoid CB1 receptor. *Addict Biol* 2008;**13**:188–195.

349. Macfarlane V, Christie G. Synthetic cannabinoid withdrawal: a new demand on detoxification services. *Drug Alcohol Rev* 2015;**34**(2):147–153.

350. Barratt MJ, Cakic V, Lenton S. Patterns of synthetic cannabinoid use in Australia. *Drug Alcohol Rev* 2013;**32** (2):141–146. https://doi.org/10.1111/j.1465-3362.2012.00519.x

351. Zimmermann US, Winkelmann PR, Pilhatsch M, Nees JA, Spanagel R, Schulz K. Withdrawal phenomena and dependence syndrome after the consumption of 'Spice Gold'. *Dtsch Arztebl Int* 2009;**106**(27):464–467. https://doi.org/10.3238/arztebl.2009.0464

352. Atwood BK, Huffman J, Straiker A, Mackie K. JWH018, a common constituent of 'Spice' herbal blends, is a potent and efficacious cannabinoid CB receptor agonist. *Br J Pharmacol* 2010;**160**(3):585–593.

353. Van Hout MC, Hearne E. User experiences of development of dependence on the synthetic cannabinoids, 5f-AKB48 and 5F-PB-22, and subsequent withdrawal syndromes *Int J Ment Health Addiction* 2017;**15**: 565. https://doi.org/10.1007/s11469-016-9650-x

354. Cooper ZD. Adverse effects of synthetic cannabinoids: management of acute toxicity and withdrawal. *Curr Psychiatry Rep* 2016;**18**:52. https://doi.org/10.1007/s11920-016-0694-1

355. Cooper ZD. Adverse effects of synthetic cannabinoids: management of acute toxicity and withdrawal. *Curr Psychiatry Rep* 2016;**18**:52. https://doi.org/10.1007/s11920-016-0694-1

356. Castaneto MS, Gorelick DA, Desrosiers NA, et al. Synthetic cannabinoids: epidemiology, pharmacodynamics, and clinical implications. *Drug Alcohol Depend* 2014;**144**:12e41.

357. Macfarlane V, Christie G. Synthetic cannabinoid withdrawal: a new demand on detoxification services. *Drug Alcohol Rev* 2015;**34**:147–153.

358. Lin CY, Wheelock AM, Morin D, et al. Toxicity and metabolism of methylnaphthalenes: comparison with naphthalene and 1-nitronaphthalene. *Toxicology* 2009;**260**(1–3):16–27. https://doi.org/10.1016/j.tox.2009.03.002

359. Hopkins CY, Gilchrist BL. A case of cannabinoid hyperemesis syndrome caused by synthetic cannabinoids. *J Emerg Med* 2013;**45**(4):544–546.

360. Armstrong F, McCurdy MT, Heavner MS. Synthetic cannabinoid-associated multiple organ failure: case series and literature review. *Pharmacotherapy* 2019;**39**:508–513.

361. Alhadi S, Tiwari A, Vohra R, Gerona R, Acharya J, Bilello K. High times, low sats: diffuse pulmonary infiltrates associated with chronic synthetic cannabinoid use. *J Med Toxicol* 2013;**9**(2):199–206.

362. Cooper ZD, Haney M. Cannabis reinforcement and dependence: role of the cannabinoid CB1 receptor. *Addict Biol* 2008;**13**:188–195.

363. Rodgman CJ, Verrico CD, Worthy RB, Lewis EE. Inpatient detoxification from a synthetic cannabinoid and control of postdetoxification cravings with naltrexone. *Prim Care Companion CNS* 2014;**16**:4.

364. Macfarlane V, Christie G. Synthetic cannabinoid withdrawal: a new demand on detoxification services. *Drug Alcohol Rev* 2015;**34**:147–153.

365. Nacca N, Vatti D, Sullivan R, Sud P, Su M, Marraffa J. The synthetic cannabinoid withdrawal syndrome. *J Addict Med* 2013;**7**:296–298.

366. Sweeney B, Talebi S, Toro D, et al. Hyperthermia and severe rhabdomyolysis from synthetic cannabinoids. *Am J Emerg Med* 2016;**34**(1):121–e1.

367. Oluwabusi OO, Lobach L, Akhtar U, Youngman B, Ambrosini PJ. Synthetic cannabinoid-induced psychosis: two adolescent cases. *J Child Adolesc Psychopharmacol* 2012;**22**:393–395.

368. Ustundag MF, Ozhan IE, Yucel A, Ozcan H. Synthetic cannabis-induced mania. *Case Rep Psychiatry* 2015;2015:310930.

369. Alvarez Y, Pérez-Mañá C, Torrens M, Farré M. Antipsychotic drugs in cocaine dependence: a systematic review and meta-analysis. *J Subst Abuse Treat* 2013;**45**(1):1–10. https://doi.org/10.1016/j.jsat.2012.12.013

370. Seeman P. Atypical antipsychotics: mechanism of action. *Can J Psychiatry* 2002;**47**(1):27–38.

371. Macfarlane V, Christie G. Synthetic cannabinoid withdrawal: a new demand on detoxification services. *Drug Alcohol Rev* 2015;**34**:147–153.

372. Nacca N, Vatti D, Sullivan R, Sud P, Su M, Marraffa J. The synthetic cannabinoid withdrawal syndrome. *J Addict Med* 2013;**7**:296–298.

373. Rodgman CJ, Verrico CD, Worthy RB, Lewis EE. Inpatient detoxification from a synthetic cannabinoid and control of postdetoxification cravings with naltrexone. *Prim Care Companion CNS* 2014;**16**:4.

374. Hermanns-Clausen M, Kneisel S, Szabo B, Auwärter V. Acute toxicity due to the confirmed consumption of synthetic cannabinoids: clinical and laboratory findings. *Addiction* 2013;**108**:534–544.

375. Ukaigwe A, Karmacharya P, Donato A. A gut gone to pot: a case of cannabinoid hyperemesis syndrome due to K2, a synthetic cannabinoid. *Case Rep Emerg Med* 2014;**2014**:167098.

376. Grigg J, Manning V, Arunogiri S, Lubman DI. Synthetic cannabinoid use disorder: an update for general psychiatrists. *Australas Psychiatry* 2019;**27**(3):279–283. https://doi.org/10.1177/1039856218822749

377. Macfarlane V, Christie G. Synthetic cannabinoid withdrawal: a new demand on detoxification services. *Drug Alcohol Rev* 2015;**34**:147–153.

378. Van Hout MC. The dynamic landscape of novel psychoactive substance (NPS) use in Ireland: results from an expert consultation. *Int J Ment Health Addict* 2017;**15**(5):985–992.

379. Van Hout MC, Hearne E. User experiences of development of dependence on the synthetic cannabinoids, 5f-AKB48 and 5F-PB-22, and subsequent withdrawal syndromes. *Int J Ment Health Addict* 2017;**15**(3):565–579.

380. Grigg J, Manning V, Arunogiri S, Lubman DI. Synthetic cannabinoid use disorder: an update for general psychiatrists. *Australas Psychiatry* 2019;**27**(3):279–283. https://doi.org/10.1177/1039856218822749

381. Musshoff F, Madea B, Kernbach-Wighton G, et al. Driving under the influence of synthetic cannabinoids ('Spice'): a case series. *Int J Legal Med* 2014;**128**(1):59–64. https://doi.org/10.1007/s00414-013-0864-1

382. Chase PB. Signs of synthetic cannabinoid vs. marijuana intoxication as determined by police drug recognition experts. *Clin Toxicol* 2013;**51**(7):667.

383. Tuv SS, Auwarter V, Vindenes V. Accidents and synthetic cannabinoids in blood of drivers. In: *Handbook of Cannabis and Related Pathologies: Biology, Pharmacology, Diagnosis, and Treatment*, pp. 848–1990. Abingdon, Elsevier, 2017.

Conclusion

Chapter

14

This is the first textbook to undertake a comprehensive, in-depth review of the literature relating to novel psychoactive substances (NPS) and club drug harms and their clinical management. The book builds on the work of the NEPTUNE project, which has been reviewing the evidence on this fast-moving area for the last decade. Some predicted that NPS would be a short-lived phenomenon; however, drug markets continue to rapidly evolve with new, and typically more harmful, substances appearing with alarming frequency. The increased role of the Internet and social media platforms to sell drugs, including NPS and club drugs, is a further example of the pace of change.

At the time of writing, the range of substances available on drug markets has never been wider. While NPS have not replaced existing illegal drugs, they are now established throughout drug markets both in terms of substances that people seek to use, as well as substances that are used to adulterate other drugs, including counterfeit medications, with sometimes catastrophic results. The mortality resulting from adulteration of illegal drugs with opioid NPS such as fentanyl analogues, is a devastating example.

Given the large number of new substances and the constantly evolving drug market, we have attempted to future proof this book by suggesting that health professionals approach unfamiliar NPS and club drugs by considering the primary psychoactive effect of the substance. The psychoactive effect should be based upon the clinical signs and symptoms at pres-

entation and these can be broadly considered as stimulant, sedative/dissociative and hallucinogenic. Using this approach, we hope that clinicians will be able to assess and manage unfamiliar substances using familiar approaches, delivering what may well be life-saving clinical interventions. We strongly suggest that all health professionals who support people who use drugs need to develop the skills to assess emerging drugs and manage their harms. This will include health staff working in drugs services, mental health, acute care settings, sexual health services and other areas in contact with populations with a high prevalence of drug use. To achieve this, appropriate training and standardised clinical competencies will be needed and these should be integrated into core curricula. We see this as an essential next step.

This book has rightly focused on clinical harms and their management; however, NPS continue to present severe challenges to researchers and policy makers. The policy challenge extends from public health to law enforcement and currently there is a limited evidence base to guide decision making. Researchers have a crucial role in improving the understanding of emerging drugs, their harms, the populations most at risk and potential new treatments. Funding for further research is a priority.

NPS and club drugs will present challenges to clinicians, researchers and policy makers for the foreseeable future and we hope that this book will play a part in the developing response.

Index

Printed in the United States
by Baker & Taylor Publisher Services